TARGETED THERAPIES in ONCOLOGY

TARGETED THERAPIES in ONCOLOGY

Edited by
Giuseppe Giaccone
Jean-Charles Soria

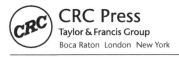

CRC Press
Taylor & Francis Group
Boca Raton London New York

CRC Press is an imprint of the
Taylor & Francis Group, an **informa** business

CRC Press
Taylor & Francis Group
6000 Broken Sound Parkway NW, Suite 300
Boca Raton, FL 33487-2742

First issued in paperback 2019

© 2014 by Taylor & Francis Group, LLC
CRC Press is an imprint of Taylor & Francis Group, an Informa business

No claim to original U.S. Government works

ISBN-13: 978-1-84214-545-6 (hbk)
ISBN-13: 978-0-367-37936-0 (pbk)

Library of Congress Cataloging-in-Publication Data

Targeted therapies in oncology / edited by Giuseppe Giaccone and Jean-Charles Soria. -- 2nd ed.
    p. ; cm.
    Includes bibliographical references and index.
    ISBN 978-1-84214-545-6 (alk. paper)
    I. Giaccone, Giuseppe. II. Soria, Jean-Charles.
    [DNLM: 1. Neoplasms--therapy. 2. Genetic Therapy. 3. Immunotherapy. 4. Molecular Targeted Therapy. QZ 266]

RC270.8
616.99'406--dc23   2013016361

Visit the Taylor & Francis Web site at
http://www.taylorandfrancis.com

and the CRC Press Web site at
http://www.crcpress.com

Contents

Preface

Rapid advances in tumor biology have led to the identification of the molecular circuitry that governs cancer cell proliferation. Better understanding of the key pathways that control tumor progression has enabled the pharmaceutical industry and academia to develop new anticancer agents targeting specific molecular events involved in the oncogenic process.

The term "targeted therapies" refers to treatment strategies directed against molecular targets considered to be involved in the process of neoplastic transformation. This is not a brand new concept in oncology, since hormonal manipulations have long been applied for the treatment of advanced and early-stage breast, prostate, and thyroid cancers.

In the past 30 years, characteristic alterations of neoplastic cells have been described, such as specific translocations, activating mutations, or gene amplifications, which have brought significant changes to the nosological classification of cancers. The molecular classification of some cancers has contributed to the development of a new class of drugs that aims at blocking, with various degrees of specificity, the activity of proteins involved in neoplastic cell development and progression. This book provides a concise and up-to-date panorama of existing targeted therapies and those being developed into valuable anticancer treatments, with an emphasis on the "clinical achievements" obtained with the aforementioned anticancer agents. The biology behind each target has also been discussed. The chapters included reflect a variety of targeted therapies aiming at blocking a wide array of "hallmarks of cancer." These therapies notably include signal-transduction inhibitors, antiangiogenic and vascular-disrupting agents, apoptosis modulators, and targeted agents of immune checkpoints; however, only the targeted agents that have already entered the clinical arena have been included. The introduction of these agents has already had a large impact across different tumor types and in early- as well as advanced-stage cancer.

Giuseppe Giaccone

Jean-Charles Soria

Acknowledgments

The authors would like to acknowledge Dr. Elena Ileana Ecaterina for providing graphical assistance for the cover page and Dr. Sophie Postel-Vinay for providing editing assistance to Professor Soria.

Editors

Giuseppe Giaccone is professor and associate director of the Lombardi Cancer Center at Georgetown University in Washington, District of Columbia. He was previously the head of the Department of Medical Oncology, Free University Medical Center, Amsterdam, the Netherlands, and most recently the chief of the Medical Oncology Branch of the National Cancer Institute in Bethesda. Professor Giaccone has written more than 500 peer-reviewed scientific papers and several books and book chapters and is a board member of several international scientific journals. His fields of research include lung cancer and the development of novel anticancer agents. He was the chair of the Lung Cancer Cooperative Group of the European Organization for Research and Treatment of Cancer until 2000. He has organized a number of international conferences, such as the Topoisomerase Symposia and the Targeted Anticancer Therapy conferences.

Jean-Charles Soria is professor of medicine at South-Paris University, France, and adjunct professor at the University of Texas MD Anderson Cancer Center. He is the chairman of the Early Drug Development Department at Institut Gustave-Roussy, Villejuif, France. He is also a member of the Thoracic Multidisciplinary Committee at this institute. Professor Soria has authored over 300 peer-reviewed scientific papers, including publications as first or last author in the *New England Journal of Medicine*, the *Journal of the National Cancer Institute*, the *Journal of Clinical Oncology*, *Clinical Cancer Research*, and *Annals of Oncology*. He is a board member of several international scientific journals. His main research interests include early clinical development across solid tumors, pharmacodynamic biomarkers, lung cancer, and personalized medicine. He is also involved in translational research related to precision medicine and tumor progression, notably in lung cancer models (INSERM unit 981).

Contributors

Fabrice Andre
Department of Medical Oncology
and
Institut National de la
   Santé et de la Recherche
   Médicale Unit
Institut Gustave Roussy
Villejuif, France
and
Faculté de Medecine
Paris Sud University
Orsay, France

Jean-Pierre Armand
Service d'Innovation
   Thérapeutique et Essais
   Précoces
Institut Gustave Roussy
Villejuif, France

Susan E. Bates
Medical Oncology Branch
National Cancer Institute
Bethesda, Maryland

Jean-Yves Blay
Department of Medicine
and
Institut National de la Santé et de la
   Recherche Médicale
Centre Leon Berard
Lyon, France

Johann de Bono
Drug Development Unit
Royal Marsden NHS Foundation Trust
and
Section of Medicine
The Institute of Cancer Research
Surrey, United Kingdom

Julie R. Brahmer
Upper Aerodigestive Malignancies
   Division
Sidney Kimmel Comprehensive Cancer
   Center at Johns Hopkins
Baltimore, Maryland

Christina Brzezniak
Department of Hematology and
   Oncology
Walter Reed National Military Medical
   Center
Bethesda, Maryland

Fatima Cardoso
Breast Unit
Champalimaud Cancer Center
Lisbon, Portugal

Corey Carter
Department of Hematology and
   Oncology
Walter Reed National Military Medical
   Center
Bethesda, Maryland

Arup R. Chakraborty
Medical Oncology Branch
National Cancer Institute
Bethesda, Maryland

Apoorva Chawla
Department of Medicine
University of Chicago
Chicago, Illinois

Janet E. Dancey
Department of Oncology
Queen's University
Kingston, Ontario, Canada

Ruggero De Maria
Scientific Direction
Regina Elena National Cancer
    Institute
Rome, Italy

Gianluca Del Conte
Department of Oncology
Ospedale San Raffaele
Milan, Italy

Olfa Derbel
Department of Medicine
Centre Leon Berard
Lyon, France

Siddhartha Devarakonda
Department of Internal Medicine
St. Luke's Hospital
Chesterfield, Missouri

Maria Vittoria Dieci
Department of Medical Oncology
and
Institut National de la
    Santé et de la Recherche
    Médicale Unit
Institut Gustave Roussy
Villejuif, France

Armelle Dufresne
Department of Medicine
Centre Leon Berard
Lyon, France

Benedetto Farsaci
National Cancer Institute
National Institutes of Health
Bethesda, Maryland

Tito Fojo
National Cancer Institute
National Institutes of Health
Bethesda, Maryland

Patrick M. Forde
Upper Aerodigestive Malignancies
    Division
Sidney Kimmel Comprehensive Cancer
    Center at Johns Hopkins
Baltimore, Maryland

Giuseppe Giaccone
Medical Oncology Branch
National Cancer Institute
Bethesda, Maryland

Ramaswamy Govindan
Department of Internal Medicine
and
Alvin J. Siteman Cancer Center
Washington University School of
    Medicine
St. Louis, Missouri

James L. Gulley
National Cancer Institute
National Institutes of Health
Bethesda, Maryland

James W. Hodge
National Cancer Institute
National Institutes of Health
Bethesda, Maryland

Pamela M. Holland
Therapeutic Innovation Unit
Amgen, Inc.
Cambridge, Massachusetts

Sahar Khan
Center for Cancer Research
National Cancer Institute
Bethesda, Maryland

Peter S. Kim
National Cancer Institute
National Institutes of Health
Bethesda, Maryland

Edina Komlodi-Pasztor
National Cancer Institute
National Institutes of Health
Bethesda, Maryland

Marcello Maugeri-Saccà
Scientific Direction
Regina Elena National Cancer
    Institute
Rome, Italy

Mehdi Mollapour
Center for Cancer Research
National Cancer Institute
Bethesda, Maryland

Daniel Morgensztern
Department of Internal Medicine
and
Alvin J. Siteman Cancer Center
Washington University School of
    Medicine
St. Louis, Missouri

Len Neckers
Center for Cancer Research
National Cancer Institute
Bethesda, Maryland

Aurelius Omlin
Drug Development Unit
Royal Marsden NHS Foundation Trust
and
The Institute of Cancer Research
Surrey, United Kingdom

Claudia Palena
National Cancer Institute
National Institutes of Health
Bethesda, Maryland

Carmel Pezaro
Drug Development Unit
Royal Marsden NHS Foundation Trust
and
The Institute of Cancer Research
London, United Kingdom

Ruth Plummer
Northern Institute for Cancer Research
Newcastle University
and
Northern Centre for Cancer Care
Freeman Hospital
Newcastle upon Tyne, United Kingdom

Sophie Postel-Vinay
Service d'Innovation
    Thérapeutique et Essais
    Précoces
Institut Gustave Roussy
Villejuif, France

Aparna Rao
Department of Medical of Oncology
Peter MacCallum Cancer Centre
Melbourne, Victoria, Australia

Isabelle Ray-Coquard
Department of Medicine
Centre Leon Berard
Lyon, France

David Reese
Department of Medical Sciences
Amgen, Inc.
Thousand Oaks, California

Antoni Ribas
Jonsson Comprehensive Cancer Center
University of California, Los Angeles
Los Angeles, California

Joana Ribeiro
Breast Unit
Champalimaud Cancer Center
Lisbon, Portugal

Lidia Robert
Jonsson Comprehensive Cancer Center
University of California, Los Angeles
Los Angeles, California

Robert W. Robey
Medical Oncology Branch
National Cancer Institute
Bethesda, Maryland

Dan L. Sackett
Eunice Kennedy Shriver National
    Institute of Child Health and Human
    Development
National Institutes of Health
Bethesda, Maryland

Ravi Salgia
Department of Medicine
University of Chicago
Chicago, Illinois

Jeffrey Schlom
National Cancer Institute
National Institutes of Health
Bethesda, Maryland

Cristiana Sessa
Istituto Oncologico della Svizzera
    Italiana
Bellinzona, Switzerland
and
Department of Oncology
Ospedale San Raffaele
Milan, Italy

Benjamin Solomon
Department of Medical Oncology
Peter MacCallum Cancer Centre
Melbourne, Victoria, Australia

Berta Sousa
Breast Unit
Champalimaud Cancer Center
Lisbon, Portugal

Peter Stephens
Northern Institute for Cancer Research
Newcastle University
Newcastle upon Tyne, United Kingdom

Anish Thomas
Medical Oncology Branch
National Cancer Institute
Bethesda, Maryland

Jane B. Trepel
Center for Cancer Research
National Cancer Institute
Bethesda, Maryland

Victoria M. Villaflor
Department of Medicine
University of Chicago
Chicago, Illinois

Simona Wagner
Department of Oncology
Queen's University
Kingston, Ontario, Canada

Annerleim Walton-Diaz
Center for Cancer Research
National Cancer Institute
Bethesda, Maryland

Jeffrey Wiezorek
Department of Global Development
Amgen, Inc.
Thousand Oaks, California

Alexandra Zimmer
Medical Oncology Branch
National Cancer Institute
Bethesda, Maryland

1 Role of Next-Generation Sequencing Technologies

Siddhartha Devarakonda
St. Luke's Hospital

Daniel Morgensztern
Washington University School of Medicine

Ramaswamy Govindan
Washington University School of Medicine

CONTENTS

INTRODUCTION

Cancer continues to be a major cause of morbidity and mortality worldwide. In the United States alone, it is estimated that one in three women and one in two men will be diagnosed with cancer during their lifetime.[1] Several targeted agents have been recently approved by the Food and Drug Administration (FDA) for the use in patients

1

with cancer (Table 1.1). Given the molecular heterogeneity of cancer and the narrow spectrum of activity with most targeted drugs, the use of molecular targeted drugs in unselected groups of patients benefits only a small percentage. Most of the success has been achieved when targeted drugs are used in molecularly defined subsets of patients, where predictable high response rates and survival can be expected.[2-5] However, virtually all patients with metastatic cancer, including those with initial dramatic responses, eventually develop secondary resistance and tumor progression. Further advances will only take place with a better understanding of molecular mechanisms underlying cancer initiation and progression. The combination of rapidly advancing sequencing technology and advanced computing power will enable us to first characterize and eventually understand the disordered cancer genome landscape in unprecedented detail. The objective of this chapter is to briefly review existing sequencing technologies and their potential impact in drug development process in oncology.

SEQUENCING TECHNOLOGIES

FIRST-GENERATION TECHNOLOGY

Fredrick Sanger won the Nobel Prize in 1980 for his work on nucleic acid sequencing. Popularly known as "Sanger sequencing" or "chain termination method," his method formed the basis for first-generation sequencing technologies that were used in the human genome project.[6,7] Briefly, the workflow in first-generation sequencing begins with fragmenting the DNA of interest with restriction endonucleases and amplifying these fragments in a bacterial host (typically *Escherichia coli*). The amplified DNA is then incubated with a mixture of deoxynucleotide triphosphates (dATP, dGTP, dCTP, dTTP) and dideoxynucleotide triphosphates (ddATP, ddGTP, ddCTP, ddTTP) in the presence of DNA polymerase. This process facilitates the synthesis of DNA complementary to the sequence of interest with incorporation of deoxynucleotides and dideoxynucleotides. However, the incorporation of a dideoxynucleotide blocks further chain elongation. Since the incorporation of ddNTPs is a random process and four different types of ddNTPs exist, the previously described process results in the synthesis of several strands of varying lengths. These fragments are then ordered by size using electrophoretic (gel-based or capillary) techniques, and the identity of terminal ddNTPs is established by detecting unique fluorescent or radioactive tags on these molecules. A computer algorithm is then used to construct the sequence. This process requires no previous knowledge of the sequence one wishes to determine and is hence a de novo sequencing technique. Greater cost of operation and low throughput (amount of DNA that can be read in a sequence reaction) are the main limitations of this method.[8] Nonetheless, Sanger sequencing is still considered the gold standard for sequence determination and is used for validating results generated by several next-generation technologies.

NEXT-GENERATION OR MASSIVELY PARALLEL SEQUENCING TECHNOLOGY

The limitations posed by Sanger sequencing have led to the development of next-generation sequencing technologies that are more efficient, parallel, cheaper, and

TABLE 1.1
FDA-Approved Novel Therapeutic Agents in Oncology
(as of December 2012)

Agent	Target	Indication for Use
Everolimus	MTOR	Renal angiomyolipoma associated with tuberous sclerosis complex (TSC)
		Hormone receptor-positive, HER2-negative breast cancer
		Renal cell carcinoma
		Pancreatic neuroendocrine tumors
Bosutinib	BCR–ABL	Philadelphia chromosome-positive CML
Cabozantinib	RET, MET, VEGFR-1, -2 and -3, KIT, TRKB, FLT-3, AXL, and TIE-2	Metastatic medullary thyroid cancer
Vismodegib	Hedgehog signaling	Basal cell carcinoma
Axitinib	VEGFR1, 2, and 3	Advanced renal cell carcinoma
Pertuzumab	HER2 and other HER family of receptors including EGFR, HER3, and HER4	HER2-positive metastatic breast cancer
Regorafenib	VEGFR2 and TIE2	Metastatic colorectal cancer
		GIST
Pazopanib	VEGFR-1, VEGFR-2, and VEGFR-3	Renal cell carcinoma
		Soft tissue sarcoma
Ziv-aflibercept	(VEGF-A) and placental growth factor (PlGF)	Metastatic colorectal cancer
Ruxolitinib	JAK1 and JAK2	Myelofibrosis
Vandetanib	EGFR, VEGFR, RET, BRK, TIE2, members of the EPH receptor kinase family, and members of the Src family of tyrosine kinases	Medullary thyroid carcinoma
Crizotinib	ALK rearrangement	ALK-rearranged NSCLC
Vemurafenib	BRAF	BRAF-mutated melanoma
Ipilimumab	CTLA-4	Metastatic melanoma
Sipuleucel	CD54+cells activated with PAP–GM–CSF	Hormone refractory prostate cancer
Bevacizumab	VEGF	Metastatic colorectal cancer
		Glioblastoma
		NSCLC
		Renal cell carcinoma
Romidepsin	HDAC	Cutaneous T-cell lymphoma and peripheral T-cell lymphomas
Plerixafor	CXCR4 chemokine receptor	NHL and multiple myeloma
Nilotinib	Bcr–Abl kinase, c-kit, and platelet-derived growth factor (PDGF)	Philadelphia chromosome-positive CML
Temsirolimus	MTOR	Renal cell carcinoma
Lapatinib	EGFR and HER2	Breast cancer

(continued)

TABLE 1.1 (continued)
FDA-Approved Novel Therapeutic Agents in Oncology
(as of December 2012)

Agent	Target	Indication for Use
Dasatinib	CR–ABL, SRC family (SRC, LCK, YES, FYN), c-KIT, EPHA2, and PDGFRß	Imatinib-resistant CML
Sunitinib	VEGFR1, 2, and 3, KIT, FLT3, CSF-1R, and RET	Kidney cancer/gastrointestinal stromal tumors (GISTs) Pancreatic NET
Vorinostat	HDAC	Cutaneous T-cell lymphoma
Panitumumab	Monoclonal antibody against EGFR	Colorectal cancer
Sorafenib	Intracellular BRAF, CRAF and extracellular KIT, FLT-3, VEGFR-2, VEGFR-3, and PDGFR-B	Renal cell carcinoma Hepatocellular carcinoma
Cetuximab	Monoclonal antibody against EGFR	Colorectal cancer
Erlotinib	EGFR	NSCLC
Imatinib	Bcr–Abl kinase, c-kit, and PDGF	GISTs Philadelphia chromosome-positive CML
Trastuzumab	HER2	HER2 overexpressing breast and gastric carcinomas
Rituximab	Monoclonal antibody against CD20	NHL, CLL

Note: List not inclusive of all FDA-approved monoclonal antibodies.

feasible for widespread application in research.[8,9] While several massively parallel sequencing technologies are currently available commercially and differ in terms of the sequencing techniques, they share a common operating principle. The workflow for next-generation sequencing always begins with the fragmentation of DNA of interest. Oligonucleotide adapter molecules are then ligated to the ends of these fragments. The DNA molecules are then immobilized on a surface that is embedded with oligonucleotide sequences complementary to the ligated adapter. Following this step, the immobilized DNA molecule undergoes amplification forming "polonies" (since these amplified, identical DNA fragments resemble colonies). The synthesis of a DNA strand complementary to the immobilized strand is then initiated using the unbound adapter (free end of the immobilized strand) as a primer. It is possible to subject several DNA libraries that contain many such polonies to this reaction simultaneously using next-generation sequencers. Nucleotide bases that are used for extending the complementary strand are fluorescent-tagged "reversible terminator" (RT) nucleotides. Once initiated, the process of chain elongation is periodically uncoupled. The process is again reinitiated after washing away unbound nucleotides and detecting fluorescence from the bound nucleotide. As one would expect, each of the four nucleotides is tagged with a unique fluorescent label. While Sanger

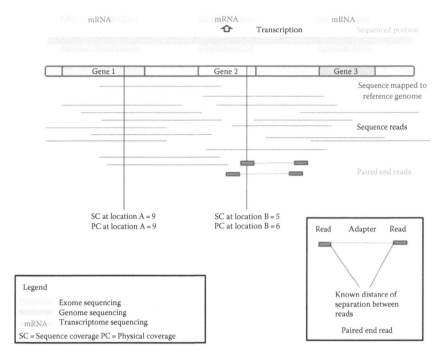

FIGURE 1.1 Schematic representation of different types of sequencing and sequence coverage. (Adapted from Meyerson, M. et al., *Nat. Rev. Genet.*, 11, 685, 2010.)

sequencing is de novo, sequencing data from next-generation sequencing are largely assembled by mapping them onto a reference genome. Apart from bringing down costs and sequencing time, next-generation sequencing also offers the ability to oversample a given sequence.[10] This allows the determination of a given sequence with greater confidence by improving coverage (number of times a particular region is sequenced) at that location (Figure 1.1). A different adaptation of the same technology is the paired-end sequencing, a strategy that involves the ligation of two different adapters to both ends of a given DNA fragment, facilitating simultaneous sequence determination from both ends.[11] A variation of this method involves linking two DNA fragments whose distance of separation on the genome is well established, using an adapter. The free ends of both these fragments are then ligated to adapters, and sequencing is performed. Because the expected distance of separation between these sequences is already known, this method allows inferring the presence structural variations (SVs) in a genome.

Commercially available popular massively parallel sequencing platforms include 454 pyrosequencing, Illumina Solexa, SOLiD, and Heliscope. Details concerning each of these platforms, advantages of using one platform over another, and their limitations have been discussed in several excellent reviews.[9–11] Depending on the extent of interest in sequencing the nucleic acid repertoire of a cell and the type of nucleic acid, sequencing can involve the whole-genome sequencing (WGS), whole-exome sequencing (WES), or transcriptome (Figure 1.1). WGS involves sequencing the entire genome of a cell. WGS can yield information pertinent to SVs (including deletions, insertions, and rearrangements), single-nucleotide variations (SNVs), and copy number alterations (CNAs). It is possible to query gene promoter, enhancer, and splice site variations using WGS as it captures sequence information from intergenic regions. On the other hand, WES only captures sequence information from exons. The exome constitutes of nearly 18,000 genes, which makes up approximately 1% of the entire genome.[12] Complementary DNA (cDNA) sequences of variable length hybridize to and capture exonic regions from isolated and fragmented DNA of interest. This custom captured DNA is then selectively sequenced. Since WES data do not capture intergenic sequences, splice site and promoter regions cannot be queried using this method. WES also misses information related to SVs that do not involve coding regions of the genome.[13] Given that the current knowledge of the genome is largely restricted to the exome and it is much cheaper to sequence the exome, WES is a useful research tool. As sequencing costs continue to decrease, it is expected that WGS will eventually replace WES. Transcriptome sequencing is different from WGS and WES in that the nucleic acid of interest is the mRNA (RNA-seq). Transcriptome sequencing largely restricts itself to the transcribed part of the genome. As mRNA is complementary to the DNA from which it is transcribed, transcriptome sequencing allows the detection of SNVs and also to an extent SVs in the exome.[10,14] Transcriptome sequencing can aid in the determination of functional consequence of alterations by accurately characterizing the level of gene expression. Transcriptome sequencing can also provide crucial insights into the mechanisms of gene regulation. WGS and WES studies require simultaneous sampling of a normal tissue sample (blood, skin, etc.) along with a tumor sample for comparison. Procuring such a control sample for transcriptome sequencing, with a level and pattern of gene expression comparable to the tumor, can be difficult.

INTERPRETATION OF GENOMIC DATA

Genome sequencing projects generate vast amounts of data with several abnormalities of unclear significance. Somatic mutations in cancer cells may be broadly subdivided into driver and passenger mutations, with only the former being implicated in oncogenesis by conferring clonal growth advantage. In contrast, passenger mutations often occur during cell division and are not associated with biological consequences. With both mutations present in the cancer cells, a key challenge in genome analysis is to identify the biologically relevant driver mutations.[15] The clinical success of a therapeutic molecule would hence depend on its capability to target driver mutations. Using many in silico tools, it is currently possible to predict the structural and functional impact of a given genetic alteration on a protein and predict its oncogenic potential and targetability. Some in silico tools also aid in assigning genes to cell-signaling pathways and gene ontologies. Functional studies will need to be done to better understand the novel pathway alterations discovered in such large-scale genomic analyses. Features of currently available cancer genomic data portals, tools for analyzing genomic data, and their limitations have been extensively reviewed elsewhere.[16] We will briefly review here the clinical implications of cancer genome sequencing.

DISCOVERY OF NOVEL THERAPEUTIC TARGETS

Lung Cancer

In a study conducted by Govindan and colleagues in which the whole genome of 17 non-small cell lung cancer (NSCLC) samples, consisting mostly of adenocarcinomas, were sequenced, potentially targetable genes were identified in all 17 samples with a median of 11 targets per patient.[17] These targetable genes included *BRAF, PIK3CG, MET, RET, FGFR1, JAK*, heat shock protein (*HSP90AA1*), and histone deacetylases. Of these, alterations in genes such as *HGF, MET, ERBB4*, and *JAK2* were recurrent. In a study carried out by Imielinski and colleagues, in which 183 NSCLC adenocarcinoma samples were sequenced, mutations deregulating RNA and epigenetic pathways were reported in nearly 10% of the samples.[18] Similarly, Govindan and colleagues also reported mutations in chromatin-associated genes *SETD2, ARID1A*, and *ARID2* and histone methyltransferases *MLL3, MLL4, WHSC1L1*, and *ASH1L*, supporting a "hallmark" role for epigenetic and RNA deregulation in the pathogenesis of adenocarcinoma. Agents capable of targeting epigenetic pathway components such as epigenetic readers,[19] DNA methyltransferases, and histone deacetylases have a potential role in the management of such tumors. Nonrecurring, potentially targetable alterations such as exon 25- and exon 26-deleted variant of *EGFR* and *ROS1* fusion were reported, along with several other novel alterations of uncertain therapeutic potential by both groups. Mutations involving the genes *U2AF1, DACH1, RELN*, and *ABCB5* were reported for the first time in lung cancer by these investigators. Particularly crucial was the observation that 8 out of 10 multiclonal tumors in the study by Govindan et al. harbored targetable alterations in the tumor subclone. Since treatment strategies centered on targeting the dominant clone can eventually fail by favoring selection of the subclone, designing regimens that target alterations in both dominant and subclone cell populations carry the potential to optimize targeted therapy.

The use of several newly developed targeted agents has improved outcomes in lung cancer patients with NSCLC.[20–22] Although no molecular targeted drug has been specifically approved for the use in squamous NSCLC, results from The Cancer Genome Atlas (TCGA) project have identified a number of potentially targetable alterations. The genomic landscape of 178 squamous cell cancer samples was characterized using next-generation sequencing technology in the TCGA project.[23] In this study, 64% of the samples were found to harbor alterations in targetable genes. At least one component of either *PI3K* or RTK signaling pathways was found altered in 47% and 26% of the samples, respectively. Amplification of *EGFR* in 7% of the cases and two mutations that conferred sensitivity to inhibition by TKIs were also observed in this study.

Frequent 3q gains affecting the *SOX2* gene locus were reported along with focal amplifications involving *CCNE1* and *FGFR1* gene loci in a study carried out by Peifer and colleagues, in which small cell lung cancer (SCLC) samples were sequenced.[24] While only *TP53* and *RB1* mutations stood out as significant on initial data analysis, further analysis suggested possible driver roles for the genes *PTEN*, *SLIT2*, *CREBBP*, *MLL*, *COBL*, *EP300*, and *EPHA7* in SCLC. Mutations in genes coding histone-modifying proteins, *EP300*, *MLL*, and *CREBBP*, were reported suggesting a role for drugs targeting epigenetic pathways. *FGFR1* amplification and *PTEN* deletions also present potential therapeutic targets (with *FGFR* and *PI3K* pathway inhibitors). Rudin and colleagues reported recurrent copy number gains in *SOX2*, *SOX4*, *MYC*, and *KIT*, in 56 SCLC samples.[25] Since SCLC cell lines with *MYC* amplifications show in vitro susceptibility to aurora kinase inhibitors, there may be a role for these agents in selected SCLC tumors.[26]

BREAST CANCER

Results from WES of tumors from 507 patients with breast cancer were reported by the investigators from TCGA.[27] Sequencing results were interpreted in the framework of expression profiling-based intrinsic subtypes of the disease. Of the tumors that tested positive for *HER2* (*HER2* +) clinically (by immunohistochemistry), 50% belonged to the *HER2*-enriched (*HER2*E) subtype, characterized by increased expression of receptor tyrosine kinases, a higher *TP53* mutation rate, and the *HER2/pHER2/EGFR/pEGFR* signature. The majority of *HER2*-positive non-*HER2*-enriched (*HER2* +/non-*HER2*E) tumors belonged to the luminal subtype, which were characterized by estrogen receptor (ER) positivity and a high rate of alterations in the transcription factor *GATA3*, a gene responsible for guiding epithelial cell differentiation in luminal cells.[28] It is possible that these intrinsic molecular differences between *HER2* +tumors guide responsiveness to *HER2*-targeted therapies and might play a critical role in biomarker-based patient selection. The role of *PIK3CA* inhibitors needs to be studied, given the high rate of *PIK3CA* mutations reported in this subset of breast cancer.

Most *HER2−/ER−/PR−* (triple-negative) breast cancers were associated with the basal-like subtype characterized by the inactivation of key tumor suppressor genes such as *TP53*, *RB1*, *PTEN*, and *BRCA1*.[27] Basal-like tumors also demonstrated greater genomic instability, higher *PIK3CA and HIF1α/ARNT* pathway activity, and features that suggest a high degree of resemblance to serous ovarian carcinomas. Molecules that target *PIK3CA*, angiogenesis (*HIF1α/ARNT* mediated), and amplified RTKs such as *FGFR*, *IGFR*, *KIT*, *MET*, and *PDGFRA* present novel therapeutic opportunities. *BRCA* gene mutations were also observed in approximately 20% of the patients with basal-like tumors. Since these alterations are known to confer sensitivity to PARP inhibitors and/or platinum agents, a role for these agents in triple-negative breast cancers has been suggested.[29] Copy number alterations involving genes that are amenable for targeting such as *IGFR1*, *cyclinD1*, *CDK4*, *CDK6*, and *EGFR* were also reported across different subtypes.

COLORECTAL CARCINOMA (CRC)

Different mutational profiles, DNA methylation, and mRNA clustering patterns for hyper and non-hypermutated colorectal tumors were reported by the

TCGA project that sequenced the exome of 224 tumors, suggesting the possibility that different molecular events guided the transformation of these tumors.[30] Mutations in *BRAF* (V600E), and *TGFBR2* were more frequent in hypermutated cancers (tumors with a mutation rate >12 per 10^6). The study showed a high degree of *WNT* pathway deregulation and 17% of the tumors overexpressed the WNT receptor *FZD10* and half of the patients had activation of the *PI3K* pathway. *PI3K* and *RAS* pathway alterations were also found to co-occur in a third of these tumors. These observations suggest a role for molecules targeting the *WNT*, *PI3K*, and *RTK-RAS* pathways in the management of CRC. Some tumors harbored the *BRAF* V600E variant, which confers sensitivity to vemurafenib in melanoma cells.[3]

Head and Neck Squamous Cell Carcinoma (HNSCC)

In a study carried out by Stransky and colleagues, 74 tumors were subjected to WES using next-generation sequencing.[31] High mutation rates were observed in non-human papillomavirus (HPV)-associated HNSCCs compared to tumors that were HPV-positive. An inverse correlation between *TP53* alteration and HPV positivity was also reported. Genes implicated in guiding squamous differentiation of cells were among the 39 significantly mutated genes in HNSCC. Alterations reported in this context included mutations in the *NOTCH1, 2,* and *3* genes; *SYNE1*; *SYNE2*; *TP63*; *IRF6*; *RIMS2*; and *PCLO*. Increased incidence of skin cancers noted in subjects receiving *NOTCH* pathway inhibitors (γ-secretase inhibitors) for other reasons supports the role of this gene in oncogenesis.[32] Targeting these tumors using synthetic lethality-based approaches by identifying tumor dependency on the inhibition of differentiation pathways may become a therapeutic strategy in HNSCC. Another strategy would be to target *DICER1*, a gene also mutated in non-epithelial ovarian cancers, which takes part in microRNA (miRNA) biogenesis.[33] The role of miRNAs in oncogenesis and therapeutic strategies has been recently reviewed.[34]

Medulloblastoma

Two studies have characterized the genomic landscape of this fatal childhood malignancy using next-generation sequencing platforms.[35,36] In the study carried out by Pugh and colleagues, 92 medulloblastoma tumors were subjected to WES.[36] As a part of the International Cancer Genome Consortium (ICGC) PedBrain Tumor project, 21 tumors were subjected to WES and 39 tumors to WGS. The findings from these studies have been interpreted in the framework of intrinsic molecular subtypes of the disease.[35] Among the WNT subgroup of tumors, *CTNNB1* and chromosome 6 losses were reported in almost all tumors. Loss of the chromosomal region 9q was more prevalent among the sonic hedgehog (SHH) subtype tumors, while group 3 and group 4 subtype tumors demonstrated extensive somatic copy number alterations. A significant rate of alteration in genes playing a role in chromatin remodeling including histone methyltransferases,

SWI/SNF group, and nuclear corepressor complex (N-CoR) members was reported across all subtypes. Mutations in genes guiding RNA processing, such as *DDX3X*, were also prevalent in WNT and SHH tumors. Group 3 and group 4 tumors that are associated with an aggressive phenotype demonstrated a high frequency of tetraploidy (54% in group 3 and 40% in group 4), and it has been suggested that tetraploidy occurs very early in the pathogenesis of these tumors. There hence exists a potential role for kinesin or checkpoint kinase inhibiting agents, which interfere with the successful transfer of tetraploidy to tumor cell progeny. Group 4 tumors that harbored isochromosome 17 (i17) also demonstrated a high rate of *KDM6A* alterations. Tumors with i17 and normal *KDM6A* demonstrated mutations in other histone-modifying genes such as *THUMPD3*, *ZMYM3*, and *MLL3*, which present a potential for targeting.[37]

OVARIAN CARCINOMA

As a part of TCGA project, 316 high-grade serous ovarian carcinoma (HGS-OvCa) tumor samples were subjected to WES.[38] *RB1* and *PIK3CA* pathway deregulation was frequent across HGS-OvCa samples. The *NOTCH* signaling pathway was also altered in 22% of the samples. Alterations in the homologous recombination repair pathway that are believed to confer sensitivity to PARP inhibitors were encountered in nearly half the samples.[29,39] These alterations included *BRCA1* mutation and hypermethylation (23%), *BRCA2* mutation (11%), amplification or mutation of *EMSY* (C11orf30) (8%), *PTEN* mutation or deletion (7%), *RAD51C* hypermethylation (3%), *ATM/ATR* mutations (1% and <1%, respectively), and mutations in Fanconi anemia core complex genes (5%). Apart from alterations in the previously mentioned pathways, 22 of the amplified or overexpressed genes were also considered targetable. This gene set included member genes such as *MECOM*, *MAPK1*, *CCNE1*, and *KRAS* that were amplified in about 10% of the samples. A 193 gene transcriptional signature comprising of 108 poor prognosis and 85 good prognosis genes was also identified by the investigators, and the predictive power of this signature was validated in a set of 255 independent samples.

MELANOMA

In a study conducted by Berger and colleagues, the whole genome of 25 metastatic melanoma samples was sequenced.[40] Apart from observing the well-characterized *BRAF* V600E mutation in 64% of these samples, mutations in *NRAS* (in a mutually exclusive fashion to *BRAF*) and the coding exons of *KIT* were also reported. The study also suggested an oncogenic role for *PREX2* gene alteration by mutation, amplification, or rearrangement. Further sequencing of an extended cohort of 107 samples estimated a prevalence of 14% for nonsynonymous *PREX2* mutations. It was speculated that *PREX2* gained oncogenic potential via mutations that disrupted normal functioning of the protein. It is possible that genes like *PREX2*, which are affected by such alterations, constitute a different category of cancer causing genes that differ from classical oncogenes or tumor suppressors, which are affected by gain-of-function or loss-of-function mutations. The therapeutic application of this finding is however uncertain at the moment.

IDENTIFICATION OF NOVEL ALTERATIONS OF KNOWN TARGETS

The ability of WGS to facilitate the process of clinical decision making was recently demonstrated in the case of a leukemic patient.[41] The investigators were able to identify a novel insertion exchange between chromosomes 15 and 17 that resulted in a *PML–RARA* gene fusion, a hallmark fusion observed in acute promyelocytic leukemia, which was missed by traditional cytogenetic assays. This information radically changed the management approach from planned bone marrow transplantation to treatment with all-trans-retinoic acid (ATRA).

CLONAL EVOLUTION

It is now possible to estimate clonality of a tumor using mutant allele frequencies within a given tumor cell population (Figure 1.2). As shown in a study conducted by Ding and colleagues, applying such an analysis to tumor samples obtained from the same patient at different stages of disease allows tracking evolution of tumor clones.[42] Tumor samples from AML patients in this study, which were sequenced at the time of diagnosis and later at the time of disease recurrence, demonstrated two patterns of disease recurrence. In the first pattern, cells from the dominant clone

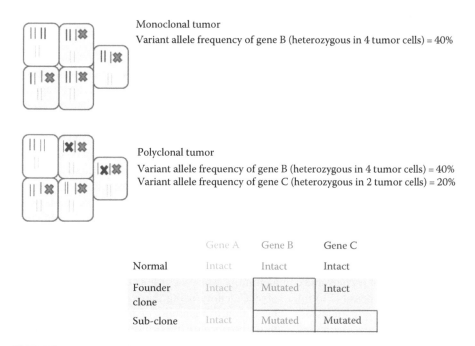

FIGURE 1.2   Schematic representation of clonal analysis using next-generation sequencing.

had acquired additional mutations. In the second pattern, cells from a minor clone were shown to survive treatment, acquire additional mutations during the course of treatment, and establish themselves as the dominant clone at the time of recurrence. A clonal analysis in lung cancer patients also indicated the presence of targetable alterations in tumor subclones.[17] These results emphasize the importance and feasibility of targeting subclones in a tumor population along with the dominant clone to ensure better disease control.

PERSONALIZING IMMUNE THERAPY

The process by which host immunity selects for tumor subclones that fail to express certain epitopes is referred to as cancer immunoediting.[43–45] This is achieved by the "elimination" of tumor clones that express highly immunogenic epitopes. These tumor subclones are also referred to as "escape" clones. Next-generation sequencing technology in conjunction with in silico analysis can aid in the identification of such epitopes, as demonstrated by Matsushita and colleagues.[45] In this study, carcinogen-induced sarcoma cell lines were transplanted into immunodeficient *Rag2–/–* and wild-type mice and shown to undergo T-cell-mediated immunoediting. Interestingly, based on an in silico analysis following next-generation sequencing of the sarcoma cell lines, the investigators were able to identify mutant spectrin-$\beta 2$ as the epitope of interest. By introducing the gene coding this mutant protein into escape tumor cells using viral vectors, the authors were also able to induce T-cell infiltration and an immune reaction against these cells. This example illustrates the possibility of using next-generation sequencing to customize personalized immunotherapy.

INCORPORATION INTO CLINICAL TRIALS

By using next-generation sequencing technologies for patient selection, trials enrolling a large number of subjects to test empiric therapies are expected to be replaced by smaller trials that test targeted agents in biomarker-selected populations. Such a paradigm shift would mandate the need for improvising the existing clinical trial machinery. The role of well-designed preclinical trials for identifying and validating biomarkers will be critical for ensuring phase III success. The conduct of such studies requires an ample amount of tissue and emphasizes the need for mandatory and efficient tissue collection and storage. As discussed earlier, tissue collection at different stages of the disease and treatment will also be necessary to better understand disease progression, treatment responsiveness, and clonal evolution. Establishing consortia that screen samples for a panel of biomarkers ("multiplex testing") to guide patient enrollment into appropriate trials would also be necessary to optimize resource and tissue utilization. Large-scale genomic studies also present challenges related to patient privacy and confidentiality when the results become publicly available, since it is possible to infer subject identity using these data.[46] Addressing the issue of notifying patients and related family members of incidentally discovered deleterious genetic alterations, without compromising privacy, is also crucial. One way of achieving this would be to implement a "movable firewall" system.[41,47] An independent third party serves as an "honest broker" in this approach. By retaining sole access to patient identifier data, the "honest broker" takes up the task of notifying patients and constantly updating de-identified patient databases. It is also unclear if alterations of uncertain clinical significance need to be discussed with patients, as such a discussion might lead to unnecessary and expensive diagnostic testing and anxiety. At the same time, withholding information from subjects can result in ethical and legal complications.

CONCLUSIONS

Ongoing large-scale genomic studies are likely to further improve our understanding of molecular underpinnings of malignant phenotype. The larger cancer research community should work together to harness fully the potential of genome sequencing to identify novel targets and use the genomic information innovatively to develop therapies uniquely suited to the given tumor. Furthermore, with diligent incorporation of genomic studies serially over time, we will understand better the clonal selection and evolution in response to therapy. The outlook for cancer research has never been brighter.

REFERENCES

1. Siegel R, Desantis C, Virgo K et al. Cancer treatment and survivorship statistics, 2012. *CA Cancer J Clin* 2012;62:220–241.
2. Kwak EL, Bang YJ, Camidge DR et al. Anaplastic lymphoma kinase inhibition in non-small-cell lung cancer. *N Engl J Med* 2010;363:1693–1703.
3. Chapman PB, Hauschild A, Robert C et al. Improved survival with vemurafenib in melanoma with BRAF V600E mutation. *N Engl J Med* 2011;364:2507–2516.
4. Lynch TJ, Bell DW, Sordella R et al. Activating mutations in the epidermal growth factor receptor underlying responsiveness of non-small-cell lung cancer to gefitinib. *N Engl J Med* 2004;350:2129–2139.
5. O'Brien SG, Guilhot F, Larson RA et al. Imatinib compared with interferon and low-dose cytarabine for newly diagnosed chronic-phase chronic myeloid leukemia. *N Engl J Med* 2003;348:994–1004.
6. Sanger F, Nicklen S, Coulson AR. DNA sequencing with chain-terminating inhibitors. *Proc Natl Acad Sci USA* 1977;74:5463–5467.
7. Lander ES, Linton LM, Birren B et al. Initial sequencing and analysis of the human genome. *Nature* 2001;409:860–921.
8. Rizzo JM, Buck MJ. Key principles and clinical applications of "next-generation" DNA sequencing. *Cancer Prev Res (Phila)* 2012;5:887–900.
9. Shendure J, Ji H. Next-generation DNA sequencing. *Nat Biotechnol* 2008;26:1135–1145.
10. Meyerson M, Gabriel S, Getz G. Advances in understanding cancer genomes through second-generation sequencing. *Nat Rev Genet* 2010;11:685–696.
11. Fullwood MJ, Wei CL, Liu ET, Ruan Y. Next-generation DNA sequencing of paired-end tags (PET) for transcriptome and genome analyses. *Genome Res* 2009;19:521–532.
12. Ng SB, Turner EH, Robertson PD et al. Targeted capture and massively parallel sequencing of 12 human exomes. *Nature* 2009;461:272–276.
13. Biesecker LG, Shianna KV, Mullikin JC. Exome sequencing: the expert view. *Genome Biol* 2011;12:128.
14. Soda M, Choi YL, Enomoto M et al. Identification of the transforming EML4-ALK fusion gene in non-small-cell lung cancer. *Nature* 2007;448:561–566.

15. Stratton MR, Campbell PJ, Futreal PA. The cancer genome. *Nature* 2009;458:719–724.
16. Chin L, Hahn WC, Getz G, Meyerson M. Making sense of cancer genomic data. *Genes Dev* 2011;25:534–555.
17. Govindan R, Ding L, Griffith M et al. Genomic landscape of non-small cell lung cancer in smokers and never-smokers. *Cell* 2012;150:1121–1134.
18. Imielinski M, Berger AH, Hammerman PS et al. Mapping the hallmarks of lung adeno-carcinoma with massively parallel sequencing. *Cell* 2012;150:1107–1120.
19. Dawson MA, Kouzarides T, Huntly BJ. Targeting epigenetic readers in cancer. *N Engl J Med* 2012;367:647–657.
20. Sandler A, Gray R, Perry MC et al. Paclitaxel-carboplatin alone or with bevacizumab for non-small-cell lung cancer. *N Engl J Med* 2006;355:2542–2550.
21. Kwak EL, Bang YJ, Camidge DR et al. Anaplastic lymphoma kinase inhibition in non-small-cell lung cancer. *N Engl J Med* 2010;363:1693–1703.
22. Pirker R, Pereira JR, Szczesna A et al. Cetuximab plus chemotherapy in patients with advanced non-small-cell lung cancer (FLEX): An open-label randomised phase III trial. *Lancet* 2009;373:1525–1531.
23. Hammerman PS, Hayes DN, Wilkerson MD et al. Comprehensive genomic character-ization of squamous cell lung cancers. *Nature* 2012;489:519–525.
24. Peifer M, Fernández-Cuesta L, Sos ML et al. Integrative genome analyses identify key somatic driver mutations of small-cell lung cancer. *Nat Genet* 2012;44:1104–1110.
25. Rudin CM, Durinck S, Stawiski EW et al. Comprehensive genomic analysis identi-fies SOX2 as a frequently amplified gene in small-cell lung cancer. *Nat Genet* 2012;44:1111–1116.
26. Sos ML, Dietlein F, Peifer M et al. A framework for identification of actionable cancer genome dependencies in small cell lung cancer. *Proc Natl Acad Sci USA* 2012;109:17034–17039.
27. Cancer Genome Atlas Network. Comprehensive molecular portraits of human breast tumours. *Nature* 2012;490:61–70.
28. Chou J, Provot S, Werb Z. GATA3 in development and cancer differentiation: Cells GATA have it! *J Cell Physiol* 2010;222:42–49.
29. Bryant HE, Schultz N, Thomas HD et al. Specific killing of BRCA2-deficient tumours with inhibitors of poly (ADP-ribose) polymerase. *Nature* 2005;434:913–917.
30. Cancer Genome Atlas Network. Comprehensive molecular characterization of human colon and rectal cancer. *Nature* 2012;487:330–337.
31. Stransky N, Egloff AM, Tward AD et al. The mutational landscape of head and neck squamous cell carcinoma. *Science* 2011;333:1157–1160.
32. Extance A. Alzheimer's failure raises questions about disease-modifying strategies. *Nat Rev Drug Discov* 2010;9:749–751.
33. Heravi-Moussavi A, Anglesio MS, Cheng SW et al. Recurrent somatic DICER1 mutations in nonepithelial ovarian cancers. *N Engl J Med* 2012;366:234–242.
34. Iorio MV, Croce CM. MicroRNA dysregulation in cancer: Diagnostics, monitoring and therapeutics. A comprehensive review. *EMBO Mol Med* 2012;4:143–159.
35. Jones DT, Jäger N, Kool M et al. Dissecting the genomic complexity underlying medulloblastoma. *Nature* 2012;488:100–115.
36. Pugh TJ, Weeraratne SD, Archer TC et al. Medulloblastoma exome sequencing uncovers subtype-specific somatic mutations. *Nature* 2012;488:106–110.
37. Esteller M. Epigenetics in cancer. *N Engl J Med* 2008;358:1148–1159.
38. Cancer Genome Atlas Research Network. Integrated genomic analyses of ovarian carci-noma. *Nature* 2011;474:609–615.
39. Curtin NJ. DNA repair dysregulation from cancer driver to therapeutic target. *Nat Rev Cancer* 2012;12:801–817.

40. Berger MF, Hodis E, Heffernan TP et al. Melanoma genome sequencing reveals frequent PREX2 mutations. *Nature* 2012;485:502–506.
41. Welch JS, Westervelt P, Ding L et al. Use of whole-genome sequencing to diagnose a cryptic fusion oncogene. *JAMA* 2011;305:1577–1584.
42. Ding L, Ley TJ, Larson DE et al. Clonal evolution in relapsed acute myeloid leukaemia revealed by whole-genome sequencing. *Nature* 2012;481:506–510.
43. Shankaran V, Ikeda H, Bruce AT et al. IFNgamma and lymphocytes prevent primary tumour development and shape tumour immunogenicity. *Nature* 2001;410:1107–1111.
44. Schreiber RD, Old LJ, Smyth MJ. Cancer immunoediting: Integrating immunity's roles in cancer suppression and promotion. *Science* 2011;331:1565–1570.
45. Matsushita H, Vesely MD, Koboldt DC et al. Cancer exome analysis reveals a T-cell-dependent mechanism of cancer immunoediting. *Nature* 2012;482:400–404.
46. Jacobs KB, Yeager M, Wacholder S et al. A new statistic and its power to infer membership in a genome-wide association study using genotype frequencies. *Nat Genet* 2009;41:1253–1257.
47. Dhir R, Patel AA, Winters S et al. A multidisciplinary approach to honest broker services for tissue banks and clinical data: A pragmatic and practical model. *Cancer* 2008;113:1705–1715.

2 Signal Transduction Inhibitors of the HER Family

Christina Brzezniak
Walter Reed National Military Medical Center

Corey Carter
Walter Reed National Military Medical Center

Anish Thomas
National Cancer Institute

Giuseppe Giaccone
National Cancer Institute

CONTENTS

INTRODUCTION

The human epidermal growth factor receptor (HER) family has been extensively investigated as a target for anticancer therapy. The HER family is composed of four transmembrane tyrosine kinase (TK) receptors, which include ErbB1 (HER1 or epidermal growth factor receptor [EGFR]), ErbB2 (HER2/neu or HER2), ErbB3 (HER3), and ErbB4 (HER4). EGFR was the first ErbB family member to be described and remains the best characterized to date [1,2]. HER kinases are overexpressed in a large number of tumors, including head and neck, colorectal, lung, breast, ovary, prostate, kidney, brain, pancreas, and bladder carcinomas [3]. Epithelial cells and malignant tumors of epithelial origin express HER kinases, but they are not expressed on mature hematopoietic cells [2,4]. The HER kinases have six known ligands: epidermal growth factor (EGF), transforming growth factor alpha (TGF-a), amphiregulin, betacellulin, heparin-binding EGF, and epiregulin [9]. These kinases bind at least one HER family member leading to receptor dimerization (homo- or heterodimerization), phosphorylation, and activation. Interestingly, HER2 has no known ligand and instead is the favored binding partner for other HER family receptors [6]. Once activated, the receptor is internalized, and its degradation or recycling can transiently downregulate signaling mediated by the receptor. Multiple signaling pathways related to cellular proliferation and survival are activated downstream of the TK, including the RAS pathway with the extracellular signal-regulated kinase (ERK)/mitogen-activated protein kinase (MAPK), the phosphatidylinositol 3-kinase/Akt (PI3K/Akt) pathway, and the signal transducer and activator of transcription (STAT) pathway. HER TK activation can also induce cell-cycle progression via various mechanisms, including the upregulation of cyclin D1 [7]. HER kinase stimulation can significantly increase the activity of c-Src, a signaling intermediate involved in cell-cycle progression, motility, angiogenesis, and survival [8] (Figure 2.1).

The overexpression of HER family kinases correlates with poor prognosis and decreased survival in several solid tumors [9–11]. Moreover, tumors that overexpress these TKs often produce their own ligands, such as TGF-a, leading to the activation of survival pathways via autocrine loops. Amplification of HER2 and EGFR mutations leads to aberrant signaling that is implicated in mediating multiple processes involved in tumor progression and metastasis, including invasion, angiogenesis, proliferation, and inhibition of apoptosis [12]. Cells harboring amplification or mutations become dependent upon the dysfunctional signaling for continued survival termed "oncogenic addiction" [13], providing a rationale for therapies targeting these receptors and their pathways.

HER TYROSINE KINASE INHIBITORS

SMALL MOLECULES

Tyrosine kinase inhibitors (TKIs) (Table 2.1) prevent autophosphorylation of the EGFR intracellular TK domain by adenosine triphosphate (ATP) competitive inhibition at the intracellular catalytic domain. EGFR TKIs fall into two broad classes:

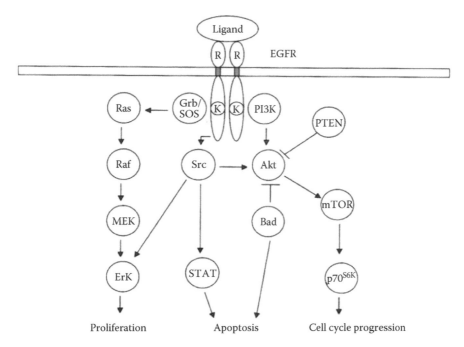

FIGURE 2.1   Schematic representation of major components of the EGF receptor pathway.

reversible inhibitors, such as gefitinib (Iressa®, AstraZeneca, London, U.K.) and erlotinib (Tarceva®, Genentech, South San Francisco, California, USA), and irreversible inhibitors, such as dacomitinib (Pfizer, New London, Connecticut, USA), neratinib (Puma Biotechnology, Los Angeles, California, USA), and afatinib (Boehringer Ingelheim, Ingelheim, Germany). Irreversible inhibitors covalently bind specific cysteine residues in the ATP binding site of EGFR. The clinical significance of reversible versus irreversible inhibition is uncertain at this point. The ability to irreversibly bind the TK domain could theoretically produce more sustained antitumor activity. Furthermore, some irreversible inhibitors have been shown to have activity against the EGFR T790M mutation, which is found in 50% of the cases of acquired resistance to reversible EGFR TKI [14]. Gefitinib and erlotinib are currently approved in many countries for clinical use in advanced non-small cell lung cancer (NSCLC) patients who failed at least one line of chemotherapy. In advanced NSCLC, erlotinib is also approved for maintenance after non-progression on first-line platinum-based chemotherapy and as first-line therapy in patients with tumors harboring EGFR-activating mutations. In addition, erlotinib is approved in pancreatic cancer patients in combination with gemcitabine (Gemzar®, Eli Lilly and Co., Indianapolis, Indiana, USA) in unresectable locally advanced or metastatic disease. Mechanistically, gefitinib is able to block MAPK and PI3K/Akt pathways, and its treatment is associated with cell-cycle arrest at G1, involving increased expression of the cyclin-dependent kinase (CDK) inhibitor p27^{KIP1} and decreased expression of CDK2, CDK4, CDK6, cyclin D1, and cyclin D3. Increased characteristics of apoptosis, such as DNA

TABLE 2.1
HER Inhibitors

Agent	Target	Characteristics	Route	Drug Company
Small molecules				
Gefitinib (Iressa®, ZD1839)	EGFR TK	Specific reversible inhibitor	Oral	AstraZeneca (London, U.K.)
Erlotinib (Tarceva®, OSI-774)	EGFR TK	Specific reversible inhibitor	Oral	OSIP (Melville, New York) Genentech (South San Francisco, California) Roche (Basel, Switzerland)
Icotinib (BPI-1096)	EGFR TK	Specific reversible inhibitor	Oral	Zhejiang Beta Pharma (Hangzhou, China)
Lapatinib (Tykerb®, GW572016)	EGFR and ErbB2 TKs	Dual reversible inhibitor	Oral	GlaxoSmithKline (Brentford, U.K.)
Neratinib (HK-1272)	EGFR and ErbB2 TKs	Irreversible inhibitor	Oral	Pfizer Puma Biotechnology (Los Angeles, California)
Dacomitinib[a] (PF-00299804)	EGFR, ErbB2, and ErbB4 TKs	Irreversible inhibitor	Oral	Pfizer (New London, Connecticut)
Afatinib[a] (BIBW 2992)	EGFR and ErbB2 TKs	Irreversible inhibitor	Oral	Boehringer Ingelheim (Ingelheim, Germany)
Vandetanib (Zactima®, AZD6474)	EGFR and VEGFR2 TKs	Inhibitor of EGFR and VGFR2	Oral	AstraZeneca
AC-480 (BMS 599626)	EGFR, ErbB2, and ErbB4 TKs	Pan-inhibitor of all ErbB members	Oral	Bristol-Myers Squibb (New York, New York), Ambit Biosciences Corporation (California)

Monoclonal antibodies

Name	Target	Type	Route	Company
Cetuximab (Erbitux®, BMS-564717)	EGFR extracellular domain	Chimeric	IV	ImClone (New York, New York), Bristol-Myers Squibb, Merck & Co. (Darmstadt, Germany)
Panitumumab (Vectibix®, ABX-EGF)	EGFR extracellular domain	Fully human	IV	Abgenix (Fremont, California), Amgen (Thousand Oaks, California)
Nimotuzumab (TheraCIM hR3)	EGFR extracellular domain	Humanized	IV	Biocon (Bangalore, India), YM BioSciences (Mississauga, Ontario)
Zalutumumab (HuMax-EGFr)	EGFR extracellular domain	Fully human	IV	Genmab (Copenhagen, Denmark)
Trastuzumab (Herceptin®, R-597)	ErbB2 extracellular domain	Humanized	IV	Roche
Pertuzumab (Perjeta®, 2C4)	Erb2 heterodimerization	Humanized	IV	Roche
CimaVax (EGF vaccine)	EGF	hrEGF bound to protein and albumin	ID	YM BioSciences (Mississauga, Ontario), Bioven (Aberdeen, Scotland)

Abbreviations: EGF, epidermal growth factor; EGFR, epidermal growth factor receptor; ID, intradermally; IV, intravenously; TK, tyrosine kinase; VEGFR2, vascular endothelial growth factor.

a Also active on the T790M-resistant mutant.

fragmentation, increased Fas protein expression, activation of initiator and effector caspases, and a change in plasma membrane phospholipids packing were also observed [15,16]. However, these effects may be limited and dependent on the tumor type [17]. Similar cell-cycle and apoptotic changes have been seen after erlotinib treatment [16,18].

MONOCLONAL ANTIBODIES

Monoclonal antibodies (mAbs) against EGFR (Table 2.1) were the first approach used in clinical studies to target EGFR signaling in malignant cells. The mAbs competitively inhibit the binding of activating ligands to the extracellular domain of EGFR, inhibiting receptor autophosphorylation and, in contrast to the TKIs, inducing its internalization and degradation. Subsequent downstream signaling events are similar to those described for the TKIs gefitinib and erlotinib. Trastuzumab (Herceptin®, Roche, Basel, Switzerland), a mAb directed against HER2, was the first mAb to be approved for the treatment of any malignancy. It has activity against HER2-positive, defined as 3+ on conventional immunohistochemistry (IHC) or gene amplification by fluorescence in situ hybridization (FISH), early stage or metastatic breast cancer. Additionally, it is approved by the Food and Drug Administration (FDA) for HER2-positive advanced or metastatic gastric cancer. Given the activity of HER2 as the favored dimerization partner for the other HER family TKs, investigating trastuzumab and HER2 overexpression is an area of considerable research. Among mAbs, both cetuximab (Erbitux®, ImClone Systems, Inc., Branchburg, New Jersey licensed to Merck & Co., Darmstadt, Germany) and panitumumab (Vectibix®, Amgen, Thousand Oaks, California) are approved for use in colorectal cancer (CRC) refractory to irinotecan (Campto®, Pfizer, Capelle aan den IJssel, the Netherlands), while cetuximab is also approved in locally advanced squamous cell carcinomas of the head and neck (SCCHN), with wild-type KRAS, in combination with radiotherapy.

OTHER EGFR INHIBITORS

Active immunization could be an attractive alternative to inhibit the HER family because it would circumvent both the need for multiple infusions and the danger of inducing an immune response typical of the antibodies. Mimotopes are small peptides that mimic a given epitope structurally, but not necessarily by amino acid sequence. The only important prerequisite is that an antibody recognizes the mimotope, for example, antibodies with proven beneficial antitumor properties, such as cetuximab. Riemer and colleagues observed that the epitope-specific immunization is feasible for active anti-EGFR immunotherapy. The in vitro biologic features of mimotope-induced antibodies are similar to those of the mAb cetuximab [19]. Bing Hu and colleagues observed that an active antitumor immunity could be induced by dendritic cells pulsed with recombinant ectodomain of mouse EGFR (DC-edMER), which may involve both humoral and cellular immunity, and may provide insight into the treatment of EGFR-positive tumors through the induction of active immunity against EGFR [20].

EGF could be another possible target. Ramos and colleagues developed an active specific immunotherapy based on EGF deprivation, observing a correlation between antibody titers, serum EGF levels, and patient survival in a phase I trial of 43 patients with NSCLC receiving the EGF vaccine [21]. The CimaVax (EGF vaccine) continues to be evaluated in preclinical and early phase I trials (Table 2.1) [22].

The use of antisense oligonucleotides inhibiting EGFR synthesis and the use of antibody-based immunoconjugates represent other interesting strategies. In preclinical studies, both treatments showed a significant inhibition of growth in EGFR-positive tumors [23,24].

PREDICTORS OF RESPONSE

Several clinical features demonstrating response to EGFR TKIs in NSCLC have been defined. Retrospective analyses of NSCLC phase II trials showed that never-smoking history, female gender, adenocarcinoma histology, and Asian origin were significantly associated with a higher response to EGFR TKIs [25–29]. Among clinical characteristics, smoking history was the most important predictor. In the TRIBUTE trial [30], median survival is significantly longer in never smokers treated with erlotinib than in never smokers treated with placebo. Similarly, in the BR21 and ISEL trials, it was shown that never smokers treated with EGFR TKIs had a significantly longer survival when compared to never smokers treated with placebo, with no survival difference in smokers irrespective of the treatment [31,32]. Thus far, there appears to be no clinical subgroup of patients with SCCHN or CRC that is more likely to respond or benefit from EGFR TKIs. Nevertheless, patients with SCCHN or CRC who develop skin rash appear to achieve greater benefit when treated with either TKIs or mAbs. Unfortunately, a clear association between signaling inhibition in skin and antitumor response has not been found, and the mechanism underlying this correlation is currently unclear [33]. Development of skin rash has been associated with sensitivity to erlotinib [34] and cetuximab [35] also in NSCLC. However, the role of rash as a marker of sensitivity to gefitinib in NSCLC is more controversial, as some trials show a correlation between rash and response [36,37], while others do not [25].

Biologic features indicative of response to EGFR TKIs in NSCLC are more clearly defined than clinical findings. Certain sensitizing EGFR mutations confer response to TKIs. The two most common mutations are the L858R point mutation on exon 21 and E746-A750 deletion on exon 19. These mutations were found to be significantly related to Asian ethnicity, female gender, adenocarcinoma histology, and never-smoking history [38–43]. Despite the success of gefitinib or erlotinib in the treatment of NSCLC with EGFR mutations, all patients ultimately develop disease progression and/or resistance. The most common, and first identified, mutation conferring resistance to first-generation EGFR TKIs is the T790M mutation. This common secondary mutation occurs in up to 50% of EGFR-mutated TKI-resistant patients and is often referred to as the "gatekeeper mutation" [44–46]. This mutation can also rarely be found as a de novo mutation seen in EGFR-mutated tumors that have not been exposed to TKIs [46–48]. This mutation in which a substitution of methionine for threonine at position 790 (T790M) alters the TKI binding site, causes an increased affinity for ATP, and reduces the efficacy of reversible TKIs [45,49]. However, there remains a portion of EGFR TKI–resistant tumors for which no secondary mutations are found, suggesting that other mechanisms of resistance must also exist. NSCLC tumors presenting EGFR mutations generally do not have KRAS mutations, which typically occur more often in smokers, are less common in East Asians, and are significantly associated with primary resistance to TKIs [50]. Mutations in KRAS are found more frequently in patients who develop disease progression with either gefitinib or erlotinib therapy and are also associated with a worse outcome when patients are treated with chemotherapy in combination with erlotinib [51]. Therefore, the presence of KRAS mutations is considered as negative selector for response to TKIs. As EGFR and KRAS mutations are mutually exclusive, this suggests a different pathogenic mechanism in smokers from never-smoker NSCLC patients [52]. However, approximately 18% of patients responding to EGFR TKIs do not have identifiable EGFR mutations. It is unclear whether this may be the result of the use of insufficiently sensitive methods of detection of the mutation (e.g., Sanger sequencing), the presence of less abundant mutant clones, or a truly different mechanism of sensitivity.

In comparison with NSCLC, EGFR TK mutations in CRC and SCCHN are very rare. In unselected SCCHN tumor specimens from Korean patients, an EGFR TK mutation was described in 7% of cases [53]. Moreover, in a North American study of tissue samples from eight SCCHN patients who responded to either gefitinib or erlotinib, no mutations were detected in the EGFR TK domain [54]. However, high EGFR gene copy number by FISH analysis is associated with a poor prognosis in SCCHN [55]. In CRC, the increased EGFR copy number detected by FISH is associated with response to the anti-EGFR mAbs cetuximab or panitumumab [56]. The polymorphism in intron 1, the CA-simple sequence repeat (CA-SSR), modulates transcriptional efficiency of the EGFR gene and subsequent EGFR expression [57]. Interestingly, shorter repeat lengths that are associated with higher EGFR expression have been shown to be predictive of response to erlotinib in SCCHN cell lines [58]. The prognostic role of EGFR expression by IHC is still controversial. In SCCHN, clinical trials with either TKIs or mAbs have not demonstrated a positive association between EGFR expression by IHC and tumor response [25].

Three major HER2 mutations are recognized, all occurring as in-frame insertions in exon 20 [59–62]. These mutations occur in a small number of NSCLC patients (2%–4%) causing constitutive activation of the HER2 receptor [63]. These mutations are similarly mutually exclusive of the KRAS mutations [64]. HER2 mutations occur with increased frequency in NSCLC tumors of female never smokers and adenocarcinoma histology. Trials evaluating therapies targeting HER2 via second-generation irreversible pan-HER inhibitors such as afatinib have demonstrated response to these therapies [65]. Overexpression of HER2, characterized by 3+ designation on standard IHC or FISH positivity for gene amplification, defines HER2 positivity in both breast and gastric/gastroesophageal cancer. This overexpression confers responsiveness to mAbs such as trastuzumab and pertuzumab. Based upon both the ToGA trial in gastric cancer and numerous trials in both early and metastatic breast cancer, addition of HER2-directed therapy to standard chemotherapy in HER2-positive tumors remains the standard of care [66–68]. In advanced-stage HER2-positive breast cancer, HER2-directed therapies may also be used as single agents. In addition to HER2-specific therapies, such as trastuzumab, all irreversible EGFR TKIs inhibit HER2; therefore, these agents may be of benefit in the NSCLC population who express HER2 mutations or amplification although more data on this population subset are needed [69] and trials are ongoing (NCT01542437).

CLINICAL DEVELOPMENT OF INHIBITORS OF THE HER FAMILY

NON-SMALL CELL LUNG CANCER

Small-molecule EGFR inhibitors gefitinib and erlotinib have been studied extensively in both selected (patients with tumors harboring EGFR-activating mutations) and unselected populations. Initial studies were preformed in unselected populations following chemotherapy failure. Gefitinib was the first molecularly targeted agent approved by the U.S. FDA in advanced unselected NSCLC based on encouraging response rates and symptomatic benefit observed in the IDEAL1 and IDEAL 2 trials [25,26,70]. These phase II studies evaluated gefitinib as a single agent following chemotherapy failure and produced objective response rates (ORRs) and median survivals ranging from 10% to 19% and 6.0 to 8.0 months, respectively (Table 2.2). In the IDEAL 1 and 2 studies, the patients were randomized to receive gefitinib 250 or 500 mg daily. There was no significant difference in response rate and survival between the two dosages. Moreover, there was a good correlation between clinical response and symptomatic improvement that was reached in approximately 40% of patients. Adverse effects were, in general, well tolerated but were more severe with the 500 mg dose in both studies [25,26]. Gefitinib, at the oral dose of 250 mg daily, was approved for patients progressing after platinum and docetaxel (Taxotere®, Sanofi-Aventis, Bridgewater, New Jersey, USA) containing chemotherapy regimens [24]. Unfortunately, a large phase III trial (ISEL) evaluating the efficacy of gefitinib as a second- or third-line therapy in unselected patients failed to show a survival advantage over placebo (5.6 vs. 5.1 months; $p=0.11$) [31] (Table 2.2), although a subset analysis demonstrated significant improvement in Asians ($n=342$) with median survival 9.5 versus 5.5 months ($p=0.01$) and in patients who never smoked ($n=375$), with median survival 8.9 versus 6.1 months ($p=0.012$) [71]. Based on the failure to provide statistically significant survival advantage, gefitinib use was restricted in the U.S. population. A further non-inferiority phase III trial (INTEREST) compared gefitinib to docetaxel in the second-line unselected population. The ORR between both arms was similar (9.1% vs. 7.6%, $p=0.33$) as was overall survival (OS) (7.6 vs. 8 months) [72] (Table 2.2).

Erlotinib has attained full approval in the United States for treatment of unselected patients, in the second- or third-line setting, based on a large phase III trial, BR.21, which demonstrated a significant survival advantage of erlotinib over placebo [32] (Table 2.2). In the BR.21 study, patients treated with erlotinib had a significant increase in progression-free survival (PFS) (2.2 vs. 1.8 months), median OS (6.7 vs. 4.7 months), and 1-year survival (31% vs. 21%) compared with patients receiving placebo [32]. Major symptoms (cough, dyspnea, and pain) were also significantly improved with erlotinib. Toxicities were acceptable and consisted mainly of skin

TABLE 2.2
Randomized Trials of First-Generation EGFR TKIs in Unselected Advanced NSCLC

Study		Regimen	No. of Patients	Response Rate (%)	Median Time to Progression (Months)	Median Survival (Months)	1-Year Survival (%)
IDEAL 1 [25]	Phase II	Gefitinib 250 mg	103	18.4	2.7	7.6	35
2nd/3rd line		Gefitinib 500 mg	105	19	2.8	8.0	29
IDEAL 2 [26]	Phase II	Gefitinib 500 mg	102	12	7.0	7.0	27
2nd/3rd line		Gefitinib 250 mg	114	10	6.0	6.0	24
BR.21 [32]	Phase III	Erlotinib 150 mg	488	9	2.2	6.7	31
2nd/3rd line		Placebo	243	<1 ($p<0.001$)	1.8 ($p<0.001$)	4.7 ($p<0.001$)	21
ISEL [31]	Phase III	Gefitinib 250 mg	1129	8.0	3.0	5.6	27
2nd/3rd line		Placebo	563	1.3	2.6	5.1	21
INTEREST [72]	Phase III	Gefitinib 250 mg	733	9.1	2.2	7.6	32
2nd/3rd line		Docetaxel 75 mg/m^2	710	7.6	2.7	8.0	34
INTACT 1 [73]	Phase III	Cisplatin–gemcitabine–placebo	363	47.2	6.0	10.9	44
1st line		Cisplatin–gemcitabine–gefitinib 250 mg	365	51.2	5.8	9.9	41
		Cisplatin–gemcitabine–gefitinib 500 mg	365	50.3	5.5	9.9	43
INTACT 2 [74]	Phase III	Carboplatin–paclitaxel–placebo	345	28.7	5.0	9.9	42
1st line		Carboplatin–paclitaxel–gefitinib 250 mg	345	30.4	5.3	9.8	41
		Carboplatin–paclitaxel–gefitinib 500 mg	347	30.0	4.6	8.7	37
TALENT [75]	Phase III	Cisplatin–gemcitabine–placebo	586	29.9	5.6	10.1	42
1st line		Cisplatin–gemcitabine–erlotinib 150 mg	586	31.5	5.4	9.9	41
TRIBUTE [73]	Phase III	Carboplatin–paclitaxel–placebo	540	19.3	4.9	10.5	43.8
1st line		Carboplatin–paclitaxel–erlotinib 150 mg	539	21.5	5.1	10.6	46.9

Abbreviations: EGFR, epidermal growth factor receptor; NSCLC, non-small cell lung cancer.

rash and diarrhea. The survival benefit observed in this study was the basis for the approval in many countries of erlotinib for patients with NSCLC who had progressed after one or two systemic chemotherapy regimens.

Gefitinib and erlotinib were also tested in combination with standard chemotherapy in the first-line setting in an unselected advanced NSCLC population (Table 2.2). Two large, randomized, placebo-controlled, double-blind phase III trials (INTACT 1 and 2) investigated the efficacy of gefitinib at the dose of 250 or 500 mg daily in combination with chemotherapy as first-line therapy. Chemotherapy was given for up to six cycles, and the EGFR TKIs were continued in patients with at minimum stable disease until progression. However, the addition of gefitinib to chemotherapy failed to improve OS, time to progression, or ORR compared with chemotherapy alone [73,74]. A subset analysis of patients with adenocarcinoma who received 90 days of chemotherapy or more in the INTACT 2 study demonstrated statistically significant prolonged OS, suggesting a gefitinib maintenance effect. In general, treatment was well tolerated and the toxicity of chemotherapy was nonoverlapping with that of gefitinib (skin rash and diarrhea). However, as expected, gefitinib 500 mg was associated with a higher degree of toxicities, as observed in the IDEAL studies, which led to more dose reductions and treatment interruptions. Two other studies employed the same combination chemotherapy regimens with erlotinib at 150 mg versus placebo (TRIBUTE and TALENT). Erlotinib was continued after termination of chemotherapy like in the INTACT studies. These combinations were well tolerated, and there was a positive correlation of survival with the degree of skin rash in the TRIBUTE study. However, these two large studies failed to demonstrate superiority of the erlotinib combinations in terms of survival, PFS, and response rate [30,75]. To summarize, the addition of EGFR TKIs to platinum-doublet chemotherapy in the unselected advanced-stage population does not provide a survival advantage.

Following the discovery of the EGFR mutations, prospective trials, as well as retrospective analysis of previously available data, have shaped our understanding of the use of these targeted therapies [76]. The subgroup analysis from the ISEL study, indicating a survival advantage in the Asian never-smoking population, motivated researchers to carry out the Iressa Pan-Asia Study (IPASS) that compared gefitinib to carboplatin plus paclitaxel (Taxol®, Bristol-Myers Squibb Co.). In this large phase III trial, all patients were in the first-line setting with a diagnosis of advanced NSCLC and an adenocarcinoma histology and were either never smokers (<100 lifetime cigarettes) or former light smokers (<10 pack-years and quit >15 years ago). The PFS interval in the overall population was statistically longer for gefitinib versus chemotherapy (HR 0.74 [95% CI 0.65–0.85], $p < 0.001$) [77]. While no statistically significant difference in OS (18.8 vs. 17.4 months) in the general population was found, a biomarker analysis for the activating EGFR mutation demonstrated significant differences. In EGFR mutation–positive patients, improvement in ORR (71.2% vs. 47.3%) and PFS (9.5 vs. 6.3 months) was demonstrated in gefitinib versus chemotherapy treatment arms, respectively, although OS was not statistically significant with median OS of 21.6 versus 21.9 months (HR 1 [95% CI 0.76–1.33], $p = 0.990$). Moreover, the EGFR wild-type population had lower ORR (1.1% vs. 23.5%) and worse PFS (1.5 vs. 5.5 months) and OS (11.2 vs. 12.7 months) when comparing gefitinib with chemotherapy, respectively [77,78]. IPASS defined the EGFR mutation–positive population as having an improved prognosis compared to its wild-type counterparts regardless of initial treatment while also illustrating benefit to TKIs only in the mutated population when used as first-line therapy. These observations were further validated through several prospective randomized trials. WJTOG3405 and NEJ002 were conducted in Japan and compared gefitinib to chemotherapy in the first-line setting for advanced-stage EGFR-mutant patients. They found significantly better ORR and improvement in PFS for the mutated patients treated with gefitinib (Table 2.3) [79,80]. Likewise, two recent trials evaluating erlotinib versus chemotherapy in the first-line setting of mutation-selected advanced-stage patients, OPTIMAL and EURTAC, also demonstrate improved ORR and significantly longer PFS (Table 2.3). The phase III OPTIMAL trial has completed enrollment and the patients remain in the follow-up period. However, analysis to date shows median PFS was 13.1 months (95% CI 10.58–16.53) in the erlotinib arm versus 4.6 months (4.21–5.42) for chemotherapy-treated patients [81]. EURTAC, also a phase III trial with interim data published in March 2012, further confirmed the findings from OPTIMAL. Here erlotinib was compared to several standard chemotherapy regimens (Table 2.3). Median PFS was 9.7 months (95% CI 8.4–12.3) in the erlotinib group, compared with 5.2 months (4.5–5.8) in the standard chemotherapy group (HR 0.37 [95% CI 0.25–0.54], $p < 0.0001$) [82]. As in previous studies of the first-generation TKIs, side effects were manageable including diarrhea and rash, and the erlotinib arms demonstrated fewer treatment-related events and dose reductions. Despite the encouraging improvement in PFS for EGFR mutation–positive patients treated with TKIs, on the whole, data have not supported improvement in OS. This may be, in part, explained by crossover of patients from chemotherapy to TKIs at progression; given the establishment of TKI activity in the second-line setting, 76% of standard chemotherapy group patients crossed over to receive a TKI. These data fundamentally establish gefitinib or erlotinib as treatment for EGFR-mutated patients with advanced NSCLC in the first-line setting and should be considered the standard of care in these patients.

A subset analyses of the INTACT 2 study suggested efficacy with maintenance gefitinib [32]. The subpopulation encompassed unselected advanced-stage adenocarcinoma patients who received at minimum 90 days of chemotherapy followed by continued gefitinib and suggested significant prolongation in survival. The idea of continued maintenance TKIs after completion of chemotherapy was specifically evaluated in two separate studies (SATURN and INFORM). In the SATURN trial, an unselected advanced-stage population was randomized to maintenance erlotinib versus placebo after completion of four cycles of platinum-based doublet if they achieved at minimum stable disease. The erlotinib arm demonstrated statistically significant improvement in PFS (12.3 vs. 11.1 months; HR 0.71, $p < 0.0001$) as well as OS (12 vs. 11 months; HR 0.81, $p = 0.0088$) [83]. The PFS and OS benefit seen in the erlotinib arm remained significant across subgroups, irrespective of tumor histology or EGFR mutation status. However, the EGFR-mutated population obtained the greatest PFS benefit. The OS benefit in the EGFR-mutant population was not as impressive, likely secondary to the 67% crossover rate in the placebo arm as well as censorship of data with most patients having not experienced an event to date [83]. The INFORM trial was designed similarly to SATURN. Unselected advanced

TABLE 2.3
Randomized Trials of First-Generation EGFR TKIs in Mutation-Selected Advanced NSCLC

Study		Regimen	No. of Patients	Response Rate (%)	Median Time to Progression (Months)	Median Survival (Months)
WJTOG3405 [79] 1st line	Phase III	Gefitinib 250 mg	86	62.1	9.2	30.9
		Cisplatin–docetaxel	86	32.2	6.3 ($p < 0.001$)	Not reached
NEJ002 [80,165] 1st line	Phase III	Gefitinib 250 mg	114	73.7	10.8	27.7
		Carboplatin–paclitaxel	110	30.7	5.4 ($p < 0.001$)	26.6
OPTIMAL [81] 1st line	Phase III	Erlotinib 150 mg	82	83	13.1	Not published to date
		Carboplatin–gemcitabine	72	36	4.6 ($p < 0.0001$)	
EURTAC [82] 1st line	Phase III	Erlotinib 150 mg	77	64	9.7	19.3
		Cisplatin–docetaxel ⎫ Cisplatin–gemcitabine ⎬ Carboplatin–gemcitabine ⎭ Carboplatin–docetaxel	76	18	5.2 ($p < 0.0001$)	19.5

Abbreviations: EGFR, epidermal growth factor receptor; NSCLC, non–small cell lung cancer.

NSCLC patients were randomized to gefitinib 250 mg daily versus placebo. Only a PFS was statistically significant in the gefitinib arm (4.8 vs. 2.6 months; HR 0.42, $p < 0.0001$), with no statistical difference in OS (18.7 vs. 16.9 months; HR 0.84, $p = 0.26$) [84]. The recently published IFCT-GFPC 0520 trial compared advanced-stage patients who did not progress after first-line platinum-based chemotherapy to either gemcitabine at 1250 mg/m^2 on days 1 and 8 of a 3-week cycle, erlotinib 150 mg daily, or observation. Four hundred sixty-four patients were enrolled and randomized to the three arms. Again, PFS was prolonged in both the gemcitabine (3.8 months, $p < 0.001$) and erlotinib (2.9 months, $p = 0.003$) compared with observation (median 1.9 months). The benefit in PFS was consistent across subgroups, irrespective of histology. A nonsignificant improvement in OS was seen in both maintenance arms compared to observation (12.1 vs. 10.8 months; HR 0.89 [95% CI 0.69–1.15], $p = 0.3867$). Of the 261 patients evaluated for EGFR IHC analysis, no significant benefit to PFS was seen with gemcitabine or erlotinib maintenance [85]. Lastly, the EORTC 08021 trial evaluating gefitinib maintenance after non-progression following platinum-based chemotherapy failed to meet their primary objective of OS after follow-up of 41 months (10.9 vs. 9.4 months; HR 0.83 [95% CI 0.6–1.15], $p = 0.2$). However, this trial was closed early secondary to poor accrual with only 178 of a planned 598 patients randomized. The secondary end point of PFS significantly favored gefitinib with median PFS of 4.1 versus 2.9 months, respectively (HR 0.61 [95% CI 0.45–0.83], $p = 0.0015$) [86]. Erlotinib is approved in the United States for maintenance therapy in locally advanced or metastatic NSLC who have not progressed after four cycles of platinum-based doublet or for treatment after failure of at least one prior chemotherapy regimen.

The activation of uncontrolled, tumor-induced angiogenesis through an increase in vascular endothelial growth factor (VEGF) secretion by cancer cells is a mechanism linked to acquired resistance to EGFR-inhibitor treatment. Early antitumor activity was obtained by combining selective anti-EGFR drugs with antiangiogenic agents. Advanced NSCLC patients pretreated with one prior chemotherapy regimen were given erlotinib and bevacizumab (Avastin®, Genentech), a recombinant anti-VEGF mAb [87] in a phase I/II study. Both agents could be given at the full dose of 150 mg/day of erlotinib and 15 mg/kg bevacizumab every 3 weeks. In the 40 patients enrolled (34 of which were in the phase II portion), the response rate was 17.5% and median survival was 9.3 months. These results appeared promising and stimulated further studies of this combination in advanced nonsquamous lung cancers. Definitive phase III trials of this combination in relapsed (BeTa trial) and in first-line nonsquamous carcinomas of the lung (ATLAS) have been preformed. In the BeTa trial, patients with recurrent or refractory NSCLC were randomized to erlotinib (150 mg daily) plus bevacizumab (15 mg/kg once every 3 weeks) versus erlotinib (150 mg daily) plus placebo. The trial did not meet its primary end point of OS benefit (9.3 vs. 9.2 months) in the bevacizumab arm. While there was a suggestion of improved PFS in the bevacizumab arm (3.4 vs. 1.7 months; HR 0.62), because of the design of the trial, this secondary end point difference could not be defined as significant. Grade 3 or 4 adverse events were greater in the bevacizumab arm compared to the control arm, respectively (60% vs. 48% of patients) [88]. The ATLAS trial has not been fully published to date; however, an abstract was presented in the

2009 ASCO annual meeting. Here, patients in the advanced-stage setting who completed first-line platinum-containing doublet plus bevacizumab without evidence of progressive disease were randomized to follow up bevacizumab plus erlotinib versus bevacizumab plus placebo on the same dosing schedule as BeTa. The PFS in the bevacizumab/erlotinib arm was statistically longer than the bevacizumab/placebo arm (4.8 vs. 3.7 months; HR 0.722, $p = 0.0012$) [89]. It is not clear if OS was affected by this treatment strategy and we await full publication of these data.

A few clinical studies have been conducted with EGFR-directed antibodies for patients with NSCLC. A large phase III trial (FLEX) has been recently completed. Patients with EGFR-expressing advanced NSCLC (stage IIIB with documented malignant pleural effusion and stage IV) were randomized in a 1:1 fashion to Group A (cetuximab 400 mg/m^2 initial dose then 250 mg/m^2 weekly, cisplatin 80 mg/m^2 on day 1, vinorelbine 30 mg/m^2 on day 1 and 8) or to Group B (cisplatin and vinorelbine as before) for a maximum of six cycles every 3 weeks. Cetuximab was administered until progression or unacceptable toxicity. Both arms had similar baseline characteristics with a total study population of 1125 patients. The trial demonstrated a very small although statistically significant OS benefit, regardless of histology (11.3 vs. 10.1 months, $p = 0.044$), in the cetuximab versus control arm, respectively [90]. This small OS advantage came with significantly increased grade 3 or 4 toxicity, specifically febrile neutropenia. Secondary to difficultly in administration and significant side effects, it is unclear if there is clinical benefit to this regimen despite the statistically significant survival advantage; controversy regarding its use exists. Cetuximab was further evaluated in the first-line setting of unselected advanced NSCLC in the BMS099 trial where chemotherapy-naive patients received paclitaxel (225 mg/m^2) or docetaxel (75 mg/m^2), at the investigator's discretion, plus carboplatin (area under the curve (AUC) 6) on day 1 every 3 weeks for a total of six cycles. In addition, they were randomized to receive cetuximab (400 mg/m^2 on day 1 then 1250 mg/m^2 weekly) versus placebo, which was continued until disease progression or unacceptable toxicity. This combination did not statistically improve RR, PFS, or OS, although OS favored the cetuximab arm (9.69 vs. 8.38 months; HR 0.890, $p = 0.169$) [91]. Cetuximab is FDA approved for use in combination with vinorelbine/cisplatin in the first-line setting of advanced or metastatic NSCLC, as well as for continuation maintenance until disease progression or unacceptable toxicity.

Pan-HER Inhibitors

Patients with EGFR-mutated lung cancer develop disease progression after a median of 10–14 months on reversible EGFR TKIs [92]. Acquired EGFR TKI resistance [93] occurs in approximately 50% of cases via the T790M mutation of the EGFR kinase domain [94,95] and much less frequently by MET amplification or other mechanisms (e.g., small cell lung cancer transition, PIK3CA mutations, and activation of parallel receptor kinases) [96–98]. The EGFR T790M mutation leads to an increase in the affinity of EGFR for ATP, thus dramatically reducing the efficacy of reversible quinazoline inhibitors like gefitinib and erlotinib [99]. Simultaneous inhibition of multiple HER receptors (pan-HER inhibition) is one of the several strategies being evaluated to overcome acquired EGFR TKI resistance.

Lapatinib (Tykerb®, GlaxoSmithKline, Brentford, Middlesex, U.K.), a reversible dual TKI of EGFR and HER2, was evaluated in a randomized phase II trial of recurrent (second line) or metastatic NSCLC (first line). Patients were randomized to receive lapatinib 1500 mg once daily or 500 mg twice daily. Despite its known efficacy in breast cancer, it did not demonstrate significant activity in chemotherapy-naive patients with advanced NSCLC [100]. Neratinib (HKI-272), another dual but irreversible TKI of EGFR and HER2, also showed no significant activity in patients with advanced NSCLC after failure of a first-generation TKI. In this phase II trial, patients with advanced NSCLC were selected for EGFR mutational status as well as for previous treatment with TKIs. Interestingly the strongest response seen to neratinib was in patients with the G719X point mutation, which incurs increased sensitivity to TKIs. Three of four patients with this mutation had a partial response (PR) and the fourth patient had stable disease (SD); median PFS in these patients was 52.7 weeks (25.6–57 weeks) [101].

Afatinib (BIBW 2992) is a small-molecule irreversible inhibitor of EGFR, HER2, and HER4 receptors. In preclinical studies, afatinib suppressed the kinase activity of wild-type and mutant EGFR and HER2 including the EGFR T790M mutation, although at a lower potency [102]. In patients with EGFR-mutant advanced lung adenocarcinoma who were previously treated with no more than one prior chemotherapy regimen ($n = 129$), a phase II trial of afatinib (LUX-Lung 2) resulted in objective responses in 79 patients (ORR 61%). The ORR was 66% among patients who had the two most common EGFR-activating mutations, deletion 19 and L858R ($n = 70$), and 39% among patients who had less common EGFR-activating mutations ($n = 23$). The number of patients with EGFR T790M mutations in this study was limited to assess the activity of afatinib in this subpopulation [103]. Afatinib was further evaluated in a phase IIB/III trial (LUX-Lung1) in patients with advanced NSCLC and disease progression after one or two lines of chemotherapy and erlotinib or gefitinib (Table 2.4). In this trial, patients were randomized ($n = 585$) in a 2:1 fashion to receive afatinib (50 mg daily) or placebo. Compared with placebo, treatment with afatinib resulted in significantly more objective responses (29 patients [7%] vs. 1 patient [0.5%]) and prolonged PFS 3.3 versus 1.1 months (HR 0.38 [95% CI 0.31–0.48], $p < 0.0001$). However, the improved efficacy of afatinib over placebo did not translate into a survival advantage, OS of 10.8 versus 12 months for afatinib versus placebo, respectively (HR 1.08 [95% CI 0.86–1.35], $p = 0.74$) [104]. A recent abstract for the phase III LUX-Lung 3 trial evaluating chemotherapy-naive patients with EGFR-mutant advanced lung adenocarcinoma ($n = 345$) randomized patients to receive afatinib or chemotherapy with cisplatin and pemetrexed (Table 2.4). The trial met its primary end point of prolonging PFS in patients who received afatinib (PFS 11.1 vs. 6.9 months; HR 0.58, $p = 0.0004$). Treatment with afatinib also led to more objective responses (ORR 56% vs. 23%; $p < 0.0001$) [105]. An ongoing phase III trial is evaluating the efficacy of afatinib versus gemcitabine and cisplatin in the first-line treatment for EGFR-mutant advanced lung adenocarcinoma (NCT01121393) (Table 2.4). Available clinical trial data suggest efficacy of afatinib as a single agent in patients with EGFR-activating mutations. However, the benefit, if any, of afatinib over the reversible EGFR TKIs and its efficacy in patients with acquired resistance EGFR inhibition are not known. Additionally, an ongoing trial (LUX-Lung 8) is evaluating

TABLE 2.4
Randomized Phase III Trials of Second-Generation (Irreversible) EGFR TKIs in Advanced NSCLC

Study	Regimen	EGFR Mutation Status	Treatment Line	Response Rate (%)	Median Time to Progression (Months)	Median Survival (Months)
JBR-26	Dacomitinib	Unselected	Second or beyond		Ongoing, recruiting (NCT01000025)	
	Placebo					
ARCHER 1009	Dacomitinib	Unselected	Second or beyond		Ongoing, recruiting (NCT01360554)	
	Erlotinib					
LUX-Lung 1 [104]	Afatinib	Unselected	Salvage	7.4	3.3	10.8
	Placebo			0.5	1.1 ($p<0.0001$)	12
LUX-Lung 3 [105]	Afatinib	Selected	First line	56	11.1	Not published to date
	Cisplatin–pemetrexed			23	6.9	
LUX-Lung 5	Paclitaxel–afatinib	Unselected	Second or beyond		Ongoing (NCT01085136)	
	Chemotherapy–investigator choice					
LUX-Lung 6	Afatinib	Selected	First line		Ongoing (NCT 01121393)	
	Cisplatin–gemcitabine					
LUX-Lung 8	Afatinib	Unselected Squamous histology	Second line		Ongoing, recruiting (NCT01523587)	
	Erlotinib					

Abbreviations: EGFR, epidermal growth factor receptor; NSCLC, non–small cell lung cancer.

the efficacy of afatinib versus erlotinib in second-line treatment of patients with advanced squamous cell lung carcinoma following platinum-based chemotherapy (NCT01523587) (Table 2.4).

Combinations with other targeted agents, with or without chemotherapy, are being studied in an attempt to improve the efficacy of afatinib. In a phase III trial (LUX-Lung 5), afatinib with weekly paclitaxel was compared with investigator's choice of single-agent chemotherapy following afatinib monotherapy in advanced NSCLC. Patients had at least one prior chemotherapy regimen and had prior failure of erlotinib or gefitinib. Interim analysis of afatinib monotherapy portion of this trial ($n=1154$) showed median PFS of 3.3 months. PFS was prolonged in patients with EGFR mutations ($n=49$) compared to wild type ($n=35$), 4.2 versus 2.6 months, respectively (NCT01085136) [106]. Afatinib has shown promising clinical activity in combination with cetuximab in advanced NSCLC patients with acquired resistance to a reversible EGFR TKI [92]. On interim analysis of a phase I study of such patients, combination of afatinib with biweekly cetuximab resulted in PRs in 8 of the 22 evaluable patients (ORR 36%; 95% CI 0.17–0.59), including 4 of 13 patients (ORR 29%) with EGFR T790M mutations (NCT01090011) (Table 2.4) [107].

Dacomitinib (PF299804) is an irreversible small-molecule inhibitor of EGFR, HER2, and HER4. In preclinical models, dacomitinib inhibited not only wild-type and the common activating mutations of the EGFR but also EGFR T790M and mutations that confer de novo resistance to reversible EGFR inhibition such as EGFR exon 20 insertion [108,109]. In a phase II study evaluating dacomitinib (45 or 30 mg daily) in chemotherapy-naive patients with advanced lung adenocarcinoma and EGFR mutation or less than a 10 pack-year smoking history, interim analysis shows that PFS at 4 months for the overall population (primary end point) was 96% (95% CI 84–99). Additionally, 34 of 46 evaluable patients with EGFR-sensitizing mutation had objective responses (ORR 74%; 95% CI 59–86) [110]. A further phase II trial randomized 188 patients with advanced NSCLC who received one or two prior chemotherapy regimens to dacomitinib (45 mg daily) or erlotinib (150 mg daily). The trial met its primary end point of improved PFS with dacomitinib versus erlotinib (median 2.8 vs. 1.9 months, $p=0.012$). However, no survival advantage was observed for dacomitinib (median 9.5 vs. 7.4 months, $p=0.205$) [111]. In a phase II study of patients with KRAS wild-type advanced NSCLC who had received at least one chemotherapy regimen and prior erlotinib, dacomitinib resulted in three PRs (3 out of 62 evaluable patients; ORR 5%) [112]. An ongoing phase III trial (ARCHER) is comparing the efficacy of dacomitinib with erlotinib in advanced NSCLC patients who have received one or two prior chemotherapy regimens (NCT01360554) and dacomitinib versus placebo (JBR-26) in a similar patient population (Table 2.4) (NCT01000025).

COLORECTAL CANCER

The overexpression of EGFR has been associated with higher staging of tumors but has not been established as a prognostic marker in CRC [120]. Both cetuximab and panitumumab are mAbs directed against EGFR that inhibit downstream signaling. Both have been approved as addition to standard chemotherapy in the first line and as monotherapy in subsequent lines of treatment in advanced CRC.

The RAS/RAF/MAPK pathway is an important downstream signaling pathway for EGFR that has been important in predicting the efficacy of these targeted therapies. Approximately 40% of CRC harbors mutations in codons 12 and 13 in exon 2 of the KRAS oncogene [121]. Tumors with KRAS mutations have demonstrated a lack of response to cetuximab or panitumumab and have led to the relabeling of these drugs to recommend against their use in KRAS-mutated tumors [122–124]. Additionally, approximately 5%–9% of CRC harbor BRAF (V600E) [125] mutations that have demonstrated a lower response to cetuximab-based therapy of 8.3% versus 38.0% (p = 0.0012) [126,127].

Cetuximab and panitumumab have been studied in combination with infusional fluorouracil, leucovorin, and irinotecan (FOLFIRI) or infusional fluorouracil, leucovorin, and oxaliplatin (FOLFOX) as initial options for the treatment of wild-type KRAS metastatic CRC. The CRYSTAL trial assigned patients to receive FOLFIRI with and without cetuximab and demonstrated an improvement in PFS with cetuximab (9.9 vs. 8.7 months; HR 0.68 [95% CI 0.50–0.94]; p = 0.02) and OS benefit (23.0 vs. 20.0 months; p = 0.0093) [128,129]. Cetuximab has not shown benefit when added to oxaliplatin-based regimens in the first-line setting. The addition of cetuximab demonstrated no benefit in OS or PFS in a randomized phase III trial, the NORDIC VII study [130]. The PRIME trial evaluated panitumumab plus FOLFOX versus FOLFOX alone in KRAS wild-type patients with advanced CRC and showed a statistically significant improvement in PFS with addition of panitumumab (HR 0.80 (95% CI, 0.67–0.95), p = 0.009) [131]. Panitumumab has also been evaluated in combination with FOLFIRI and in wild-type KRAS tumors. Panitumumab demonstrated an improvement in PFS with median 5.9 months for panitumumab arm versus 3.9 months for the FOLFIRI arm (HR 0.73 [95% CI 0.59–0.90], p = 0.004). A nonsignificant trend toward increased OS was observed; median OS was 14.5 versus 12.5 months, respectively (HR 0.85 [95% CI 0.70–1.04], p = 0.12) [132].

Bevacizumab is a humanized mAb that blocks the activity of VEGF. Bevacizumab has been shown to be effective in first-line chemotherapy in advanced CRC. Both cetuximab and panitumumab have been evaluated in combination with bevacizumab and chemotherapy in phase III trials (CAIRO2 and PACCE). Both trials demonstrated that combination therapy with multiple biologic agents is associated with decreased outcomes and increased toxicity [133,134].

The use of cetuximab or panitumumab is approved as monotherapy upon progression after initial chemotherapy. Cetuximab has been studied as a single agent and in combination with irinotecan in this setting. The EPIC trial demonstrated that adding cetuximab to irinotecan does not prolong survival in patients with metastatic CRC previously treated with fluoropyrimidine and oxaliplatin. The median OS was comparable between treatments; cetuximab arm was 10.7 months (95% CI 9.6–11.3) and irinotecan arm was 10.0 months (95% CI 9.1–11.3) (HR 0.975 [95% CI 0.854–1.114], p = 0.71) [135]. Panitumumab has been studied as a single agent in the setting of metastatic CRC for patients with disease progression on oxaliplatin- and irinotecan-based therapy [136]. Later, a retrospective analysis of the subset of patients in this trial with known KRAS tumor status showed that the benefit of panitumumab versus best supportive care was enhanced in patients with KRAS wild-type tumors (PFS 12.3 vs. 7.3 weeks) [123].

Breast Cancer

Trastuzumab is the first targeted mAb against ErbB2 to be approved for the treatment of any cancer. Trastuzumab was first approved for the treatment of HER2–neu overexpressing breast cancer and now has become the standard of care for treatment of both early stage and advanced metastatic and recurrent breast cancer that overexpresses HER2–neu. Trastuzumab is also the first targeted therapy to be approved in the adjuvant setting. There have been five randomized trials demonstrating the benefit of trastuzumab when added to adjuvant chemotherapy [14–152]. The North Central Cancer Treatment Group (NCCTG) N9831 trial and the B-31 trial were analyzed via meta-analysis to determine the efficacy of adjuvant trastuzumab in patients with HER2-positive breast cancer. There were 4045 patients included in the joint analysis demonstrating a 48% reduction in the risk of recurrence (HR 0.52 [95% CI 0.45–0.60], $p<0.001$) and a 39% reduction in the risk of death (HR 0.61 [95% CI 0.50–0.75], $p=0.001$) [153].

Pertuzumab has also been recently approved by the U.S. FDA. It is a recombinant humanized mAb that inhibits the ligand-dependent dimerization of HER2 and its downstream signaling. Pertuzumab and trastuzumab bind to different epitopes of HER2 receptor and have complementary mechanisms of action. Tumor modeling has demonstrated that when these two mAbs are administered together, they provide a greater overall antitumor effect than either alone [154]. A randomized, double-blinded, phase III study compared the efficacy and safety of pertuzumab in combination with trastuzumab and docetaxel versus trastuzumab and docetaxel alone in the first-line treatment for HER2–neu-positive metastatic breast cancer [155]. The primary end point of the study was PFS, and secondary end points included ORR, OS, and safety. A total of 808 patients were enrolled. The trial demonstrated that the addition of pertuzumab provided an improvement in the median PFS by 6.1 months (12.4 vs. 18.5 months) in the pertuzumab group (HR 0.62 [95% CI 0.51–0.75], $p<0.001$). Interim analysis of OS when 43% of prespecified events occurred did not meet statistical significance yet favored the pertuzumab-containing regimen with more deaths in the control group (23.6%) compared to the pertuzumab (17.2%) arm (HR 0.64 [95% CI 0.47–0.88], $p=0.005$). The most common adverse reactions in the pertuzumab group were diarrhea, rash, mucositis, febrile neutropenia, and dry skin [155]. Several trials have demonstrated benefit of continuation of trastuzumab therapy following disease progression on a trastuzumab-containing regimen [156,157].

Lapatinib is a small-molecule EGFR and HER2–neu TKI. Lapatinib has been approved by the U.S. FDA in combination with capecitabine. The use of lapatinib is an option for patients with HER2-positive disease following progression on a trastuzumab-containing regimen. A phase III study compared lapatinib plus capecitabine with capecitabine alone in women with advanced or metastatic breast cancer refractory to trastuzumab [158]. Time to progression was increased in patients receiving the combination (8.4 vs. 4.4 months; HR 0.49 [95% CI 0.34–0.71], $p<0.001$). Lapatinib has also been studied in estrogen receptor–positive and HER2–neu-positive metastatic breast cancer in combination with letrozole. The combination therapy improved PFS over letrozole alone (8.2 vs. 3.0 months; HR 0.71 [95% CI 0.53–0.96], $p=0.019$) without statistical OS benefit. Although with less than 50%

of OS events recorded at publication, there was a trend toward OS benefit (HR 0.74 [95% CI 0.5–1.1], $p = 0.113$) [159]. Lapatinib has also been evaluated in a phase III trial in which patients with heavily pretreated metastatic breast cancer and disease progression on trastuzumab therapy were randomly assigned to monotherapy with lapatinib or trastuzumab plus lapatinib. PFS was increased from 8.1 to 12 weeks ($p = 0.008$) with the combination. Likewise, the secondary end point of OS was not statistically significant, yet there was a trend toward improved OS in the combination arm (HR 0.75 [95% CI 0.53–1.07], $p = 0.106$) [34].

HEAD AND NECK CANCER

Inhibition of EGFR signaling by small molecules, mAbs directed against ligands or the receptor, immunotoxin conjugates, or antisense oligonucleotides have demonstrated robust activity in preclinical models of SCCHN [139]. Cetuximab has received U.S. FDA approval for the treatment of patients with locally advanced SCCHN on the basis of a phase III trial where patients were randomly assigned to treatment with high-dose radiotherapy alone (213 patients) or high-dose radiotherapy plus weekly cetuximab (211 patients) [144]. The median duration of locoregional control was 24.4 months for patients treated with combined therapy versus 14.9 months for those treated with radiotherapy alone (HR 0.68; $p = 0.005$). Radiotherapy plus cetuximab significantly prolonged PFS (HR 0.70; $p = 0.006$) and OS (HR 0.74; $p = 0.03$). With the exception of acneiform rash and infusion reactions, the incidence of grade 3 or greater toxic effects, including mucositis, did not differ significantly between the two groups.

In phase I trials in recurrent/metastatic (R/M) disease, cetuximab combined with platinum agents with or without fluorouracil was found to be safe and tolerable at full doses of the cytotoxic agents [140]. The Eastern Cooperative Oncology Group performed a placebo-controlled, randomized phase III trial of cisplatin with or without cetuximab, enrolling 117 assessable patients who had not been treated previously for R/M disease [141]. More than 95% of the participants had received prior therapy for locally advanced disease, and approximately two-thirds of the patients in each arm had metastatic disease at study entry. Patients in the experimental arm were allowed to cross over and received cetuximab on progression. The cisplatin–cetuximab arm achieved an ORR of 26% versus 10% in the cisplatin-alone group ($p = 0.03$). However, the primary end point of PFS did not reach statistical significance for the cisplatin–cetuximab group (4.2 vs. 2.7 months; $p = 0.09$) nor did OS (9.2 vs. 8 months; $p = 0.21$).

Cetuximab also shows activity in patients with platinum-refractory disease. In a phase II trial [142], 96 patients who had progressed while receiving a platinum-based regimen were treated with cetuximab alone. On progression during treatment with cetuximab, patients were offered combination therapy with cetuximab and a platinum agent. An overall response rate of 10% with five patients achieving a complete response and a median survival of 294 days was reported. Two phase II studies have evaluated cetuximab in combination with either cisplatin or carboplatin in patients who progressed while receiving platinum-based regimens [142,143]. The efficacy of cetuximab as a single agent in platinum-refractory patients suggests that the activity in these trials can be attributed mostly to the addition of cetuximab and that the agent alone may achieve the same results.

Erlotinib has been tested in patients with R/M disease as monotherapy [145] and in combination with chemotherapy [146] and has achieved disappointing results. However, erlotinib has been combined with bevacizumab in a phase I/II trial in patients with R/M disease [147]. Median time of OS and PFS were 7.1 months (95% CI 5.7–9.0) and 4.1 months (2.8–4.4). This combination appeared well tolerated, without dose-limiting toxicities observed in the phase I portion of the trial, and the recommended phase II dose of erlotinib 150 mg daily and bevacizumab 15 mg/kg every 3 weeks was administered to an expansion cohort of 48 patients.

GASTRIC CANCER

The overexpression of EGFR, VEGFR, and HER2–neu has been associated with a poor prognosis in gastric cancer [113]. Trastuzumab is a humanized mAb to the extracellular domain of the HER2–neu [114]. The results of the ToGA trial [66] have led to all gastric cancer being tested for overexpression of HER2–neu. This trial enrolled 594 patients and randomly assigned them to study treatment, trastuzumab plus cisplatin and fluoropyrimidine ($n=298$), or chemotherapy alone, cisplatin and fluoropyrimidine ($n=296$). Of this, 584 patients were included in the primary analysis ($n=294$; $n=290$). Median OS was 13.8 months (95% CI 12–16) in those assigned to trastuzumab plus chemotherapy compared with 11.1 months [10–13] in those assigned to chemotherapy alone (HR 0.74 [95% CI 0.60–0.91], $p=0.0046$). Safety profiles were similar between the two arms and no unexpected adverse events occurred in the trastuzumab arm. Trastuzumab is not recommended in combination with any anthracycline regimen. The overexpression of HER2–neu occurs between 10% and 27% in gastric cancer [115,116]. Therefore, patients with inoperable, metastatic or recurrent adenocarcinoma of the stomach or gastroesophageal junction should be evaluated for HER2–neu overexpression using IHC and/or FISH. Trastuzumab should be considered in all patients with 3+ overexpression by IHC or FISH positive (HER2/CEP17 ratio > 2) [117]. The current reported rate of overexpression is between 10% and 18% [118]. The evaluation of bevacizumab, erlotinib, and cetuximab is currently being evaluated in phase III trials.

PANCREATIC CANCER

Pancreatic tumors often overexpress EGFR and this overexpression has been associated with a worse prognosis. Erlotinib has been studied in a phase III trial when added with gemcitabine in patients with unresectable, locally advanced, or metastatic pancreatic cancer. Patients were randomly assigned 1:1 to receive standard gemcitabine plus erlotinib (100 or 150 mg/day orally) or gemcitabine plus placebo in a double-blind, international phase III trial. A total of 569 patients were randomly assigned. OS was prolonged in the erlotinib plus gemcitabine arm (HR 0.82 [95% CI, 0.69–0.99], $p=0.038$; median OS 6.24 months vs. 5.91 months). One-year survival was also greater with erlotinib plus gemcitabine (23% vs. 17%; $p=0.023$). There is a higher incidence of adverse events when adding erlotinib to standard gemcitabine [119].

CENTRAL NERVOUS SYSTEM TUMORS

Glioblastomas are the most common primary malignant brain tumors in adults. The use of erlotinib and gefitinib has shown limited activity in clinical trials. Gefitinib has showed no objective tumor responses in this patient population [137]. Erlotinib has been studied in a phase II trial enrolling 65 newly diagnosed glioblastomas. Erlotinib was given at a dose of 100 mg per day with whole-brain radiation therapy in addition to temozolomide (Temodar®, Merck & Co.). Erlotinib was then increased to 150 mg per day after completion of radiation therapy. Molecular markers of EGFR, EGFRvIII, phosphatase and tensin homolog (PTEN), and methylation status of the promotor region of the MGMT gene were analyzed from tumor tissue. Survival was compared with outcomes from two historical phase II trials. Median survival was 19.3 months in the current study and 14.1 months in the combined historical control studies, with a hazard ratio for survival (treated/control) of 0.64 (95% CI 0.45–0.91) [138]. Treatment was well tolerated with study finding a strong correlation between MGMT promotor methylation and survival, as well as an association between MGMT promoter methylated tumors and PTEN positivity shown by IHC with improved survival [138].

MEDULLARY THYROID CANCER

Vandetanib (Zactima®, AstraZeneca) is a once-daily oral inhibitor of RET kinase, VEGFR, and EGFR TK that has undergone phase III testing and has been recently approved by the U.S. FDA for treatment of advanced medullary thyroid cancer (MTC). Patients with advanced MTC were randomly assigned in a 2:1 ratio to receive vandetanib 300 mg per day ($n=231$) or placebo ($n=100$). The study demonstrated prolongation PFS with vandetanib versus placebo (HR 0.46 [95% CI, 0.31–0.69], $p<0.001$). Statistically significant advantages for vandetanib were also seen for ORR ($p<0.001$), disease control rate ($p=0.001$), and biochemical response ($p<0.001$) [148].

FUTURE DIRECTIONS

Further improvement to identify predictors of response will help to better select patients who are most likely to benefit from EGFR TKIs and define appropriate use of combination therapies targeting multiple expression pathways. On the other hand, the mechanisms of resistance also need to be elucidated. Data suggest that EGFR inhibition may not be effective in the presence of independently activated proteins (e.g., MAPK, KRAS, PI3K/Akt, and STAT3), tumor cell dedifferentiation (e.g., epithelial–mesenchymal transition), or the expression of other cell surface receptors (e.g., insulin-like growth factor-1 receptor (IGF-1R) or an increase in VEGF). If these mechanisms underlie resistance in the clinic, then the emerging therapeutics targeting these processes or proteins are expected to synergize and provide wider applicability of the EGFR inhibitors. The continued study and use of pan-HER inhibitors in an effort to provide more complete signaling blockade and longer suppression of the signaling pathway may provide keys to overcoming both acquired and inherent resistance. Furthermore, to exploit the concept of oncogenic addiction, combinations of targeted therapies with chemotherapy in an effort to suppress both mutated as well as unmutated clones appear promising.

There are already clinical trials underway combining an EGFR inhibitor with different target inhibitors for signaling downstream from the HER kinase receptor. The RAS–RAF–MEK–ERK cascade is constitutively activated via mutation of HRAS, KRAS, or NRAS causing dysregulation of cell growth, differentiation, and apoptosis. While KRAS mutations are generally mutually exclusive of EGFR mutations, they will occasionally occur together. These patients do not respond to EGFR TKIs [163]. Mutations and inhibition of MEK in combination with HER family inhibition are being studied in several tumor types including NSCLC and CRC. Likewise, the PI3K/Akt pathway mutations prolong survival and growth. Rapamycin analogs inhibit a downstream activator of Akt, mammalian target of rapamycin (mTOR), or antiangiogenesis agents. Combination of mTOR inhibitors plus EGFR small molecules or mAbs is being studied in both breast and prostate cancer.

Combining EGFR inhibitors with suppression of parallel signaling pathways is also an area of vested interest. The mesenchymal–epithelial transition (MET) factor pathway is an oncogenic mediator that is activated by the ligand hepatocyte growth factor (HGF). Activation of this pathway results in tumorigenesis. Upward of 20% of tumors exposed to EGFR TKIs acquire MET amplification, which is uncommon at initial diagnosis, providing a rationale for a combination MET/EGFR inhibitory approach [160]. Preclinical data demonstrate activity of both anti-MET mAbs and small molecules (TKIs) to restore or enhance activity of EGFR kinase inhibitors in NSCLC [161,162]. There are several ongoing trials with both first- and second-generation TKIs in combination with MET inhibition. In fact, crizotinib (Xalkori®, Pfizer, New London, Connecticut), an oral ALK plus cMET/HGF receptor TK, is FDA approved as a single agent for the treatment of advanced NSCLC demonstrating EML4-ALK translocation. Activation of the VEGF receptor or IGF-1R can stimulate tumor growth or bypass the HER and activate downstream signaling [164]. Bevacizumab and other VEGF inhibitors are being studied in combination with various HER family inhibitors in several tumor types including NSCLC, glioma, thymoma, and breast cancer.

Pan-HER inhibition via second-generation irreversible inhibitors continues to be an area of much promise. The simultaneous blockade of EGFR as well as its dimerization partners has the potential to offer a more complete downstream signal blockade. Not to mention, given their irreversible nature, one would expect a prolonged suppression of the HER family pathways. Evaluation of these new compounds in patients with acquired EGFR mutations, such as the T790M gatekeeper mutation, may help change the paradigm on treatment of EGFR-mutated malignancies.

Finally, the combination of HER inhibitors with standard or novel chemotherapy approaches may take advantage of the concept of oncogenic addiction. As the targeted therapy suppresses mutated or amplified TK signaling, systemic chemotherapy would hope to eliminate the wild-type clones. Although the addition of first-generation TKIs to up-front chemotherapy in NSCLC has not provided encouraging results, continued suppression of the mutated clone is being studied in this disease. Furthermore, the combination of mAbs and small molecules such as erlotinib with standard chemotherapy is seen in metastatic CRC, breast cancer, and pancreatic cancer. Novel approaches such as immunotherapy (CimaVax), combinations, and use of second-generation irreversible TKIs with chemotherapy are likely to be of continued investigational and therapeutic interest.

REFERENCES

1. Cohen S, Carpenter G, King L Jr. Epidermal growth factor-receptor-protein kinase interactions. Co-purification of receptor and epidermal growth factor-enhanced phosphorylation activity. *J Biol Chem* 1980; 255:4834–4842.
2. Carpenter G. Receptors for epidermal growth factor and other polypeptide mitogens. *Annu Rev Biochem* 1987; 56:881–914.
3. Kim ES, Khuri FR, Herbst RS. Epidermal growth factor receptor biology (IMC-C225). *Curr Opin Oncol* 2001; 13:506–513.
4. Gullick WJ. Prevalence of aberrant expression of the epidermal growth factor receptor in human cancers. *Br Med Bull* 1991; 47:87–98.
5. Yarden Y. The EGFR family and its ligands in human cancer. Signaling mechanisms and therapeutic opportunities. *Eur J Cancer* 2001; 37(Suppl 4):S3–S8.
6. Olayioye MA, Neve RM, Lane HA et al. The ErbB signaling network: Receptor heterodimerization in development and cancer. *EMBO J* 2000; 19:3159–3167.
7. Marmor MD, Skaria KB, Yarden Y. Signal transduction and oncogenesis by ErbB/HER receptors. *Int J Radiat Oncol Biol Phys* 2004; 58:903–913.
8. Dehm SM, Bonham K. SRC gene expression in human cancer: The role of transcriptional activation. *Biochem Cell Biol* 2004; 82:263–274.
9. Laskin JJ, Sandler AB. Epidermal growth factor receptor: A promising target in solid tumours. *Cancer Treat Rev* 2004; 30:1–17.
10. Salomon DS, Brandt R, Ciardiello F et al. Epidermal growth factor-related peptides and their receptors in human malignancies. *Crit Rev Oncol Hematol* 1995; 19:183–232.
11. Nicholson RI, Gee JM, Harper ME. EGFR and cancer prognosis. *Eur J Cancer* 2001; 37(Suppl 4):S9–S15.
12. Normanno N, Bianco C, De LA et al. The role of EGF-related peptides in tumor growth. *Front Biosci* 2001; 6:D685–D707.
13. Sharma SV, Bell DW, Settleman J, Haber DA. Epidermal growth factor receptor mutations in lung cancer. *Nat Rev Cancer* 2007; 7:169–181.
14. Kwak EL, Sordella R, Bell DW et al. Irreversible inhibitors of the EGF receptor may circumvent acquired resistance to gefitinib. *Proc Natl Acad Sci USA* 2005; 102:7665–7670.
15. Chang GC, Hsu SL, Tsai JR et al. Molecular mechanisms of ZD1839-induced G1-cell cycle arrest and apoptosis in human lung adenocarcinoma A549 cells. *Biochem Pharmacol* 2004; 68:1453–1464.
16. Huang S, Armstrong EA, Benavente S et al. Dual-agent molecular targeting of the epidermal growth factor receptor (EGFR): Combining anti-EGFR antibody with tyro- sine kinase inhibitor. *Cancer Res* 2004; 64:5355–5362.
17. Janmaat ML, Kruyt FA, Rodriguez JA et al. Response to epidermal growth factor receptor inhibitors in non-small cell lung cancer cells: Limited antiproliferative effects and absence of apoptosis associated with persistent activity of extracellular signal- regulated kinase or Akt kinase pathways. *Clin Cancer Res* 2003; 9:2316–2326.
18. Bulgaru AM, Mani S, Goel S et al. Erlotinib (Tarceva): A promising drug targeting epidermal growth factor receptor tyrosine kinase. *Expert Rev Anticancer Ther* 2003; 3:269–279.

19. Riemer AB, Kurz H, Klinger M et al. Vaccination with cetuximab mimotopes and biological properties of induced anti-epidermal growth factor receptor antibodies. *J Natl Cancer Inst* 2005; 97:1663–1670.

20. Hu B, Wei Y, Tian L et al. Active antitumor immunity elicited by vaccine based on recombinant form of epidermal growth factor receptor. *J Immunother* 2005; 28:236–244.

21. Ramos TC, Vinageras EN, Ferrer MC et al. Treatment of NSCLC patients with an EGF-based cancer vaccine: Report of a Phase I trial. *Cancer Biol Ther* 2006; 5:145–149.

22. Rodriguez PC, Neninger E, García B et al. Safety, immunogenicity and preliminary efficacy of multiple-site vaccination with an epidermal growth factor (EGF) based cancer vaccine in advanced non small cell lung cancer (NSCLC) patients. *J Immune Based Ther Vaccines* 2011; 9:7.

23. Ciardiello F, Caputo R, Troiani T et al. Antisense oligonucleotides targeting the epidermal growth factor receptor inhibit proliferation, induce apoptosis, and co- operate with cytotoxic drugs in human cancer cell lines. *Int J Cancer* 2001; 93:172–178.

24. Azemar M, Schmidt M, Arlt F et al. Recombinant antibody toxins specific for ErbB2 and EGF receptor inhibit the in vitro growth of human head and neck cancer cells and cause rapid tumor regression in vivo. *Int J Cancer* 2000; 86:269–275.

25. Fukuoka M, Yano S, Giaccone G et al. Multi-institutional randomized phase II trial of gefitinib for previously treated patients with advanced non-small-cell lung cancer (The IDEAL 1 Trial) [corrected]. *J Clin Oncol* 2003; 21:2237–2246.

26. Kris MG, Natale RB, Herbst RS et al. Efficacy of gefitinib, an inhibitor of the epidermal growth factor receptor tyrosine kinase, in symptomatic patients with non- small cell lung cancer: A randomized trial. *JAMA* 2003; 290:2149–2158.

27. Perez-Soler R, Chachoua A, Hammond LA et al. Determinants of tumor response and survival with erlotinib in patients with non-small-cell lung cancer. *J Clin Oncol* 2004; 22:3238–3247.

28. Miller VA, Kris MG, Shah N et al. Bronchioloalveolar pathologic subtype and smoking history predict sensitivity to gefitinib in advanced non-small-cell lung cancer. *J Clin Oncol* 2004; 22:1103–1109.

29. Kim YH, Ishii G, Goto K et al. Dominant papillary subtype is a significant predictor of the response to gefitinib in adenocarcinoma of the lung. *Clin Cancer Res* 2004; 10:7311–7317.

30. Herbst RS, Prager D, Hermann R et al. TRIBUTE: A phase III trial of erlotinib hydrochloride (OSI-774) combined with carboplatin and paclitaxel chemotherapy in advanced non-small-cell lung cancer. *J Clin Oncol* 2005; 23:5892–5899.

31. Thatcher N, Chang A, Parikh P et al. Gefitinib plus best supportive care in previously treated patients with refractory advanced non-small-cell lung cancer: Results from a randomized, placebo-controlled, multicentre study (Iressa Survival Evaluation in Lung Cancer). *Lancet* 2005; 366:1527–1537.

32. Shepherd FA, Rodrigues PJ, Ciuleanu T et al. Erlotinib in previously treated non- small-cell lung cancer. *N Engl J Med* 2005; 353:123–132.

33. Saltz L, Kies M, Abbruzzese JL et al. The presence and intensity of the cetuximab-induced acne-like rash predicts increased survival in studies across multiple malignancies. *Abstr 817, 39th Annual Meeting of American Society of Clinical Oncology*, Chicago, IL, May 31–June 3, 2003. Alexandria, VA: American Society of Clinical Oncology (ASCO), 1964.

34. Blackwell KL, Burstein HJ, Storniolo AM et al. Randomized study of Lapatinib alone or in combination with trastuzumab in women with ErbB2-positive, trastuzumab-refractory metastatic breast cancer. *J Clin Oncol* 2010; 28:1124–1130.

35. Thienelt CD, Bunn PA, Jr, Hanna N et al. Multicenter phase I/II study of cetuximab with paclitaxel and carboplatin in untreated patients with stage IV non-small-cell lung cancer. *J Clin Oncol* 2005; 23:8786–8793.

36. Janne PA, Gurubhagavatula S, Yeap BY et al. Outcomes of patients with advanced non-small cell lung cancer treated with gefitinib (ZD1839, "Iressa") on an expanded access study. *Lung Cancer* 2004; 44:221–230.

37. Mohamed MK, Ramalingam S, Lin Y et al. Skin rash and good performance status predict improved survival with gefitinib in patients with advanced non-small cell lung cancer. *Ann Oncol* 2005; 16:780–785.

38. Lynch TJ, Bell DW, Sordella R et al. Activating mutations in the epidermal growth factor receptor underlying responsiveness of non-small-cell lung cancer to gefitinib. *N Engl J Med* 2004; 350:2129–2139.

39. Paez JG, Janne PA, Lee JC et al. EGFR mutations in lung cancer: Correlation with clinical response to gefitinib therapy. *Science* 2004; 304:1497–1500.

40. Pao W, Miller V, Zakowski M et al. EGF receptor gene mutations are common in lung cancers from "never smokers" and are associated with sensitivity of tumors to gefitinib and erlotinib. *Proc Natl Acad Sci USA* 2004; 101:13306–13311.

41. Miller VA, Kris MG, Shah N et al. Bronchioloalveolar pathologic subtype and smoking history predict sensitivity to gefitinib in advanced non-small-cell lung cancer. *J Clin Oncol* 2004; 22(6):1103–1109.

42. Jänne PA, Gurubhagavatula S, Yeap BY et al. Outcomes of patients with advanced non-small cell lung cancer treated with gefitinib (ZD1839, "Iressa") on an expanded access study. *Lung Cancer* 2004; 44(2):221–230.

43. Heist RS, Christiani D. EGFR-targeted therapies in lung cancer: Predictors of response and toxicity. *Pharmacogenomics* 2009; 10(1):59–68.

44. Fukui T, Mitsudomi T. Mutations in the epidermal growth factor receptor gene and effects of EGFR-tyrosine kinase inhibitors on lung cancers. *Gen Thorac Cardiovasc Surg* 2008; 56:97–103.

45. Yun CH, Mengwasser KE, Toms AV et al. The T790M mutation in EGFR kinase causes drug resistance by increasing the affinity for ATP. *Proc Natl Acad Sci USA* 2008; 105:2070–2075.

46. Sequist LV, Waltman BA, Dias-Santagata D et al. Genotypic and histological evolution of lung cancers acquiring resistance to EGFR inhibitors. *Sci Transl Med* 2011; 3:75ra26.

47. Sequist LV, Martins RG, Spigel D et al. First-line gefitinib in patients with advanced non-small-cell lung cancer harboring somatic EGFR mutations. *J Clin Oncol: Off J Am Soc Clin Oncol* 2008; 26:2442–2449.

48. Bell DW, Gore I, Okimoto RA et al. Inherited susceptibility to lung cancer may be associated with the T790M drug resistance mutation in EGFR. *Nat Genet* 2005; 37:1315–1316.

49. Engelman JA, Janne PA. Mechanisms of acquired resistance to epidermal growth factor receptor tyrosine kinase inhibitors in non-small cell lung cancer. *Clin Cancer Res: Off J Am Assoc Cancer Res* 2008; 14:2895–2899.

50. Pao W, Wang TY, Riely GJ et al. KRAS mutations and primary resistance of lung adeno-carcinomas to gefitinib or erlotinib. *PLoS Med* 2005; 2:e17.

51. Eberhard DA, Johnson BE, Amler LC et al. Mutations in the epidermal growth factor receptor and in KRAS are predictive and prognostic indicators in patients with non-small-cell lung cancer treated with chemotherapy alone and in combination with erlotinib. *J Clin Oncol* 2005; 23:5900–5909.

52. Shigematsu H, Lin L, Takahashi T et al. Clinical and biological features associated with epidermal growth factor receptor gene mutations in lung cancers. *J Natl Cancer Inst* 2005; 97:339–346.

53. Lee JW, Soung YH, Kim SY et al. Somatic mutations of EGFR gene in squamous cell carcinoma of the head and neck. *Clin Cancer Res* 2005; 11:2879–2882.

54. Cohen EE, Lingen MW, Martin LE et al. Response of some head and neck cancers to epidermal growth factor receptor tyrosine kinase inhibitors may be linked to mutation of ERBB2 rather than EGFR. *Clin Cancer Res* 2005; 11:8105–8108.

55. Chung CH, Ely K, McGavran L et al. Increased epidermal growth factor receptor gene copy number is associated with poor prognosis in head and neck squamous cell carcinomas. *J Clin Oncol* 2006; 24:4170–4176.

56. Moroni M, Veronese S, Benvenuti S et al. Gene copy number for epidermal growth factor receptor (EGFR) and clinical response to antiEGFR treatment in colorectal cancer: A cohort study. *Lancet Oncol* 2005; 6:279–286.

57. Liu W, Innocenti F, Chen P et al. Interethnic difference in the allelic distribution of human epidermal growth factor receptor intron 1 polymorphism. *Clin Cancer Res* 2003; 9:1009–1012.

58. Amador ML, Oppenheimer D, Perea S et al. An epidermal growth factor receptor intron 1 polymorphism mediates response to epidermal growth factor receptor inhibitors. *Cancer Res* 2004; 64:9139–9143.

59. Stephens P, Hunter C, Bingell G et al. Lung cancer: Intragenic ERBB2 kinase mutations in tumours. *Nature* 2004; 431:525–526.

60. Shigematsu H, Takahashi T, Nomura M et al. Somatic mutations of the GER2 kinase domain in lung adenocarcinoma. *Cancer Res* 2005; 65:1642–1646.

61. Sonobe M, Manabe T, Wada H et al. Lung adenocarcinoma harboring mutations in the ERBB2 kinase domain. *J Mol Diagn* 2006; 8:351–356.

62. Buttitta F, Barassi F, Fresu G et al. Mutational analysis of the HER2 gene in lung tumors from Caucasian patients: Mutations are mainly present in adenocarcinomas with bronchioloalveolar features. *Int J Cancer* 2006; 119:2586–2591.

63. Pao W, Girard N. New driver mutations in non-small-cell lung cancer. *Lancet Oncol* 2011; 12:175–180.

64. Vijayalakshmi R, Krishnamurthy A. Targetable "driver" mutations in non small cell lung cancer. *Indian J Surg Oncol* 2011; 2(3):178–188.

65. De Greve J, Teugels E, De Mey J et al. Clinical activity of BIBW2992, an irreversible inhibitor of EGFR and HER2 in adenocarcinoma of the lung with mutations in the kinase domain of HER2neu. *J Thorac Oncol* 2009; 4:S307 (Abstr).

66. Bang YJ, Van Cutsem E, Feyereislova A et al: Trastuzumab in combination with chemotherapy versus chemotherapy alone for treatment of HER2-positive advanced gastric or gastro-oesophageal junction cancer (ToGA): A phase 3, open-label, randomised controlled trial. *Lancet* 2010; 376:687–697.

67. Wolff AC, Hammond ME, Schwartz JN et al. American Society of Clinical Oncology/ College of American Pathologists guideline recommendations for human epidermal growth factor receptor 2 testing in breast cancer. *J Clin Oncol* 2007; 25(1):118–145.

68. Seidman AD, Berry D, Cirrincione C et al. Randomized phase III trial of weekly compared with every-3-weeks paclitaxel for metastatic breast cancer, with trastuzumab for all HER-2 overexpressors and random assignment to trastuzumab or not in HER-2 non-overexpressors: Final results of Cancer and Leukemia Group B protocol 9840. *J Clin Oncol* 2008; 26(10):1642–1649.

69. De Greve J, Decoster L, De Mey J et al. Clinical activity of BINW2992, an irreversible inhibitor of EGFR and HER2 in adenocarcinoma of the lung with mutations in the kinase domain of HER2neu. Presented at: *The 2nd European Lung Cancer Conference*, Geneva, Switzerland, 2010.

70. Cohen MH, Williams GA, Sridhara R et al. United States Food and Drug Administration drug approval summary: Gefitinib (ZD1839; Iressa) tablets. *Clin Cancer Res* 2004; 10:1212–1218.

71. Chang A, Parikh P, Thongprasert S et al. Gefitinib (IRESSA) in patients of Asian origin with refractory advanced non-small cell lung cancer: Subset analysis from the ISEL study. *J Thorac Oncol* 2006; 1(8):847–855.

72. Kim ES, Hirsh V, Mok T et al. Gefitinib versus docetaxel in previously treated non-small-cell lung cancer (INTEREST): A randomized phase III trial. *Lancet* 2008; 372(9652):1809–1818.

73. Giaccone G, Herbst RS, Manegold C et al. Gefitinib in combination with gemcitabine and cisplatin in advanced non-small-cell lung cancer: A phase III trial–INTACT 1. *J Clin Oncol* 2004; 22:777–784.

74. Herbst RS, Giaccone G, Schiller JH et al. Gefitinib in combination with paclitaxel and carboplatin in advanced non-small-cell lung cancer: A phase III trial–INTACT 2. *J Clin Oncol* 2004; 22:785–794.

75. Gatzemeier U, Pluzanska A, Szczesna A et al. Phase III study of erlotinib in combination with cisplatin and gemcitabine in advanced non-small-cell lung cancer: The Tarceva lung cancer investigation trial. *J Clin Oncol* 2007; 25(12):1545–1552.

76. Pao W, Chmielecki J. Rational, biologically based treatment of EGFR-mutant non-small-cell lung cancer. *Nat Rev Cancer* 2010; 10(11):760–774.

77. Mok TS, Wu YL, Thongprasert S et al. Gefitinib or carboplatin-paclitaxel in pulmonary adenocarcinoma. *N Engl J Med* 2009; 361(10):947–957.

78. Fukuoka M, Wu YL, Thongprasert S et al. Biomarker analyses and final overall survival results from a phase III, randomized, open-label, first-line study of gefitinib versus carboplatin/paclitaxel in clinically selected patients with advanced non-small-cell lung cancer in Asia (IPASS). *J Clin Oncol* 2011; 29(21):2866–2874.

79. Mitsudomi T, Morita S, Yatabe Y et al. Gefitinib versus cisplatin plus docetaxel in patients with non-small-cell lung cancer harbouring mutations of the epidermal growth factor receptor (WJTOG3405): An open label, randomized phase 3 trial. *Lancet Oncol* 2010; 11(2):121–128.

80. Maemondo M, Inoue A, Kobayashi K et al. Gefitinib or chemotherapy for non-small-cell lung cancer with mutated EGFR. *N Engl J Med* 2010; 362(25):2380–2388.

81. Zhou C, Wu YL, Chen G et al. Erlotinib versus chemotherapy as first-line treatment for patients with advanced EGFR mutation-positive non-small-cell lung cancer (OPTIMAL, CTONG-0802): A multicentre, open-label, randomized, phase 3 study. *Lancet Oncol* 2011; 12(8):735–742.

82. Rosell R, Carcereny E, Gervais R et al. Erlotinib versus standard chemotherapy as first-line treatment for European patients with advanced EGFR mutation-positive non-small-cell lung cancer (EURTAC): A multicentre, open-label, randomized phase 3 trial. *Lancet Oncol* 2012; 13(3):239–246.

83. Cappuzzo F, Ciuleanu T, Stelmakh L et al. Erlotinib as maintenance treatment in advanced non-small-cell lung cancer: A multicentre, randomized, placebo-controlled phase 3 study. *Lancet Oncol* 2010; 11(6):521–529.

84. Zhang L, Ma S, Song X et al. Gefitinib versus placebo as maintenance therapy in patients with locally advanced or metastatic non-small-cell lung cancer (INFORM; C-TONG 0804): A multicentre, double-blind randomized phase 3 trial. *Lancet Oncol* 2012; 13(5):466–475.

85. Perol M, Chouaid C, Milleron BJ et al. A randomized, phase iii study of gemcitabine or erlotinib maintenance therapy versus observation, with predefined second-line treatment, after cisplatin-gemcitabine induction chemotherapy in advanced non-small-cell lung cancer. *J Clin Oncol* 2012; 30(28):3516–3524.

86. Gaafar RM, Surmont VF, Scagliotti GV et al. A double-blind, randomised, placebo-controlled phase III intergroup study of gefitinib in patients with advanced NSCLC, non-progressing after first line platinum-based chemotherapy (EORTC 08021/ILCP 01/03). *Eur J Cancer* 2011; 47(15):2331–2340.

87. Herbst RS, Johnson DH, Mininberg E et al. Phase I/II trial evaluating the anti- vascular endothelial growth factor monoclonal antibody bevacizumab in combination with the HER-1/epidermal growth factor receptor tyrosine kinase inhibitor erlotinib for patients with recurrent non-small-cell lung cancer. *J Clin Oncol* 2005; 23:2544–2555.

88. Herbst RS, Ansari R, Bustin F et al. Efficacy of bevacizumab plus erlotinib versus erlotinib alone in advanced non-small-cell lung cancer after failure of standard first-line chemotherapy (BeTa): A double-blind, placebo-controlled, phase 3 trial. *Lancet* 2011; 377(9780):1846–1854.

89. Miller VA, O'Connor P, Soh C et al. A randomized, double-blind, placebo-controlled, phase IIIb trial (ATLAS) comparing bevacizumab (B) therapy with or without erlotinib (E) after completion of chemotherapy with B for first-line treatment of locally advanced, recurrent, or metastatic non-small cell lung cancer (NSCLC). *Abstr LBA8002, 45nd Annual Meeting of American Society of Clinical Oncology*, Orlando, FL, May 29–June 2, 2009. Alexandria, VA: American Society of Clinical Oncology (ASCO), 1964.

90. Pirker R, Pereira JR, Szczesna A et al. Cetuximab plus chemotherapy in patients with advanced non-small-cell lung cancer (FLEX): An open-label randomized phase III trial. *Lancet* 2009; 373(9674):1525–1531.

91. Lynch TJ, Patel T, Dreisbach L et al. Cetuximab and first-line taxane/carboplatin chemotherapy in advanced non-small-cell lung cancer: Results of the randomized multicenter phase III trial BMS099. *J Clin Oncol* 2010; 28(6):911–917.

92. Rosell R, Moran T, Queralt C et al. Screening for epidermal growth factor receptor mutations in lung cancer. *N Engl J Med* 2009; 361(10):958–967.

93. Jackman D, Pao W, Riely GJ et al. Clinical definition of acquired resistance to epidermal growth factor receptor tyrosine kinase inhibitors in non-small-cell lung cancer. *J Clin Oncol* 2010; 28(2):357–360.

94. Kobayashi S, Ji H, Yuza Y et al. An alternative inhibitor overcomes resistance caused by a mutation of the epidermal growth factor receptor. *Cancer Res* 2005; 65(16):7096–7101.

95. Pao W, Miller VA, Politi KA et al. Acquired resistance of lung adenocarcinomas to gefitinib or erlotinib is associated with a second mutation in the EGFR kinase domain. *PLoS Med* 2005; 2(3):e73.

96. Engelman JA, Zejnullahu K, Mitsudomi T et al. MET amplification leads to gefitinib resistance in lung cancer by activating ERBB3 signaling. *Science* 2007; 316(5827):1039–1043.

97. Bean J, Brennan C, Shih JY et al. MET amplification occurs with or without T790M mutations in EGFR mutant lung tumors with acquired resistance to gefitinib or erlotinib. *Proc Natl Acad Sci USA* 2007; 104(52):20932–20937.

98. Sequist LV, Waltman BA, Dias-Santagata D et al. Genotypic and histological evolution of lung cancers acquiring resistance to EGFR inhibitors. *Sci Transl Med* 2011; 3(75):75ra26.

99. Yun CH, Mengwasser KE, Toms AV et al. The T790M mutation in EGFR kinase causes drug resistance by increasing the affinity for ATP. *Proc Natl Acad Sci USA* 2008; 105(6):2070–2075.

100. Ross HJ, Blumenschein GR, Aisner J et al. Randomized phase ii multicenter trial of two schedules of lapatinib as first- or second-line monotherapy in patients with advanced or metastatic non-small cell lung cancer. *Clin Cancer Res* 2010; 16(6):1938–1949.

101. Sequist LV, Besse B, Lynch TJ et al. Neratinib, an irreversible pan-ErbB receptor tyrosine kinase inhibitor: Results of a phase II trial in patients with advanced non-small-cell lung cancer. *J Clin Oncol* 2010; 28(18):3076–3083.

102. Li D, Ambrogio L, Shimamura T et al. BIBW2992, an irreversible EGFR/HER2 inhibitor highly effective in preclinical lung cancer models. *Oncogene* 2008; 27(34):4702–4711.

103. Yang JC, Shih JY, Su WC et al. Afatinib for patients with lung adenocarcinoma and epidermal growth factor receptor mutations (LUX-Lung 2): A phase 2 trial. *Lancet Oncol* 2012; 13(5):539–548.

104. Miller VA, Hirsh V, Cadranel J et al. Afatinib versus placebo for patients with advanced, metastatic non-small-cell lung cancer after failure of erlotinib, gefitinib, or both, and one or two lines of chemotherapy (LUX-Lung 1): A phase 2b/3 randomised trial. *Lancet Oncol* 2012; 13(5):528–538.

105. James Chih-Hsin Yang MHS, Nobuyuki Yamamoto. LUX-Lung 3: A randomized, open-label, phase III study of afatinib versus pemetrexed and cisplatin as first-line treatment for patients with advanced adenocarcinoma of the lung harboring EGFR-activating mutations. *J Clin Oncol* 2012; 30:15s (Abstr LBA7500).

106. Martin H, Schuler DP, James C-HY. Interim analysis of afatinib monotherapy in patients with metastatic NSCLC progressing after chemotherapy and erlotinib/gefitinib (E/G) in a trial of afatinib plus paclitaxel versus investigator's choice chemotherapy following progression on afatinib monotherapy. *J Clin Oncol* 2012; 30:15s (Abstr 7557).

107. Janjigian YY, Horn L. Activity and tolerability of afatinib (BIBW 2992) and cetuximab in NSCLC patients with acquired resistance to erlotinib or gefitinib. *J Clin Oncol* 2011; 29:15s (Abstr 7525).

108. Engelman JA, Zejnullahu K, Gale CM et al. PF00299804, an irreversible pan-ERBB inhibitor, is effective in lung cancer models with EGFR and ERBB2 mutations that are resistant to gefitinib. *Cancer Res* 2007; 67(24):11924–11932.

109. Wu JY, Wu SG, Yang CH et al. Lung cancer with epidermal growth factor receptor exon 20 mutations is associated with poor gefitinib treatment response. *Clin Cancer Res* 2008; 14(15):4877–4882.

110. Mark G, Kris TM, Sai-Hong Ignatius Ou. First-line dacomitinib (PF-00299804), an irreversible pan-HER tyrosine kinase inhibitor, for patients with EGFR-mutant lung cancers. *J Clin Oncol* 2012; 30:15s (Abstr 7530).

111. Ramalingam SS, Blackhall F, Krzakowski M et al. Randomized phase II study of dacomitinib (pf-00299804), an irreversible pan-human epidermal growth factor receptor inhibitor, versus erlotinib in patients with advanced non-small-cell lung cancer. *J Clin Oncol* 2012; 30(27):3337–3344.

112. Campbell A RKL, Camidge DR, Giaccone G, Gadgeel SM, Khuri FR et al. PF-00299804 (PF299) patient (pt)-reported outcomes (PROs) and efficacy in adenocarcinoma (adeno) and nonadeno non-small cell lung cancer (NSCLC): A phase (P) II trial in advanced NSCLC after failure of chemotherapy (CT) and erlotinib (E). *J Clin Oncol* 2010; 28:15s (Abstr 7596).

113. Wagner AD, Moehler M. Development of targeted therapies in advanced gastric cancer: Promising exploratory steps in a new era. *Curr Opin Oncol* 2009; 21:381–385.

114. Molecule of the month: Trastuzumab. *Drug News Perspect* 1998; 11(5):305.

115. Yano T, Doi T, Ohtsu A et al. Comparison of HER2 gene amplification assessed by fluorescence in situ hybridization and HER2 protein expression assessed by immuno-histochemistry in gastric cancer. *Oncol Rep* 2006; 15:65–71.

116. Gravalos C, Jimeno A. HER2 in gastric cancer: A new prognostic factor and a novel therapeutic target. *Ann Oncol* 2008; 19:1523–1529.

117. Hofmann M, Stoss O, Shi D et al. Assessment of a HER2 scoring system for gastric cancer: Results from a validation study. *Histopathology* 2008; 52:797–805.

118. Gomez-Martin C, Garralda E, Echarri MJ et al. HER2/neu testing for anti-HER2-based therapies in patients with unresectable and/or metastatic gastric cancer. *J Clin Pathol* 2012; 65:751–757.

119. Moore MJ, Goldstein D, Hamm J et al. Erlotinib plus gemcitabine compared with gemcitabine alone in patients with advanced pancreatic cancer: A phase III trial of the National Cancer Institute of Canada Clinical Trials Group. *J Clin Oncol* 2007; 25:1960–1966.

120. Spano JP, Lagorce C, Atlan D et al. Impact of EGFR expression on colorectal cancer patient prognosis and survival. *Ann Oncol* 2005; 16:102–108.

121. Roth AD, Tejpar S, Delorenzi M et al. Prognostic role of KRAS and BRAF in stage II and III resected colon cancer: Results of the translational study on the PETACC-3, EORTC 40993, SAKK 60–00 trial. *J Clin Oncol* 2010; 28:466–474.
122. Lievre A, Bachet JB, Le Corre D et al. KRAS mutation status is predictive of response to cetuximab therapy in colorectal cancer. *Cancer Res* 2006; 66:3992–3995.
123. Amado RG, Wolf M, Peeters M et al. Wild-type KRAS is required for panitumumab efficacy in patients with metastatic colorectal cancer. *J Clin Oncol* 2008; 26:1626–1634.
124. Karapetis CS, Khambata-Ford S, Jonker DJ et al. K-ras mutations and benefit from cetuximab in advanced colorectal cancer. *N Engl J Med* 2008; 359:1757–1765.
125. Di Nicolantonio F, Martini M, Molinari F et al. Wild-type BRAF is required for response to panitumumab or cetuximab in metastatic colorectal cancer. *J Clin Oncol* 2008; 26:5705–5712.
126. Loupakis F, Ruzzo A, Cremolini C et al. KRAS codon 61, 146 and BRAF mutations predict resistance to cetuximab plus irinotecan in KRAS codon 12 and 13 wild-type metastatic colorectal cancer. *Br J Cancer* 2009; 101:715–721.
127. De Roock W, Claes B, Bernasconi D et al. Effects of KRAS, BRAF, NRAS, and PIK3CA mutations on the efficacy of cetuximab plus chemotherapy in chemotherapy-refractory metastatic colorectal cancer: A retrospective consortium analysis. *Lancet Oncol* 2010; 11:753–762.
128. Van Cutsem E, Kohne CH, Hitre E et al. Cetuximab and chemotherapy as initial treatment for metastatic colorectal cancer. *N Engl J Med* 2009; 360:1408–1417.
129. Van Cutsem E, Kohne CH, Lang I et al. Cetuximab plus irinotecan, fluorouracil, and leucovorin as first-line treatment for metastatic colorectal cancer: Updated analysis of overall survival according to tumor KRAS and BRAF mutation status. *J Clin Oncol* 2011; 29:2011–2019.
130. Tveit KM, Guren T, Glimelius B et al. Phase III trial of cetuximab with continuous or intermittent fluorouracil, leucovorin, and oxaliplatin (Nordic FLOX) versus FLOX alone in first-line treatment of metastatic colorectal cancer: The NORDIC-VII study. *J Clin Oncol* 2012; 30:1755–1762.
131. Douillard JY, Siena S, Cassidy J et al. Randomized, phase III trial of panitumumab with infusional fluorouracil, leucovorin, and oxaliplatin (FOLFOX4) versus FOLFOX4 alone as first-line treatment in patients with previously untreated metastatic colorectal cancer: The PRIME study. *J Clin Oncol* 2010; 28:4697–4705.
132. Peeters M, Price TJ, Cervantes A et al. Randomized phase III study of panitumumab with fluorouracil, leucovorin, and irinotecan (FOLFIRI) compared with FOLFIRI alone as second-line treatment in patients with metastatic colorectal cancer. *J Clin Oncol* 2010; 28:4706–4713.
133. Tol J, Koopman M, Cats A et al. Chemotherapy, bevacizumab, and cetuximab in metastatic colorectal cancer. *N Engl J Med* 2009; 360:563–572.
134. Hecht JR, Mitchell E, Chidiac T et al. A randomized phase IIIB trial of chemotherapy, bevacizumab, and panitumumab compared with chemotherapy and bevacizumab alone for metastatic colorectal cancer. *J Clin Oncol* 2009; 27:672–680.
135. Sobrero AF, Maurel J, Fehrenbacher L et al. EPIC: Phase III trial of cetuximab plus irinotecan after fluoropyrimidine and oxaliplatin failure in patients with metastatic colorectal cancer. *J Clin Oncol* 2008; 26:2311–2319.
136. Van Cutsem E, Peeters M, Siena S et al. Open-label phase III trial of panitumumab plus best supportive care compared with best supportive care alone in patients with chemotherapy-refractory metastatic colorectal cancer. *J Clin Oncol* 2007; 25:1658–1664.
137. Rich JN, Reardon DA, Peery T et al. Phase II trial of gefitinib in recurrent glioblastoma. *J Clin Oncol* 2004; 22:133–142.

138. Prados MD, Chang SM, Butowski N et al. Phase II study of erlotinib plus temozolomide during and after radiation therapy in patients with newly diagnosed glioblastoma multiforme or gliosarcoma. *J Clin Oncol* 2009; 27:579–584.

139. Pomerantz RG, Grandis JR. The epidermal growth factor receptor signaling network in head and neck carcinogenesis and implications for targeted therapy. *Semin Oncol* 2004; 31:734–743.

140. Baselga J, Pfister D, Cooper MR et al. Phase I studies of anti-epidermal growth factor receptor chimeric antibody C225 alone and in combination with cisplatin. *J Clin Oncol* 2000; 18:904–914.

141. Burtness B, Goldwasser MA, Flood W et al. Phase III randomized trial of cisplatin plus placebo compared with cisplatin plus cetuximab in metastatic/recurrent head and neck cancer: An Eastern Cooperative Oncology Group study. *J Clin Oncol* 2005; 23:8646–8654.

142. Baselga J, Trigo JM, Bourhis J et al. Phase II multicenter study of the antiepidermal growth factor receptor monoclonal antibody cetuximab in combination with platinum-based chemotherapy in patients with platinum-refractory metastatic and/or recurrent squamous cell carcinoma of the head and neck. *J Clin Oncol* 2005; 23:5568–5577.

143. Herbst RS, Arquette M, Shin DM et al. Phase II multicenter study of the epidermal growth factor receptor antibody cetuximab and cisplatin for recurrent and refractory squamous cell carcinoma of the head and neck. *J Clin Oncol* 2005; 23:5578–5587.

144. Bonner JA, Harari PM, Giralt J et al. Radiotherapy plus cetuximab for squamous-cell carcinoma of the head and neck. *N Engl J Med* 2006; 354:567–578.

145. Soulieres D, Senzer NN, Vokes EE et al. Multicenter phase II study of erlotinib, an oral epidermal growth factor receptor tyrosine kinase inhibitor, in patients with recurrent or metastatic squamous cell cancer of the head and neck. *J Clin Oncol* 2004; 22:77–85.

146. Siu LL, Soulieres D, Chen EX et al. Phase I/II trial of erlotinib and cisplatin in patients with recurrent or metastatic squamous cell carcinoma of the head and neck: A Princess Margaret Hospital phase II consortium and National Cancer Institute of Canada Clinical Trials Group Study. *J Clin Oncol* 2007; 25:2178–2183.

147. Cohen EE, Davis DW, Karrison TG et al. Erlotinib and bevacizumab in patients with recurrent or metastatic squamous-cell carcinoma of the head and neck: A phase I/II study. *Lancet Oncol* 2009; 10:247–257.

148. Wells SA, Jr., Robinson BG, Gagel RF et al. Vandetanib in patients with locally advanced or metastatic medullary thyroid cancer: A randomized, double-blind phase III trial. *J Clin Oncol* 2012; 30:134–141.

149. Joensuu H, Kellokumpu-Lehtinen PL, Bono P et al. Adjuvant docetaxel or vinorelbine with or without trastuzumab for breast cancer. *N Engl J Med* 2006; 354:809–820.

150. Piccart-Gebhart MJ, Procter M, Leyland-Jones B et al. Trastuzumab after adjuvant chemotherapy in HER2-positive breast cancer. *N Engl J Med* 2005; 353:1659–1672.

151. Romond EH, Perez EA, Bryant J et al. Trastuzumab plus adjuvant chemotherapy for operable HER2-positive breast cancer. *N Engl J Med* 2005; 353:1673–1684.

152. Slamon D, Eiermann W, Robert N et al. Adjuvant trastuzumab in HER2-positive breast cancer. *N Engl J Med* 2011; 365:1273–1283.

153. Perez EA, Romond EH, Suman VJ et al. Four-year follow-up of trastuzumab plus adjuvant chemotherapy for operable human epidermal growth factor receptor 2-positive breast cancer: Joint analysis of data from NCCTG N9831 and NSABP B-31. *J Clin Oncol* 2011; 29:3366–3373.

154. Scheuer W, Friess T, Burtscher H et al. Strongly enhanced antitumor activity of trastuzumab and pertuzumab combination treatment on HER2-positive human xenograft tumor models. *Cancer Res* 2009; 69:9330–9336.

155. Baselga J, Cortes J, Kim SB et al. Pertuzumab plus trastuzumab plus docetaxel for metastatic breast cancer. *N Engl J Med* 2012; 366:109–119.

156. Bartsch R, Wenzel C, Altorjai G et al. Capecitabine and trastuzumab in heavily pre-treated metastatic breast cancer. *J Clin Oncol* 2007; 25:3853–3858.
157. von Minckwitz G, du Bois A, Schmidt M et al. Trastuzumab beyond progression in human epidermal growth factor receptor 2-positive advanced breast cancer: A German breast group 26/breast international group 03–05 study. *J Clin Oncol* 2009; 27:1999–2006.
158. Geyer CE, Forster J, Lindquist D et al. Lapatinib plus capecitabine for HER2-positive advanced breast cancer. *N Engl J Med* 2006; 355:2733–2743.
159. Johnston S, Pippen J, Jr., Pivot X et al. Lapatinib combined with letrozole versus letrozole and placebo as first-line therapy for postmenopausal hormone receptor-positive metastatic breast cancer. *J Clin Oncol* 2009; 27:5538–5546.
160. Chen HJ, Mok TS, Chen ZH et al. Clinicopathologic and molecular features of epidermal growth factor receptor T790M mutation and c-MET amplification in tyrosine kinase inhibitor-resistant Chinese non-small cell lung cancer. *Pathol Oncol Res* 2009; 15(4):651–658.
161. Zucali PA, Ruiz MG, Giovannetti E et al. Role of cMET expression in non-small-cell lung cancer patients treated with EGFR tyrosine kinase inhibitors. *Ann Oncol* 2008; 19(9):1605–1612.
162. Engelman JA, Zejnullahu K, Mitsudomi T et al. MET amplification leads to gefitinib resistance in lung cancer by activating ERBB3 signaling. *Science* 2007; 316(5827): 1039–1043.
163. Eberhard DA, Johnson BE, Amler LC et al. Mutations in the epidermal growth factor receptor and in KRAS are predictive and prognostic indicators in patients with non-small-cell lung cancer treated with chemotherapy alone and in combination with erlotinib. *J Clin Oncol* 2005; 23(25):5900–5909.
164. Guix M, Faber AC, Wang SE et al. Acquired resistance to EGFR tyrosine kinase inhibitors in cancer cells is mediated by loss of IGF-binding proteins. *J Clin Invest* 2008; 118(7):2609–2619.
165. Inoue A, Kobayashi K, Maemondo M et al. Updated overall survival results from a randomized phase III trial comparing gefitinib with carboplatin-paclitaxel for chemo-naive non-small cell lung cancer with sensitive EGFR gene mutations (NEJ002). *Ann Oncol* 2013; 24(1):54–59.

3 HER2 Inhibition and Clinical Achievements

Berta Sousa
Champalimaud Cancer Center

Joana Ribeiro
Champalimaud Cancer Center

Fatima Cardoso
Champalimaud Cancer Center

CONTENTS

PATHOPHYSIOLOGY OF HER2 IN BREAST CANCER

HER2 IN THE PATHOGENESIS OF BREAST CANCER

Human epidermal growth factor receptor 2 (HER2/neu) is a proto-oncogene that encodes the HER2 protein. HER2 is a type I transmembrane glycoprotein that contains an N-terminal extracellular domain (ECD), a single transmembrane helix, a TK domain, and an intracellular regulatory domain whose activation represents an initiating event in signal transduction that results in cell proliferation and inhibits apoptosis.

HER2 is a member of the epidermal growth factor receptor (EGFR) or HER family that contains three additional members that are HER1 (EGFR/ErbB1), HER3, and HER4. In order to become activated, the receptor must first interact with a ligand and then interact with another receptor in a process known as dimerization. Dimerization, which can happen with a like member (homodimerization) or a different member of the family (heterodimerization), will then trigger phosphorylation and activate downstream signaling cascades. HER2 is the preferred heterodimerization partner of each of the other HER receptors [1]. Heterodimers with HER2 are more stable [2,3], and their signaling is more potent [4] than combinations without HER2, the most potent of which is HER2–HER3.

HER2 gene amplification and/or protein overexpression has been identified in 10%–34% of invasive breast cancer (BC) [5] with a decreased of incidence in more recent series. In BC, activation of HER2 results primarily from the amplification of the HER2 gene; at a lesser degree, it can occur through transcriptional/translational mechanism without gene amplification that appears to account for less than 10% of HER2-overexpressing BC [6].

HER2 MEASUREMENT IN BREAST CANCER

HER2 testing should be routinely performed in patients with a new diagnosis of invasive BC. A joint consensus panel convened by the American Society of Clinical Oncology (ASCO) and the College of American Pathologists (CAP) developed testing algorithms for tumor HER2 status [7,8].

The benefit from trastuzumab treatment has been seen in patients with immunohistochemistry (IHC) 3+ staining and/or HER2 gene amplification by FISH [9], as opposed to patients with IHC 0/+1 and/or nonamplified HER2 status [10].

IHC remains the most frequent initial test for determination of HER2 status. The recommended algorithm defining positive, equivocal, and negative values for HER2 protein expression according to the ASCO/CAP guidelines is IHC 3+ (HER2 positive) when tumor exhibits uniform and intense membrane staining in more than 30% of the invasive tumor cells, IHC 2+ (HER2 equivocal) defined by weak or nonuniform but complete membrane staining in more than 10% of the tumor cells, and IHC 0/1+ (HER2 negative) defined by weak, incomplete membrane staining in any portion of the tumor cells (1+) or by the absence of any staining (0). Studies have shown that when a standardized IHC assay is performed on specimens that are carefully fixed, processed, and embedded, there is good to excellent correlation between gene copy status and protein expression levels [11–13].

The fluorescent in situ hybridization (FISH) technique identifies the number of copies of the HER2 gene, often in conjunction with the number of chromosome 17 centromere (CEP17) copies. The algorithm defining positive, equivocal, and negative values for gene amplification recommended is the following: positive, a FISH result of more than six *HER2* gene copies per nucleus or a FISH ratio (*HER2* gene signals to chromosome 17 signals) of more than 2.2, and negative, a FISH result of less than 4.0 *HER2* gene copies per nucleus or FISH ratio of less than 1.8.

Chromogenic in situ hybridization (CISH) technique is another technique approved by the FDA to define patient eligibility for trastuzumab therapy. There are two types of CISH assay: standard CISH, which uses an HER2 probe only, and dual-color CISH (dc-CISH), which uses an HER2 probe and a CEP17 probe. Inclusion of a CEP17 probe in dc-CISH allows the *HER2*/CEP17 ratio to be calculated, enabling exclusion of chromosome 17 polysomy.

The silver-enhanced in situ hybridization (SISH) method employs both HER2 and CEP17 probes hybridized on separate slides and is currently under review by the FDA.

MECHANISMS OF ACTION OF HER2-TARGETED AGENTS

Trastuzumab is a monoclonal antibody (mAb) directed against the ECD of HER2. It is still unclear how trastuzumab wields its effects [14,15]. However, several mechanisms of action have been proposed, including (1) cytostatic effect associated with G1 phase cell-cycle arrest due to trastuzumab-induced upregulation of the cyclin-dependent kinase (CDK) inhibitor p27kip1; (2) reduction of the phosphatidylinositol-3 kinase (PI3K)/Akt signaling pathway, by reducing PTEN phosphorylation via Src inhibition, which increases PTEN membrane localization and activity, ultimately leading to abrogation of cell proliferation and apoptosis [16]; (3) inhibition of proteolytic cleavage of the ECD of the HER2 protein, which results in a ~95 kDa truncated membrane-bound fragment (p95HER2) with ligand-independent kinase activity; (4) antiangiogenic effect, either indirectly through modulation of pro- and antiangiogenic factors or directly via inhibition of endothelial cell survival and capillary tube formation [17]; (5) cytotoxic effect via antibody-dependent cellular cytotoxicity (ADCC); and ultimately, (6) interference with DNA repair and synthesis after chemotherapy (CT) or radiotherapy, respectively, through HER2 translocation to the nucleus (Figure 3.1) [18].

Lapatinib is an oral small molecule that reversibly inhibits the intracellular tyrosine kinase activity of both HER2 and EGFR (also known as HER1), suppressing tyrosine autophosphorylation and thereby downstream pathways, such as the MAPK/Erk1/2 and PI3K/Akt pathways [19,20].

Neratinib is a small molecule, irreversible, pan-HER tyrosine kinase inhibitor (TKI).

Pertuzumab is a humanized mAb that binds to the ECD II of HER2 [21] that inhibits interactions of HER2 with other receptors (heterodimerization with EGFR and HER3).

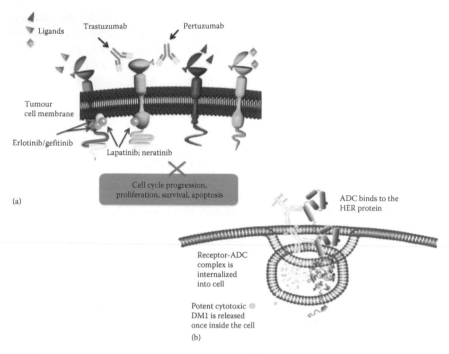

FIGURE 3.1 (a) Mechanism of action of anti-HER2 agents. (Adapted from Lang, I. (ed.), ErbB2-positive breast cancer medical education programme: 2011 update, Part of the Oncology Academy series. With permission. Copyright 2011 GlaxoSmithKline.) (b) Mechanism of action of T-DM1.

Trastuzumab emtansine (T-DM1) is an antibody drug conjugate of anti-HER2-targeted antitumor properties of trastuzumab with the potent cytotoxic agent DM1 (derivative of maytansine) [22]. Both drugs are conjugated with a stable linker and the particular features of this drug compared to trastuzumab are the following: (1) following internalization by HER2-overexpressing tumor cells, T-DM1 delivers the potent cytotoxic agent DM1 directly to the tumor cell cytoplasm, disrupting microtubule assembly/disassembly dynamics and inducing apoptosis after G2/M cell-cycle arrest [23–26]; (2) lower trastuzumab equivalent dose (3.6 mg/kg every 3 weeks for T-DM1 vs. 6 mg/kg every 3 weeks for trastuzumab) and lower half-life (4 days for conjugated T-DM1 vs. 3–4 weeks for trastuzumab) [27,28]; and (3) inhibition of PI3K signaling by the DM1 component in preclinical models potentially implicated in trastuzumab resistance [29].

Afatinib is a novel small molecule, TKI, irreversible, and targets EGFR/HER1 and HER2.

CLINICAL ACHIEVEMENTS OF HER2-TARGETED AGENTS IN BREAST CANCER

The introduction of trastuzumab, the first anti-HER2 mAb, has significantly changed the prognosis of this subset of patients in adjuvant and metastatic setting. In this section, available data on adjuvant, neoadjuvant, and metastatic therapy will be reviewed; ongoing trials and new therapeutic options will be discussed.

ANTI-HER2 TREATMENT IN THE ADJUVANT SETTING

Clinical and Pathological Criteria for Treatment

Newly diagnosed BC should all be tested for HER2 overexpression.

Based on the results of several adjuvant randomized trials, trastuzumab in combination with CT is the standard of care for patients with early HER2-positive cancer [30–35].

Patients eligible for these trials had node-positive disease or high-risk node-negative disease with usual tumor size cutoff of 1 cm. Although the benefit of trastuzumab in subcentimeter node-negative disease has not been directly addressed in clinical trials, we know today that (a) beyond HER2 status itself, there are no clinical or pathological factors that can identify which patients selectively benefit from adjuvant trastuzumab; (b) proportional risk reduction with trastuzumab is observed regardless of age, nodal status, tumor size, tumor grade, or tumor hormone receptor expression [33,36]; and (c) retrospective studies suggest a higher risk of recurrence for patients with HER2-positive node-negative tumors compared to those with HER2-negative tumors of the same size [37–39].

The National Comprehensive Cancer Network (NCCN) and the updated European Society for Medical Oncology (ESMO) guidelines recommend trastuzumab and CT for women with HER2-positive node-negative tumors measuring 0.6–1.0 cm (i.e., T1b) and for smaller tumors that have ≤2 mm axillary node metastases (pN1mi) [40,41].

Efficacy of Trastuzumab-Based Therapy

Results are now available from six adjuvant trastuzumab randomized clinical trials involving more than 13,000 women and in 2012 a meta-analysis has been published [42].

National Surgical Adjuvant Breast and Bowel Project B-31
and North Central Cancer Treatment Group N9831

The National Surgical Adjuvant Breast and Bowel Project (NSABP) B-31 and North Central Cancer Treatment Group (NCCTG) N9831 trials were jointly analyzed due to their similarities in design, combining data from the control arms of each study and data from the concurrent treatment arm. Both studies randomized 3351 women with early BC and HER2+ disease to four cycles of doxorubicin 60 mg/m^2 and cyclophosphamide 600 mg/m^2 (AC) 3 weekly (3wk) followed by paclitaxel (B-31, 175 mg/m^2 3wk for four cycles; N9831 and optional for B-31, 80 mg/m^2 weekly [wk] for 12 doses) with or without 1 year of concurrent trastuzumab given as a wk regimen (4 mg/m^2 followed by 2 mg/m^2 wk) [33,43].

Regarding patients and methods, we must emphasize that both trials were initially designed to recruit women with involved lymph nodes at the time of surgery. Near the completion of accrual, the N9831 trial was expanded to include women with high-risk node-negative disease (primary tumor size > 1 cm if estrogen receptor (ER)-negative or tumor size > 2 cm if ER-positive). Initially, both studies used local pathologic testing for

HER2 positivity to enroll patients. However, 18% of central testing results were discordant when the first 104 patients were reviewed in the B-31 trial [44]. The protocol was amended to require that HER2 determinations were made by NSABP-approved laboratories or by FISH. Similar discrepancies between local and central HER2 testing in the N9831 trial led to mandatory central HER2 testing before randomization [45].

Trastuzumab therapy was associated with significant increase in disease-free survival (DFS) and a 33% reduction in the risk of death ($p = 0.015$) [33]. After these findings, crossover from control group to trastuzumab therapy was allowed. The third interim analysis has shown a 48% reduction in the risk of relapse ($p < 0.001$) and a 39% reduction in the risk of death ($p = 0.001$), despite 21% of the patients in the control crossed to trastuzumab [46]. These results are confirmed in the recent updated final analysis (median follow-up of 8.4 years), where a 40% reduction in risk of relapse was seen [adjusted HR: 0.60 (95% CI: 0.53–0.68), $p < 0.0001$] together with substantial improvement in overall survival (OS) [adjusted HR: 0.63 (95% CI: 0.54–0.73), $p < 0.0001$] [47].

Herceptin Adjuvant Trial

The Herceptin adjuvant (HERA) trial randomized 5102 women with early HER2+ BC to 1 of 3 arms: ≥ 4 cycles of CT alone or CT followed by 1 year of adjuvant trastuzumab in a 3wk regimen (8 mg/m² loading dose followed by 6 mg/m²) or CT followed by 2 years of adjuvant trastuzumab [48]. Unlike B-31 and N9831, central pathologic assessment of HER2 status was mandatory at the start and a greater proportion of patients had high-risk node-negative disease (T > 1.0 cm, any ER status) (33% vs. 7%). The choice of CT was left to the discretion of investigators and only 26% patients received taxane therapy. It should also be noted that normal left ventricular ejection fraction (LVEF) (defined as $\geq 55\%$) after the completion of CT was mandatory, unlike for the B-31/N9831 trials where baseline cardiac assessment was done prior to initiate CT.

After a median follow-up of 12 months, the first interim analysis showed a significantly better DFS for 1-year trastuzumab compared to observation [HR 0.54 (95% CI: 0.43–0.67)]. At this time, patients in the observation group were allowed to cross over to trastuzumab arm and to choose between 1 and 2 years of treatment. The second analysis with 23.5 months of median follow-up and median time from crossover of 2.8 months has shown significant increase in OS for the trastuzumab arm [HR 0.66 (95% CI: 0.47–0.91), $p = 0.115$] [30]. The last analysis, after a median follow-up of 96 months, demonstrated a persistent significant improvement of DFS for 1 year of trastuzumab versus observation. Even with 52% of crossover rate, the HR was 0.76 for both DFS ($p < 0.0001$) and OS ($p = 0.0005$) [49].

BCIRG 006

The Breast Cancer International Research Group (BCIRG) 006 trial randomized 3222 women with HER2+ disease to (a) four cycles of AC followed by four cycles of 3wk docetaxel 100 mg/m² (AC → T), (b) AC → T concurrently with trastuzumab wk regimen followed by trastuzumab 3wk till complete 1 year of treatment, and (c) six cycles of the docetaxel 75 mg/m² and carboplatin (AUC6) 3wk and trastuzumab wk regimen (TCH) followed by trastuzumab 3wk till 1 year (34). Regarding patients and methods, we must emphasize that in comparison with B-31/N9831 and HERA, patients were eligible for the BCIRG 006 only if HER2+ disease was demonstrated centrally by HER2 gene amplification on FISH. Additionally, 29% of patients in BCIRG 006 had high-risk node-negative disease at diagnosis compared to 7% and 33% in the previous studies, respectively.

At a median follow-up of 65 months, 656 events triggered this protocol-specified analysis. Both trastuzumab arms demonstrated statistically significant advantages in either DFS or OS versus the control group; no statistically significant difference between the two trastuzumab arms was observed but there was a numerical advantage for the anthracycline-based group albeit with more cardiac events [34]. It is important to consider that the trial hypothesis was that the non-anthracycline-containing arm was superior to the anthracycline arm, which was not demonstrated, and therefore, the study was negative for this secondary question. The study was not powered to test the equivalence between these two types of CT and therefore cannot be used to consider non-anthracycline-based CT for HER2-positive early BC as efficacious as anthracycline-based CT. Among the four major trials, BCIRG 006 registered the lowest rate of crossover (2.1%).

FinHER

In the Finland Herceptin (FinHER) study, 1040 women with node-positive or high-risk node-negative (defined as tumor size > 2 cm and progesterone receptor [PgR] expression absent) early-stage BC were randomized to receive three cycles of 3wk docetaxel (T) 100 mg/m^2 followed by three cycles of 3wk 5-fluorouracil (5-FU) 600 mg/m^2, epirubicin 60 mg/m^2, and cyclophosphamide 600 mg/m^2 (FEC) or 9 wk injection of vinorelbine (V) 25 mg/m^2 followed by three cycles of FEC [31]. The planned dose of docetaxel was reduced to 80 mg/m^2 during the course of the study due to an unexpectedly high observed rate of febrile neutropenia. All women randomized to T $\rightarrow$ FEC versus V $\rightarrow$ FEC underwent local IHC assessment for HER2 status. Patients with 2+ or 3+ HER2 IHC staining were centrally assessed for HER2 gene amplification using CISH. CISH-positive patients ($n = 232$) underwent a second randomization to nine injections of wk trastuzumab coadministered with docetaxel or vinorelbine before FEC therapy or no trastuzumab therapy.

At a median follow-up of 36 months, the inclusion of trastuzumab in the adjuvant CT regimen resulted in a significantly better DFS [HR 0.42 (95% CI: 0.21–0.83), $p = 0.01$]; also, OS tended to be better, although not significant ($p = 0.07$) [31]. The last update of the study, at a median follow-up of 5 years, confirmed the benefits of adding a short course of concurrent trastuzumab to docetaxel followed by FEC versus CT alone in the subgroup of HER2-positive disease [HR for DDFS = 0.65 (95% CI: 0.38–1.12), $P = .12$] [50]. However, these results need to be confirmed in a larger series because of the limited sample size and low number of events.

PACS-04

In the PACS-04 study, 3050 women with node-positive early BC were first randomized between epirubicin–docetaxel and FEC, and then HER2-positive patients ($n = 528$) were randomly assigned to receive sequential trastuzumab (1 year, 3wk) or to observation [32]. Like in the HERA trial, HER2 status was centrally assessed (IHC 3+ or IHC 2+ and FISH positive).

At a median follow-up of 4 years, the addition of sequential trastuzumab was not associated with a significant difference in the risk of recurrence or death [32]. In the intent-to-treat (ITT) analysis, the rate of HER2+ untreated patients with trastuzumab was 10%. Many attempts have been made to understand why PACS-04 is the only negative trastuzumab adjuvant trial but no definite explanation can be given: A sequential instead of concomitant use of trastuzumab with CT was used but that was also the case in HERA trial; it could be an underpowered study but it is still larger than the FinHER trial; it was the trial with the longest follow-up at first presentation but benefits have been maintained in other trials with longer follow-up.

Meta-Analysis

A 2012 meta-analysis of eight studies involving 11,991 patients assessed the benefits of adding trastuzumab to adjuvant CT in patients with HER2+ BC(42). The inclusion of trastuzumab resulted in an improvement in DFS with an HR = 0.60 (95% CI: 0.50–0.71), regardless of trastuzumab treatment duration or administration schedule (i.e., concurrent with CT or sequentially following CT) and an improvement in OS [HR 0.66 (95% CI: 0.57–0.77)].

Several CT regimens used with trastuzumab have been evaluated in large prospective studies. Historically, anthracyclines have been considered critical for the management of HER2+ BC. A number of studies from the pre-trastuzumab era support this concept. Retrospective subset analyses of anthracycline-based adjuvant CT studies have suggested that the major benefit for these regimens is seen in HER2-overexpressing tumors [51]. The value of HER2 and TOP2A as predictive markers of response to anthracycline-based therapy has been extensively studied. In the meta-analysis by Di Leo et al. [52] although HER2 amplification and combined TOP2A amplification and deletion had some value in prediction of responsiveness to anthracycline-based therapy, the overall findings did not support the use of TOP2A to select the adjuvant CT regimen in this patient population.

With the advent of trastuzumab, concerns have been raised regarding the use of anthracycline-based regimens in HER2-positive early BC due to potential cardiotoxicity. Previous or concurrent anthracyclines are a risk factor for trastuzumab-related cardiotoxicity. Notwithstanding the increased incidence of cardiac events, these still remain in very acceptable ranges for all types of CT regimens used in the adjuvant setting. Rate of severe congestive heart failure in adjuvant trials ranged between 0.4% and 3.5%, depending on the regimen and schedule used.

Combining trastuzumab with a non-anthracycline-containing CT regimen was evaluated in the BCIRG 006 trial with the aim to investigate whether the association of trastuzumab, carboplatin, and docetaxel could be better tolerated without any loss in terms of efficacy versus the anthracycline-based schedule. At a median follow-up of 65 months, the difference in DFS and OS between ACTH and TCH although not statically significant was numerically different, with a trend favoring the anthracycline-containing regimen. The trial hypothesis that TCH was superior to ACTH was not proven and, since the study was not powered to detect equivalence between ACTH and TCH, this conclusion cannot be taken. With respect to adverse events, the differences were significantly lower rates of severe (grade ¾) neutropenia (66% vs. 63%) and leukopenia (48% vs. 60%) but significantly higher rates of anemia (6% vs. 3%) and thrombocytopenia (6% vs. 2%) for TCH and a higher incidence of congestive heart failure (2% vs. 0.4%) and subclinical and sustained loss of mean LVEF (18.6% vs. 9.4%) for ACTH. Based on this trial alone, TCH can only be considered an alternative treatment for patients with contraindications to anthracyclines (preexisting cardiac conditions, borderline ejection fraction at baseline, or prior anthracycline exposure), while anthracycline-based regimens remain the standard of care.

Findings suggest that the more dramatic risk reduction when adding trastuzumab to CT is observed when using some concurrent CT and trastuzumab and employing both anthracycline and a taxane. Whether in some patients anthracyclines can be safely avoided is a matter of intense research and validated predictive biomarkers are eagerly awaited.

Timing of Trastuzumab Initiation

An important decision for clinicians is whether trastuzumab should be administered concurrently or sequentially after the completion of adjuvant CT. In early disease setting, the NSABP B-31, BCIRG 006, and FinHER trials used combination designs, whereas the HERA and PACS-04 trials used a sequential approach.

The only trial to address this question directly was the N9831. The second planned interim analysis, with a median follow-up of 6 years, indicates that although trastuzumab added sequentially to CT improves DFS, there is a strong trend toward a better outcome with concurrent trastuzumab relative to sequential administration [53].

In the 2012 meta-analysis [42] that confirmed the benefits of adding trastuzumab to adjuvant CT in patients with HER2-positive BC, the benefit in OS was associated with concurrent administration [HR 0.64 (95% CI: 0.53–0.76)] but not with sequential treatment of CT followed by single-agent trastuzumab [HR 0.85 (95% CI: 0.43–1.67)]. BCIRG 006 also supports the use of trastuzumab administered concurrently with CT in the adjuvant setting [34].

Duration of Trastuzumab Treatment

Results from two studies presented at the 2012 ESMO and a 2012 meta-analysis support one year of trastuzumab as the standard of care in the adjuvant therapy for patients with HER2-positive early BC.

In the *HERA trial*, a comparison between 1 and 2 years of adjuvant trastuzumab after CT concluded that 2 years of treatment was not better than 1 year [49]. DFS at 8 years was 75.8% with 2 years of trastuzumab and 76.0% with 1 year (HR = 0.99, P = .86). OS was 86.4% and 87.6%, respectively (P = .63). The same pattern held true for both hormone receptor–positive and hormone receptor–negative subgroups.

The *PHARE trial* recruited over 3380 HER2-positive patients and randomly assigned them to receive either 6 months or 1 year of adjuvant trastuzumab. The trial results were reported as unable to prove the non-inferiority hypothesis of 6 months versus 1 year of adjuvant trastuzumab. Nevertheless, there is a trend in favor of 12-month treatment for the overall population albeit with higher incidence of cardiotoxicity [54]. The median follow-up in the trial was 42.5 months and at the time of the analysis, 395 DFS events were reported. According to the design of this trial, which allowed for a non-inferiority hazard ratio margin of 1.15, the 6-month trastuzumab arm (arm B) was not demonstrated to be significantly inferior to 12-month trastuzumab (arm A), since the confidence interval contains the 1.15 non-inferiority margin [HR = 1.28 (95% CI: 1.04–1.56), $p = 0.29$].

In the *2012 meta-analysis*, trastuzumab administered for 12 months was associated with an improvement in OS [HR 0.67 (95% CI: 0.57–0.80)]; while trastuzumab treatment for ≤6 months also showed a trend toward an improvement in OS, it did not reach statistical significance [HR 0.55 (95% CI: 0.27–1.11)] [42].

Based on these results, the standard duration of treatment in this setting remains, for the moment, 1 year. However, several trials are still ongoing evaluating the optimal duration and regimen of adjuvant trastuzumab and might lead to a different conclusion in the future. Additionally, at this time, there are no predictive markers allowing us to determine which patients could derive the same benefit from a shorter duration of adjuvant trastuzumab and further research is needed.

The relative benefit of 6 months versus 1 year of trastuzumab is being evaluated in the PERSEPHONE trial (which also evaluates sequential vs. concurrent trastuzumab) and the HELLENIC trial (using only concurrent therapy). The SHORT-HER and SOLD trials are evaluating 9 weeks versus 12 months of trastuzumab given concomitantly with a taxane, similar to the FinHER trial.

Other Anti-HER2 Agents

Lapatinib: The two major adjuvant trials of lapatinib are ALLTO and TEACH. The ALLTO trial is a large phase III randomized adjuvant study comparing the activity trastuzumab alone versus trastuzumab followed by lapatinib versus the combination of lapatinib administered concomitantly with trastuzumab, which included around 8400 patients.

In the TEACH trial, patients are eligible if (a) recent diagnosis of early-stage HER2+ BC and unable or unwilling to receive trastuzumab or (b) remote diagnosis HER2+ BC with no evidence of disease relapse and no prior trastuzumab treatment. The study will be a phase III randomized, double-blind, multicenter, placebo-controlled trial that will evaluate the efficacy of lapatinib monotherapy in the adjuvant setting (Table 3.1).

Neratinib: A large randomized, double-blind, placebo-controlled adjuvant study—ExteNET enrolled 2842 patients who have completed adjuvant trastuzumab for no longer than 2 years and free of recurrence, randomly assigned to neratinib versus placebo for one year; results are expected in 2013.

Pertuzumab: Ongoing studies are investigating pertuzumab plus trastuzumab in the adjuvant setting for HER2+ BC. The APHINITY trial (NCT01358877) is a randomized multicenter, double-blind, placebo-controlled study comparing CT plus trastuzumab plus placebo versus CT plus trastuzumab plus pertuzumab.

Trastuzumab emtansine: T-DM1 is being investigated in a multicenter, international phase II, single-arm study of patients with early-stage HER2+ BC, following anthracycline-based adjuvant or neoadjuvant CT (TDM4874g, NCT01196052) with cardiotoxicity as primary end point.

TABLE 3.1

Phase III Randomized Trials of Adjuvant Trastuzumab in Patients with HER2+ BC

Study	Population	Median Follow-up (Months)	Treatment	DFS (P value)	OS (P value)
HERA [41]	Node-positive or node-negative high-risk EBC after completion of standard CT (n=5.090)	96	No additional therapy H 1 year H 2 year	HR=0.76, p<0.0001	HR=0.76, p=0.0005
NSABP B-31/ NCCTG N9831 [39]	Node-positive node-negative high-risk EBC (n=4046)	100.8	AC→Pac AC→Pac→H	62.2% 73.7% (p<0.001)	75.2% 84.0% (p<0.0001)
NCCTG N9831 [61]	Node-positive node-negative high-risk EBC (n=1.944)	63.6	AC→PacH AC→Pac→H	84% (5 years) 80% (p=0.0216)	NR NR
BCIRG 006 [28]	Node-positive node-negative high-risk EBC (n=3222)	65	AC→Doc AC→Doc–H Doc–Carb–H	75% 84% (p<0.001 vs. chemotherapy) 81% (p<0.04 vs. CT)	87% 92% (p<0.001 vs. chemotherapy) 87% (p<0.038 vs. CT)
PACS-04 [26]	Node-positive EBC	47	FEC or Epi–Doc FEC or Epi–Doc→H 1 year	78% (3 years) 81% (p=0.41)	96% (3 years) 95% (p=2.38)
FinHER [43]	Node-positive node-negative high-risk EBC (n=232)	62	Doc or Vin →FEC Doc or Vin →FEC–H	73.3% 83% (p=0.12)	82.3% 91.3% (5 years) (p=0.094)
Meta-analysis 2012 [51]	All trials included			HR: 0.60, 95% p<0.00001	HR: 0.66, 95% p<0.00001

AC, doxorubicin and cyclophosphamide; Carb, carboplatin; Doc, docetaxel; Epi, epirubicin; FEC, 5-fluorouracil, epirubicin, and cyclophosphamide; H, trastuzumab; Pac, paclitaxel; Vin, vinorelbine.

Neoadjuvant Anti-HER2 Treatment

Neoadjuvant therapy (NT) also called primary systemic treatment (PST) is the standard of care for women with locally advanced, inflammatory, or inoperable primary BC [55–58]. The demonstration by the landmark NSABP B-18 trial [59,60] that NT offered the same survival benefits as postoperative treatment has moved NT to the context of operable disease, looking for the surgical advantages of tumor downstaging. Subsequently, the NSABP B-27 [61] trial and other studies [62–64] have shown that patients with pathologic complete response (pCR) to NT have improved DFS and OS, suggesting its use as a surrogate marker for trials comparing different schedules of primary systemic therapy. Currently, NT is generally used to improve the surgical options, to determine the response to systemic therapy, and to obtain long-term DFS.

An integrated meta-analysis [65] on individual data from the German Breast Group (GBG) and the AGO Breast Group, including 6402 patients enrolled in neoadjuvant trials containing doxorubicin or epirubicin and docetaxel or paclitaxel, with or without trastuzumab, has identified predictive markers of pCR: ER-negative status compared to ER+ [OR 3.2 (95% CI: 2.7–3.8), $p < 0.0001$], HER2+ disease [OR 2.2 (95% CI: 1.8–2.5), $p < 0.0001$], higher grade [OR 1.8 (95% CI: 1.5–2.2), $p < 0.0001$], younger age [OR 1.3 (95% CI: 1.2–1.6), $p = 0.0001$], non-lobular-type tumors [OR 1.7 (95% CI: 1.2–2.3), $p = 0.001$], and smaller tumor size [OR 1.5 (95% CI: 1.2–1.9), $p = 0.0006$].

The recent international panel on NT recommended that trastuzumab should be incorporated into the NT CT regimen in patients with HER2+ disease [66].

Trastuzumab

The first reported randomized trial from the MDACC showed a very high pCR rate of 65.2% in patients treated with trastuzumab (vs. 26%) [67,68] and these results led to a premature closure of the study. However, such high pCR rates have not been reproduced in other studies. In this study, no safety concerns were raised related to concurrent treatment with anthracycline, with no cases of cardiac clinical dysfunction or cardiac deaths.

Additional data on neoadjuvant trastuzumab come from the NOAH trial [69] where 228 HER2+ BC patients were randomized to a neoadjuvant CT regimen consisting of doxorubicin, paclitaxel, cyclophosphamide, methotrexate, and fluorouracil with or without H given concurrently. Patients further received adjuvant trastuzumab for a total of 1 year. A parallel cohort of 99 patients with HER2-negative disease was included and treated with the same CT regimen. Trastuzumab-treated patients had a significant improvement of event-free survival at 3 years, with a hazard ratio (HR) of 0.59 (95% CI: 0.38–0.90). Only two patients (2%) developed symptomatic cardiac failure that responded to treatment and no cardiac deaths were reported. The German GeparQuattro study [70,71] also evaluated neoadjuvant trastuzumab. This randomized phase III trial assessed the incorporation of capecitabine in an anthracycline/taxane–based regimen and the concurrent use of trastuzumab with these CT regimens in HER2 overexpressing patients. Of 1509 patients included, 445 patients had HER2+ BC and received trastuzumab (6 mg/kg) every 3 weeks concomitant with all CT cycles. pCR rate was higher in HER2-positive disease compared to HER2-negative group (31.7% vs. 15.7%). In the subgroup of patients that did not responded to epirubicin/cyclophosphamide, pCR rate was also higher in HER2+ versus HER2-negative tumors (16.7% vs. 3.3%). Higher grade 3 and 4 neutropenia as well as conjunctivitis were seen in trastuzumab-treated group, but there were no cardiac safety concerns. There are no trials comparing the trastuzumab given as neoadjuvant to trastuzumab given as adjuvant therapy. However, since the magnitude of benefit seems to be the same and since response rates are clearly increased with the use of neoadjuvant trastuzumab, one might infer that for patients with HER2-positive BC and an indication for neoadjuvant systemic therapy, trastuzumab should be offered as early as possible and hence in the neoadjuvant setting.

Lapatinib

Lapatinib is an oral dual TKI that targets EGFR and HER2 and has been tested in the NT setting, both as single agent and in combination with trastuzumab. In the Neoadjuvant Lapatinib and/or Trastuzumab Treatment Optimisation (NeoALTTO) study [72], 455 patients were randomly assigned to oral lapatinib (1500 mg), intravenous trastuzumab (loading dose 4 mg/kg, subsequent doses 2 mg/kg), or lapatinib (1000 mg) plus trastuzumab. Patients received anti-HER2 therapy alone for 6 weeks initially and then combined to wk paclitaxel (80 mg/m^2) for 12 weeks before surgery. After surgery, patients received adjuvant CT followed by the same targeted therapy as in the neoadjuvant phase for 52 weeks. Combination of lapatinib and trastuzumab yielded a significantly higher pCR rate than the monotherapy arms. The response to lapatinib was numerically lower than to trastuzumab, although the difference did not reach statistical significance. The dual combination was associated with higher toxicity, mainly diarrhea (grade 3 in 23.4% patients) and liver-enzyme alterations consisting mainly of transient and reversible rise in transaminases (grade 3 in 17.5% patients and treatment discontinuation in 30 patients). This trial also confirmed the finding from previous studies of higher pCR rate in ER-negative tumors compared with ER-positive ones.

Lapatinib has also been compared to trastuzumab as neoadjuvant treatment in the GeparQuinto trial [73], a phase III randomized trial that enrolled 620 untreated HER2+ patients with operable or locally advanced BC. Patients were randomized to four cycles of epirubicin (90 mg/m^2) plus cyclophosphamide (600 mg/m^2) and four cycles of docetaxel (100 mg/m^2), every 3 weeks, with either trastuzumab 3wk (6 mg/kg/loading dose of 8 mg/kg) or lapatinib (1000–1250 mg) throughout all cycles before surgery. Main results have shown a significantly higher pCR rate for trastuzumab treatment arm (30.3%) compared to lapatinib (22.7%). Trastuzumab treatment was more associated to edema (39.1% vs. 28.7%) and dyspnea (29.6% vs. 21.4%), and lapatinib with more diarrhea (75.0% vs. 47.4%) and skin rash (54.9% vs. 31.9%).

Taken together, the results of these two studies have led to the recommendation that lapatinib should not be used as single (neo)adjuvant anti-HER2 target outside clinical trials. Additionally, based on these results and on a preplanned interim analysis of the large adjuvant ALTTO trial, patients treated with lapatinib monotherapy in this study were informed and proposed to receive adjuvant trastu-zumab, which, although necessary, will impact in the long-term results of this study. The reasons for these disappointing results of lapatinib monotherapy in early BC are not yet fully understood. Several hypotheses have been speculated such as lower capacity to block the HER2 pathway compared to trastuzumab, a higher efficacy of trastuzumab due to the additional tumor effect by the antitumor anti-body–derived cellular cytotoxicity process, or a lower drug exposure of lapatinib related to dose reductions and low adherence linked to its higher toxicity. Finally an important finding of this study is related to the cardiac safety of the concurrent administration of trastuzumab and anthracyclines, with only one patient experienc-ing congestive heart failure.

In the similarly designed phase II randomized CHER-LOB study, patients were randomized between wk trastuzumab, lapatinib (1500 mg orally daily), or trastu-zumab plus lapatinib (1000 mg PO), concurrently with CT. The CT regimen used was wk paclitaxel (80 mg/m^2) for 12 weeks followed by FEC for four courses. Results were recently published [74] showing higher pCR for the combination of trastuzumab and lapatinib (46.7%). Diarrhea, dermatologic toxicities, and hepatic toxicities were observed more frequently in patients receiving lapatinib. No cases of congestive heart failure were noticed.

Pertuzumab

The new anti-HER2 humanized mAb pertuzumab acts through inhibition of recep-tor dimerization and was tested in the NT setting through the NeoSphere trial [75]. This was a phase II randomized trial designed to test the antitumor activity and toler-ability of the combination of docetaxel, trastuzumab, and pertuzumab (THP), com-pared to trastuzumab plus pertuzumab (HP), docetaxel and pertuzumab (TP), and docetaxel and trastuzumab (TH). Cycles were given intravenously q3w: pertuzumab, 840 mg loading dose and 420 mg maintenance; trastuzumab, 8 mg/kg loading dose and 6 mg/kg maintenance; and docetaxel, 75 mg/m^2 with escalation to 100 mg/m^2 if the starting dose was well tolerated. After surgery, all patients received trastuzumab to complete 1 year and three cycles of FEC; in case of neoadjuvant HP, they also received trastuzumab before FEC. The pCR was significantly higher ($p = 0.014$) for the combination of docetaxel with both anti-HER2 target agents (THP), with good tolerability, namely, cardiac safety.

These studies, together with important evidence from two trials in the metastatic setting [76,77], provide evidence that the dual blockage of the HER2 receptor has superior efficacy and this strategy is currently being evaluated in the large adjuvant phase III trial APHINITY, as well as in the ALTTO trial. The results of these two important adjuvant trials may lead to a change in clinical practice. Nevertheless, many questions remain unanswered such as (1) Which is the optimal combination of anti-HER2 agents? (2) Which is the best CT regimen to use with these agents? (3) Can CT be avoided in some patients when a dual blockade strategy is used? (4) What is the role of dual HER2 blockade in combination with endocrine therapy for HER2+ and ER+ BC? (5) Can we identify reliable biomarkers predictive of response to each specific anti-HER2 agent or combination?

Anti-HER2 Treatment in Metastatic Breast Cancer

Trastuzumab-Based Therapy

Trastuzumab was first approved by the FDA in 1998 for first-line treatment of metastatic breast cancer (MBC). In the randomized phase III study conducted by Slamon et al. [9], 469 patients received first-line treatment for MBC with CT (anthracyclines or taxanes) plus or minus trastuzumab. The addition of trastuzumab to CT was associated with longer survival, with a 5 month increase of median survival time (25.1 vs. 20.3 months, $p=0.046$) and a 20% reduction in the risk of death. Longer time to disease progression (7.4 vs. 4.6 months, $p<0.001$), higher response rate (50% vs. 32%, $p<0.001$), and longer duration of response (9.1 vs. 6.1 months, $p<0.001$) were also observed. This trial raised the concern of combination of anthracyclines and trastuzumab, as cardiac dysfunction was the main adverse effect of the combination: 27% in anthracycline (epirubicin and cyclophosphamide) and trastuzumab arm, 13% in taxane (paclitaxel) and trastuzumab, 8% anthracycline alone arm, and 1% for the taxane alone arm (Table 3.2).

As monotherapy, trastuzumab has shown response rates of 19%–26% in first-line treatment and 15% beyond first-line [78–80].

Several combinations of CT and trastuzumab have been tested in phase III and phase II trials, mainly as first-line treatment, with response rates ranging from 30% to 70% [81–91]. Single agents have included taxanes (docetaxel or paclitaxel), capecitabine, and vinorelbine, mainly associated with a wk schedule of trastuzumab but a 3wk one was also showed to be effective [79,92]. CT duplets have also been tested as taxanes (paclitaxel or docetaxel) plus carboplatin, capecitabine and docetaxel, ixabepilone plus carboplatin, and gemcitabine plus carboplatin. Regarding these studies, the only phase III data are provided from the BCIRG007 trial comparing the combination of docetaxel, carboplatin, and trastuzumab to docetaxel alone plus trastuzumab [89] and the Robert et al. study [86] comparing paclitaxel and carboplatin with paclitaxel alone plus trastuzumab. Incorporation of carboplatin in the taxane–trastuzumab therapy yield no increase in response rate, time to progression (TTP), and OS in the BCIRG007 study, and in the Robert et al. study, it was associated with increased response rate and TTP, but no improvement of OS. Furthermore, the population of this study was heterogeneous regarding HER2 status, as it included both HER2 IHC 3+ and 2+.

Head-to-head comparisons have been tested between combination of docetaxel and trastuzumab versus vinorelbine and trastuzumab in the HERNATA and TRAVIOTA study [81,82]. These trials showed no difference of efficacy between the two regimens with a more favorable toxicity profile for the vinorelbine arm. The full published report [81] describes higher rates of grade 3 and grade 4 febrile neutropenia (36.0% vs. 10.1%), leukopenia (40.3% vs. 21.0%), infection (25.1% vs. 13.0%), fever (4.3% vs. 0%), neuropathy (30.9% vs. 3.6%), nail changes (7.9% vs. 0.7%), and edema (6.5% vs. 0%) for the combination of docetaxel with trastuzumab. These data, together with the meta-analysis of Piccart et al. [93], show that there is no reason to consider a taxane as the preferred first-line cytotoxic agent for MBC and that drugs with a better toxicity profile, namely, much less alopecia, such as vinorelbine and capecitabine should be considered.

TABLE 3.2
Overview of Main Anti-HER2 Trials in MBC

Study	Population	Treatment	Primary End point	Time to Progression/ Progression-Free Survival	Overall Survival
Slamon et al. [51]	469 pts 1st-line treatment	CT+H CT	TTP	7.4 v 4.6 m RR=0.51 (95% CI, 0.47–0.70)	25.1 v 20.3 m RR=0.80 (95% CI, 0.64–1.00)
Kaufman et al. [66]	207 pts 1st-line treatment	Ana+H Ana	PFS	4.8 v 2.4 m HR=0.63 (95% CI, 0.47–0.84)	28.5 v 23.9 m ns
Von Minckwitz et al. [68]	156 pts Progression on H (2nd-line CT)	Cap+H Cap	TTP	8.2 v 5.6 m HR=0.69 (95% CI, 0.48–0.97)	25.5 v 20 m ns
Valero et al. [63]	263 pts 1st-line treatment	Doc+H Doc+Carbo+H	TTP	11.1 v 10.4 m HR=0.9 (95% CI, 0.69–1.2)	37.1 v 37.4 m HR=0.9 (95% CI, 0.88–0.92)
Robert et al. [60]	196 pts 1st-line treatment	Pac+Carbo+H Pac+H	RR	10.7 v 7.1 m HR=0.66 (95% CI, 0.59–0.73)	35.7 v 32.2 m HR=1.01 (95% CI, 0.76–1.36)
Andersson et al. [55]	284 pts 1st-line treatment	Doc+H Vin+H	TTP	12.4 v 15.3 m HR=0.94 (95% CI, 0.71–1.25)	35.7 v 38.8 m HR=1.01 (95% CI, 0.71–1.42)
Burstein et al. [56]	41 pts 1st-line treatment	Vin+H Tax+H	RR	8.5 v 6 m $p=0.09$	—

Study	Patients	Details	Treatment	Endpoint	Result	Second result
Geyer et al. [75]	324pts	Progression on H (≥2nd-line CT)	Cap+L / Cap	PFS	8.4 v 4.4m HR=0.49 (95% CI, 0.34–0.71)	N36/35 HR=0.92 (95% CI, 0.58–1.46)
Johnston et al. [76]	219 pts	1st-line treatment	Let+L / L	PFS inv	8.2 v 3M HR=0.71 (95% CI, 0.53–0.96)	33.3 v 32.3 m HR=0.74 (95% C, 0.5–1.1)
Gelmon et al. [78]	600 pts	1st-line treatment	Tax+H / Tax+L	PFS	13.7 v 9m HR=1.48 (95% CI, 1.15–1.92)	HR=1.25 (95% CI, 0.85–1.93) —
Blackwell et al. [50]	296 pts	(≥2nd-line CT)	L / L+H	PFS inv	8.1 v 12 wks HR=0.73 (95% CI, 0.57–0.93)	9.5 vs 14 m HR=0.75 (95% CI, 0.53–1.07)
Verma et al. [79]	991 pts	(≥2nd-line CT)	TDM-1 / Cap+L	PFS OS Toxicity	9.6 v 6.4 m HR=0.65 (95% CI, 0.55–0.77)	30.9 v 25.1m HR=0.68 (95% CI, 0.55–0.85)
Baselga et al. [49]	808 pts	1st-line treatment	Doc+H+P / Doc+P	PFS ind	18.5 v 12.4 m HR=0.62 (95% CI, 0.51–0.75)	— HR=0.64 (95% CI, 0.47–0.88)

Ana, anastrozole; CT, chemotherapy; Carbo, carboplatin; Cap, capecitabine; Doc, docetaxel; H, trastuzumab; HR, hazard ratio; L, lapatinib; Let, letrozole; ns, nonsignificant; OS, overall survival; P, pertuzumab; Pac, paclitaxel; pts, patients; PFS, progression-free survival; PFS inv, progression-free survival by investigator review; PFS ind, progression-free survival independently assessed; Tax, taxane-based therapy (docetaxel or paclitaxel); RR, relative risk; m, months; TTP, time to progression; Vin, vinorelbine; wks, weeks.

Trastuzumab has also been studied in combination with endocrine therapy for first-line treatment of HER2+ and ER-positive MBC. The randomized phase III TAnDEM study [94] enrolled 207 patients to anastrozole plus or minus trastuzumab, with patients in the anastrozole arm alone allowed to cross over to the combination at the time of progression. The combination was associated to prolonged PFS of 4.8 versus 2.4 months (HR = 0.63, CI 95% 0.47–8.84, log-rank $p = 0.006$) and increased TTP, CBR, and ORR. No difference was seen in OS, but it is important to highlight that there was a 70% of crossover rate to the combination arm. Toxicity was also higher for the combination with grade 3 and grade 4 events in 23% versus 5% and 15 versus 1%, respectively. The PFS of this trial was shorter than expected, emphasizing the more aggressive nature of HER2+/hormonal receptor–positive disease compared to HER2-negative/hormonal receptor–positive disease. The main message from this study is that in patients adequately selected, such as more indolent disease and non-extensive metastatic disease, hormonal therapy plus trastuzumab can postpone the initiation of CT in this setting.

Lapatinib

Lapatinib was developed after trastuzumab, presenting a complementary mechanism of action. It is an oral agent that inhibits the tyrosine kinases of HER2 and EGFR, showing preclinically non-cross-resistance with trastuzumab [19]. Phase II studies have tested lapatinib in monotherapy [95–98], both in trastuzumab-treated and naive patients with non-enthusiastic ORR ranging from 1.4% to 24%. Combination of lapatinib with both CT and endocrine therapy has been studied in randomized phase III trials [99–102]. The combination of capecitabine and lapatinib compared to capecitabine alone [100] in patients progressing on previous treatment with anthracycline, taxane, and trastuzumab yielded increased TTP (6.2 vs. 4.3 months, HR = 0.57, CI 95%: 0.43–0.77, $p < 0.001$) as well as increased ORR (23.7% vs. 13.9%, OR: 1.9, CI 95% 1.1–1.4, $p = 0.017$) and CBR (29.3% vs. 17.4%, OR: 2.0, 95% CI: 1.2–3.3, $p = 0.008$). These results led to FDA approval of lapatinib in MBC setting as a second-line treatment. The final OS analysis [99] did not show a statistically significant increase of OS although a trend was seen; this is most probably related to the lack of power of the study due to its early termination as well as to the impact of crossover.

Data on lapatinib use in the first-line setting come from a trial evaluating lapatinib plus paclitaxel versus paclitaxel plus placebo in patients with MBC negative or untested for HER2 overexpression [102]. In this trial, 580 patients were enrolled and no difference for the primary end point TTP was seen between the two treatment arms in the overall population. However, for the 15% of patients ($n = 86$) defined as HER2-positive (49 in paclitaxel–lapatinib arm and 37 in paclitaxel–placebo arm), the TTP was significantly longer in lapatinib-treated patients versus patients receiving placebo (36.4 vs. 25.1 weeks, HR = 0.53, 95% CI:0.31–0.89, $p = 0.005$).

Lapatinib was also combined with letrozole and compared to letrozole and placebo in a phase III randomized trial in HER2+ and HER2-negative disease [101]. While in the HER2-negative patients there was no benefit from the addition of lapatinib, the HER2+ population ($n = 219$) had significantly improved

PFS (3.0–8.2 months, HR=0.71, CI 95%: 0.53–0.96, p=0.019), ORR (15%–28%, OR=0.4, CI 95%: 0.2–0.9, p=0.021), and CBR (29%–48%, OR=0.4, CI 95%: 0.2–0.8, p=0.003), but no significant improvement of OS. Interestingly, a subgroup analysis of the HER2-negative patients revealed that in the subgroup with resistance to tamoxifen, the addition of lapatinib led to a similar 5-month improvement in PFS; although coming from an unplanned subgroup analysis and hence needing confirmation, these are the first clinical data supporting the hypothesis that an important mechanism of resistance to endocrine therapy is the activation of the HER pathway.

As is the case for trastuzumab, also for lapatinib, there are no trials comparing the endocrine therapy plus lapatinib approach to CT–lapatinib combinations nor there are biomarkers to best select the candidates to one of the two approaches.

The combination of lapatinib and trastuzumab was tested in heavily pretreated MBC patients in the study EGF104900 [77]. The trial enrolled 296 patients progressing on trastuzumab-containing regimens and randomized to receive lapatinib alone or in combination with trastuzumab. In the ITT population, 31% patients had ≥6 lines of CT and received a median of three prior trastuzumab-containing regimens. The update analysis revealed a significant benefit in terms of PFS (HR 0.74 [CI 95%: 0.58–0.94]) and OS (HR=0.74 [95% CI: 0.57–0.97]), with improvements of OS rates of 10% at 6 months and 15% at 12 months. Adverse events were similar in both treatment groups, and only diarrhea was more common in the combination arm.

Trastuzumab versus Lapatinib

Some recent data were present from the phase III randomized MA.31 trial [103] designed to compare first-line treatment with taxane plus trastuzumab (wk paclitaxel or 3wk docetaxel) or the same combination of taxane plus lapatinib, in 636 HER2-positive MBC patients, with the primary end point being PFS. With a median follow-up of 13.6 months, the taxane–lapatinib arm had inferior PFS compared to the taxane–trastuzumab: 8.8 versus 11.4 months, HR=1.33 (CI 95%: 1.06–1.67). There was no difference in OS. In terms of toxicity, there were more grade 3–4 diarrhea and rash in taxane–lapatinib arm, leading to significant dose reductions/delays, which may had an impact in the overall results.

Additional data are available from the phase III CEREBEL trial [104] that randomized HER2+ MBC patients, with no evidence of CNS disease, previously treated with anthracyclines and taxanes to lapatinib plus capecitabine or trastuzumab plus capecitabine. The study was looking for the incidence of CNS as first site of relapse, defined as the primary endpoint, and enrolled 475 patients. The trial was terminated based on the results of the first interim analysis, due to a low number of CNS events (3% and 5% respectively), which deemed the study not feasible. Additionally, the PFS was lower in the lapatinib combined arm versus the trastuzumab one: 6.6 versus 8.0 months, respectively, HR=1.3 (95% CI: 1.04–1.64).

TDM-1 and Pertuzumab

Two new agents have recently appeared targeting HER2, T-DM1 and pertuzumab [76,105]. Phase II studies of TDM1 [106,107] had promising results, with reports of CBR 48.2% and median PFS of 6.9 months in patients previously treated with trastuzumab, lapatinib, and multiple CT lines. A phase III study that compared TDM1 to lapatinib+capecitabine [105], as first-, second-, or third-line therapy fasted recruited 991 MBC HER2+ patients, previously treated with trastuzumab and taxanes in the metastatic setting or progressing in the locally advanced setting. T-DM1 increased OS (primary end point) in the second interim analysis of 25.1–30.9 months and HR=0.69 (95% CI: 0.55–0.85). There was also an increase of PFS of 6.4–9.6 months HR=0.65 (95% CI: 0.55–0.77). T-DM1 also had a favorable toxicity profile with lower grade 3 and 4 events (41% vs. 57%), and there was only higher incidence compared to lapatinib and capecitabine of thrombocytopenia and increased serum aminotransferase levels, whereas diarrhea, nausea, vomiting, and palmoplantar erythrodysesthesia were higher in the comparator. T-DM1 is waiting for FDA and EMA approval and will be certainly a new agent to incorporate in the treatment of MBC. These results highlight the benefit of continuing suppression of the HER2 pathway through evolution of MBC. Questions need to be answered about the best sequencing of anti-HER targets, which CT and endocrine therapy combinations and their sequencing, as well as monotherapy. Several ongoing trials are trying to address these questions.

Pertuzumab complementary action in targeting HER2 also showed significant clinical activity in phase II studies [108,109], which led to a randomized phase III trial, where 808 patients [76] were treated with trastuzumab and docetaxel plus or minus pertuzumab as first-line treatment for HER2-positive MBC. The inclusion of pertuzumab improved PFS (primary endpoint) from 12.4 to 18.5 months and HR 0.62 (95% CI: 0.51–0.77, $p<0.001$). A trend to increased OS was seen but more mature data are still needed. Additionally, the characteristics of the enrolled patient population (i.e., 54.2% and 52.7% of trastuzumab-naive patients in pertuzumab and no pertuzumab arm, respectively) make the extrapolation of these results to trastuzumab-pretreated patients challenging. The efficacy of dual blocking with trastuzumab and pertuzumab is being evaluated in the adjuvant setting through the large phase III APHINITY trial.

Neratinib has been evaluated in MBC in an open-label phase II study [110] that included two cohorts of patients, one (cohort *a*) with previous trastuzumab treatment and another (cohort *b*) with no prior treatment. Oral neratinib was administered once daily to 136 patients, 66 in cohort *a* (median previous trastuzumab treatment of 14.3 months) and 70 in cohort *b*. Median PFS was 22.3 and 39.6 weeks in cohort *a* and *b*, respectively, whereas 16-week PFS rates (primary endpoint) were 59% and 78%. ORR and CBR were 24% and 33% among patients with prior trastuzumab and 56% and 69% in trastuzumab-naive ones. Main adverse events were diarrhea, nausea, vomiting, and fatigue. Diarrhea was the most frequent grade 3/4 adverse event (29 patients) and led to dose reductions in 24% patients in cohort *a* and 4% in cohort *b*. The data suggest clinical activity of neratinib in HER2+ BC, with manageable toxicity leading to the incorporation of this agent in ongoing research. The combination of neratinib and temsirolimus in HER2+ MBC or triple-negative disease is being evaluated in a phase II study (NCT01111825, www.clinicaltrials. gov). In the neoadjuvant setting, two studies are actively recruiting: I-SPY 2 TRIAL (*Neoadjuvant and Personalized Adaptive Novel Agents to Treat Breast Cancer*) is comparing neratinib with several other targeted agents and trastuzumab-based therapy; another phase II study is evaluating neratinib plus or minus trastuzumab, followed by postoperative trastuzumab in locally advanced HER2+ BC (NCT01008150, www.clinicaltrials.gov).

Afatinib is a novel potent TKI targeting HER1 and HER2, tested in phase II studies in HER2+ and [111] HER2-negative MBC [112]. In a phase II open-label study [111], 43 patients with HER2+ MBC or locally advanced disease progressing following trastuzumab treatment were treated with oral afatinib 50 mg once daily. Patients received a median of three prior CT lines (range 0–15) and 68.3% had trastuzumab treatment for more than 1 year. The primary end point was response rate. Four patients (10%) achieved partial response, 15 (37%) had stable disease, and 19 (46%) had clinical benefit. Median PFS was 15.1 weeks (CI 95%: 8.1–16.7). The most frequent grade 3 adverse events were diarrhea (24.4%) and rash (9.8%), which were manageable with dose reduction (40 and 30 mg) and treatment pause. The authors highlight the importance of preemptive management of diarrhea under afatinib treatment to prevent complications. Although a small study, it is interesting to note that there were no cardiotoxicity issues or changes in LVEF measurements during treatment. A similar phase II study conducted in 50 patients with MBC HER2-negative disease [112] revealed limited activity for afatinib in this setting, but the results in the HER2+ heavily pretreated population have moved this agent to further research. Several ongoing trials are evaluating (a) afatinib in patients whose tumors progress after trastuzumab treatment, (b) the safety of the combination with trastuzumab and the efficacy of dual blocking, (c) afatinib versus other anti-HER2 agents, (d) treatment of metastatic CNS disease, and (e) treatment of inflammatory BC: (a1) The *LUX-Breast-1* trial is a phase III study assessing the efficacy of afatinib combined with vinorelbine in MBC patients whose tumors progress after first-line trastuzumab treatment, compared to trastuzumab beyond progression plus vinorelbine (NCT01125566, www.clinicaltrials.gov). (a2) The *LUX-Breast-2* trial is a phase II study of afatinib alone or combined with wk paclitaxel or vinorelbine (if progression on afatinib within the trial) in patients relapsing after adjuvant or neoadjuvant anti-HER2 treatment (NCT01271725, www.clinicaltrials.gov). (b1) A phase I trial is assessing the safety of afatinib in combination with 3wk trastuzumab in HER2+ MBC patients (NCT01649271, www.clinicaltrials.gov). (b2) A Phase II study is testing the neoadjuvant treatment with afatinib plus trastuzumab given for 6 weeks, followed by the combination of afatinib, trastuzumab, and paclitaxel given for 11–12 weeks, followed by EC plus trastuzumab given for 12 weeks (NCT01594177, www.clinicaltrials.gov). (c) A phase II randomized trial of afatinib versus lapatinib versus trastuzumab as neoadjuvant treatment of stage IIIa HER2+ BC has completed accrual (NCT00826267, www.clinicaltrials.gov). (d) The *LUX-Breast-3* trial is a randomized phase II study of afatinib alone or in combination with vinorelbine, versus investigator's choice, in patients with progressive CNS disease after trastuzumab and/or lapatinib treatment (NCT01441596; www.clinicaltrials.gov). (e) A phase II study is being conducted in patients with inflammatory BC, progressing or not on prior trastuzumab treatment, who are treated with afatinib, or afatinib plus wk vinorelbine if afatinib progression within the study (NCT01325428, www.clinicaltrials.gov).

Anti-HER2 Treatment beyond Progression

There is growing evidence for continuing anti-HER2-based therapy after progression on trastuzumab [113–115]. A randomized study from the GBG [114] assessed in 156 patients progressing on first-line treatment with trastuzumab and CT to capecitabine and trastuzumab versus capecitabine. The capecitabine and trastuzumab arm had higher TTP (median TTP 8.2 vs. 5.6 months, HR=0.69, CI 95%: 0.48–0.97) and ORR (48.1% vs. 27%, OR=2.5, p=0.0115). This study was stopped at 156 patients failing the target accrual of 482 patients due to slow enrollment and revealing the final analysis [115] no statistically significant difference in OS (HR=0.94, 95% CI: 0.65–1.35, p=0.73) although a trend for better OS was seen. A post hoc analysis of patients continuing or not trastuzumab in third-line treatment revealed significant increase in post-progression OS for the group receiving trastuzumab (HR=0.63, p=0.02). These results, together with the trial of capecitabine + lapatinib versus capecitabine alone led to the standard of care of continuing anti-HER2 treatment beyond progression. This is a landmark change in oncology where usually a treatment is stopped at progression. The recent results with TDM1 treatment give additional evidence for the benefit of continuing suppression of the HER2 pathway. Crucial questions remain unanswered such as: (1) For how long should the HER2 pathway be blocked? (2) Which is the best sequence of anti-HER2 agents? (3) Which CT and endocrine therapy combinations as well as their sequencing?

CONCLUSIONS

The clinical achievements of anti-HER2 agents in the treatment of HER2+ BC are one of the major advances in anticancer treatment and led to a change in the natural history of this subtype of BC. Together with imatinib, trastuzumab is the paradigm of the new targeted agents, proving that blocking a crucial pathway in the development of a cancer can led to benefits of significant magnitude. However, just like with endocrine therapy (the first form of targeted therapy), it has also shown that even in a situation where the target is known and the drug blocks the target, the efficacy rate does not reach 100% and that resistance still occurs. Research efforts must continue to be focused not only on the development of new anti-HER2 agents, with better efficacy and/or less toxicity, but also on the discovery and validation of predictive biomarkers that may allow us to better define which patients can benefit from each drug or combination of drugs, both in the adjuvant and metastatic settings.

REFERENCES

1. Graus-Porta D, Beerli RR, Daly JM, Hynes NE. ErbB-2, the preferred heterodimerization partner of all ErbB receptors, is a mediator of lateral signaling. *EMBO J.* 1997 April 1;16(7):1647–1655.
2. Roskoski R, Jr. The ErbB/HER receptor protein-tyrosine kinases and cancer. *Biochem Biophys Res Commun.* 2004 June 18;319(1):1–11.
3. Tzahar E, Waterman H, Chen X, Levkowitz G, Karunagaran D, Lavi S et al. A hierarchical network of interreceptor interactions determines signal transduction by Neu differentiation factor/neuregulin and epidermal growth factor. *Mol Cell Biol.* 1996 October;16(10):5276–5287.

4. Karunagaran D, Tzahar E, Beerli RR, Chen X, Graus-Porta D, Ratzkin BJ et al. ErbB-2 is a common auxiliary subunit of NDF and EGF receptors: Implications for breast cancer. *EMBO J*. 1996 January 15;15(2):254–264.

5. Schechter AL, Stern DF, Vaidyanathan L, Decker SJ, Drebin JA, Greene MI et al. The neu oncogene: An erb-B-related gene encoding a 185,000-Mr tumour antigen. *Nature*. 1984 December 6–12;312(5994):513–516.

6. Ross JS, Fletcher JA. HER-2/neu (c-erb-B2) gene and protein in breast cancer. *Am J Clin Pathol*. 1999 July;112(1 Suppl 1):S53–S67.

7. Wolff AC, Hammond ME, Schwartz JN, Hagerty KL, Allred DC, Cote RJ et al. American Society of Clinical Oncology/College of American Pathologists guideline recommendations for human epidermal growth factor receptor 2 testing in breast cancer. *J Clin Oncol*. 2007 January 1;25(1):118–145.

8. Hammond ME, Hayes DF, Wolff AC. Clinical Notice for American Society of Clinical Oncology/College of American Pathologists guideline recommendations on ER/PgR and HER2 testing in breast cancer. *J Clin Oncol*. 2011 May 20;29(15):e458.

9. Slamon DJ, Leyland-Jones B, Shak S, Fuchs H, Paton V, Bajamonde A et al. Use of chemotherapy plus a monoclonal antibody against HER-2 for metastatic breast cancer that overexpresses HER-2. *N Engl J Med*. 2001 March 15;344(11):783–792.

10. Seidman AD BD, Cirrincione C et al. CALGB 9840: Phase III study of weekly (W) paclitaxel (P) via 1-hour(h) infusion versus standard (S) 3h infusion every third week in the treatment of metastatic breast cancer (MBC), with trastuzumab (T) for HER2 positive MBC and randomized for T in HER2 normal MBC. *J Clin Oncol*. 22: 6s, 2004 (abstr 512).

11. Hayes DF, Thor AD. c-erbB-2 in breast cancer: Development of a clinically useful marker. *Semin Oncol*. 2002 June;29(3):231–245.

12. Masood S, Bui MM. Prognostic and predictive value of HER2/neu oncogene in breast cancer. *Microsc Res Tech*. 2002 October 15;59(2):102–118.

13. Cuadros M, Villegas R. Systematic review of HER2 breast cancer testing. *Appl Immunohistochem Mol Morphol*. 2009 January;17(1):1–7.

14. Fiszman GL, Jasnis MA. Molecular mechanisms of trastuzumab resistance in HER2 overexpressing breast cancer. *Int J Breast Cancer*. 2011;2011:352182.

15. Wong AL, Lee SC. Mechanisms of resistance to trastuzumab and novel therapeutic strategies in HER2-positive breast cancer. *Int J Breast Cancer*. 2012;2012:415170.

16. Nagata Y, Lan KH, Zhou X, Tan M, Esteva FJ, Sahin AA et al. PTEN activation contributes to tumor inhibition by trastuzumab, and loss of PTEN predicts trastuzumab resistance in patients. *Cancer Cell*. 2004 August;6(2):117–127.

17. Damiano V, Garofalo S, Rosa R, Bianco R, Caputo R, Gelardi T et al. A novel toll-like receptor 9 agonist cooperates with trastuzumab in trastuzumab-resistant breast tumors through multiple mechanisms of action. *Clin Cancer Res*. 2009 November 15;15(22):6921–6930.

18. Tagliabue E, Campiglio M, Pupa SM, Menard S, Balsari A. Activity and resistance of trastuzumab according to different clinical settings. *Cancer Treat Rev*. 2012 May;38(3):212–217.

19. Konecny GE, Pegram MD, Venkatesan N, Finn R, Yang G, Rahmeh M et al. Activity of the dual kinase inhibitor lapatinib (GW572016) against HER-2-overexpressing and trastuzumab-treated breast cancer cells. *Cancer Res*. 2006 February 1;66(3): 1630–1639.

20. Spector NL, Xia W, Burris H, 3rd, Hurwitz H, Dees EC, Dowlati A et al. Study of the biologic effects of lapatinib, a reversible inhibitor of ErbB1 and ErbB2 tyrosine kinases, on tumor growth and survival pathways in patients with advanced malignancies. *J Clin Oncol*. 2005 April 10;23(11):2502–2512.

21. Franklin MC, Carey KD, Vajdos FF, Leahy DJ, de Vos AM, Sliwkowski MX. Insights into ErbB signaling from the structure of the ErbB2-pertuzumab complex. *Cancer Cell.* 2004 April;5(4):317–328.

22. Lewis Phillips GD, Li G, Dugger DL, Crocker LM, Parsons KL, Mai E et al. Targeting HER2-positive breast cancer with trastuzumab-DM1, an antibody-cytotoxic drug conjugate. *Cancer Res.* 2008 November 15;68(22):9280–9290.

23. Barok M, Tanner M, Koninki K, Isola J. Trastuzumab-DM1 causes tumour growth inhibition by mitotic catastrophe in trastuzumab-resistant breast cancer cells in vivo. *Breast Cancer Res.* 2011;13(2):R46.

24. Lopus M, Oroudjev E, Wilson L, Wilhelm S, Widdison W, Chari R et al. Maytansine and cellular metabolites of antibody-maytansinoid conjugates strongly suppress microtubule dynamics by binding to microtubules. *Mol Cancer Ther.* 2010 October;9(10):2689–2699.

25. Oroudjev E, Lopus M, Wilson L, Audette C, Provenzano C, Erickson H et al. Maytansinoid-antibody conjugates induce mitotic arrest by suppressing microtubule dynamic instability. *Mol Cancer Ther.* 2010 October;9(10):2700–2713.

26. Remillard S, Rebhun LI, Howie GA, Kupchan SM. Antimitotic activity of the potent tumor inhibitor maytansine. *Science.* 1975 September 19;189(4207):1002–1005.

27. Bruno R, Washington CB, Lu JF, Lieberman G, Banken L, Klein P. Population pharmacokinetics of trastuzumab in patients with HER2+ metastatic breast cancer. *Cancer Chemother Pharmacol.* 2005 October;56(4):361–369.

28. Gupta M, Lorusso PM, Wang B, Yi JH, Burris HA, 3rd, Beeram M et al. Clinical implications of pathophysiological and demographic covariates on the population pharmacokinetics of trastuzumab emtansine, a HER2-targeted antibody-drug conjugate, in patients with HER2-positive metastatic breast cancer. *J Clin Pharmacol.* 2012 May;52(5):691–703.

29. Li G FC, Parsons KL, Guo J, Lewis Phillips GD. Trastuzumab-DM1: mechanisms of action and mechanisms of resistance. *Eur J Cancer.* 2010;8(suppl):73.

30. Smith I, Procter M, Gelber RD, Guillaume S, Feyereislova A, Dowsett M et al. 2-Year follow-up of trastuzumab after adjuvant chemotherapy in HER2-positive breast cancer: A randomised controlled trial. *Lancet.* 2007 January 6;369(9555):29–36.

31. Joensuu H, Kellokumpu-Lehtinen PL, Bono P, Alanko T, Kataja V, Asola R et al. Adjuvant docetaxel or vinorelbine with or without trastuzumab for breast cancer. *N Engl J Med.* 2006 February 23;354(8):809–820.

32. Spielmann M, Roche H, Delozier T, Canon JL, Romieu G, Bourgeois H et al. Trastuzumab for patients with axillary-node-positive breast cancer: Results of the FNCLCC-PACS 04 trial. *J Clin Oncol.* 2009 December 20;27(36):6129–6134.

33. Romond EH, Perez EA, Bryant J, Suman VJ, Geyer CE, Jr., Davidson NE et al. Trastuzumab plus adjuvant chemotherapy for operable HER2-positive breast cancer. *N Engl J Med.* 2005 October 20;353(16):1673–1684.

34. Slamon D, Eiermann W, Robert N, Pienkowski T, Martin M, Press M et al. Adjuvant trastuzumab in HER2-positive breast cancer. *N Engl J Med.* 2011 October 6;365(14):1273–1283.

35. Perez E SV, Davidson N, Gralow J, Kaufman P, Ingle J, Dakhil S, Zujewski J, Pisansky T, Jenkins R. Results of chemotherapy alone, with sequential or concurrent addition of 52 weeks of trastuzumab in the NCCTG n9831 her2-positive adjuvant breast cancer trial. *Cancer Res.* 2010 July 1;70:5640–5645.

36. Untch M, Gelber RD, Jackisch C, Procter M, Baselga J, Bell R et al. Estimating the magnitude of trastuzumab effects within patient subgroups in the HERA trial. *Ann Oncol.* 2008 June;19(6):1090–1096.

37. Curigliano G, Viale G, Bagnardi V, Fumagalli L, Locatelli M, Rotmensz N et al. Clinical relevance of HER2 overexpression/amplification in patients with small tumor size and node-negative breast cancer. *J Clin Oncol.* 2009 December 1;27(34):5693–5699.

38. Gonzalez-Angulo AM, Litton JK, Broglio KR, Meric-Bernstam F, Rakkhit R, Cardoso F et al. High risk of recurrence for patients with breast cancer who have human epidermal growth factor receptor 2-positive, node-negative tumors 1 cm or smaller. *J Clin Oncol.* 2009 December 1;27(34):5700–5706.

39. Chia S, Norris B, Speers C, Cheang M, Gilks B, Gown AM et al. Human epidermal growth factor receptor 2 overexpression as a prognostic factor in a large tissue microarray series of node-negative breast cancers. *J Clin Oncol.* 2008 December 10;26(35): 5697–5704.

40. National Comprehensive Cancer Network (NCCN) guidelines. Available at: www.nccn. org (Accessed on May 15).

41. Aebi S, Davidson T, Gruber G, Cardoso F. On behalf of the ESMO guidelines working group primary breast cancer: ESMO clinical practice guidelines for diagnosis, treatment and follow-up. *Ann Oncol.* 2011;22 (Suppl 6):vi12–vi24.

42. Moja L, Tagliabue L, Balduzzi S, Parmelli E, Pistotti V, Guarneri V et al. Trastuzumab containing regimens for early breast cancer. *Cochrane Database Syst Rev.* 2012;4: CD006243.

43. Perez E RE, Suman V et al. Updated results of the combined analysis of NCCTG N9831 and NSABP B-31 adjuvant chemotherapy with/without trastuzumab in patients with HER2-positive breast cancer. *J Clin Oncol* 2007;25 (suppl 18):512, 6s.

44. Paik S, Bryant J, Tan-Chiu E, Romond E, Hiller W, Park K et al. Real-world performance of HER2 testing—National Surgical Adjuvant Breast and Bowel Project experience. *J Natl Cancer Inst.* 2002 June 5;94(11):852–854.

45. Roche PC SV, Jenkins RB, Davidson NE, Martino S, Kaufman PA, Addo FK, Murphy B, Ingle JN, Perez EA. Concordance between local and central laboratory HER2 testing in the breast intergroup trial N9831. *J Natl Cancer Inst.* 2002;94(11):855–857.

46. Perez EA, Romond EH, Suman VJ, Jeong JH, Davidson NE, Geyer CE, Jr. et al. Four-year follow-up of trastuzumab plus adjuvant chemotherapy for operable human epidermal growth factor receptor 2-positive breast cancer: Joint analysis of data from NCCTG N9831 and NSABP B-31. *J Clin Oncol.* 2011 September 1;29(25):3366–3373.

47. Romond EVS, Jeong J-H, Sledge GW, Jr., Geyer CE, Jr., Martino S, Rastogi P, Gralow J et al., and National Surgical Adjuvant Breast and Bowel Project (NSABP) Operations and Biostatistical Centers. Trastuzumab plus adjuvant chemotherapy for HER2-positive breast cancer: Final planned joint analysis of overall survival (OS) from NSABP B-31 and NCCTG N9831. *Cancer Res.* 2012;72(24):Suplement 3.

48. Piccart-Gebhart MJ, Procter M, Leyland-Jones B, Goldhirsch A, Untch M, Smith I et al. Trastuzumab after adjuvant chemotherapy in HER2-positive breast cancer. *N Engl J Med.* 2005 October 20;353(16):1659–1672.

49. Gelber RD GA, Piccart M et al. HERA Trial: 2 years versus 1 year of trastuzumab after adjuvant chemotherapy in women with HER2-positive early breast cancer at 8 years of median follow up. 2012 ESMO Congress. 2012 Presented October 1, 2012.

50. Joensuu H, Bono P, Kataja V, Alanko T, Kokko R, Asola R et al. Fluorouracil, epirubicin, and cyclophosphamide with either docetaxel or vinorelbine, with or without trastuzumab, as adjuvant treatments of breast cancer: Final results of the FinHer Trial. *J Clin Oncol.* 2009 December 1;27(34):5685–5692.

51. Gennari A, Sormani MP, Pronzato P, Puntoni M, Colozza M, Pfeffer U et al. HER2 status and efficacy of adjuvant anthracyclines in early breast cancer: A pooled analysis of randomized trials. *J Natl Cancer Inst.* 2008 January 2;100(1):14–20.

52. Di Leo A, Desmedt C, Bartlett JM, Piette F, Ejlertsen B, Pritchard KI et al. HER2 and TOP2A as predictive markers for anthracycline-containing chemotherapy regimens as adjuvant treatment of breast cancer: A meta-analysis of individual patient data. *Lancet Oncol.* 2011 November;12(12):1134–1142.

53. Perez EA, Suman VJ, Davidson NE, Gralow JR, Kaufman PA, Visscher DW et al. Sequential versus concurrent trastuzumab in adjuvant chemotherapy for breast cancer. *J Clin Oncol.* 2011 December 1;29(34):4491–4497.
54. Pivot X RG, Bonnefoi H et al. PHARE trial results of subset analysis comparing 6 to 12 months of trastuzumab in adjuvant early breast cancer. *Program and abstracts of the 35th Annual San Antonio Breast Cancer Symposium.* [Abstract S5-3]. 2012 December 4–8, 2012; San Antonio, TX.
55. Bear HD. Indications for neoadjuvant chemotherapy for breast cancer. *Semin Oncol.* 1998 April;25(2 Suppl 3):3–12.
56. Hortobagyi GN. Comprehensive management of locally advanced breast cancer. *Cancer.* 1990 September 15;66(6 Suppl):1387–1391.
57. Hortobagyi GN, Ames FC, Buzdar AU, Kau SW, McNeese MD, Paulus D et al. Management of stage III primary breast cancer with primary chemotherapy, surgery, and radiation therapy. *Cancer.* 1988 December 15;62(12):2507–2516.
58. Hortobagyi GN, Blumenschein GR, Spanos W, Montague ED, Buzdar AU, Yap HY et al. Multimodal treatment of locoregionally advanced breast cancer. *Cancer.* 1983 March 1;51(5):763–768.
59. Fisher B, Bryant J, Wolmark N, Mamounas E, Brown A, Fisher ER et al. Effect of preoperative chemotherapy on the outcome of women with operable breast cancer. *J Clin Oncol.* 1998 August;16(8):2672–2685.
60. Wolmark N, Wang J, Mamounas E, Bryant J, Fisher B. Preoperative chemotherapy in patients with operable breast cancer: Nine-year results from National Surgical Adjuvant Breast and Bowel Project B-18. *J Natl Cancer Inst Monogr.* 2001;(30):96–102.
61. Bear HD, Anderson S, Brown A, Smith R, Mamounas EP, Fisher B et al. The effect on tumor response of adding sequential preoperative docetaxel to preoperative doxorubicin and cyclophosphamide: Preliminary results from National Surgical Adjuvant Breast and Bowel Project Protocol B-27. *J Clin Oncol.* 2003 November 15;21(22):4165–4174.
62. Mieog JS, van der Hage JA, van de Velde CJ. Preoperative chemotherapy for women with operable breast cancer. *Cochrane Database Syst Rev.* 2007 Apr 18;(2):CD005002.
63. Kuerer HM, Newman LA, Smith TL, Ames FC, Hunt KK, Dhingra K et al. Clinical course of breast cancer patients with complete pathologic primary tumor and axillary lymph node response to doxorubicin-based neoadjuvant chemotherapy. *J Clin Oncol.* 1999 February;17(2):460–469.
64. van der Hage JA, van de Velde CJ, Julien JP, Tubiana-Hulin M, Vandervelden C, Duchateau L. Preoperative chemotherapy in primary operable breast cancer: Results from the European Organization for Research and Treatment of Cancer trial 10902. *J Clin Oncol.* 2001 November 15;19(22):4224–4237.
65. von Minckwitz GMK, Kümmel S et al. Integrated meta-analysis on 6402 patients with early breast cancer receiving neoadjuvant anthracycline-taxane +/− trastuzumab containing chemotherapy. *Cancer Res.* 2009;69(2 Suppl):79.
66. Kaufmann M, Hortobagyi GN, Goldhirsch A, Scholl S, Makris A, Valagussa P et al. Recommendations from an international expert panel on the use of neoadjuvant (primary) systemic treatment of operable breast cancer: An update. *J Clin Oncol.* 2006 April 20;24(12):1940–1949.
67. Buzdar AU, Ibrahim NK, Francis D, Booser DJ, Thomas ES, Theriault RL et al. Significantly higher pathologic complete remission rate after neoadjuvant therapy with trastuzumab, paclitaxel, and epirubicin chemotherapy: Results of a randomized trial in human epidermal growth factor receptor 2-positive operable breast cancer. *J Clin Oncol.* 2005 June 1;23(16):3676–3685.
68. Buzdar AU, Valero V, Ibrahim NK, Francis D, Broglio KR, Theriault RL et al. Neoadjuvant therapy with paclitaxel followed by 5-fluorouracil, epirubicin, and cyclophosphamide chemotherapy and concurrent trastuzumab in human epidermal growth

factor receptor 2-positive operable breast cancer: An update of the initial randomized study population and data of additional patients treated with the same regimen. *Clin Cancer Res.* 2007 January 1;13(1):228–233.

69. Gianni L, Eiermann W, Semiglazov V, Manikhas A, Lluch A, Tjulandin S et al. Neoadjuvant chemotherapy with trastuzumab followed by adjuvant trastuzumab versus neoadjuvant chemotherapy alone, in patients with HER2-positive locally advanced breast cancer (the NOAH trial): A randomised controlled superiority trial with a parallel HER2-negative cohort. *Lancet.* 2010 January 30;375(9712):377–384.

70. Untch M, Rezai M, Loibl S, Fasching PA, Huober J, Tesch H et al. Neoadjuvant treatment with trastuzumab in HER2-positive breast cancer: Results from the GeparQuattro study. *J Clin Oncol.* 2010 April 20;28(12):2024–2031.

71. von Minckwitz G, Rezai M, Loibl S, Fasching PA, Huober J, Tesch H et al. Capecitabine in addition to anthracycline- and taxane-based neoadjuvant treatment in patients with primary breast cancer: Phase III GeparQuattro study. *J Clin Oncol.* 2010 April 20;28(12):2015–2023.

72. Baselga J, Bradbury I, Eidtmann H, Di Cosimo S, de Azambuja E, Aura C et al. Lapatinib with trastuzumab for HER2-positive early breast cancer (NeoALTTO): A randomised, open-label, multicentre, phase 3 trial. *Lancet.* 2012 February 18;379(9816):633–640.

73. Untch M, Loibl S, Bischoff J, Eidtmann H, Kaufmann M, Blohmer JU et al. Lapatinib versus trastuzumab in combination with neoadjuvant anthracycline-taxane-based chemotherapy (GeparQuinto, GBG 44): A randomised phase 3 trial. *Lancet Oncol.* 2012 February;13(2):135–144.

74. Guarneri V, Frassoldati A, Bottini A, Cagossi K, Bisagni G, Sarti S et al. Preoperative chemotherapy plus trastuzumab, lapatinib, or both in human epidermal growth factor receptor 2-positive operable breast cancer: Results of the randomized phase II CHER-LOB study. *J Clin Oncol.* 2012 June 1;30(16):1989–1995.

75. Gianni L PT, Im Y-H et al. Neoadjuvant Pertuzumab (P) and Trastuzumab (H): Antitumor and safety analysis of a randomized phase II study ('NeoSphere'). *Cancer Res.* 2010;70(24 Suppl)Abstr S3–S2.

76. Baselga J, Cortes J, Kim SB, Im SA, Hegg R, Im YH et al. Pertuzumab plus trastuzumab plus docetaxel for metastatic breast cancer. *N Engl J Med.* 2012 January 12;366(2):109–119.

77. Blackwell KL, Burstein HJ, Storniolo AM, Rugo HS, Sledge G, Aktan G et al. Overall survival benefit with lapatinib in combination with trastuzumab for patients with human epidermal growth factor receptor 2-positive metastatic breast cancer: Final results from the EGF104900 Study. *J Clin Oncol.* 2012 July 20;30(21):2585–2592.

78. Cobleigh MA, Vogel CL, Tripathy D, Robert NJ, Scholl S, Fehrenbacher L et al. Multinational study of the efficacy and safety of humanized anti-HER2 monoclonal antibody in women who have HER2-overexpressing metastatic breast cancer that has progressed after chemotherapy for metastatic disease. *J Clin Oncol.* 1999 September;17(9):2639–2648.

79. Baselga J, Carbonell X, Castaneda-Soto NJ, Clemens M, Green M, Harvey V et al. Phase II study of efficacy, safety, and pharmacokinetics of trastuzumab monotherapy administered on a 3-weekly schedule. *J Clin Oncol.* 2005 April 1;23(10):2162–2171.

80. Vogel CL, Cobleigh MA, Tripathy D, Gutheil JC, Harris LN, Fehrenbacher L et al. Efficacy and safety of trastuzumab as a single agent in first-line treatment of HER2-overexpressing metastatic breast cancer. *J Clin Oncol.* 2002 February 1;20(3):719–726.

81. Andersson M, Lidbrink E, Bjerre K, Wist E, Enevoldsen K, Jensen AB et al. Phase III randomized study comparing docetaxel plus trastuzumab with vinorelbine plus trastuzumab as first-line therapy of metastatic or locally advanced human epidermal growth factor receptor 2-positive breast cancer: The HERNATA study. *J Clin Oncol.* 2011 January 20;29(3):264–271.

82. Burstein H, Keshaviah A, Baron A et al. Trastuzumab and vinorelbine or taxane chemotherapy for HER2+ metastatic breast cancer: The TRAVIOTA study. *ASCO Annual Meeting 2006.* 2006; Baltimore, MD.

83. Marty M, Cognetti F, Maraninchi D, Snyder R, Mauriac L, Tubiana-Hulin M et al. Randomized phase II trial of the efficacy and safety of trastuzumab combined with docetaxel in patients with human epidermal growth factor receptor 2-positive metastatic breast cancer administered as first-line treatment: The M77001 study group. *J Clin Oncol.* 2005 July 1;23(19):4265–4274.

84. Michalaki V, Fotiou S, Gennatas S, Gennatas C. Trastuzumab plus capecitabine and docetaxel as first-line therapy for HER2-positive metastatic breast cancer: Phase II results. *Anticancer Res.* 2010 July;30(7):3051–3054.

85. Moulder S, Li H, Wang M, Gradishar WJ, Perez EA, Sparano JA et al. A phase II trial of trastuzumab plus weekly ixabepilone and carboplatin in patients with HER2-positive metastatic breast cancer: An Eastern Cooperative Oncology Group Trial. *Breast Cancer Res Treat.* 2010 February;119(3):663–671.

86. Robert N, Leyland-Jones B, Asmar L, Belt R, Ilegbodu D, Loesch D et al. Randomized phase III study of trastuzumab, paclitaxel, and carboplatin compared with trastuzumab and paclitaxel in women with HER-2-overexpressing metastatic breast cancer. *J Clin Oncol.* 2006 June 20;24(18):2786–2792.

87. Tripathy D. Capecitabine in combination with novel targeted agents in the management of metastatic breast cancer: Underlying rationale and results of clinical trials. *Oncologist.* 2007 April;12(4):375–389.

88. Untch M, Muscholl M, Tjulandin S, Jonat W, Meerpohl HG, Lichinitser M et al. First-line trastuzumab plus epirubicin and cyclophosphamide therapy in patients with human epidermal growth factor receptor 2-positive metastatic breast cancer: Cardiac safety and efficacy data from the Herceptin, Cyclophosphamide, and Epirubicin (HERCULES) trial. *J Clin Oncol.* 2010 March 20;28(9):1473–1480.

89. Valero V, Forbes J, Pegram MD, Pienkowski T, Eiermann W, von Minckwitz G et al. Multicenter phase III randomized trial comparing docetaxel and trastuzumab with docetaxel, carboplatin, and trastuzumab as first-line chemotherapy for patients with HER2-gene-amplified metastatic breast cancer (BCIRG 007 study): Two highly active therapeutic regimens. *J Clin Oncol.* 2011 January 10;29(2):149–156.

90. Wardley AM, Pivot X, Morales-Vasquez F, Zetina LM, de Fatima Dias Gaui M, Reyes DO et al. Randomized phase II trial of first-line trastuzumab plus docetaxel and capecitabine compared with trastuzumab plus docetaxel in HER2-positive metastatic breast cancer. *J Clin Oncol.* 2010 February 20;28(6):976–983.

91. Yardley DA, Burris HA, 3rd, Simons L, Spigel DR, Greco FA, Barton JH et al. A phase II trial of gemcitabine/carboplatin with or without trastuzumab in the first-line treatment of patients with metastatic breast cancer. *Clin Breast Cancer.* 2008 October;8(5):425–431.

92. Leyland-Jones B, Gelmon K, Ayoub JP, Arnold A, Verma S, Dias R et al. Pharmacokinetics, safety, and efficacy of trastuzumab administered every three weeks in combination with paclitaxel. *J Clin Oncol.* 2003 November 1;21(21):3965–3971.

93. Piccart-Gebhart MJ, Burzykowski T, Buyse M, Sledge G, Carmichael J, Luck HJ et al. Taxanes alone or in combination with anthracyclines as first-line therapy of patients with metastatic breast cancer. *J Clin Oncol.* 2008 April 20;26(12):1980–1986.

94. Kaufman B, Mackey JR, Clemens MR, Bapsy PP, Vaid A, Wardley A et al. Trastuzumab plus anastrozole versus anastrozole alone for the treatment of postmenopausal women with human epidermal growth factor receptor 2-positive, hormone receptor-positive metastatic breast cancer: Results from the randomized phase III TAnDEM study. *J Clin Oncol.* 2009 November 20;27(33):5529–5537.

95. Blackwell KL, Pegram MD, Tan-Chiu E, Schwartzberg LS, Arbushites MC, Maltzman JD et al. Single-agent lapatinib for HER2-overexpressing advanced or metastatic breast cancer that progressed on first- or second-line trastuzumab-containing regimens. *Ann Oncol.* 2009 June;20(6):1026–1031.

96. Burstein HJ, Storniolo AM, Franco S, Forster J, Stein S, Rubin S et al. A phase II study of lapatinib monotherapy in chemotherapy-refractory HER2-positive and HER2-negative advanced or metastatic breast cancer. *Ann Oncol.* 2008 June;19(6):1068–1074.

97. Gomez HL, Doval DC, Chavez MA, Ang PC, Aziz Z, Nag S et al. Efficacy and safety of lapatinib as first-line therapy for ErbB2-amplified locally advanced or metastatic breast cancer. *J Clin Oncol.* 2008 June 20;26(18):2999–3005.

98. Toi M, Iwata H, Fujiwara Y, Ito Y, Nakamura S, Tokuda Y et al. Lapatinib monotherapy in patients with relapsed, advanced, or metastatic breast cancer: Efficacy, safety, and biomarker results from Japanese patients phase II studies. *Br J Cancer.* 2009 November 17;101(10):1676–1682.

99. Cameron D, Casey M, Oliva C, Newstat B, Imwalle B, Geyer CE. Lapatinib plus capecitabine in women with HER-2-positive advanced breast cancer: Final survival analysis of a phase III randomized trial. *Oncologist.* 2010;15(9):924–934.

100. Geyer CE, Forster J, Lindquist D, Chan S, Romieu CG, Pienkowski T et al. Lapatinib plus capecitabine for HER2-positive advanced breast cancer. *N Engl J Med.* 2006 December 28;355(26):2733–2743.

101. Johnston S, Pippen J, Jr., Pivot X, Lichinitser M, Sadeghi S, Dieras V et al. Lapatinib combined with letrozole versus letrozole and placebo as first-line therapy for post-menopausal hormone receptor-positive metastatic breast cancer. *J Clin Oncol.* 2009 November 20;27(33):5538–5546.

102. Di Leo A, Gomez HL, Aziz Z, Zvirbule Z, Bines J, Arbushites MC et al. Phase III, double-blind, randomized study comparing lapatinib plus paclitaxel with placebo plus paclitaxel as first-line treatment for metastatic breast cancer. *J Clin Oncol.* 2008 December 1;26(34):5544–5552.

103. Karen A. Gelmon FB, Bella Kaufman et al. Open-label phase III randomized controlled trial comparing taxane-based chemotherapy (Tax) with lapatinib (L) or trastuzumab (T) as first-line therapy for women with HER2+ metastatic breast cancer: Interim analysis (IA) of NCIC CTG MA.31/GSK EGF 108919. 2012 ASCO Annual Meeting, *J Clin Oncol.* 2012 June 20;30(Suppl 18):LBA671.

104. Pivot X SV, Zurawski V et al. CEREBEL (EGF111438): An open label randomized phase III study comparing the incidence of CNS metastases in patients with HER2+ metastatic breast cancer, treated with lapatinib plus capecitabine versus trastuzumab plus capecitabine. *Ann Oncol.* 2012;23 (Suppl 9): ixe1–ixe30.

105. Verma S, Miles D, Gianni L, Krop IE, Welslau M, Baselga J et al. Trastuzumab emtansine for HER2-positive advanced breast cancer. *N Engl J Med.* 2012 November 8;367(19):1783–1791.

106. Burris HA, 3rd, Rugo HS, Vukelja SJ, Vogel CL, Borson RA, Limentani S et al. Phase II study of the antibody drug conjugate trastuzumab-DM1 for the treatment of human epidermal growth factor receptor 2 (HER2)-positive breast cancer after prior HER2-directed therapy. *J Clin Oncol.* 2011 February 1;29(4):398–405.

107. Krop IE, LoRusso P, Miller KD, Modi S, Yardley D, Rodriguez G et al. A phase II study of trastuzumab emtansine in patients with human epidermal growth factor receptor 2-positive metastatic breast cancer who were previously treated with trastuzumab, lapatinib, an anthracycline, a taxane, and capecitabine. *J Clin Oncol.* 2012 September 10;30(26):3234–3241.

108. Baselga J, Gelmon KA, Verma S, Wardley A, Conte P, Miles D et al. Phase II trial of pertuzumab and trastuzumab in patients with human epidermal growth factor receptor 2-positive metastatic breast cancer that progressed during prior trastuzumab therapy. *J Clin Oncol.* 2010 March 1;28(7):1138–1144.

109. Gianni L, Llado A, Bianchi G, Cortes J, Kellokumpu-Lehtinen PL, Cameron DA et al. Open-label, phase II, multicenter, randomized study of the efficacy and safety of two dose levels of Pertuzumab, a human epidermal growth factor receptor 2 dimerization inhibitor, in patients with human epidermal growth factor receptor 2-negative metastatic breast cancer. *J Clin Oncol.* 2010 March 1;28(7):1131–1137.

110. Burstein HJ, Sun Y, Dirix LY, Jiang Z, Paridaens R, Tan AR et al. Neratinib, an irreversible ErbB receptor tyrosine kinase inhibitor, in patients with advanced ErbB2-positive breast cancer. *J Clin Oncol.* 2010 March 10;28(8):1301–1307.

111. Lin NU, Winer EP, Wheatley D, Carey LA, Houston S, Mendelson D et al. A phase II study of afatinib (BIBW 2992), an irreversible ErbB family blocker, in patients with HER2-positive metastatic breast cancer progressing after trastuzumab. *Breast Cancer Res Treat.* 2012 June;133(3):1057–1065.

112. Schuler M, Awada A, Harter P, Canon JL, Possinger K, Schmidt M et al. A phase II trial to assess efficacy and safety of afatinib in extensively pretreated patients with HER2-negative metastatic breast cancer. *Breast Cancer Res Treat.* 2012 August;134(3):1149–1159.

113. Gelmon KA, Mackey J, Verma S, Gertler SZ, Bangemann N, Klimo P et al. Use of trastuzumab beyond disease progression: Observations from a retrospective review of case histories. *Clin Breast Cancer.* 2004 April;5(1):52–58; discussion 9–62.

114. von Minckwitz G, du Bois A, Schmidt M, Maass N, Cufer T, de Jongh FE et al. Trastuzumab beyond progression in human epidermal growth factor receptor 2-positive advanced breast cancer: A German breast group 26/breast international group 03–05 study. *J Clin Oncol.* 2009 April 20;27(12):1999–2006.

115. von Minckwitz G, Schwedler K, Schmidt M, Barinoff J, Mundhenke C, Cufer T et al. Trastuzumab beyond progression: Overall survival analysis of the GBG 26/BIG 3–05 phase III study in HER2-positive breast cancer. *Eur J Cancer.* 2011 October;47(15):2273–2281.

116. Lang, I. (ed.). ErbB2-positive breast cancer medical education programme: 2011 update. Part of the Oncology Academy series.

4 Inhibiting the Phosphoinositide 3-Kinase/AKT/ Mammalian Target of Rapamycin Pathway

Simona Wagner
Queen's University

Janet E. Dancey
Queen's University

CONTENTS

INTRODUCTION

The phosphatidylinositol 3-kinase (PI3K)–AKT–mammalian target of rapamycin complex (mTORC) signal axis is critically important for normal and cancerous cell functions and an important target for cancer therapeutics development. The pathway is activated by cell surface receptor stimulation and sends signals to downstream effector molecules that control the cell cycle proliferation, growth, survival, protein synthesis, and glucose metabolism.[1] Aberrant activation of the pathway is one of the most frequent occurrences in human cancer and plays an important role in multiple aspects of tumorigenesis.[2] Among the mechanisms of aberrant activation are (1) mutation or gene amplification of receptor tyrosine kinases (RTKs), or oncogenes in the pathway (PI3K or AKT), and (2) deletion or epigenetic silencing and loss of function of tumor suppressors, such as the phosphatidylinositol 3,4,5-trisphosphate (PtdIns (3,4,5)) phosphatase and tensing homologue deleted on chromosome 10 (PTEN).[3] Aberrant activation is linked to uncontrolled proliferation, resistance to apoptosis, angiogenesis, and metastasis that may be reversed by targeted inhibition. Given the frequency of pathway abnormalities in cancer and responsiveness to pathway inhibition, there is considerable interest in the development of new therapeutics targeting the PI3K, AKT, and mTOR kinases. In this chapter, we will review the biology of the PI3K/AKT/mTOR pathway and the progress made in the development of novel agents targeting this pathway for cancer treatment.

BIOLOGY OF THE PI3K PATHWAY

PI3K proteins are heterodimers composed of regulatory and kinase subunits. There are three classes of PI3K family of enzymes based on biochemical and structural characteristics: class I are receptor-regulated phosphatidylinositol 4,5-bisphosphate PtdIns (4, 5) P2 kinases, class II are PI3K-C2 kinases (which have an additional C-terminal C2 domain), and class III is composed of the PtdIns-specific enzyme Vps34. There is also PI3K-related protein kinase (PIKK) family, containing enzymes with a catalytic core similar to the PI3Ks, such as mTOR, and DNA damage response, such as ataxia telangiectasia mutated (ATM).[4] PI3K enzymes form a family of proteins with distinct tissue distributions, substrate specificities, and biological functions.

Most cancer therapeutics are directed at class I PI3Ks. Class I PI3Ks are divided into class IA enzymes, which are activated by RTK, G-protein–coupled receptors (GPCR), and some oncogenes (e.g., Ras) and class IB enzymes, which are activated

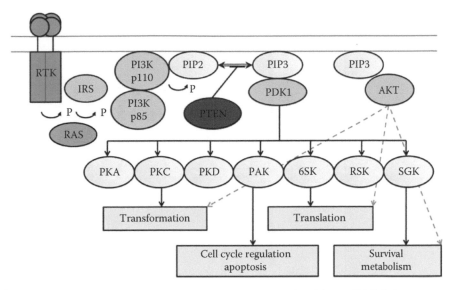

FIGURE 4.1 PI3K signaling via phosphoinositide-dependent kinase (PDK1). In response to extracellular signaling through membrane receptors and through IRS or Ras, PI3K phosphorylates the 3′-hydroxyl of phosphatidylinositol 4,5-bisphosphate (PIP2) to generate phosphatidylinositol 3,4,5-trisphosphate (PIP3). The tumor suppressor phosphatase and tensin homologue deleted on chromosome 10 (PTEN) opposes the action of PI3K by dephosphorylating 3′-phosphoinositides. PIP3 recruits proteins that have a pleckstrin homology domain to the cell membrane including AKT and the PDK1. PDK1 activates AKT and other proteins such as protein kinase A (PKA), protein 21-activated kinase (PAK), isoforms of p70 ribosomal S6 kinase (S6K), serum- and glucocorticoid-responsive kinases (SGK) and p90 ribosomal S6 kinase (p90RSK), atypical and novel PKC isoforms (PKD), protein C-related kinase (PRK 1 and 2), and others. Activation of these substrates leads to an increase in protein translation and regulation of cell cycle, apoptosis, survival, motility, and cell metabolism. *Note*: Oncogenes are colored in green and tumor suppressors in red.

by GPCRs. The class I PI3K kinases consist of a p110 catalytic subunit and p85 regulatory subunit[5] (Figure 4.1 and Table 4.1). The regulatory subunit mediates receptor binding, activation, and localization of the enzyme. Class I PI3K generate the PtdIns (3,4,5) P3 lipid that is dephosphorylated into PtdIns (3,4) P2 and PtdIns (4,5) P2 by phosphatidyl-3- and 5-phosphatases, respectively. There are four isoforms of the catalytic subunit and each isoform has unique signaling functions and tissue distribution. Generally, the ubiquitously expressed p110α and p100β influence cellular proliferation and insulin signaling, whereas p110γ and p100δ, expressed in leukocytes, are involved in immune function and inflammation. Isoform specificity of PI3K inhibitors is relevant to therapeutics development as it determines both the clinical indication and anticipated toxicity of the inhibitor.[6,7] The PtdIns (3,4,5) P3 and PtdIns (3,4) P2 regulate the localization and function of multiple effector proteins, which bind these lipids through their pleckstrin homology (PH) domains causing translocation of the target protein to the plasma membrane.[1,8] Mutations in the PH domain of the target protein can lead to constitutive

TABLE 4.1

Members of the PI3K–AKT–mTOR Pathway

Activators Components in the PI3K Pathway	Function	Tissue Distribution	Activators	Selective Substrates and Downstream Effectors
Class I PI3K				PtdIns(4,5)P2
Class IA Isoforms: alpha, beta, gamma, delta	Bind to the p85 regulatory subunit	All cell types, with p110delta and p110 gamma enriched in leukocytes	RTK and GPCR either directly or indirectly through Ras	AKT, BTK, GAB2, and others
Class IB	Do not bind the p85 regulatory subunit			
Class II PI3K 3 isoform: (C2α, C2β, C2γ)	Cell migration, glucose metabolism, exocytosis, smooth muscle cell contraction, and apoptosis	PI3K-C2α and PI3K-C2β are expressed in differentiated epithelial and mesenchymal cells of origin; PI3K-C2γ is present in most tissue.	RTK, GPCR, GTPases, calcium	FAB1, SGK3, SNX13, NADPH oxidase, and proteins with sorting and scaffolding functions in membrane transport, kinesins and nexin family members
Class III PI3K (Vps34)	Endocytosis, autophagy and nutrient signaling	Ubiquitously expressed	Amino acids, glucose, and GPCR	Many effectors suggesting a scaffolding function for Vps34
AKT 1	Proliferation, survival, motility, angiogenesis, metabolism glucose homeostasis	Most tissues	PDK1, mTORC2	>100 substrates identified
AKT2		Most tissues		
AKT 3		Neuronal tissue and testes		

	Function	Tissue Distribution	Activators	Selective Substrates and Downstream Effectors
mTORC1 (mTOR, raptor, PRAS40, GβL, deptor)	Protein synthesis, ribosome biogenesis, and angiogenesis. Cell growth and proliferation	Ubiquitously expressed	AKT through TSC, Rheb	S6K1, 4EBP1
mTORC2 (mTOR, rictor, mLST8, deptor, Sin1)	Organization of actin cytoskeleton, cell cycle progression and survival	Ubiquitously expressed	AKT through TSC, Rheb	SGK, PKC, AKT
Suppressors Components into the PI3K Pathway	**Function**	**Tissue Distribution**	**Activators**	**Selective Substrates and Downstream Effectors**
PTEN	Negative regulator of PI3K signaling	Ubiquitously expressed	PtdIns	CENP-C1, APC, E-cadherin
TSC 1 and 2	Negative regulator of mTORC1	Ubiquitously expressed	AKT	mTORC1, mTORC2

FAB1, 1-phosphatidylinositol-3-phosphate 5-kinase; APC, adenomatous polyposis coli; BTK, Bruton's tyrosine kinase; CENP, centromere proteins; eIF4E, eukaryotic initiation factor 4E; 4EBP1, eukaryotic initiation factor 4E-binding protein 1; GPCR, G-protein coupled receptors; GAB2, GRB2-associated binding protein 2; GTP, guanosine-5′-triphosphate; INPP4B, inositol polyphosphate 4-phosphatase type II; AKT, mammalian homologue of the retroviral transforming protein v-AKT; mTOR, mammalian target of rapamycin; mTORC, mammalian target of rapamycin complex; NADPH, nicotinamide adenine dinucleotide phosphate; PTEN, phosphatase and tensing homologue deleted on chromosome 10; PtdIns, phosphatidylinositol; PI3K, phosphatidylinositol 3-kinase; PIK3CA, phosphatidylinositol 3-kinase catalytic subunit; PIK3R, phosphatidylinositol 3-kinase regulatory subunit; PDK1, phosphoinositide-dependent protein kinase 1;PKC, protein kinase C; Rheb, Ras homologue enriched in brain; RTKs, receptor tyrosine kinases; S6K1, S6 Kinase 1; STK11, serine/threonine kinase 11; SGK3, serum/glucocorticoid regulated kinase family; member; SNX13, sorting nexin 13; SHIP, Src-homology 2–containing inositol 5′-phosphatase; TSC1, tuberous sclerosis 1; TSC2, tuberous sclerosis 2.

activation, redistribution to the cell membrane, and altered sensitivity to different targeted anticancer agents.[9]

Two key proteins with PH domains are AKT and 3-phosphoinositide–dependent protein kinase 1(PDK1). AKT is a serine/threonine kinase (the mammalian homologue of the retroviral transforming protein v-AKT or protein kinase B, PKB). The AKT is expressed as three isoforms—AKT1, AKT2, and AKT3—which are encoded by three different genes. Both PDK1 and AKT activation is initiated by translocation to the plasma membrane. A conformational change in AKT exposes two important amino acid residues for phosphorylation: threonine 308 (Thr308) and serine 473 (Ser473).[5] The phosphorylation at Thr308 by PDK1 is critical for AKT activation, but additional phosphorylation of Ser473 by the mTOR complex 2 (mTORC2) enhances AKT activity.[10] AKT signaling is complex, involving multiple substrates and positive and negative feedback loops. AKT phosphorylates more than 100 substrates and modulates a variety of cellular functions including cellular proliferation[11] and metabolism[12,13] (Figure 4.2 and Table 4.1). One recently identified AKT substrate is the tuberous sclerosis 2 (TSC2) tumor suppressor, which is a GTPase-activating protein (GAP) for the monomeric guanosine triphosphate (GTP) that antagonize mTORC1

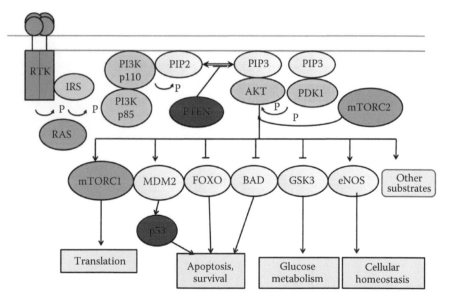

FIGURE 4.2 AKT signaling: AKT kinases are activated by phosphorylation at threonine 308 and serine 473 through the action of PDK1 and mTOR–rictor complex (mTORC2), respectively. AKT signaling controls key cellular processes of transcription, translation, cell cycle regulation, cytoskeletal reorganization, survival, and apoptosis. AKT substrates consist of the mTOR–raptor complex (mTORC1) preapoptotic proteins, BCL2-associated agonist of cell death (BAD) and caspase 9, the growth-inhibitory proteins, glycogen synthase 3 beta (GSK3β) and the forkhead box O transcription factors (FOXO), endothelial nitric oxide (eNOS) involved in angiogenesis and cell homeostasis, and the murine double minute 2 (MDM2) ubiquitin ligase involved in apoptosis. Note oncogenes are colored in green and tumor suppressors in red.

signaling through the inhibition of Ras homologue enriched in brain (Rheb). AKT phosphorylates and inhibits TSC2, allowing Rheb to activate mTORC1, which in turn phosphorylates its downstream targets, S6 kinase 1 (S6K1) and eukaryotic initiation factor 4E-binding protein 1 (4EBP1). AKT is one of the main regulators of mTORC1 complex, which is involved in protein translation and ribosome biogenesis.[14]

mTOR integrates growth factor, nutrients, and energy signaling to coordinate cell growth and proliferation.[14] mTOR forms two different protein complexes. The mTOR complex-1 (mTORC1) contains regulatory-associated protein of mTOR (Raptor), mammalian ortholog of LST8 (mLST8/GβL), DEP domain–containing mTOR-interacting protein (deptor), and proline-rich AKT substrate 40 (PRAS40), whereas mTOR complex-2 (mTORC2) contains rapamycin-insensitive companion of mTOR (Rictor), GβL, protein with rictor, deptor, and mammalian stress-activated protein kinase–interacting protein 1 (mSin1). The two complexes are activated in different ways and have distinct substrate specificity and functions.[14] mTORC1 responds to energy, amino acid, growth factors, and oxygen levels, whereas mTORC2 is activated by growth factors. Activated mTORC1 phosphorylates S6K1 and 4EBP1, which are two proteins involved in the regulation of translation initiation, protein synthesis, and cell growth. (Figure 4.3 and Table 4.1). mTORC1 is more sensitive than mTORC2 to rapamycin.

PI3K, AKT, and mTORC1 and 2 activities are controlled by multiple regulatory feedback loops. mTORC2 phosphorylates AKT providing a positive feedback loop on this pathway.[15] Negative feedback regulation of AKT can occur through S6K1, which catalyzes an inhibitory phosphorylation on insulin receptor substrate protein 1 (IRS1), abrogating activation of PI3K.[3] Inhibition of mTORC1 by deptor activates AKT indirectly, by relieving the inhibitory loop on PI3K triggered by S6K1.[16] Thus, deptor has both tumor-suppressive (by the inhibition of mTORC1 and 2) and oncogenic roles (by the activation of AKT). Tuberous sclerosis complex (TSC) is composed of two proteins TSC1 and TSC2. TSC1/2 complex inhibits mTORC1 and positively regulates mTORC2 kinase activity by an unknown mechanism.[17] All the regulatory loops describe a cellular mechanism that prevents simultaneous activation of mTORC1 and mTORC2 and sustained activation of the PI3K pathway.[14]

PI3K–AKT–mTOR PATHWAY IN CANCER

Aberrant activation of PI3K–AKT–mTOR pathway is linked to cancer development and is frequently detected in malignancies (Table 4.2). The best-known genetic alterations of this pathway are activating point mutation of PI3K, amplification of genomic region containing AKT, and the loss of the tumor suppressor PTEN.[18]

Although amplification and point mutations have been described in PI3K kinase and regulatory genes, *PIK3CA* mutations are the most common and best described. The *PIK3CA* point mutations detected in cancer are somatic and heterozygous mutations and can be divided into four classes defined by the four domains of the catalytic subunit in which they occur: the adaptor-binding domain, C2 domain, helical domain, and catalytic domain. Analysis of *PIK3CA* gene in human tumor samples has identified somatic mutations that affect 38 residues.[19] The majority of the mutations map to three sites, E542 and E545 in the helical domain (exon 9)

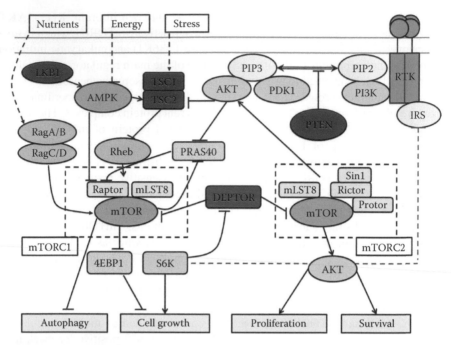

FIGURE 4.3 mTOR signaling: mTOR is functional in two protein complexes: mTORC1, containing raptor, mammalian lethal with Sec 13 protein 8 (mLST8), and deptor; and mTORC2, containing rictor, protor, mLST8, mammalian stress–activated protein kinase–interacting protein (Sin1), and deptor. Critical inputs regulating mTORC1 include growth factors, amino acids, stress, energy levels, and oxygen. mTOR regulates cytoskeletal organization, cell survival, autophagy, and metabolism. mTORC1 is phosphorylated via AKT through inactivation of tuberous sclerosis complex (TSC 1 and 2).TSC2 is a GAP toward Ras homologue enriched in brain (Rheb) that activates mTORC1. AKT also signals to mTORC1 by phosphorylating proline-rich AKT substrate 40 kDa (PRAS). The energy sensing pathway is linked to mTOR through LKB1 (or STK11, serine–threonine kinase 11) and AMP-activated protein kinase (AMPK1). Amino acids also activate mTORC1 through the 4 Rag proteins (Rag A, B, C, D). mTORC1 regulates many biological processes through the phosphorylation of proteins involved in translation, such as p70 ribosomal S6Kinase (S6K1) and eukaryotic initiation factor 4E-binding protein 1 (4EBP1). mTORC2 complex phosphorylates many AGC kinases including AKT, serum, and glucocorticoid-induced protein kinase 1 (SGK1) and protein kinase C (PKC). Depicted in red dashed line is the negative feedback loop between 6SK and insulin receptor substrate (IRS), resulting in increased phosphorylation of AKT and its subsequent activation. *Note*: Oncogenes are colored in green and tumor suppressors in red.

and H1047 in the kinase domain (exon20). The E542 and E545 are commonly changed to lysine, whereas H1047 is frequently substituted with arginine. These mutations are of functional importance as they result in gain of enzymatic function and induce oncogenic transformation.[20,21] Since p110α is a critical component of cellular physiology, small-molecule inhibitors that discriminate the mutated and wild-type form of PIK3CA might minimize undesirable effects that could arise from interference with the wild-type protein.[18,22]

TABLE 4.2
Oncogenes and Tumor Suppressor Genes in the PI3K–AKT–mTOR Pathway

Alterations in Cancer	Tumor Type
Proto-oncogenes	
PIK3CA mutations	Breast, colorectal, gastric, lung, thyroid, endometrial, esophageal, liver, and lung carcinomas; acute leukemia, GBM, and pituitary tumors
PI3Kα amplification	Breast, cervical, uterine, ovarian, gastric, thyroid, lung, and head and neck squamous cell carcinomas, pituitary tumor
PI3Kβ amplification	Bladder and colon carcinomas, GBM
PI3Kδ amplification	Acute myeloid leukemia, colon and bladder carcinoma, and GBM
PI3Kγ amplification	Medulloblastoma, pancreatic ductal carcinoma, neuroblastoma
PIK3R1 mutation (p85α subunit)	Colon and ovarian carcinoma, GBM
AKT1 amplification	Gastric carcinoma, GBM, gliosarcoma
AKT2 amplification	Breast, ovarian, pancreatic, gastric, and head and neck carcinoma
AKT1 mutation	Breast, ovarian, pancreatic, and head and neck carcinoma
Increased AKT3 mRNA	Breast, prostate carcinomas
Increased 4EBP1 expression	Breast, colon, ovarian, and prostate carcinomas
eIF4E overexpression	Breast, colon, and head and neck carcinoma, non-Hodgkin's lymphoma, myelogenous leukemia
S6K1 amplification and overexpression	Lung, ovarian, breast, kidney, and liver carcinomas
Rheb overexpression	Breast, head and neck, and squamous carcinomas
Tumor suppressors	
PTEN mutation	Breast, colorectal, prostate, gastric, lung, kidney, ovarian, uterine, thyroid, endometrial, and head and neck carcinomas, GBM, melanoma
PTEN deletion/LOH	Bladder, breast, colorectal, gastric carcinomas, GBM, melanoma, T-cell acute lymphoblastic leukemia
SHIP-1 mutation	Acute myeloid leukemia
SHIP-1 deletion	Acute myeloid leukemia, T-cell lymphoblastic leukemia
SHIP-2 overexpression	Breast carcinoma
INPP4B LOH	Breast, ovarian carcinoma
TSC1/TSC2	Lymphangioleiomyomatosis
STK11 (LKB1)	Peutz–Jeghers syndrome

eIF4E, Eukaryotic initiation factor 4E; 4EBP1, eukaryotic initiation factor 4E-binding protein 1; GPCR, G-protein–coupled receptors; INPP4B, inositol polyphosphate 4-phosphatase type II; AKT, mammalian homologue of the retroviral transforming protein v-AKT; mTOR, mammalian target of rapamycin; mTORC, mammalian target of rapamycin complex; PTEN, phosphatase and tensing homologue deleted on chromosome 10; PtdIns, phosphatidylinositol; PI3K, phosphatidylinositol 3-kinase; PIK3CA, phosphatidylinositol 3-kinase catalytic subunit; PI3KR, phosphatidylinositol 3-kinase regulatory subunit; PDK1, phosphoinositide-dependent protein kinase 1; Rheb, Ras homologue enriched in brain; RTKs, tyrosine kinases; S6K1, S6 kinase 1; STK11, serine/threonine kinase 11; SHIP, Src-homology 2–containing inositol 5′-phosphatase; TSC1, tuberous sclerosis 1; TSC2, tuberous sclerosis 2.

The roles that AKT plays in cancer are complex. AKT isoforms can be activated by genetic mutations or genome amplifications and by mutations in upstream signaling components. *AKT2* is not mutated frequently in human cancer, but *AKT2* amplification was reported in human ovarian carcinoma and breast carcinomas.[23,24] A mutation of *AKT3* was reported in melanoma samples.[25] *AKT1* has been reported to be mutated in breast, colorectal, melanoma, and ovarian cancers.[26] A transforming E17K PH domain mutation in AKT1 has been reported in breast, colorectal, and ovarian cancers.[26] The mutant exhibits transforming activity in vitro and in vivo due to PIP3-independent recruitment to the membrane. This PH domain mutation in *AKT1* gene does not alter its sensitivity to ATP-competitive inhibitors, but does alter its sensitivity to allosteric kinase inhibitors.[26]

The pathway can also be activated through loss of function of tumor suppressor genes PTEN, TSC1/2, and serine/threonine kinase 11 (STK11). Aberrant expression and function of these tumor suppressors is common in human cancers. STK11 is an inhibitor of the mTOR pathway in response to energy starvation through its activation of 5′-AMP-activated protein kinase (AMPK).[27] STK11 is a tumor suppressor inactivated in Peutz–Jeghers syndrome, which includes the occurrence of gastrointestinal tract hamartomas.[28] PTEN is important in tumor suppression.[29,30] PTEN loss or mutation leads to accumulation of PtdIns (3,4,5) P3 that mimics the effect of PI3K activation and stimulates effectors such as AKT and mTOR[31,32] and to centromere breakage and chromosome instability.[33,34] PTEN loss of function occurs in 25%–30% of human cancers, particularly those of the endometrium, central nervous system, skin, prostate, and breast, and certain hematologic malignancies.[29,35–37] Loss of function may occur through mutations, deletions, and transcriptional silencing through hypermethylation, protein instability[38], or microRNA regulation of its expression.[39,40] In general, germ-line mutation in *PTEN*, *TSC1/2*, and *STK11* is associated with neoplastic syndromes and increased risk of developing invasive cancers. In vitro and in vivo models suggest that loss of function is associated with aberrant activation of the PI3K pathway and neoplastic transformation that is amenable to pharmacological inhibition that may result in an anticancer effect.

In addition to PTEN, there are two additional inositol polyphosphate phosphatases that are involved in regulating the PI3K pathway through the degradation of phosphoinositols: Src-homology 2 (SH2)–containing inositol 5′-phosphatase (SHIP) and inositol polyphosphate 4-phosphatase type II (INPP4B). There are two SHIP phosphatases, SHIP-1 and SHIP-2, and they play a key role in the negative regulation of AKT activity within the hematopoietic cells.[41,42] Evidence suggests that INPP4B is a tumor suppressor gene involved in several epithelial carcinomas, including breast, ovarian, and prostate cancer.[43–46]

There is now extensive evidence that various components of this pathway play critical roles in normal and neoplastic cell functions. Key to successful clinical development of small-molecule inhibitors will be identifying whether the agents will have acceptable therapeutic window given the role the pathway plays in normal cell physiology, how the activity of specific agents to targets in the pathway are determined by the specific genetic events leading to aberrant pathway activation, and whether biomarkers can be identified that allow for selection of patients likely to respond to treatment.

AGENTS TARGETING PI3K–AKT–mTOR PATHWAY

PI3K INHIBITORS

PI3K inhibitors can be grouped into the two classes: lipid analogs that interfere with membrane binding through the PH domain and small-molecule kinase inhibitors that bind in the ATP binding-pocket of the catalytic domain of PI3K kinase and inhibit its activity.[47–49] PI3K class I inhibitors have antiproliferative, antiangiogenic effects and are modifiers of glucose methabolism.[47–49] They also are therapeutic agents that are broadly active in preclinical models, particularly tumor models with specific pathway mutations. Clinical trial results indicate that PI3K inhibitors have similar toxicity profiles. Rash, GI, thrombocytopenia, and liver enzyme elevations are the most significant toxicities in terms of frequency and severity. Hyperglycemia has been noted in preclinical and clinical studies and is expected given the role of the pathway in cellular metabolism and glucose/insulin regulation.[47–49] Objective tumor responses were uncommon but have been reported.[47,50] Tumor response may be linked to the presence of specific activation mutations in PI3K and whether agents effectively inhibit the mutant forms of the protein. Pharmacodynamic (PD) studies have shown inhibition of pathway components in tumor and surrogate normal tissue such as AKT, S6K1, the proliferation marker Ki67, and uptake of fluorodeoxyglucose (FDG) measured by positron emission tomography (PET). Currently, there are a number of PI3K and PI3K–mTOR dual inhibitors in clinical development that are summarized in Table 4.3. A selection of these agents is described in the succeeding text (Figure 4.4).

BKM120 (NVP-BKM120; Novartis)

BKM120 (NVP-BKM120; Novartis) is an orally bioavailable, reversible inhibitor of PI3K. This compound inhibits all four class I PI3K isoforms in biochemical assays with at least 50-fold selectivity against other protein kinases.[51] Tested in a panel of 353 cell lines, BKM120 exhibited preferential inhibition of tumor cell bearing PIK3CA mutations.[51] BKM120 also showed dose-dependent in vivo PD activity, as measured by inhibition of pAKT and tumor growth inhibition in xenograft models.[51]

Overall, there are approximately 40 ongoing phase I and II single-agent or in combination trials with BKM120. In a clinical phase I dose-escalation study of BKM120, the agent was well tolerated with an acceptable dose-dependent safety profile.[47] Toxicities reported were rash, hyperglycemia, and mood alteration that may reflect on-target effect of PI3K inhibition in normal tissue. A single partial response (triple-negative breast cancer) and a number of patients with prolonged stable disease of at least 8 months duration[47] were seen among the 35 patients. BKM120 demonstrated dose-dependent PD effects based on changes in FDG-PET, fasting insulin C-peptide, fasting blood glucose, and pS6K1.[47] Phase II trials of BKM120 are ongoing in endometrial cancer, castration-resistant metastatic prostate cancer, recurrent glioblastoma (GBM), metastatic breast and colorectal cancers, and non-small cell lung cancer (NSCLC).

TABLE 4.3
Selective Inhibitors in Clinical Development

Inhibitor	Company	Target	Phase of Clinical Development	Tumor Type	References
BKM120	Novartis	Class I PI3Ks	Phase I, II	Solid tumors	[47,51]
XL 147	Exelixis/Sanofi-Aventis	Class I PI3Ks	Phase I, II	Solid tumors	[52,53]
GDC0941	Genentech	Class I PI3Ks	Phase I, II	Lymphoma, lung, breast, cancer, other solid tumor	[50,54]
PX866	Oncothyreon	Class I PI3Ks	Phase I, II	Glioma, breast, colon, prostate, lung, pancreatic cancers	[55,56]
GSK2126458 (GSK 458)	GlaxoSmithKline	Class I PI3Ks	Phase I	Lymphoma and solid tumors	[57]
BAY 80–6946	Bayer	Class I PI3Ks	Phase I	Solid tumors, hematologic malignancies	[58,59]
BYL719	Novartis	PI3Kα	Phase I	Solid tumors	[60]
CAL 101 (GS-1101)	Gilead/Calistoga	PI3Kδ	Phase II	Leukemia, lymphoma, and solid tumors	[61–63]
UCN-01	Keryx Biopharmaceuticals	PDK1, PKC isoforms	Phase I, II	Leukemia, lymphoma, ovarian, melanoma	[64]
MK 2206	Merck	Pan AKT	Phase I, II	Solid tumors	[65–67]

RX-0201	Rexahn Pharmaceuticals	Pan AKT	Phase I, II	Kidney and pancreatic cancer	[68,69]
PBI-05204 (oleandrin)	Phoenix Biotechnology	Pan AKT, FGF-2, NF-kB, and S6K	Phase I	Solid tumors	[70]
GSK2110183	GlaxoSmithKline	Pan AKT	Phase I, II	Hematologic malignancies, Langerhans cell histiocytosis, ovarian cancer	www.clinicaltrails.gov
GSK2141795	GlaxoSmithKline	Pan AKT	Phase I	Lymphoma, ovarian and other solid tumors	www.clinicaltrails.gov
GDC-0068	Genentech	Pan AKT	Phase I	Pancreatic cancer and solid tumors	www.clinicaltrails.gov
VD-0002	VioQuest Pharmaceuticals	Pan AKT	Phase I	Solid tumors and hematologic malignancies	www.clinicaltrails.gov
MKC-1	EntreMed	AKT, mTOR	Phase I, II	Ovarian, breast, lung, pancreatic, colorectal carcinoma	[71,72]
AZD8055	AstraZeneca	mTORC1/mTORC2	Phase I, II	GBM, liver, other solid tumors, lymphomas	[73,74]
AZD20114	AstraZeneca	mTORC1/mTORC2	Phase I	Solid tumors	www.clinicaltrails.gov
OSI-027	Astellas/OSI Pharmaceuticals	mTORC1/mTORC2	Phase I	Solid tumors, Lymphomas	[75]
INK-128	Intellikine	mTORC1/mTORC2	Phase I	Myeloma, Waldenström macroglobulinemia	[76]
CC-223	Celgene	mTORC1/mTORC2	Phase I	lymphoma, myeloma	[77]

(continued)

TABLE 4.3 (continued)
Selective Inhibitors in Clinical Development

Inhibitor	Company	Target	Phase of Clinical Development	Tumor Type	References
BEZ235, NVP-BEZ235	Novartis	PI3K/mTOR	Phase I, II	Solid tumors, breast cancer	[78,79]
BGT226 (CBGT226A1101)	Novartis	PI3K/mTOR	Phase I, II	Solid tumors	[80–82]
XL-765 (SAR245409)	Exelixis	PI3K/mTOR	Phase I, II	GBM, lung, lymphoma, other solid tumors	[83–85]
GDC0980	Genentech	PI3K/mTOR	Phase I, II	breast cancer, lymphoma and solid tumors	[86,87]
SF1126	Semafore Pharmaceuticals	PI3K/mTOR	Phase I	Solid tumors and B-cell malignancies	[88–90]
PF-4691502	Pfizer	PI3K/mTOR	Phase I	Breast cancer and other solid tumors	www.clinicaltrails.gov

FGF-2, fibroblast growth factor; AKT, mammalian homologue of the retroviral transforming protein v-AKT; mTORC, mammalian target of rapamycin complex; NF-κB, nuclear factor kappa-light-chain-enhancer of activated B cells; PI3K, phosphatidylinositol 3-kinase; PDK1, phosphoinositide-dependent protein kinase 1; PKC, protein kinase C; S6K1, S6 kinase 1.

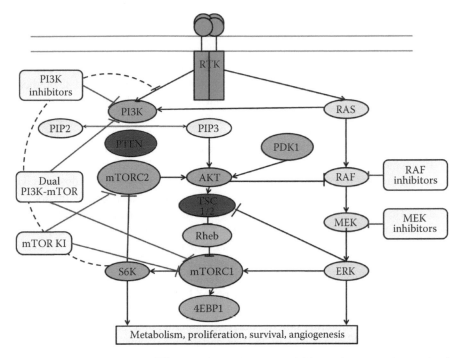

FIGURE 4.4 Targeting the PI3K pathway in cancer: Inhibitors that target key nodes in the PI3K signaling pathway, including RTK, PI3K, AKT, and mTOR, have reached clinical trials. There are four groups of PI3K pathway inhibitors: (1) PI3K inhibitors, (2) AKT inhibitors, (3) dual PI3K/mTOR inhibitors that inhibits both PI3K and mTOR kinases, and (4) rapalogs and mTOR kinase inhibitors that inhibit both mTORC1 and mTORC2 complexes. Combination of PI3K inhibitors, with growth factors, other PI3K pathway inhibitors, and mitogen-activated protein kinase (RAF, MEK, and ERK) inhibitors may achieve more effective clinical results. *Note*: Oncogenes are colored in green and tumor suppressors in red.

XL147 (SAR245408; Exelixis and Sanofi-Aventis)

XL147 (SAR245408; Exelixis and Sanofi-Aventis) is another selective PI3K inhibitor that has shown single-agent preclinical activity in human breast cancer cell lines and xenograft models with an IC_{50} of approximately 6 μM and has demonstrated synergistic activity with other therapeutics.[91–93] In an open-label, phase I dose-escalation study of XL147 in patients with advanced solid tumors and lymphomas, the agent reduced PI3K pathway signaling and phosphorylation of MEK and ERK in tumor tissue associated with reductions in Ki67 and increase in apoptosis.[52] The MTD of XL147 was 600 mg/day with either intermittent or continuous dosing schedules. The DLT for the intermittent dosing schedule was rash. Of the 75 evaluable patients, 13 (17%) patients had stable disease and 1 (1%) patient with NSCLC had a partial response.[52]

GDC-0941 (Genentech)

GDC-0941 (Genentech) is a specific inhibitor of class I PI3K with demonstrated selectivity against a large panel of protein kinases, including mTOR and DNA-PK.

In preclinical models, GDC-0941 led to cell cycle arrest and induced apoptosis in a panel of tumor cell lines and also blocks endothelial cell growth.[94] Oral dosing of GDC-0941 inhibited human tumor growth in xenograft models, including those with mutations in PIK3CA, PTEN, and K-Ras genes.[95] A recent study used a large panel of breast cancer cell lines and in vivo xenograft models to identify candidate predictive biomarkers for GDC-0941. The study found that models harboring mutations in PI3KCA and amplification of HER2 were more likely to be sensitive to the inhibitor. However, some models that do not harbor these alterations were also sensitive to the antitumor effects of GDC-0941, suggesting a need for additional diagnostic markers.[96]

Two phase I dose-escalation studies, evaluating GDC-0941 in patients with advanced tumors, reported encouraging results. In one study, a single dose of GDC-0941 was administrated followed by a 1 week washout and then QD dosing for 21 of 28 days. Drug-related adverse events (AEs) were nausea, diarrhea, vomiting, dysgeusia, and decreased appetite. Signs of clinical activity included a partial response by RECIST in a patient with melanoma and an 80% decrease in CA-125 in an ovarian cancer patient. Reductions in FDG-PET were seen in a small-bowel GIST patient and an ovarian cancer patient. Additional PD studies showed 56% decrease in pS6K1 staining in paired biopsies.[50] In another phase I study, GDC-0941 was dosed QD and BID for 21/28 day schedule. Drug-related AEs were similar in both arms with nausea, diarrhea, vomiting, fatigue, decrease appetite, and rash. Two patients have exhibited partial response by RECIST: an endocervical cancer patient and an ER+, HER2- breast cancer patient. Additional signs of antitumor activity include CA-125 responses in three patients with ovarian cancer.[54] The MTD was exceeded at 450 mg.

PX-866 (Oncothyreon)

PX-866 (Oncothyreon) is a semisynthetic derivative of wortmannin and irreversibly inhibits PI3K through the formation of a covalent bond with PI3K.[55] The primary metabolite of PX-866, 17-OH wortmannin, is even more potent than the parent compound.[55] In a panel of human tumor xenografts, the presence of PIK3CA mutations and the loss of PTEN activity were positive predictors of response to PX-866, whereas oncogenic Ras mutations were a predictor for resistance.[55] In glioma cells, PX-866 inhibited proliferation in a variety of cell lines, with greater sensitivity seen in PTEN-negative cell lines. PX-866 also increased autophagy and decreased the invasive and angiogenic potential of tumor cells.[97]

Results from a single-agent, phase I open-label, dose-escalation study of PX-866 in patients with advanced solid tumors demonstrated that PX-866 was well tolerated using both intermittent and continuous dosing schedule.[56,98] The most common AEs were diarrhea, nausea, vomiting, fatigue, and ALT and AST level elevation. The MTD for the intermittent schedule was 12 mg. Overall, 13 of 60 (22%) patients treated with PX-866 have stable disease after a median 57 days on study.[56] Phase II studies are ongoing, enrolling patients with relapsed GBM and castration-resistant prostate carcinoma.

CAL-101 (Calistoga Pharmaceuticals)

CAL-101 (Calistoga Pharmaceuticals) is an oral p110δ isoform-specific PI3K inhibitor and potent in inhibitor of PI3K signaling in hematologic malignancies in laboratory and clinical studies. Preclinical studies of CAL-101 as a single agent and in combination with other drugs demonstrate efficacy in chronic lymphocytic leukemia (CLL), B-cell lymphoproliferative disorders, and multiple myeloma.[63,99] Early results from two phase I trials have been promising. In an interim analysis of phase I trial in patients with relapsed or refractory CLL or B-cell non-Hodgkin lymphoma (NHL) treated at 50–350 mg BID, the dose-limiting toxicity was a reversible elevation in serum AST and ALT seen in 21% of patients treated at the two highest dose levels.[63,100] Objective responses were seen in 9 of 15 of indolent NHL, 6 of 7 mantle cell lymphoma (MCL), and 4 of 17 CLL patients. Similarly promising clinical activity was seen in a second study of previously treated CLL patients evaluating CAL-101 doses of 50–350 mg BID and 300 mg QD. The overall intention to treat response rate was 26%. Medians for duration of response and progression-free survival had not been reached at 11 months of follow-up.[62,63] Reported AEs included pneumonia, neutropenia, thrombocytopenia, anemia, and ALT/AST increase. Results support the 150 mg BID dose for future single-agent and combination studies.

DUAL PI3K/mTOR INHIBITORS

There are pragmatic and scientific reasons for the development of dual inhibitors of PI3K and mTOR. Identifying PI3K or mTOR-specific inhibitors with appropriate pharmacological properties is challenging due to the structural similarities of the catalytic domain of p110 and mTOR. In addition, PI3K/AKT pathway activating mutation also activate the mTOR pathway, a validated cancer therapeutic target. Thus, dual inhibition of these targets may be a more effective therapeutic approach. In general, the dual PI3K/mTOR–targeting agents induce reversible ATP-competitive inhibition. Preclinical and clinical studies results to date suggest that these inhibitors may be more active but also more toxic that rapamycin and its derivatives.

BEZ235 (NVP-BEZ235; Novartis)

BEZ235 (NVP-BEZ235; Novartis) is an imidazo (4,5-c)quinoline derivative that inhibits PI3K and mTOR kinase activity by binding to the ATP-binding cleft of these enzymes. It has been extensively studied in preclinical models, including glioma, sarcoma, and breast, renal cell, and lung carcinomas.[101–104] BEZ235 treatment of glioma cell lines led to G_1 cell cycle arrest, induced autophagy, and decreased the expression of vascular endothelial growth factor (VEGF).[105] In vivo, BEZ235 significantly prolonged the survival of tumor-bearing mice.[105]

Several trials of BEZ235, either as a single agent or in combination, in patients with advanced solid tumors are ongoing. Two formulations have been assessed. A phase I multicenter, single-agent, dose-escalation study of BEZ 235 administrated once daily as a gelatin capsule was conducted in advanced solid tumors patients.[78] Among 59 patients, two partial responses (one Cowden syndrome patient and one breast carcinoma patient) and 16 minor responses were observed. There were no DLTs and AEs included nausea, vomiting, diarrhea, fatigue, anemia, and anorexia. BEZ235 exhibited dose-dependent PI3K inhibition as measured by elevation of plasma C-peptide level.[78] In a phase I/II b study, 28 patients with advanced solid tumors were treated with a special delivery system (SDS) capsule formulation of BEZ235 as a single agent and in combination with trastuzumab.[79] The MTD for BEZ235 SDS was 1600 mg/day. BEZ235 was well tolerated and the most AEs considered to be related to the study drug included nausea, diarrhea, vomiting, and fatigue.[79] Six (40%) of the 15 evaluable patients had stable disease; four of whom were treated for longer than 12 weeks.

NVP-BGT226 (Novartis)

NVP-BGT226 (Novartis) is a small-molecule inhibitor of all class I PI3Ks and mTOR. BGT226 specifically inhibits p110α, β, δ, and γ with a preference for wild-type and mutated α-isoform and mTOR.[81] Preclinical studies showed that BGT226 inhibited growth in myeloma, pancreatic, and head and neck cancer cell lines in a time- and dose-dependent manner.[80,106,107] Fifty-seven patients were enrolled on a phase I trial of BGT226 administered at 2.5–125 mg/day three times weekly (TIW).[81] Three patients treated at 125 mg had DLTs (grade 3 nausea, vomiting, diarrhea). Other BGT226 AEs included nausea, diarrhea, vomiting, and fatigue. Seventeen patients (30%) had stable disease as best RECIST response, and thirty patients (53%) achieved stable metabolic disease as assessed by FDG-PET. No correlation between metabolic response and tumor shrinkage was observed.[81]

XL765 (SAR245409; Exelixis and Sanofi-Aventis)

XL765 (SAR245409; Exelixis and Sanofi-Aventis) exhibits specific PI3K inhibition with nanomolar IC_{50} values against α-, β-, γ-, and δ-isoforms. XL765 dose-dependent cytotoxicity in GBM cell lines has been reported.[84,108] In a phase I single-agent study in 79 patients, XL765 was well tolerated.[85] The maximum administrated dose (MAD) is 120 mg BID. On the QD schedule, the MAD is 100 mg and the preliminary MTD is 90 mg. The most common related AEs with XL765 were nausea, diarrhea, anorexia, elevated liver enzymes, rash, and vomiting. Currently, phase 1 combinations studies of XL765 with erlotinib[109] and temozolomide[108,110] in patients with malignant glioma are underway.

GDC-0980 (Genentech)

GDC-0980 (Genentech) is a selective, orally bioavailable inhibitor of class I PI3K and mTOR kinase.[111] In contrast to mTOR inhibitors, GDC-0980 induced apoptosis in several cancer cell lines, including those with direct pathway activation via PI3K and PTEN.[111] In a phase I dose-escalation trial, the agent was administered in a 21/28-day schedule in patients with solid tumors and NHL.[86] The MTD was 70 mg with DLT of maculopapular rash. Of the 33 patients enrolled, 3 patients with mesothelioma demonstrated 23%–28% decreases in tumor activity by RECIST and 5 of 6 patients had 29%–64% decreases in maximal standardized uptake value by FDG-PET.[87]

SF1126 (Semaphore Pharmaceuticals)

SF1126 (Semaphore Pharmaceuticals) is an intravenous small-molecule pan-isoform PI3K and mTOR dual inhibitor. SF126 is LY294002 linked to a peptide inhibitor of αVβ3 and αVβ5-integrins, transmembrane cell adhesion proteins that are expressed in tumor vasculature. SF1126 induces cytostasis in tumor xenografts models, associated with the pharmacokinetic accumulation of the agent in tumor tissue and the PD knockdown of phosphorylated AKT in vivo.[112] Unlike LY294002, SF126 is water-soluble and suitable for clinical use. In a phase I trial for patients with advanced solid tumors, SF1126 was given as a twice weekly intravenous infusion. The drug was well tolerated and just one patient had grade 3 diarrhea. Stable disease was reported in 11 of 26 patients, and a significant inhibition of pS6K by immunohistochemistry in a tumor biopsy of a pancreatic cancer patient was measured.[89] Current clinical studies include a phase I trial in advanced solid tumors and a phase I trial in B-cell malignancies.[88,90]

In summary, a number of selective PI3K and dual PI3K–mTOR inhibitors have entered clinical development. The agents appear to be well tolerated and most agents have been shown to inhibit PI3K in tumor and/or normal tissues. The extent of pathway inhibition has been variable across the trials with different agents. This variability may reflect different effects of the agents on targets or in the techniques and technologies used. The degree of target and pathway inhibition required for antitumor effect is uncertain. Whether dual inhibitors will be superior to specific PI3K or mTOR inhibitors will require further evaluation. RECIST responses are uncommon with pan-PI3K inhibitors. A number of trials have assessed antitumor effects in patients with tumors harboring mutations in PI3K, Ras, and PTEN. Results suggest that objective tumor responses may correlate with the presence of these markers; however, further clinical evaluation is needed to clarify the correlation between antitumor activity and the presence of specific mutations. The most dramatic activity has been reported with CAL-101 that is a specific inhibitor of p110δ isoform expressed in blood cells. The activity may be due to the particular sensitivity of malignant lymphoproliferative cells to PI3K inhibitors or due to the wider therapeutic window achieved with a delta isoform–specific inhibitor.

AKT INHIBITORS

Small-molecule inhibitor of AKT can be organized in several chemical classes: phosphatidylinositol analogs, ATP-competitive small-molecule, pseudosubstrate compounds, and allosteric inhibitors.[69,113] AKT inhibitors exhibit antiproliferative activity in most in vitro models and antiapoptotic activities in some models. Most of the more specific AKT inhibitors have demonstrated target modulation by assessing the phosphorylation status of AKT, PRAS40, and other substrates in surrogate normal tissue and/or tumor. Early clinical trials have shown that objective responses are uncommon, and results from trials of relatively nonspecific agents such as perifosine have not been promising.[114,115] Results from recent trials of small-molecule inhibitors are summarized in this section.

MK-2206 (Merck)

MK-2206 (Merck) is an oral agent that allosterically and selectively inhibits phosphorylation of both Thr308 and Ser473 residues of all AKT isoforms.[116] MK-2206 caused 60% growth inhibition and inhibited all AKT isoforms in mouse xenograft studies of the A2780 ovarian cancer cell line.[117] Combination studies of MK-2206 and other targeted therapies in preclinical models demonstrated synergistic inhibition of cell proliferation in different human cancer cell lines.[118]

Recently, a first-in-man phase I trial of MK-2206 in patients with advanced solid tumors showed that MK-2206 was well tolerated and inhibited AKT in normal and tumor tissue samples.[66] The MTD of MK-2206 was 60 mg on alternate days. Dose-limiting toxicities were skin rash, stomatitis, nausea, pruritus, hyperglycemia, and diarrhea.[66] Demonstrated PD effects of targeted inhibition included suppression of AKT Ser473 phosphorylation in tumor biopsies, suppression of phosphorylated threonine-246 PRAS40 in hair follicles, and reversible hyperglycemia associated with increased in insulin c-peptide.[66] A patient with pancreatic adenocarcinoma had a 23% reduction in tumor measurements.[66] Other phase I studies assessing the combinations of MK-2206 with erlotinib, carboplatin, paclitaxel, and docetaxel and trastuzumab and lapatinib in HER2-amplified tumors are ongoing.[69]

PBI-05204 (Oleandrin; Phoenix Biotechnology)

PBI-05204 (oleandrin; Phoenix Biotechnology) is a derivative of *Nerium oleander* and is an inhibitor of several kinases, including AKT, fibroblast growth factor 2 (FGF2), NF-κB, and S6K.[119] A recent report of a phase I clinical trial of the agent in advanced solid tumor patients stated that 15 patients had received doses ranging from 0.6 to 10.2 mg oral daily and that PBI-05204 was well tolerated with few toxicities.[70] Three patients with bladder, colorectal, and fallopian tube carcinomas had stable disease lasting more than 4 months. PBI-05204 reduced pAKT, pS6K, and pS6 in PBMCs from four patients.

GSK690693 (GlaxoSmithKline)

GSK690693 (GlaxoSmithKline) is an ATP-competitive inhibitor of all AKT isoforms at nanomolar concentrations. Daily administration of GSK690693 produced antitumor activity in mice bearing established human SKOV-3 ovarian, LNCaP prostate, and BT474 and HCC1954 breast carcinoma xenografts[120] and in myr-AKT mice expressing a constitutively activated membrane-bound form of AKT.[121] Preclinical studies showed that dosing was associated with reduction in the phosphorylation of AKT substrates, inhibition of glycogen synthesis, activation of glycogenolysis,[48] and induction of peripheral insulin resistance. A phase I clinical study of GSK690693 intravenous formulation was terminated due to drug-related toxicities (ClinicalTrial.gov.identifier: NCT00493818). GlaxoSmithKline is developing an alternate orally administered agent, GSK2141795.

In summary, among AKT inhibitors in development, results to date suggest that the allosteric inhibitor MK-2206 is the most advanced agent that has demonstrated acceptable tolerability, PD effects on target and pathway, and good pharmacology. Additional studies will be required to define antitumor activity, preferred combination regimens, and markers of sensitivity or resistance for patient selection.

Mammalian Target of Rapamycin Kinase Inhibitors

mTOR is a validated cancer therapeutic target. Preclinical investigation of mTOR signaling network has deciphered important mechanisms contributing to human tumorigenesis and stimulated development of mTOR targeted anticancer therapies. There are two classes of mTOR inhibitors: rapalogs and mTOR kinase inhibitors (TOR-KI). The rapalogs improve cancer patient outcomes in a number of settings. TOR-KIs appear to be more active than rapalogs in preclinical studies and are currently in early clinical trials. Recent results are highlighted in this section.

Rapalogs

Rapalogs include rapamycin (sirolimus, Rapamune®, Wyeth), temsirolimus (CCI-779, Torisel®, Wyeth), everolimus (RAD001, Afinitor®, Novartis), and ridaforolimus (AP23473, MK-8669, deforolimus, Ariad, Merck).[122] Rapalogs have antiproliferative and immunosuppressive activity that is mediated by allosteric inhibition of mTORC1. Rapalogs complex with the immunophilin, FK506-binding protein 12, (FKBP12), and bind to the TORC1 C-terminus at the FKBP12–rapamycin–binding domain, causing a conformational change that inhibits the catalytic function of the protein.[123,124] mTORC2 is less sensitive to rapalogs: in a minority of cell lines, a prolonged exposure to rapamycin also inhibits mTORC2 activation of AKT. The mechanism through which rapamycin inhibits mTORC2 is not fully known but may be related to the intracellular scavenging of mTOR.[125]

Phase III trials have been conducted for three rapalogs. These agents have been well tolerated. Mucositis, thrombocytopenia, infection, and rarely pneumonitis have been reported AEs. Temsirolimus and everolimus have been approved for the treatment of metastatic renal cell carcinoma (RCC).[126,127] Temsirolimus is also approved for the treatment of MCL[128] and everolimus has been approved for treatment of neuroendocrine tumors and, in combination with exemestane, in breast cancer.[129] Ridaforolimus was shown to improve progression-free survival in patients with soft tissue sarcoma.[130,131] Rapalogs have shown promising activity in endometrial carcinoma.[132] Although rapalogs have a role as cancer therapeutics, overall their impact on patient benefit has been relatively modest, and results suggest that only a subset of patients are likely to have tumors that are sensitive to rapalogs. Unfortunately, there are no markers that clearly identify which patients are likely to benefit from treatment.

Both preclinical and clinical studies have shown that rapalogs are primarily cytostatic.[133] A number of reasons have been proposed for the modest activity of rapalogs. The effects of rapalogs in cancer may be limited by feedback activation of PI3K, MAPK, mTORC2, and downstream AGC kinases, all of which circumvent the rapalog effects on protein biosynthesis and cell cycle. The presence of these feedback loops supports two approaches to improve clinical outcomes with mTOR inhibitors: (1) developing agents that more effectively inhibit mTOR and (2) developing combination regimens with targeted agents such as IGF1R, PI3K, AKT, or MAPK inhibitors or standard hormonal agents and chemotherapy. Clinical trials in a variety of tumors and hematologic malignancies are testing these approaches.

mTOR Kinase Inhibitors

The recognition that rapalogs suboptimally inhibit mTOR substrates and cause feedback activation of several oncogenic pathways has prompted the development of TOR-KIs. mTOR kinase inhibitors inhibit both TORC1 and TORC2 functions and have the potential to more profoundly inhibit protein and lipid biosynthesis, cell growth, and cell cycle progression than rapalogs.[134] TOR-KIs suppress not only mTORC1 activation on 4EBP1 but also mTORC2 activation of AKT/GSK3β and PKC pathways[135] and AKT/SGK1/RSK1-mediated p27-RhoA effects on tumor cell motility and metastasis.[136] TOR-KIs may oppose glycolysis more strongly than rapamycin due to the lack of feedback activation of PI3K, direct inhibition of mTORC2, and loss of AKT-dependent glutamate-1 accumulation.[137] TOR-KIs also block cell lipid biosynthetic processes that contribute to the selective loss of rapidly proliferating tumor cells.[138,139] Collectively, these data indicate that TOR-KIs may more effectively oppose tumor proliferation, invasion, metastasis, angiogenesis, and survival compared to rapalogs. TOR-KIs in preclinical and clinical development include WYE354 and WYE132 (Pfizer),[137] PP30 and PP242 (INK-128, Intellikine),[140] AZD8055 (AstraZeneca),[141] OSI-027(OSI Pharmaceuticals), and Torin1.[142]

AZD8055 (AstraZeneca)

AZD8055 (AstraZeneca) is an orally administered, specific mTOR kinase inhibitor with growth-inhibitory effect in vitro and antitumor activity in vivo.[143] AZD8055 inhibited the phosphorylation of S6K, 4EBP1, AKT, and other downstream proteins.[141] AZD8055 induced p21 and p27 resulting in G1-phase arrest and inhibition of proliferation to a greater extent than rapamycin.[144] Interestingly, cell lines resistant to rapamycin and AKT inhibition remained sensitive to AZD8055.[141,145] A phase I trial of AZD8055 in patients with advanced solid tumors reported that the recommended phase 2 dose for AZD8055 is 90 mg BD.[73] DLTs were elevations in hepatic transaminases that occurred between day 35 and 45 and with no clear relationship with plasma concentration of AZD8055. Toxicities frequently associated with administration of rapalogs, such as rash and mucositis, were not dose limiting.

OSI-027 (OSI Pharmaceuticals)

OSI-027 (OSI Pharmaceuticals) is a selective and potent mTORC1 and mTORC2 inhibitor.[146] OSI-027 inhibited phosphorylation of 4E-BP1, S6K1, and AKT as well as cell proliferation and tumor growth in diverse in vitro and in vivo cancer cell models.[146] In a phase I single-agent trial, patients received escalating doses of OSI-027 in three schedules (S1: days 1–3q7d, S2: once weekly, and S3: continuous once daily). S1 and S2 patients were dosed at 10, 15, and 20 mg and S3 patients at 5, 10, and 20 mg. OSI-027 administration led to reduced phosphorylation of 4EBP1in PBMCs from 13 of 23 patients.[75] Eight patients have had stable disease lasting more than 12 weeks. The MTD has not been reached and dose-escalation studies are ongoing.

In summary, it is too early to determine whether TOR-KIs will result in superior clinical outcomes compared to rapalogs. Although preclinical efficacy evaluations have identified very promising antitumor activity, a key question is whether TOR-KIs will have a favorable therapeutic index as effects on proliferative and metabolic pathways in normal cells may lead to enhanced toxicity. Similar to other agents targeting the PI3K pathway, identifying predictive markers of sensitivity and resistance, optimal dose/schedule, and partners in combination regimens may be key to the successful clinical development of TOR-KIs.

BIOMARKERS FOR PI3K/AKT/mTOR INHIBITORS

PI3K–AKT–mTOR–targeted therapeutics translation to the clinic depends in the identification and application of a number of types of biomarkers, ranging from proof-of-mechanisms PD markers to predictive markers of drug activity.[147] PD biomarkers that assess for target and pathway inhibition have been evaluated in readily obtainable tissues, such as skin, hair, and peripheral blood mononuclear cells and tumor tissue.[148] The commonly used molecular markers of PI3K inhibition have been phosphorylated AKT and phosphorylated S6K1 in biopsies of the surrogate tissue and tumor tissue.[149] In addition, inhibition of the PI3K pathway in tumors can be measured by FDG-PET[150] or insulin C-peptide plasma levels due to pathway effects on glucose homeostasis, transport, and metabolism.[143] To date, these markers can be used to demonstrate proof of mechanism and target inhibition to support decisions regarding the selection of dose and schedule for further evaluation. However, there does not appear to be a strong correlation between changes in these PD markers and the occurrence of antitumor activity within patients.

Markers that identify patients likely to benefit from therapy are predictive markers. Such markers should distinguish sensitive from refractory tumors. Currently, candidate predictive biomarkers such as the presence of activating mutations or other genomic alterations within the pathway that lead to aberrant pathway activation are under investigation.[151] These markers include assessing for gain of function mutations and/or amplification in upstream growth factors such as HER2, as well as PIK3CA, AKT, and KRAS, and loss of function mutations or protein expression in PTEN. Other marker strategies are focused on the expression of PI3K pathway substrates and gene expression patterns purported to correlate with aberrant pathway activations.[152] It is too early to determine whether these markers sufficiently distinguish between patients with tumors that are sensitive versus insensitive to the agents.[153] It is likely that a predictive gene expression signature or a collection of markers will prove to be more helpful than a single biomarker in predicting responses to specific PI3K pathway inhibitors. Deciphering which tumors will respond to PI3K, AKT, or mTOR inhibition via mutation analysis or other techniques will not only aid the development of the investigational agents but also optimize their use in clinical practice.

COMBINATIONS OF TARGETED THERAPIES

The PI3K pathway is highly interconnected with multiple feedback loops and with complex cross talk with other signaling networks. As a result, combination strategies with either cytotoxic chemotherapies or other targeted agents will be necessary for the optimal use of these inhibitors. Combination therapy strategies could involve either vertical or horizontal (or parallel) pathway blockade[113] in tumor and endothelial cells.[154] Ideally, these combinations result in synergistic effects on tumor growth and acceptable toxicity.

The vertical blockade strategy involves combining one or more agents that target components within a specific pathway and is useful in overcoming negative feedback loops. Examples of this approach are the dual PI3K/mTOR inhibitors and the combination of everolimus with IGF-1R inhibitors that test this proof of concept.[155] Vertical blockade through combining PI3K/AKT/mTOR inhibitors with growth factor receptor inhibitors may also overcome mechanisms of resistance to growth factor inhibitors. There are preclinical data supporting the combinations PI3K pathway inhibitors with EGFR,[109] HER2,[156,157] or IGF-1R inhibitors.[155] For example, the presence of PIK3CA mutations and loss of PTEN in HER2-overexpressing cancer correlates with a lower response to trastuzumab[156] and lapatinib.[157] Treatment with the PI3K/mTOR dual inhibitors BEZ235 or GDC-0941 restored the action of trastuzumab and lapatinib in vitro and in vivo.[157,158] Multiple clinical trials evaluating the addition of growth factor and PI3K/AKT/mTOR pathway inhibitors are underway.[159]

Horizontal blockade involves the use of targeted agents to inhibit two or more signaling pathways. Recent data have demonstrated that deregulation of the Ras pathway is an important factor of tumor resistance to PIK3 inhibitors.[55,160] A number of studies with human cancer cell line and transgenic models that harbor both PI3K pathway and Ras mutations showed additive or synergistic effects when inhibitors of these pathways are combined.[55,160] The combination of BKM120 and GSK1120212, a MEK inhibitor, is being tested in phase I clinical trials in patients with advanced solid tumors.[51]

CONCLUSIONS

Progress in the development of PI3K, AKT, and mTOR inhibitors has been remarkable. Results of PI3K inhibitors in early preclinical studies and clinical trials have been promising. Laboratory studies have shown tumor growth inhibition in vitro and in vivo in multiple cancer models. Early clinical trials have reported favorable tolerability profiles. However, antitumor activity reported to date has been modest. Even when tested in patients with tumors harboring mutations in PI3K pathway, the degree of activity is considerably less than that seen with BRAF and ALK inhibitors. Possible reasons for the lack of activity are multiple: (1) the pathway is complex and feedback loops and cross talk can compensate for targeted inhibition, (2) biomarker(s) to select the patient population most likely to respond to inhibitors have not yet been identified, and (3) agents to date may be unable to sufficiently inhibit the PI3K pathway due to normal tissue toxicity. Clearly, target-related DLTs of hyperglycemia, diarrhea, and rash limit the ability to increase doses of pan-PI3K inhibitors. However, PI3Kδ inhibitors have less normal tissue toxicity due to limited normal tissue expression of the delta isoform. Tissue distribution results in a greater ability to escalate dose to inhibit PI3K isoform in malignant hematopoietic cells. In solid tumors, the ability to preferentially inhibit mutant forms of PI3K may similarly increase therapeutic window and allow greater target inhibition in tumor relative to normal tissue if such agents can be identified. Perhaps the greatest therapeutic efficacy of agents targeting the PI3K pathway will lay in their targeted administration to patients with cancer most likely to benefit and to the development of rational combination with drugs that block nodal pathways in cancer signaling and prevent feedback pathway activation. Thus, identification of reliable biomarkers to assist in patient selection and effective combination regimens are key priority areas of further research.

REFERENCES

1. Vanhaesebroeck B, Stephens L, Hawkins P. PI3K signalling: The path to discovery and understanding. *Nature Reviews* 2012;13:195–203.
2. Samuels Y, Wang Z, Bardelli A et al. High frequency of mutations of the PIK3CA gene in human cancers. *Science (New York)* 2004;304:554.
3. Chandarlapaty S, Sawai A, Scaltriti M et al. AKT inhibition relieves feedback suppression of receptor tyrosine kinase expression and activity. *Cancer Cell* 2011;19:58–71.
4. Keith CT, Schreiber SL. PIK-related kinases: DNA repair, recombination, and cell cycle checkpoints. *Science (New York)* 1995;270:50–51.
5. Liu P, Cheng H, Roberts TM et al. Targeting the phosphoinositide 3-kinase pathway in cancer. *Nature Reviews* 2009;8:627–644.
6. Ihle NT, Powis G. Take your PIK: Phosphatidylinositol 3-kinase inhibitors race through the clinic and toward cancer therapy. *Molecular Cancer Therapeutics* 2009;8:1–9.
7. Ihle NT, Powis G. The biological effects of isoform-specific PI3-kinase inhibition. *Current Opinion in Drug Discovery & Development* 2010;13:41–49.
8. Vanhaesebroeck B, Guillermet-Guibert J, Graupera M et al. The emerging mechanisms of isoform-specific PI3K signalling. *Nature Reviews* 2010;11:329–341.
9. Vanhaesebroeck B, Vogt PK, Rommel C. PI3K: From the bench to the clinic and back. *Current Topics in Microbiology and Immunology* 2010;347:1–19.
10. Sarbassov DD, Guertin DA, Ali SM et al. Phosphorylation and regulation of Akt/PKB by the rictor-mTOR complex. *Science (New York)* 2005;307:1098–1101.
11. Manning BD, Cantley LC. AKT/PKB signaling: Navigating downstream. *Cell* 2007;129:1261–1274.
12. Fujita N, Sato S, Katayama K et al. Akt-dependent phosphorylation of p27Kip1 promotes binding to 14–3–3 and cytoplasmic localization. *The Journal of Biological Chemistry* 2002;277:28706–28713.
13. Vivanco I, Sawyers CL. The phosphatidylinositol 3-kinase AKT pathway in human cancer. *Nature Reviews Cancer* 2002;2:489–501.
14. Efeyan A, Sabatini DM. mTOR and cancer: Many loops in one pathway. *Current Opinion in Cell Biology* 2010;22:169–176.
15. Carracedo A, Pandolfi PP. The PTEN-PI3K pathway: Of feedbacks and cross-talks. *Oncogene* 2008;27:5527–5541.
16. Peterson TR, Laplante M, Thoreen CC et al. DEPTOR is an mTOR inhibitor frequently overexpressed in multiple myeloma cells and required for their survival. *Cell* 2009;137:873–886.
17. Huang J, Dibble CC, Matsuzaki M et al. The TSC1-TSC2 complex is required for proper activation of mTOR complex 2. *Molecular and Cellular Biology* 2008;28:4104–4115.
18. Hafsi S, Pezzino FM, Candido S et al. Gene alterations in the PI3K/PTEN/AKT pathway as a mechanism of drug-resistance (review). *International Journal of Oncology* 2012;40:639–644.
19. Huang CH, Mandelker D, Gabelli SB et al. Insights into the oncogenic effects of PIK3CA mutations from the structure of p110alpha/p85alpha. *Cell Cycle (Georgetown, Tex.)* 2008;7:1151–1156.
20. Huang CH, Mandelker D, Schmidt-Kittler O et al. The structure of a human p110alpha/p85alpha complex elucidates the effects of oncogenic PI3Kalpha mutations. *Science (New York)* 2007;318:1744–1748.
21. Kang S, Bader AG, Vogt PK. Phosphatidylinositol 3-kinase mutations identified in human cancer are oncogenic. *Proceedings of the National Academy of Sciences of the United States of America* 2005;102:802–807.
22. Vogt PK, Hart JR, Gymnopoulos M et al. Phosphatidylinositol 3-kinase: the oncoprotein. *Current Topics in Microbiology and Immunology* 2010;347:79–104.

23. Bellacosa A, de Feo D, Godwin AK et al. Molecular alterations of the AKT2 oncogene in ovarian and breast carcinomas. *International Journal of Cancer* 1995;64:280–285.

24. Cheng JQ, Godwin AK, Bellacosa A et al. AKT2, a putative oncogene encoding a member of a subfamily of protein-serine/threonine kinases, is amplified in human ovarian carcinomas. *Proceedings of the National Academy of Sciences of the United States of America* 1992;89:9267–9271.

25. Davies MA, Stemke-Hale K, Tellez C et al. A novel AKT3 mutation in melanoma tumours and cell lines. *British Journal of Cancer* 2008;99:1265–1268.

26. Carpten JD, Faber AL, Horn C et al. A transforming mutation in the pleckstrin homology domain of AKT1 in cancer. *Nature* 2007;448:439–444.

27. Corradetti MN, Inoki K, Bardeesy N et al. Regulation of the TSC pathway by LKB1: evidence of a molecular link between tuberous sclerosis complex and Peutz-Jeghers syndrome. *Genes & Development* 2004;18:1533–1538.

28. Inoki K, Corradetti MN, Guan KL. Dysregulation of the TSC-mTOR pathway in human disease. *Nature Genetics* 2005;37:19–24.

29. Chow LM, Baker SJ. PTEN function in normal and neoplastic growth. *Cancer Letters* 2006;241:184–196.

30. Myers MP, Pass I, Batty IH et al. The lipid phosphatase activity of PTEN is critical for its tumor suppressor function. *Proceedings of the National Academy of Sciences of the United States of America* 1998;95:13513–13518.

31. Salmena L, Carracedo A, Pandolfi PP. Tenets of PTEN tumor suppression. *Cell* 2008;133:403–414.

32. Carracedo A, Alimonti A, Pandolfi PP. PTEN level in tumor suppression: HOW much is too little? *Cancer Research* 2011;71:629–633.

33. Gupta A, Yang Q, Pandita RK et al. Cell cycle checkpoint defects contribute to genomic instability in PTEN deficient cells independent of DNA DSB repair. *Cell Cycle (Georgetown, Tex.)* 2009;8:2198–2210.

34. Alimonti A, Carracedo A, Clohessy JG et al. Subtle variations in Pten dose determine cancer susceptibility. *Nature Genetics* 2010;42:454–458.

35. Sakr RA, Barbashina V, Morrogh M et al. Protocol for PTEN expression by immunohistochemistry in formalin-fixed paraffin-embedded human breast carcinoma. *Applied Immunohistochemistry & Molecular Morphology: AIMM/Official Publication of the Society for Applied Immunohistochemistry* 2010;18:371–374.

36. Vitolo MI, Weiss MB, Szmacinski M et al. Deletion of PTEN promotes tumorigenic signaling, resistance to anoikis, and altered response to chemotherapeutic agents in human mammary epithelial cells. *Cancer Research* 2009;69:8275–8283.

37. Mirmohammadsadegh A, Marini A, Nambiar S et al. Epigenetic silencing of the PTEN gene in melanoma. *Cancer Research* 2006;66:6546–6552.

38. Liu W, Zhou Y, Reske SN et al. PTEN mutation: Many birds with one stone in tumorigenesis. *Anticancer Research* 2008;28:3613–3619.

39. Huse JT, Brennan C, Hambardzumyan D et al. The PTEN-regulating microRNA miR-26a is amplified in high-grade glioma and facilitates gliomagenesis in vivo. *Genes & Development* 2009;23:1327–1337.

40. Tay Y, Kats L, Salmena L et al. Coding-independent regulation of the tumor suppressor PTEN by competing endogenous mRNAs. *Cell* 2011;147:344–357.

41. Lo TC, Barnhill LM, Kim Y et al. Inactivation of SHIP1 in T-cell acute lymphoblastic leukemia due to mutation and extensive alternative splicing. *Leukemia Research* 2009;33:1562–1566.

42. Locke NR, Patterson SJ, Hamilton MJ et al. SHIP regulates the reciprocal development of T regulatory and Th17 cells. *Journal of Immunology* 2009;183:975–983.

43. Murray D, Honig B. Electrostatic control of the membrane targeting of C2 domains. *Molecular Cell* 2002;9:145–154.

44. Munday AD, Norris FA, Caldwell KK et al. The inositol polyphosphate 4-phosphatase forms a complex with phosphatidylinositol 3-kinase in human platelet cytosol. *Proceedings of the National Academy of Sciences of the United States of America* 1999;96:3640–3645.
45. Fedele CG, Ooms LM, Ho M et al. Inositol polyphosphate 4-phosphatase II regulates PI3K/Akt signaling and is lost in human basal-like breast cancers. *Proceedings of the National Academy of Sciences of the United States of America* 2010;107:22231–22236.
46. Gewinner C, Wang ZC, Richardson A et al. Evidence that inositol polyphosphate 4-phosphatase type II is a tumor suppressor that inhibits PI3K signaling. *Cancer Cell* 2009;16:115–125.
47. Bendell JC, Rodon J, Burris HA et al. Phase I, dose-escalation study of BKM120, an oral pan-class I PI3K inhibitor, in patients with advanced solid tumors. *Journal of Clinical Oncology* 2012;30:282–290.
48. Crouthamel MC, Kahana JA, Korenchuk S et al. Mechanism and management of AKT inhibitor-induced hyperglycemia. *Clinical Cancer Research* 2009;15:217–225.
49. Duran I, Kortmansky J, Singh D et al. A phase II clinical and pharmacodynamic study of temsirolimus in advanced neuroendocrine carcinomas. *British Journal of Cancer* 2006;95:1148–1154.
50. Moreno Garcia V, Baird RD, Shah KJ et al. A phase I study evaluating GDC-0941, an oral phosphoinositide-3 kinase (PI3K) inhibitor, in patients with advanced solid tumors or multiple myeloma. *ASCO Meeting Abstracts* 2011;29:3021.
51. Maira SM, Pecchi S, Huang A et al. Identification and characterization of NVP-BKM120, an orally available pan-class I PI3-kinase inhibitor. *Molecular Cancer Therapeutics* 2012;11:317–328.
52. Edelman G, Bedell C, Shapiro G et al. A phase I dose-escalation study of XL147 (SAR245408), a PI3K inhibitor administered orally to patients (pts) with advanced malignancies. *ASCO Meeting Abstracts* 2010;28:3004.
53. Shapiro G, Kwak E, Baselga J et al. Phase I dose-escalation study of XL147, a PI3K inhibitor administered orally to patients with solid tumors. *ASCO Meeting Abstracts* 2009;27:3500.
54. Von Hoff DD, LoRusso P, Demetri GD et al. A phase I dose-escalation study to evaluate GDC-0941, a pan-PI3K inhibitor, administered QD or BID in patients with advanced or metastatic solid tumors. *ASCO Meeting Abstracts* 2011;29:3052.
55. Ihle NT, Lemos R, Jr., Wipf P et al. Mutations in the phosphatidylinositol-3-kinase pathway predict for antitumor activity of the inhibitor PX-866 whereas oncogenic Ras is a dominant predictor for resistance. *Cancer Research* 2009;69:143–150.
56. Jimeno A, Hong DS, Hecker S et al. Phase I trial of PX-866, a novel phosphoinositide-3-kinase (PI-3K) inhibitor. *ASCO Meeting Abstracts* 2009;27:3542.
57. Munster PN, van der Noll R, Voest EE et al. Phase I first-in-human study of the PI3 kinase inhibitor GSK2126458 (GSK458) in patients with advanced solid tumors (study P3K112826). *ASCO Meeting Abstracts* 2011;29:3018.
58. Patnaik A, Appleman LJ, Mountz JM et al. A first-in-human phase I study of intravenous PI3K inhibitor BAY 80-6946 in patients with advanced solid tumors: Results of dose-escalation phase. *ASCO Meeting Abstracts* 2011;29:3035.
59. Jeffers M, Dubowy RL, Lathia CD et al. Evaluation of the PI3K inhibitor BAY 80-6946 in hematologic malignancies. *ASCO Meeting Abstracts* 2012;30:e13576.
60. Juric DRJ, Gonzalez-Angulo A, Burris H, Bendell J. BYL719, a next generation PI3K alpha specific inhibitor: Preliminary safety, PK, and efficacy results from the first-in-human study. *Proc AACR 103 Annual Meetings*, Chicago, IL, 2012.
61. Furman RR, Byrd JC, Brown JR, et al. CAL-101, An isoform-selective inhibitor of phosphatidylinositol 3-kinase P110-delta, demonstrates clinical activity and pharmacodynamic effects in patients with relapsed or refractory chronic lymphocytic leukemia. *ASH Annual Meeting Abstracts* 2010;116:55.

62. Coutre SE, Byrd JC, Furman RR et al. Phase I study of CAL-101, an isoform-selective inhibitor of phosphatidylinositol 3-kinase P110d, in patients with previously treated chronic lymphocytic leukemia. *ASCO Meeting Abstracts* 2011;29:6631.

63. Castillo JJ, Furman M, Winer ES. CAL-101: A phosphatidylinositol-3-kinase p110-delta inhibitor for the treatment of lymphoid malignancies. *Expert Opinion on Investigational Drugs* 2012;21:15–22.

64. Li T, Christensen SD, Frankel PH et al. A phase II study of cell cycle inhibitor UCN-01 in patients with metastatic melanoma: A California Cancer Consortium trial. *Investigational New Drugs* 2012;30:741–748.

65. Tolcher AW, Yap TA, Fearen I et al. A phase I study of MK-2206, an oral potent allosteric Akt inhibitor (Akti), in patients (pts) with advanced solid tumor (ST). *ASCO Meeting Abstracts* 2009;27:3503.

66. Yap TA, Yan L, Patnaik A et al. First-in-man clinical trial of the oral pan-AKT inhibitor MK-2206 in patients with advanced solid tumors. *Journal of Clinical Oncology* 2011;29:4688–4695.

67. Tolcher AW, Baird RD, Patnaik A et al. A phase I dose-escalation study of oral MK-2206 (allosteric AKT inhibitor) with oral selumetinib (AZD6244; MEK inhibitor) in patients with advanced or metastatic solid tumors. *ASCO Meeting Abstracts* 2011;29:3004.

68. Marshall J, Posey J, Hwang J et al. A phase I trial of RX-0201 (AKT anti-sense) in patients with an advanced cancer. *ASCO Meeting Abstracts* 2007;25:3564.

69. Pal SK, Reckamp K, Yu H et al. Akt inhibitors in clinical development for the treatment of cancer. *Expert Opinion on Investigational Drugs* 2010;19:1355–1366.

70. Bidyasar S, Kurzrock R, Falchook GS et al. A first-in-human phase I trial of PBI-05204 (oleandrin), an inhibitor of Akt, FGF-2, NF-Kb, and p70S6K in advanced solid tumor patients. *ASCO Meeting Abstracts* 2009;27:3537.

71. Tevaarwerk A, Wilding G, Eickhoff J et al. Phase I study of continuous MKC-1 in patients with advanced or metastatic solid malignancies using the modified Time-to-Event Continual Reassessment Method (TITE-CRM) dose escalation design. *Investigational New Drugs* 2012;30:1039–1045.

72. Faris JE, Arnott J, Zheng H et al. A phase 2 study of oral MKC-1, an inhibitor of importin-beta, tubulin, and the mTOR pathway in patients with unresectable or metastatic pancreatic cancer. *Investigational New Drugs* 2012;30:1614–1620.

73. Banerji U, Aghajanian C, Raymond E et al. First results from a phase I trial of AZD8055, a dual mTORC1 and mTORC2 inhibitor. *ASCO Meeting Abstracts* 2011;29:3096.

74. Willems L, Chapuis N, Puissant A et al. The dual mTORC1 and mTORC2 inhibitor AZD 8055 has anti-tumor activity in acute myeloid leukemia. *Leukemia* 2012;26:1195–1202.

75. Tan DS, Dumez H, Olmos D et al. First-in-human phase I study exploring three schedules of OSI-027, a novel small molecule TORC1/TORC2 inhibitor, in patients with advanced solid tumors and lymphoma. *ASCO Meeting Abstracts* 2010;28:3006.

76. Hsieh AC, Liu Y, Edlind MP et al. The translational landscape of mTOR signalling steers cancer initiation and metastasis. *Nature* 2012;485:55–61.

77. Shih KC, Bendell JC, Reinert A et al. Phase I trial of an oral TORC1/TORC2 inhibitor (CC-223) in advanced solid and hematologic cancers. *ASCO Meeting Abstracts* 2012;30:3006.

78. Burris H, Rodon J, Sharma S et al. First-in-human phase I study of the oral PI3K inhibitor BEZ235 in patients (pts) with advanced solid tumors. *ASCO Meeting Abstracts* 2010;28:3005.

79. Peyton JD, Rodon Ahnert J, Burris H et al. A dose-escalation study with the novel formulation of the oral pan-class I PI3K inhibitor BEZ235, solid dispersion system (SDS) sachet, in patients with advanced solid tumors. *ASCO Meeting Abstracts* 2011;29:3066.

80. Chang KY, Tsai SY, Wu CM et al. Novel phosphoinositide 3-kinase/mTOR dual inhibitor, NVP-BGT226, displays potent growth-inhibitory activity against human head and neck cancer cells in vitro and in vivo. *Clinical Cancer Research* 2011;17:7116–7126.

81. Markman B, Tabernero J, Krop I et al. Phase I safety, pharmacokinetic, and pharmacodynamic study of the oral phosphatidylinositol-3-kinase and mTOR inhibitor BGT226 in patients with advanced solid tumors. *Annals of Oncology: Official Journal of the European Society for Medical Oncology/ESMO* 2012;23:2399–2408.

82. Fokas E, Yoshimura M, Prevo R et al. NVP-BEZ235 and NVP-BGT226, dual phosphatidylinositol 3-kinase/mammalian target of rapamycin inhibitors, enhance tumor and endothelial cell radiosensitivity. *Radiation Oncology* 2012;7:48.

83. Papadopoulos KP, Markman B, Tabernero J et al. A phase I dose-escalation study of the safety, pharmacokinetics (PK), and pharmacodynamics (PD) of a novel PI3K inhibitor, XL765, administered orally to patients (pts) with advanced solid tumors. *ASCO Meeting Abstracts* 2008;26:3510.

84. LoRusso P, Markman B, Tabernero J et al. A phase I dose-escalation study of the safety, pharmacokinetics (PK), and pharmacodynamics of XL765, a PI3K/TORC1/TORC2 inhibitor administered orally to patients (pts) with advanced solid tumors. *ASCO Meeting Abstracts* 2009;27:3502.

85. Brana I, LoRusso P, Baselga J et al. A phase I dose-escalation study of the safety, pharmacokinetics (PK), and pharmacodynamics of XL765 (SAR245409), a PI3K/TORC1/TORC2 inhibitor administered orally to patients (pts) with advanced malignancies. *ASCO Meeting Abstracts* 2010;28:3030.

86. Dolly S, Wagner AJ, Bendell JC et al. A first-in-human, phase 1 study to evaluate the dual PI3K/mTOR inhibitor GDC-0980 administered QD in patients with advanced solid tumors or non-Hodgkin's lymphoma. *ASCO Meeting Abstracts* 2010;28:3079.

87. Wagner AJ, Bendell JC, Dolly S et al. A first-in-human phase I study to evaluate GDC-0980, an oral PI3K/mTOR inhibitor, administered QD in patients with advanced solid tumors. *ASCO Meeting Abstracts* 2011;29:3020.

88. Schwertschlag US, Chiorean EG, Anthony SP et al. Phase 1 pharmacokinetic (PK) and pharmacodynamic(PD) evaluation of SF1126 a vascular targeted pan phosphoinositide 3- kinase (PI3K) inhibitor in patients with solid tumors. *ASCO Meeting Abstracts* 2008;26:14532.

89. Chiorean EG, Mahadevan D, Harris WB et al. Phase I evaluation of SF1126, a vascular targeted PI3K inhibitor, administered twice weekly IV in patients with refractory solid tumors. *ASCO Meeting Abstracts* 2009;27:2558.

90. Mahadevan D, Chiorean EG, Harris W et al. Phase I study of the multikinase prodrug SF1126 in solid tumors and B-cell malignancies. *ASCO Meeting Abstracts* 2011;29:3015.

91. Foster P. Potentiating the antitumor effects of chemotherapy with the selective PI3K inhibitor XL147. *AACR Meeting Abstracts* 2007;2007:C199.

92. Shapiro G, Edelman G, Calvo E et al. Targeting aberrant PI3K pathway signaling with XL147, a potent, selective and orally bioavailable PI3K inhibitor. *AACR Meeting Abstracts* 2007;2007:C205.

93. Chakrabarty A, Sanchez V, Kuba MG et al. Feedback upregulation of HER3 (ErbB3) expression and activity attenuates antitumor effect of PI3K inhibitors. *Proceedings of the National Academy of Sciences of the United States of America* 2012;109:2718–2723.

94. Folkes AJ, Ahmadi K, Alderton WK et al. The identification of 2-(1H-indazol-4-yl)-6-(4-methanesulfonyl-piperazin-1-ylmethyl)-4-morpholin-4-yl-thieno[3,2-d]pyrimidine (GDC-0941) as a potent, selective, orally bioavailable inhibitor of class I PI3 kinase for the treatment of cancer. *Journal of Medicinal Chemistry* 2008;51:5522–5532.

95. Raynaud FI, Eccles SA, Patel S et al. Biological properties of potent inhibitors of class I phosphatidylinositide 3-kinases: From PI-103 through PI-540, PI-620 to the oral agent GDC-0941. *Molecular Cancer Therapeutics* 2009;8:1725–1738.

96. O'Brien C, Wallin JJ, Sampath D et al. Predictive biomarkers of sensitivity to the phosphatidylinositol 3′ kinase inhibitor GDC-0941 in breast cancer preclinical models. *Clinical Cancer Research* 2010;16:3670–3683.

97. Koul D, Shen R, Kim YW et al. Cellular and in vivo activity of a novel PI3K inhibitor, PX-866, against human glioblastoma. *Neuro-Oncology* 2010;12:559–569.

98. Jimeno A, Herbst RS, Falchook GS et al. Final results from a phase I, dose-escalation study of PX-866, an irreversible, pan-isoform inhibitor of PI3 kinase. *ASCO Meeting Abstracts* 2010;28:3089.

99. Norman P. Selective PI3Kdelta inhibitors, a review of the patent literature. *Expert Opinion on Therapeutic Patents* 2011;21:1773–1790.

100. Furman RR, Byrd JC, Flinn IW et al. Interim results from a phase I study of CAL-101, a selective oral inhibitor of phosphatidylinositol 3-kinase p110d isoform, in patients with relapsed or refractory hematologic malignancies. *ASCO Meeting Abstracts* 2010;28:3032.

101. Maira SM, Stauffer F, Brueggen J et al. Identification and characterization of NVP-BEZ235, a new orally available dual phosphatidylinositol 3-kinase/mammalian target of rapamycin inhibitor with potent in vivo antitumor activity. *Molecular Cancer Therapeutics* 2008;7:1851–1863.

102. Serra V, Markman B, Scaltriti M et al. NVP-BEZ235, a dual PI3K/mTOR inhibitor, prevents PI3K signaling and inhibits the growth of cancer cells with activating PI3K mutations. *Cancer Research* 2008;68:8022–8030.

103. Cao P, Maira SM, Garcia-Echeverria C et al. Activity of a novel, dual PI3-kinase/mTOR inhibitor NVP-BEZ235 against primary human pancreatic cancers grown as orthotopic xenografts. *British Journal of Cancer* 2009;100:1267–1276.

104. Bhende PM, Park SI, Lim MS et al. The dual PI3K/mTOR inhibitor, NVP-BEZ235, is efficacious against follicular lymphoma. *Leukemia* 2010;24:1781–1784.

105. Liu TJ, Koul D, LaFortune T et al. NVP-BEZ235, a novel dual phosphatidylinositol 3-kinase/mammalian target of rapamycin inhibitor, elicits multifaceted antitumor activities in human gliomas. *Molecular Cancer Therapeutics* 2009;8:2204–2210.

106. Baumann P, Schneider L, Mandl-Weber S et al. Simultaneous targeting of PI3K and mTOR with NVP-BGT226 is highly effective in multiple myeloma. *Anti-Cancer Drugs* 2012;23:131–138.

107. Glienke W, Maute L, Wicht J et al. The dual PI3K/mTOR inhibitor NVP-BGT226 induces cell cycle arrest and regulates Survivin gene expression in human pancreatic cancer cell lines. *Tumour Biology: The Journal of the International Society for Oncodevelopmental Biology and Medicine* 2012;33:757–765.

108. Prasad G, Sottero T, Yang X et al. Inhibition of PI3K/mTOR pathways in glioblastoma and implications for combination therapy with temozolomide. *Neuro-Oncology* 2011;13:384–392.

109. Cohen RB, Janne PA, Engelman JA et al. A phase I safety and pharmacokinetic (PK) study of PI3K/TORC1/TORC2 inhibitor XL765 (SAR245409) in combination with erlotinib (E) in patients (pts) with advanced solid tumors. *ASCO Meeting Abstracts* 2010;28:3015.

110. Nghiemphu PL, Omuro AM, Cloughesy T et al. A phase I safety and pharmacokinetic study of XL765 (SAR245409), a novel PI3K/TORC1/TORC2 inhibitor, in combination with temozolomide (TMZ) in patients (pts) with newly diagnosed malignant glioma. *ASCO Meeting Abstracts* 2010;28:3085.

111. Wallin JJ, Edgar KA, Guan J et al. GDC-0980 is a novel class I PI3K/mTOR kinase inhibitor with robust activity in cancer models driven by the PI3K pathway. *Molecular Cancer Therapeutics* 2011;10:2426–2436.

112. Garlich JR, De P, Dey N et al. A vascular targeted pan phosphoinositide 3-kinase inhibitor prodrug, SF1126, with antitumor and antiangiogenic activity. *Cancer Research* 2008;68:206–215.

113. Yap TA, Garrett MD, Walton MI et al. Targeting the PI3K-AKT-mTOR pathway: progress, pitfalls, and promises. *Current Opinion in Pharmacology* 2008;8:393–412.

114. Van Ummersen L, Binger K, Volkman J et al. A phase I trial of perifosine (NSC 639966) on a loading dose/maintenance dose schedule in patients with advanced cancer. *Clinical Cancer Research* 2004;10:7450–7456.

115. Cho DC, Hutson TE, Samlowski W et al. Two phase 2 trials of the novel Akt inhibitor perifosine in patients with advanced renal cell carcinoma after progression on vascular endothelial growth factor-targeted therapy. *Cancer* 2012;118:6055–6062.

116. Yan L. Abstract #DDT01–1: MK-2206: A potent oral allosteric AKT inhibitor. *AACR Meeting Abstracts* 2009;2009:DDT01–1.

117. Lu W, Defeo-Jones D, Davis L et al. Abstract #3714: In vitro and in vivo antitumor activities of MK-2206, a new allosteric Akt inhibitor. *AACR Meeting Abstracts* 2009;2009:3714.

118. Hirai H, Sootome H, Nakatsuru Y et al. MK-2206, an allosteric Akt inhibitor, enhances antitumor efficacy by standard chemotherapeutic agents or molecular targeted drugs in vitro and in vivo. *Molecular Cancer Therapeutics* 2010;9:1956–1967.

119. Yang P, Menter DG, Cartwright C et al. Oleandrin-mediated inhibition of human tumor cell proliferation: Importance of Na,K-ATPase alpha subunits as drug targets. *Molecular Cancer Therapeutics* 2009;8:2319–2328.

120. Rhodes N, Heerding DA, Duckett DR et al. Characterization of an Akt kinase inhibitor with potent pharmacodynamic and antitumor activity. *Cancer Research* 2008;68:2366–2374.

121. Altomare DA, Zhang L, Deng J et al. GSK690693 delays tumor onset and progression in genetically defined mouse models expressing activated Akt. *Clinical Cancer Research* 2010;16:486–496.

122. Huang S, Bjornsti MA, Houghton PJ. Rapamycins: Mechanism of action and cellular resistance. *Cancer Biology & Therapy* 2003;2:222–232.

123. Kim DH, Sarbassov DD, Ali SM et al. mTOR interacts with raptor to form a nutrient-sensitive complex that signals to the cell growth machinery. *Cell* 2002;110:163–175.

124. Populo H, Lopes JM, Soares P. The mTOR signalling pathway in human cancer. *International Journal of Molecular Sciences* 2012;13:1886–1918.

125. Sarbassov DD, Ali SM, Sengupta S et al. Prolonged rapamycin treatment inhibits mTORC2 assembly and Akt/PKB. *Molecular Cell* 2006;22:159–168.

126. Hudes G, Carducci M, Tomczak P et al. Temsirolimus, interferon alfa, or both for advanced renal-cell carcinoma. *The New England Journal of Medicine* 2007;356:2271–2281.

127. Motzer RJ, Escudier B, Oudard S et al. Efficacy of everolimus in advanced renal cell carcinoma: A double-blind, randomised, placebo-controlled phase III trial. *Lancet* 2008;372:449–456.

128. Hess G, Herbrecht R, Romaguera J et al. Phase III study to evaluate temsirolimus compared with investigator's choice therapy for the treatment of relapsed or refractory mantle cell lymphoma. *Journal of Clinical Oncology* 2009;27:3822–3829.

129. Villarreal-Garza C, Cortes J, Andre F et al. mTOR inhibitors in the management of hormone receptor-positive breast cancer: The latest evidence and future directions. *Annals of Oncology: Official Journal of the European Society for Medical Oncology/ESMO* 2012;23:2526–2535.

130. Chawla SP, Staddon AP, Baker LH et al. Phase II study of the mammalian target of rapamycin inhibitor ridaforolimus in patients with advanced bone and soft tissue sarcomas. *Journal of Clinical Oncology* 2012;30:78–84.

131. Chawla SP, Blay J, Ray-Coquard IL et al. Results of the phase III, placebo-controlled trial (SUCCEED) evaluating the mTOR inhibitor ridaforolimus (R) as maintenance therapy in advanced sarcoma patients (pts) following clinical benefit from prior standard cytotoxic chemotherapy (CT). *ASCO Meeting Abstracts* 2011;29:10005.

132. Oza AM, Elit L, Tsao MS et al. Phase II study of temsirolimus in women with recurrent or metastatic endometrial cancer: A trial of the NCIC Clinical Trials Group. *Journal of Clinical Oncology* 2011;29:3278–3285.

133. Meric-Bernstam F, Gonzalez-Angulo AM. Targeting the mTOR signaling network for cancer therapy. *Journal of Clinical Oncology* 2009;27:2278–2287.

134. Willems L, Tamburini J, Chapuis N et al. PI3K and mTOR signaling pathways in cancer: new data on targeted therapies. *Current Oncology Reports* 2012;14:129–138.

135. Wander SA, Hennessy BT, Slingerland JM. Next-generation mTOR inhibitors in clinical oncology: How pathway complexity informs therapeutic strategy. *The Journal of Clinical Investigation* 2011;121:1231–1241.

136. Larrea MD, Hong F, Wander SA et al. RSK1 drives p27Kip1 phosphorylation at T198 to promote RhoA inhibition and increase cell motility. *Proceedings of the National Academy of Sciences of the United States of America* 2009;106:9268–9273.

137. Laplante M, Sabatini DM. An emerging role of mTOR in lipid biosynthesis. *Current Biology* 2009;19:R1046–R1052.

138. Laplante M, Sabatini DM. mTOR signaling in growth control and disease. *Cell* 2012;149:274–293.

139. Yu K, Toral-Barza L, Shi C et al. Biochemical, cellular, and in vivo activity of novel ATP-competitive and selective inhibitors of the mammalian target of rapamycin. *Cancer Research* 2009;69:6232–6240.

140. Feldman ME, Apsel B, Uotila A et al. Active-site inhibitors of mTOR target rapamycin-resistant outputs of mTORC1 and mTORC2. *PLoS Biology* 2009;7:e38.

141. Chresta CM, Davies BR, Hickson I et al. AZD8055 is a potent, selective, and orally bioavailable ATP-competitive mammalian target of rapamycin kinase inhibitor with in vitro and in vivo antitumor activity. *Cancer Research* 2010;70:288–298.

142. Thoreen CC, Kang SA, Chang JW et al. An ATP-competitive mammalian target of rapamycin inhibitor reveals rapamycin-resistant functions of mTORC1. *The Journal of Biological Chemistry* 2009;284:8023–8032.

143. Fasolo A, Sessa C. Current and future directions in mammalian target of rapamycin inhibitors development. *Expert Opinion on Investigational Drugs* 2011;20:381–394.

144. O'Reilly KE, Rojo F, She QB et al. mTOR inhibition induces upstream receptor tyrosine kinase signaling and activates Akt. *Cancer Research* 2006;66:1500–1508.

145. Marshall G, Howard Z, Dry J et al. Benefits of mTOR kinase targeting in oncology: Pre-clinical evidence with AZD8055. *Biochemical Society Transactions* 2011;39:456–459.

146. Bhagwat SV, Gokhale PC, Crew AP et al. Preclinical characterization of OSI-027, a potent and selective inhibitor of mTORC1 and mTORC2: Distinct from rapamycin. *Molecular Cancer Therapeutics* 2011;10:1394–1406.

147. Dancey J. mTOR signaling and drug development in cancer. *Nature Reviews Clinical Oncology* 2010;7:209–219.

148. Dowling RJ, Topisirovic I, Fonseca BD et al. Dissecting the role of mTOR: Lessons from mTOR inhibitors. *Biochimica Et Biophysica Acta* 2010;1804:433–439.

149. Dan S, Okamura M, Seki M et al. Correlating phosphatidylinositol 3-kinase inhibitor efficacy with signaling pathway status: In silico and biological evaluations. *Cancer Research* 2010;70:4982–4994.

150. Schwarz JK, Payton JE, Rashmi R et al. Pathway-specific analysis of gene expression data identifies the PI3k/Akt pathway as a novel therapeutic target in cervical cancer. *Clinical Cancer Research* 2012;18:1464–1471.

151. Ghigo A, Damilano F, Braccini L et al. PI3K inhibition in inflammation: Toward tailored therapies for specific diseases. *BioEssays: News and Reviews in Molecular, Cellular and Developmental Biology* 2010;32:185–196.
152. Yap TA, Sandhu SK, Workman P et al. Envisioning the future of early anticancer drug development. *Nature Reviews Cancer* 2010;10:514–523.
153. Ellis LM, Hicklin DJ. Resistance to targeted therapies: Refining anticancer therapy in the era of molecular oncology. *Clinical Cancer Research* 2009;15:7471–7478.
154. Schnell CR, Stauffer F, Allegrini PR et al. Effects of the dual phosphatidylinositol 3-kinase/mammalian target of rapamycin inhibitor NVP-BEZ235 on the tumor vasculature: Implications for clinical imaging. *Cancer Research* 2008;68:6598–6607.
155. Di Cosimo S, Scaltriti M, Val D et al. The PI3-K/AKT/mTOR pathway as a target for breast cancer therapy. *ASCO Meeting Abstracts* 2007;25:3511.
156. Berns K, Horlings HM, Hennessy BT et al. A functional genetic approach identifies the PI3K pathway as a major determinant of trastuzumab resistance in breast cancer. *Cancer Cell* 2007;12:395–402.
157. Eichhorn PJ, Gili M, Scaltriti M et al. Phosphatidylinositol 3-kinase hyperactivation results in lapatinib resistance that is reversed by the mTOR/phosphatidylinositol 3-kinase inhibitor NVP-BEZ235. *Cancer Research* 2008;68:9221–9230.
158. Junttila TT, Akita RW, Parsons K et al. Ligand-independent HER2/HER3/PI3K complex is disrupted by trastuzumab and is effectively inhibited by the PI3K inhibitor GDC-0941. *Cancer Cell* 2009;15:429–440.
159. Bauman JE, Arias-Pulido H, Lee S-J et al. Phase II study of temsirolimus and erlotinib in patients (pts) with recurrent/metastatic (R/M), platinum-refractory head and neck squamous cell carcinoma (HNSCC). *ASCO Meeting Abstracts* 2012;30:5549.
160. Engelman JA. Targeting PI3K signalling in cancer: Opportunities, challenges and limitations. *Nature Reviews Cancer* 2009;9:550–562.

5 BRAF and MEK Inhibitors

Lidia Robert
University of California, Los Angeles

Antoni Ribas
University of California, Los Angeles

CONTENTS

INTRODUCTION

The mitogen-activated protein kinase (MAPK) pathway is an intracellular signaling pathway regulating cell cycle and other cellular functions, which is commonly aberrant in human tumors.[1] This activated kinase cascade drives a serial phosphorylation of the MEK and ERK kinases that concludes in proliferation and survival. The activated MAPK pathway plays a critical role in proliferation, cell motility, and cell survival. Downstream substrates of *ERK* include nuclear targets such as ETS and AP-1, which are transcription factors and apoptotic regulators.[2] With respect to cell proliferation, ERK1/2 is specially important in the expression of cyclin D1 to promote progression through the G1 phase of the cell cycle.[3]

A paradigmatic example of this activation is melanoma, where deregulation of the MAPK pathway is evident in over 90% of the cases. In approximately 50% of cases, this is due to the *BRAF^{V600}* mutation; an additional 20% of melanomas carry *NRAS^{Q61}* mutations, and additional less frequent mutations in *KIT* and *KRAS* have also been identified constitutively activating the RAS–RAF–MEK–ERK cascade. Mutations in *BRAF* are, in general, mutually exclusive with mutations of other proteins in the MAPK pathway,[4] though recently, exceptions have been reported.[5] This fact creates an addictive relationship between melanoma and MAPK pathway and arises as a very tempting target.

BRAF^{V600} mutations are present in approximately 7% of all cancers in general, which makes them the most prevalent single-nucleotide point mutation in a protein kinase in cancer.[6] Interestingly, high frequencies of this mutation have also been reported in 50% of papillary thyroid carcinoma, 100% of hairy-cell leukemias, and a small fraction (less than 5%) of colon, lung, ovarian, and other cancer histologies. The *BRAF* gene is located in the chromosome 7q24. It is in the exon 15 of the B isoform of the RAF kinase. The most common *BRAF^{V600}* mutation is a single-nucleotide change that results in a valine-to-glutamic acid substitution at amino acid 600 (*BRAF^{V600E}*). Approximately 5%–12% of V600 BRAF mutations are V600K[7], and in a smaller percentage, single-nucleotide changes have also been reported. This subtle change causes negative charges in the phosphorylation site enhancing the kinase activity[8] and driving the pathway to a constant activation regardless of the dimerization complexes.[9] This is hypothesized to occur because mutant *BRAF* is locked in this activated conformational state, which leads to a 500-fold increase in BRAF kinase activity compared to the wild-type kinase.[10]

This chapter will discuss new compounds targeting this pathway, deepening in mechanism of action, evidence of benefit, and mechanisms of resistance described so far. The ultimate challenge remains on how to block the pathway and reduce and/or delay the onset of acquired resistance.

TARGETING THE MAPK PATHWAY

Under normal signaling conditions, the binding of a growth factor to a receptor tyrosine kinase (RTK), such as c-KIT, activates RAS that then activates the RAF kinases. There are three RAF serine/threonine kinases, ARAF, BRAF, and CRAF. Homologous and heterologous dimer complexes between BRAF and CRAF act as key point regulators of the activated cascade. RAF activation phosphorylates MEK, and MEK phosphorylates ERK. However, the functional relationship between BRAF and CRAF is nonreciprocal: BRAF can activate CRAF, but not vice versa.[11]

Overall, inhibitors of RAF have been divided into type I inhibitors, which selectively inhibit the activated RAF kinase (vemurafenib and dabrafenib), and type II inhibitors, which inhibit the resting RAF (sorafenib). Attempts at blocking oncogenic signaling through the MAPK pathways started some years ago with tyrosine kinase inhibitors (TKIs) as sorafenib. This small molecule was originally designed to inhibit CRAF and was only later shown to also block BRAF.[12] This TKI inhibits multiple signaling kinases including Raf family members, platelet-derived growth factor receptor (PDGFR), vascular endothelial growth factor receptors 1 and 2 (VEGF1 and VEGF2), c-Kit, and Fms-like tyrosine kinase 3. The clinical testing of sorafenib in patients with metastatic melanoma did not support a mutated

$BRAF^{V600}$ inhibitor function since sorafenib has activity against the inactive form of the RAF kinases (type II kinase inhibitor). It also inhibits the VEGF kinase resulting in dose-limiting toxicities before the BRAF inhibitor function is evident in humans. Currently, sorafenib tosylate has Food and Drug Association (FDA) and European Medicine Agency (EMA) approval for non-resectable hepatocellular carcinoma (HCC) and advanced renal cell carcinoma (RCC).

Recognizing this interesting target, the first specific BRAF inhibitor with activity against the active kinase (type I kinase inhibitor), vemurafenib, entered clinical testing in late 2006 reporting promising effects in melanoma, inducing cell cycle arrest and apoptosis exclusively in $BRAF^{V600E}$-positive cells.[13] To this effect, two compounds, vemurafenib and dabrafenib, have offered outstanding results in terms of response rates in patients with $BRAF^{V600}$ mutant metastatic melanoma.

BRAF INHIBITORS

VEMURAFENIB

Vemurafenib (formerly PLX4032) belongs to a family of mutant BRAF kinase inhibitors that were discovered using a scaffold-based drug design approach. The first studies in vitro demonstrated that this ATP-competitive RAF inhibitor decreases $BRAF^{V600E}$ kinase activity at 10-fold lower concentration than wild-type BRAF. It showed as well activity in melanomas with homozygous and heterozygous BRAF mutations.[14] Translating this interesting compound into the clinic, BRAF inhibitor in melanoma (BRIM)-1, a multicenter phase I trial, enrolled 55 patients with solid tumors to receive a dose escalation of vemurafenib, including an extension cohort of 32 patients with $BRAF^{V600}$ mutant metastatic melanoma.[15] After a period of initial low exposure due to poor oral bioavailability of the initial formulation, reformulated capsules of microprecipitated bulk powder (MBP) led to establishing a maximum tolerated dose at 960 mg twice daily and set itself apart by the unprecedented objective response rate.

BRIM-2 was the phase II trial, which enrolled 132 patients with $BRAF^{V600}$ mutant metastatic melanoma who had previously received standard of care therapy for this disease.[16] The results showed an overall response rate of 53% by Response Evaluation Criteria in Solid Tumors (RECIST) 1.1, with a median duration of response of 6.7 months and an unexpected long median overall survival of 15.9 months.

The phase III trial, BRIM-3, published in 2011, included 675 patients with unresectable, treatment-naïve stage IIIC or stage IV metastatic melanoma with the $BRAF^{V600E}$ mutation.[17] The trial was designed as a two-arm randomized clinical trial comparing vemurafenib, 960 mg orally twice daily, versus the FDA-approved chemotherapy for metastatic melanoma, dacarbazine, at 1000 mg/m^2 administered every 3 weeks. The results confirmed the high response rate previously reported in phases I and II, with an estimated overall survival (OS) for vemurafenib arm of 13.2 months compared to 9.9 months in the dacarbazine arm (update in October 2011). The duration of response ranged from 2 to over 18 months, with a mean duration of response of 6.7 months. In the initial report, the response rate was 48% for the vemurafenib group compared to 5% for the dacarbazine group, consistent with the previous experience with both agents. Additionally, the best tumor response (not requiring to meet RECIST) was observed in over 80% of patients. This clinical trial demonstrated statistically significant improvements in progression-free survival and overall survival, meeting its primary efficacy endpoints. Common adverse events associated with vemurafenib were arthralgia, maculopapular rash, fatigue, alopecia, keratoacanthoma or cutaneous squamous-cell carcinoma (cuSCC), photosensitivity, nausea, and diarrhea. Overall, the group of patients that required dose reduction in the vemurafenib arm was 38%.

On August 17, 2011, vemurafenib was FDA approved based on the results of BRIM-3. On December 15, 2011, the EMA also gave approval for the treatment of patients with unresectable metastatic melanoma harboring $BRAF^{V600E}$ mutation.

It is unclear whether this clinical efficacy can be extrapolated to other cancers. Hairy-cell leukemia has been found to be a $BRAF^{V600}$ mutant in 100% of the cases. It is commonly treated with purine analogues or rituximab. So far only sporadic cases of outstanding responses in previously refractory hairy-cell leukemia have been reported,[18] supporting the idea of BRAF as a key driver mutation in this disease.

DABRAFENIB

Dabrafenib (formerly GSK2118436) is a potent adenosine triphosphate (ATP)-competitive inhibitor of BRAF kinase and is selective for mutant BRAF. In mutated *BRAF* cell lines, it shows dose-dependent inhibition of MEK and ERK phosphorylation. The phase I study of dabrafenib demonstrated tumor decrease in 18 of 30 patients (60%) and a >20% tumor decrease by RECIST at first restaging, similar to that observed for vemurafenib.

BREAK-3[19] was the phase III trial comparing dabrafenib with dacarbazine in patients with $BRAF^{V600E}$ mutant metastatic melanoma who were previously untreated. This study had a crossover design, with patients in the chemotherapy arm allowing receiving dabrafenib upon progression, since the primary endpoint was progression-free survival. Results demonstrated superiority of dabrafenib in progression-free survival, 5.1 months for dabrafenib versus 2.7 months for dacarbazine, with an overall response rate of 50% versus 6%. Toxicities included skin changes, low-grade cuSCC, headache, nausea, fatigue, and vomiting. When compared to vemurafenib, the available data suggest that dabrafenib may result in a higher frequency of pyrexia and a lower incidence of photosensitivity and epithelial skin lesions.

Brain metastases are present in 20% of patients at diagnosis, in 40%–45% of patients overall, and in 73% of the autopsies performed on patients who died from metastatic melanoma.[20] However, most studies used to exclude patients with brain metastases from clinical trials. Clinical experience and a completed clinical trial (BREAK-MB) demonstrate that dabrafenib has significant antitumor activity in this subset of patients. The putative mechanism for this surprising intracranial effect has been related to the disruption of the blood–brain barrier once macrometastases have penetrated through.

Effects of BRAF Inhibitors in Non-BRAF Mutant Cells

BRAF inhibitors in the context of BRAF wild type with strong upstream signaling induce a paradoxical activation on the MAPK pathway. This mechanism obeys to a conformational change and activation of CRAF induced by the BRAF inhibitor bound to BRAF facilitated by the dimerization and interaction with activated RAS. If we consider this phenomenon in metastatic melanoma, wild type or *RAS* mutated, the result will drive toward progression and stimulation of cell survival. This limits the usage of BRAF inhibitors in *BRAF*-mutated tumors.

Paradoxical MAPK activation explains the development of nonmelanoma skin cancers—well-differentiated cuSCCs and keratoacanthomas—appearing in 20%–30% of patients receiving BRAF inhibitors.[21–25] These lesions are confined in the skin and are easily removable by surgical resection, curettage, or cryotherapy. These cells have preexisting *RAS* mutations (particularly in *HRAS*) or have upstream upregulated RTK signaling. After an initial carcinogenic event inducing these genetic alterations, the exposure to the BRAF inhibitor induces paradoxical increases in MAPK signaling and proliferation of cells harboring mutated HRAS. These lesions develop early after BRAF inhibitor exposure and only in a subset of patients, which supports the idea that BRAF inhibitors do not initiate tumorigenesis but rather accelerate the progression of preexisting subclinical cancerous lesions. This fact has also pointed to the usefulness of combining a BRAF inhibitor with a MEK inhibitor to prevent this toxic effect,[26] avoiding the development of cancerous lesions in mouse models[21] and in clinical trials.[27]

Considering melanoma as an immuno-responsive tumor, the effects of vemurafenib on immune cells have been studied to explore the feasibility of future combinatorial approaches with immunotherapy for melanoma.[28] The MAPK pathway is critical in signaling for T cell receptor (TCR) and B cell receptor (BCR), just as it is also indispensable once lymphocyte response to antigen is activated.[29] Laboratory testing and samples from patients treated with BRAF inhibitors confirm that these agents allow adequate function of lymphocytes,[28,30] supporting their testing in combination.

Mechanisms of Resistance to BRAF Inhibitors

When first exposing patients to BRAF inhibitors, an overall response rate in metastatic melanoma of more than 50%[17] has been reported but only 5% of BRAF mutant colon cancer. In the melanoma setting, minor responses with clinical improvement are also experienced in some patients. The development of resistance to single-agent vemurafenib or dabrafenib occurs in most patients within months. The mechanisms underlying primary resistance and acquired resistance are the subject of intense research.

Mechanisms related with acquired resistance to BRAF inhibitors have been classified into two groups: reactivation of the MAPK pathway or enhanced cell signaling through pathways other than the MAPK pathway.

The MAPK pathway-dependent mechanism is the most usual way to develop resistance. Mutations in NRAS such as Q61[5,31] are the most frequent ones. Although

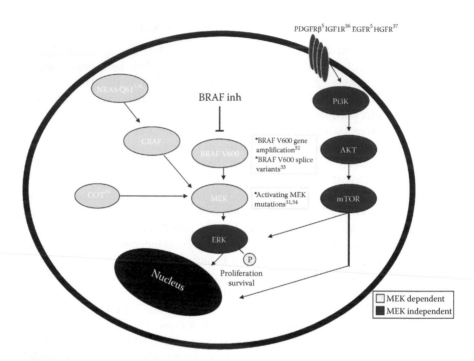

FIGURE 5.1   Mechanisms of acquired resistance to BRAF inhibitors.

no secondary mutations in the BRAF[V600] kinase have been identified, the amplification of the mutant gene itself is another well-known mechanism.[32] Splice variants of BRAF allow the homodimerization and re-signal downstream.[33] Mutations in MEK1[31,34] have also been described. In addition, some resistant tumors have been reported to upregulate cancer Osaka thyroid (COT or MAP3K8) signaling, putatively reactivating the MAPK pathway.[35]

Other acquired resistance pathways bypass the BRAF inhibition through non-MAPK reactivation. Upregulation of membrane receptors with tyrosine kinase such as the platelet-derived growth factor beta (PDGFRβ),[5] the insulin growth factor receptor 1 (IGF1R),[36] or hepatocyte growth factor (HGF),[37] ends up activating MAPK-redundant signaling.[5] These mechanisms of acquired resistance appear to develop in a mutually exclusive manner. Thus, mechanisms of acquired resistance to BRAF inhibitors remain the principal challenge in the clinical use of selective BRAF inhibitors (Figure 5.1).

MEK INHIBITORS

Targeting MEK is a downstream strategy that is currently being tested in monotherapy and in combination with a broad range of tumors. More than 10 MEK inhibitors have been tested in the clinic with this aim. Most of them are noncompetitive allosteric inhibitors, which work outside of the ATP-binding site and lock the kinase in a closed and catalytically inactive conformation.[38]

MEK is a special appealing inhibition point, considering the critical position of it as a funnel in the MAPK pathway downstream of the three RAS isoforms and the three RAF isoforms. Inhibiting it may result in blocking MAPK signaling from multiple upstream oncogenes.[39]

In vitro studies have shown extreme sensitivity in cells harboring $BRAF^{V600}$ mutations with IC50 values around 100 nM or less.[40] These data also showed inhibition of pERK in RAS mutant cells, but with lower sensitivity. This pointed the possibility that RAS and BRAF may have differential dependence to MAPK pathway.

MEK INHIBITION AGAINST BRAF MUTANT MELANOMA

In vitro studies demonstrated that the $BRAF^{V600}$ mutation confers high sensitivity to MEK inhibitors in melanoma cell lines, correlated with both downregulation of cyclin D1 protein expression and the induction of G1 arrest.[40]

MEK INHIBITION AGAINST BRAF WILD-TYPE MELANOMA

So far, $BRAF$ wild-type melanoma cell lines have been more difficult to treat. However, the exposure of different oncogenic mutations to MEK inhibition has shown cytotoxic activity against cell lines with $NRAS$, $GNAQ$, $or GNA11$ driver mutations.[39] In general, higher sensitivity to $BRAF$ mutant cell lines has been reported compared to $NRAS$ mutants.[40] However, half of the melanoma cell lines carrying $NRAS$-activating mutations were found sensitive to the MEK inhibitor TAK733.[39] For those resistant to MEK inhibition, there was overactivation of the PI3K/AKT pathway providing a rationale to explore the combination with PI3K and AKT inhibitors. In uveal melanoma, mutually exclusive mutations in $GNAQ$ $or GNA11$ result in upregulation of MAPK pathway signaling, among others. Data have shown sensitivity to TAK733 in vitro with decreases in pERK. However, correlation with clinical results will have to be obtained.

CLINICAL TESTING OF MEK INHIBITORS IN MELANOMA

Despite the effective inhibition of the pathway in the in vitro context, translating the benefits of MEK inhibitors into the clinic has encountered the obstacle of a narrow therapeutic window. Fixing the tolerable dose in monotherapy has meant a decrease in response power. The most remarkable results have been in the metastatic melanoma $BRAF^{V600}$ mutant context. METRIC was a phase III trial comparing trametinib (formerly GSK1120212) against dacarbazine or paclitaxel in patients with metastatic melanoma with $BRAF^{V600}$ mutations.[41] This study was conducted before the data demonstrating the overall survival advantage of vemurafenib had not been yet reported. Although the overall response rate was lower than that with BRAF inhibitors, the study demonstrated improvements in the primary endpoints of progression-free survival and overall survival. Main toxicities included diarrhea, fatigue, papulopustular rash, vomiting, nausea, and reversible visual disturbances. cuSCCs were not reported, consistent with the lack of paradoxical MAPK activation with MEK inhibitors. Mild to moderate anemia is the most usual hematological toxicity, without neutropenia.

TABLE 5.1

MEK Inhibitors Tested in the Metastatic Melanoma Setting

MEK Inhibitor	Setting	Intervention	Results
Selumetinib (AZD6244)	BRAF- or NRAS-mutated stage IV melanomas	Monotherapy	Ongoing
	BRAF mutant MM	Combination with AKTi	Ongoing
	Uveal MM	Against TMZ	Ongoing
GDC-0973	BRAF mutant MM progressing to BRAFi	Combination with vemurafenib (BRIM-7)	Ongoing
MEK162	BRAF or NRAS mutant MM	Monotherapy[42]	Preliminary results
MSC1936369B	Solid tumors	Combination with PI3K/mTOR inhibitors	Ongoing
PD-0325901	Solid tumors	Monotherapy	Completed
TAK-733	Solid tumors	Monotherapy	Ongoing
Trametinib (GSK1120212)	BRAF mutant MM	Monotherapy	Preliminary results
	BRAF mutant MM	Combination DTIC/paclitaxel (METRIC)[41]	Preliminary results
	BRAF mutant MM	Combination dabrafenib[27]	Preliminary results
	Uveal melanoma GNA11 and GNAQ mutant	Monotherapy	Ongoing
	BRAF mutant MM	Combination with dabrafenib versus vemurafenib	Ongoing

AKTi, AKT inhibitors; BRAFi, BRAF inhibitor; MM, metastatic melanoma; DTIC, dacarbazine; TMZ, temozolomide.

MEK162, another allosteric MEK inhibitor, demonstrated antitumor activity in a phase II trial in patients with both *BRAF* and *NRAS* mutant advanced melanoma. This was the first demonstration of benefit in patients with *NRAS* mutant melanoma, with a 21% overall response rate and 46% disease stabilization.[42]

Other ongoing clinical trials are evaluating combinations of type I RAF inhibitors with MEK inhibitors. Table 5.1 summarizes the different MEK inhibitor compounds tested clinically so far.

So far, the efficacy of MEK inhibitors in monotherapy seems to be confined to a subset of patients, which may have predictive markers such as genetic alterations. Sequencing order or combination strategies will be the challenge with respect to determining the role of trametinib in the treatment of patients with BRAF mutant melanoma. Inhibition of MEK and ERK or combining inhibition of RAF with inhibitors of these downstream kinases may also be an effective strategy for tumors that are MAPK driven in a BRAF-independent fashion. These compounds give way to expand the treatment possibilities to patients.

Co-treatment with BRAF inhibitors is the rational approach to suppress the ERK pathway in those MAPK-dependent resistance mechanisms and attenuating skin toxicities. This dual inhibition of the MAPK pathway may help circumvent a common adverse event seen with monotherapy with BRAF inhibitors.

MECHANISMS OF RESISTANCE TO BRAF AND MEK INHIBITORS

The major finding is that MEK-inhibitor-resistant cells frequently maintain their addiction to the MAPK pathway, referring to alterations inside the upstream pathway. Mutations in MEK1 and MEK2 have been described as heterozygous and amplifications in *KRAS* and *BRAF* were also detected in resistant cell lines.[43,44] The combination of strategies or downstream targeting will attempt to revert these mechanisms. ERK inhibitors are currently a subject of preclinical studies[43] and early phase clinical trials.

Data evaluating the susceptibility of cell lines derived from melanomas with acquired resistance to BRAF inhibitors demonstrated that sensibility to a MEK inhibitor was dependent on the mechanism of resistance.[45,46] While initial *BRAF^V600* melanoma cell lines were sensitive to both BRAF and MEK inhibitors, many developed cross-resistance to both inhibitors. However, cell lines with the acquired *NRAS^Q61* mutations remained sensitive to MEK inhibitors, demonstrating the continued dependence on the MAPK pathway for driver oncogenic signaling. The cell lines with RTK upregulation as the mechanism of acquired resistance did not respond to the addition of the MEK inhibitor because they use an alternative survival pathway through PI3K/AKT/mTOR. These RTK-mediated acquired resistance cell lines were indeed sensitive to the addition of an AKT inhibitor or rapamycin in combination with vemurafenib. Thus, these data suggest that acquired resistance to BRAF inhibitors may be overcome or partially overcome in vitro by addition of either a MEK inhibitor or an inhibitor of the AKT/mTOR pathway, depending on the mechanism of resistance. Similarly, cell lines resistant to dabrafenib remain sensitive to an inhibitor of PI3K/AKT/mTOR.[31]

Considering the rapid recovery of pERK signal after BRAF inhibitor, the combination of BRAF and MEK inhibitors to prevent the onset of resistance has also been explored.[47] Dual BRAF/MEK inhibition effectively blocked colony formation in vitro supporting the combination. These effects were not achieved in either of the compounds alone, suggesting that despite targeting two points in the same pathway seem redundant, these may counteract the feedback inhibition.

COMBINATIONS OF BRAF AND MEK INHIBITORS

The combination of BRAF and MEK inhibitors is predicted to increase the antitumor activity in BRAF mutant melanoma by having two sequential levels of blocking of the oncogenic MAPK signaling, and at the same time, it would avoid side effects related to paradoxical MAPK activation in cells with upstream mutations, such as the ones that lead to cuSCCs. Furthermore, it may prevent the development of acquired resistance mechanisms that are mediated by reactivation of MEK signaling, as what happens when there are secondary *NRAS^Q61* mutations or *BRAF^V600* amplification or splice variants. Outcomes of a phase I/II trial combining dabrafenib (GSK2118436) with trametinib (GSK1120212) have shown encouraging results in patients with *BRAF*[V600E/K] mutant metastatic melanoma.[27] This study concluded that a combination approach at full dose was feasible and safe and lowers incidence of hyperproliferative skin lesions in the combination group compared to dabrafenib alone. Clinical activity will have to be confirmed in future ongoing trials, but early data demonstrate benefits with delay on the resistance onset and raising the median duration of treatment to 10.7 months. BRIM-7 is the phase Ib trial testing a combination between vemurafenib and GDC-0973, an oral MEK inhibitor for patients with *BRAF*[V600] mutant melanoma, for patients who have progressed on single-agent vemurafenib.

CONCLUSIONS

The metastatic melanoma context has been enriched with new targeted therapies according to specific oncogenic events in the MAPK pathway. In the *BRAF* mutant setting, BRAF inhibitors—vemurafenib and dabrafenib—have opened the door to new hopes and treatments. However, the relatively rapid onset of resistance and the appearance of cuSCC have demanded a better understanding of the biology. Underlying the cuSCC, the paradoxical activation of the MAPK, which can be prevented with the combination of MEK inhibitors, has been described. The addiction to the pathway has focused most on the efforts to maintain blockade of oncogenic MAPK signaling. MEK inhibitors show effective results in monotherapy and promising results in combination, potentially with efficacy in the *NRAS* mutant context.

REFERENCES

1. Hanahan D, Weinberg RA. Hallmarks of cancer: The next generation. *Cell* 2011; 144:646–674.
2. Balmanno K, Cook SJ. Tumour cell survival signalling by the ERK1/2 pathway. *Cell Death and Differentiation* 2009;16:368–377.
3. Meloche S, Pouyssegur J. The ERK1/2 mitogen-activated protein kinase pathway as a master regulator of the G1- to S-phase transition. *Oncogene* 2007;26:3227–3239.
4. Curtin JA, Fridlyand J, Kageshita T et al. Distinct sets of genetic alterations in melanoma. *The New England Journal of Medicine* 2005;353:2135–2147.
5. Nazarian R, Shi H, Wang Q et al. Melanomas acquire resistance to B-RAF(V600E) inhibition by RTK or N-RAS upregulation. *Nature* 2010;468:973–977.
6. Greenman C, Stephens P, Smith R et al. Patterns of somatic mutation in human cancer genomes. *Nature* 2007;446:153–158.
7. Rubinstein JC, Sznol M, Pavlick AC et al. Incidence of the V600K mutation among melanoma patients, and potential response to the specific BRAF inhibitor PLX4032. *Journal of Translational Medicine* 2010;8:67.
8. Ikenoue T, Hikiba Y, Kanai F et al. Functional analysis of mutations within the kinase activation segment of B-Raf in human colorectal tumors. *Cancer Research* 2003;63:8132–8137.
9. Davies H, Bignell GR, Cox C et al. Mutations of the BRAF gene in human cancer. *Nature* 2002;417:949–954.
10. Sondergaard JN, Nazarian R, Wang Q et al. Differential sensitivity of melanoma cell lines with BRAFV600E mutation to the specific Raf inhibitor PLX4032. *Journal of Translational Medicine* 2010;8:39.

11. Garnett MJ, Rana S, Paterson H, Barford D, Marais R. Wild-type and mutant B-RAF activate C-RAF through distinct mechanisms involving heterodimerization. *Molecular Cell* 2005;20:963–969.
12. Wilhelm SM, Carter C, Tang L et al. BAY 43–9006 exhibits broad spectrum oral antitumor activity and targets the RAF/MEK/ERK pathway and receptor tyrosine kinases involved in tumor progression and angiogenesis. *Cancer Research* 2004;64:7099–7109.
13. Tsai J, Lee JT, Wang W et al. Discovery of a selective inhibitor of oncogenic B-Raf kinase with potent antimelanoma activity. *Proceedings of the National Academy of Sciences of the United States of America* 2008;105:3041–3046.
14. Bollag G, Hirth P, Tsai J et al. Clinical efficacy of a RAF inhibitor needs broad target blockade in BRAF-mutant melanoma. *Nature* 2010;467:596–599.
15. Flaherty KT, Puzanov I, Kim KB et al. Inhibition of mutated, activated BRAF in metastatic melanoma. *The New England Journal of Medicine* 2010;363:809–819.
16. Sosman JA, Kim KB, Schuchter L et al. Survival in BRAF V600-mutant advanced melanoma treated with vemurafenib. *The New England Journal of Medicine* 2012; 366:707–714.
17. Chapman PB, Hauschild A, Robert C et al. Improved survival with vemurafenib in melanoma with BRAF V600E mutation. *The New England Journal of Medicine* 2011;364:2507–2516.
18. Dietrich S, Glimm H, Andrulis M, von Kalle C, Ho AD, Zenz T. BRAF inhibition in refractory hairy-cell leukemia. *The New England Journal of Medicine* 2012;366:2038–2040.
19. Hauschild A, Grob JJ, Demidov LV et al. Dabrafenib in BRAF-mutated metastatic melanoma: A multicentre, open-label, phase 3 randomised controlled trial. *Lancet* 2012,380:358–365.
20. de la Monte SM, Moore GW, Hutchins GM. Patterned distribution of metastases from malignant melanoma in humans. *Cancer Research* 1983;43:3427–3433.
21. Su F, Viros A, Milagre C et al. RAS mutations in cutaneous squamous-cell carcinomas in patients treated with BRAF inhibitors. *The New England Journal of Medicine* 2012;366:207–215.
22. Poulikakos PI, Zhang C, Bollag G, Shokat KM, Rosen N. RAF inhibitors transactivate RAF dimers and ERK signalling in cells with wild-type BRAF. *Nature* 2010;464:427–430.
23. Hatzivassiliou G, Song K, Yen I et al. RAF inhibitors prime wild-type RAF to activate the MAPK pathway and enhance growth. *Nature* 2010;464:431–435.
24. Heidorn SJ, Milagre C, Whittaker S et al. Kinase-dead BRAF and oncogenic RAS cooperate to drive tumor progression through CRAF. *Cell* 2010;140:209–221.
25. Hall-Jackson CA, Eyers PA, Cohen P et al. Paradoxical activation of Raf by a novel Raf inhibitor. *Chemistry and Biology* 1999;6:559–568.
26. Falchook GS, Long GV, Kurzrock R et al. Dabrafenib in patients with melanoma, untreated brain metastases, and other solid tumours: A phase 1 dose-escalation trial. *Lancet* 2012;379:1893–1901.
27. Weber JS, Flaherty K, J.R I. Updated safety and efficacy results from a phase I/II study of the oral BRAF inhibitor dabrafenib (GSK2118436) combined with the oral MEK1/2 inhibitor trametinib (GSK1120212) in patients with BRAFi-naive metastatic melanoma. *Journal of Clinical Oncology* 2012; 30(suppl; abstr 8510).
28. Comin-Anduix B, Chodon T, Sazegar H et al. The oncogenic BRAF kinase inhibitor PLX4032/RG7204 does not affect the viability or function of human lymphocytes across a wide range of concentrations. *Clinical Cancer Research: An Official Journal of the American Association for Cancer Research* 2010;16:6040–6048.
29. Berridge MJ. Lymphocyte activation in health and disease. *Critical Reviews in Immunology* 1997;17:155–178.

30. Hong DS, Vence L, Falchook G et al. BRAF(V600) inhibitor GSK2118436 targeted inhibition of mutant BRAF in cancer patients does not impair overall immune competency. *Clinical Cancer Research: An Official Journal of the American Association for Cancer Research* 2012;18:2326–2335.

31. Greger JG, Eastman SD, Zhang V et al. Combinations of BRAF, MEK, and PI3K/mTOR inhibitors overcome acquired resistance to the BRAF inhibitor GSK2118436 dabrafenib, mediated by NRAS or MEK mutations. *Molecular Cancer Therapeutics* 2012;11:909–920.

32. Shi H, Moriceau G, Kong X et al. Melanoma whole-exome sequencing identifies (V600E)B-RAF amplification-mediated acquired B-RAF inhibitor resistance. *Nature Communications* 2012;3:724.

33. Poulikakos PI, Persaud Y, Janakiraman M et al. RAF inhibitor resistance is mediated by dimerization of aberrantly spliced BRAF(V600E). *Nature* 2011;480:387–390.

34. Wagle N, Emery C, Berger MF et al. Dissecting therapeutic resistance to RAF inhibition in melanoma by tumor genomic profiling. *Journal of Clinical Oncology: Official Journal of the American Society of Clinical Oncology* 2011;29:3085–3096.

35. Johannessen CM, Boehm JS, Kim SY et al. COT drives resistance to RAF inhibition through MAP kinase pathway reactivation. *Nature* 2010;468:968–972.

36. Villanueva J, Vultur A, Lee JT et al. Acquired resistance to BRAF inhibitors mediated by a RAF kinase switch in melanoma can be overcome by cotargeting MEK and IGF-1R/PI3K. *Cancer Cell* 2010;18:683–695.

37. Straussman R, Morikawa T, Shee K et al. Tumour micro-environment elicits innate resistance to RAF inhibitors through HGF secretion. *Nature* 2012:487:500–504.

38. Adjei AA, Cohen RB, Franklin W et al. Phase I pharmacokinetic and pharmacodynamic study of the oral, small-molecule mitogen-activated protein kinase kinase 1/2 inhibitor AZD6244 (ARRY-142886) in patients with advanced cancers. *Journal of Clinical Oncology: Official Journal of the American Society of Clinical Oncology* 2008;26:2139–2146.

39. von Euw E, Atefi M, Attar N et al. Antitumor effects of the investigational selective MEK inhibitor TAK733 against cutaneous and uveal melanoma cell lines. *Molecular Cancer* 2012;11:22.

40. Solit DB, Garraway LA, Pratilas CA et al. BRAF mutation predicts sensitivity to MEK inhibition. *Nature* 2006;439:358–362.

41. Flaherty KT, Robert C, Hersey P et al. Improved survival with MEK inhibition in BRAF-mutated melanoma. *The New England Journal of Medicine* 2012;367:107–114.

42. Ascierto P. Efficacy and safety of oral MEK162 in patients with locally advanced and unresectable or metastatic cutaneous melanoma harboring BRAF V600 or NRAS MUTATIONS. *Journal of Clinical Oncology* 2012; 30(suppl; abstr 8511).

43. Hatzivassiliou G, Liu B, O'Brien C et al. ERK inhibition overcomes acquired resistance to MEK inhibitors. *Molecular Cancer Therapeutics* 2012;11:1143–1154.

44. Poulikakos PI, Solit DB. Resistance to MEK inhibitors: Should we co-target upstream? *Science Signaling* 2011;4:pe16.

45. Atefi M, von Euw E, Attar N et al. Reversing melanoma cross-resistance to BRAF and MEK inhibitors by co-targeting the AKT/mTOR pathway. *PloS One* 2011;6:e28973.

46. Shi H, Kong X, Ribas A, Lo RS. Combinatorial treatments that overcome PDGFRbeta-driven resistance of melanoma cells to V600EB-RAF inhibition. *Cancer Research* 2011;71:5067–5074.

47. Paraiso KH, Fedorenko IV, Cantini LP et al. Recovery of phospho-ERK activity allows melanoma cells to escape from BRAF inhibitor therapy. *British Journal of Cancer* 2010;102:1724–1730.

6 *KIT* and KIT Inhibitors

Jean-Yves Blay
Centre Leon Berard

Armelle Dufresne
Centre Leon Berard

Olfa Derbel
Centre Leon Berard

Isabelle Ray-Coquard
Centre Leon Berard

CONTENTS

INTRODUCTION

The *KIT* gene is mutated in several hematological malignancies and solid tumors in humans. The identification of the specific genetic alterations in the KIT gene (translocations, deletions, point mutations, amplifications) enables now to distinguish specific nosological groups within tumor types (gastrointestinal stromal tumor [GIST], melanoma, thymic carcinoma). Beyond the identification of these mutations as diagnostic tools, the nature of these driver mutations in tyrosine kinases enables to guide the administration of inhibitors of KIT, such as imatinib, sunitinib, and others in clinical setting. GIST, melanoma, and rare subsets of thymic carcinomas are known to be sensitive to these targeted therapies in advanced stage. Adjuvant treatment was found to improve survival in GIST patients with high risk of relapse. Yet, the emergence of multiclonal secondary resistance mutations encoding for a resistant form of the receptor within tumor cell masses remains a therapeutic challenge in advanced stage. The role of KIT inhibitors in other diseases in which no such mutations have been identified, such as aggressive fibromatosis (AF) or cystic adenoid carcinomas where a contribution of KIT is suspected, is unclear. The D816 mutations observed in mastocytosis, leukemia, and germ cell tumors result in intrinsic resistance to most tyrosine kinase inhibitors (TKIs) and represent a therapeutic challenge. Clinical research must include translational research programs to evaluate the response of the molecular target in vivo in the clinical setting and the mechanisms of resistance.

Targeted therapies against oncogene products are directed against proteins involved in neoplastic transformation as the result of genomic alterations, such as specific translocations, activating mutations, or gene amplifications. These treatments can be applied in two different situations: (1) when the genomic alteration is directly contributing to the initiation of the malignant transformation (the term "driver mutation" is often used in this situation) and (2) when the genomic alteration is involved in tumor progression as a cofactor and not in the onset of malignant transformation [1–3]. The KIT protein was among the first described as activated through gene mutations and, as a driver, in specific tumor types in humans [4–9]. Several TKIs available for clinical use inhibit KIT [10–14]. In this chapter, we will review the molecular basis and clinical activity of TKIs targeting the KIT receptor.

KIT GENE AND THE KIT PROTEIN

The human *KIT* proto-oncogene is located on the long arm of chromosome 4 (4 q11–q12). It contains 21 exons, which are transcribed and then translated into a protein of 976 amino acids with a molecular weight of 145 kDa. The KIT protein is a type III transmembrane tyrosine kinase receptor whose extracellular portion binds a ligand known as stem-cell factor (SCF), also called steel factor [4].

The extracellular portion is composed of 5 immunoglobulin-like domains, the first 3 involved in ligand binding and the 4th and 5th, encoded by exon 6–9, are responsible for dimerization. The intracellular portion of KIT contains the juxtamembrane domain, encoded by exon 11, and 2 kinase domains separated by the kinase insert domain. The structure of KIT is close to that of other receptor tyrosine kinases (RTKs) with oncogenic properties, including platelet-derived growth factor receptors (PDGFRs) A and B, CSF-1R, and FLT3. KIT activation normally occurs when two adjacent receptors are brought together, after binding to ligands, causing receptor dimerization. Homodimerization is accompanied by structural changes in the receptors, resulting in the activation of the kinase domains. The activated kinase then cross-phosphorylates tyrosine residues in the homodimer partner. The phosphotyrosines also serve as binding sites for various substrates, many of which are phosphorylated by KIT. The Src family kinases (SFKs), the p85 subunit of phosphatidylinositol 3-kinase (PI3K), phospholipase C-gamma, and adaptors that lead to the activation of MAP kinase pathways are directly recruited and activated by binding to phospho-Y residues on the receptor [15].

KIT expression is widely distributed on a variety of cell types in humans including the hematopoietic lineage, neural crest cells, as well as in their malignant counterparts. KIT function is essential for normal hematopoiesis, for melanogenesis, for the development and function of mast cells in many tissues, and for the differentiation and proliferation of interstitial cells of Cajal (ICCs) in the gut [4]. As for most growth factor RTKs, multiple physiological functions have been ascribed to KIT as well, which include cell survival, proliferation, differentiation, adhesion, and apoptosis [16]. These functions are accomplished once the normal receptor binds the ligand and also by the mutated activated forms of the receptor, even though each mutated form of the receptor may activate specifically distinct pathways [4,8,16].

Six different isoforms of KIT resulting from alternative splicing of the mRNA have been identified. The variants with or without an additional glutamine at position 252 have not been reported to have a differential biological activity, nor do the 2 variants with or without a serine residue in position 715 [10]. Conversely, two isoforms characterized by the presence or absence of the tetrapeptide sequence glycine–asparagine–asparagine–lysine (GNNK) in the extracellular part of the juxtamembrane region differ functionally, with the GNNK isoform showing tumorigenic potency [17,18].

Rare allelic variants of the KIT protein are also observed and have been suggested to play a role in the physiopathology of several neoplastic diseases. The M541L variant, resulting from a codon variant in exon 10, has been reported as a possible mutation in systemic mastocytosis or AF, as well as a biomarker for response to KIT TKIs in AF, but is actually an SNP [10,19,20]. Its incidence is actually similar in the general population and in patients with AF [21]. Several publications have suggested that this represents a constitutively active form of KIT with specific biological activities [10].

KIT MUTANTS

Mutations in the KIT gene are reported in a variety of malignant diseases, as reported in the COSMIC database (Table 6.1). The topography of the mutation of *KIT* varies across tumor types. KIT mutations have been described in almost all portions of the genes [4–10]:

1. In the ligand (SCF)-binding domain exons (from 1 to 5, encoding amino acid 1–308), mostly in mastocytosis [22,23].
2. In the dimerization domain (exons 6–7, aa 309–410) in mastocytosis [22,24].
3. In the proteolytic cleavage site (exons 8–9, aa 411–513) in GIST and mastocytosis [22–30].
4. In the transmembrane region (exon 10, aa 514–549) in mastocytosis and possibly in AF [20–26].
5. In the auto-inhibition domain (exon 11, aa 550–591) in GIST, melanoma, thymoma, mastocytosis, and AML [28–40].
6. In the signal transduction domain (exons 12–21, aa 592–976), within this last portion in the kinase 1 or 2 domains, or in the kinase insert domain. These latter mutations are often observed in hematological malignancies, including systemic mastocytosis and AML, but also in germ cell tumors of the testis, GIST, melanoma, and thymic carcinoma. These mutations may also often be identified as secondary mutations arising from the selection pressure induced by imatinib in GIST [22–40].

In general, KIT mutations result in ligand-independent kinase activation and confer an oncogenic role to the protein. In solid tumors, the most common mutations of KIT affect the juxtamembrane domain encoded by exon 11. Secondary resistance mutations in *KIT* exons 13 and 14 affect the drug-binding residues of imatinib.

In hematological malignancies, as well as in germ cell tumors, most mutations occur in *KIT* exon 17, frequently on codon 816. These mutations favor the active

TABLE 6.1
KIT Mutations in Solid Tumors and Hematological Malignancies in the COSMIC Database

Primary Tissue	Unique Mutated Samples	% Mutated	No. of Samples
Adrenal gland	0	0	3
Autonomic ganglia	1	0	319
Biliary tract	0	0	32
Bone	18	5	339
Breast	6	1	831
Central nervous system	4	0	1,019
Cervix	0	0	16
Endometrium	12	9	136
Eye	10	3	310
Fallopian tube	0	0	3
Genital tract	13	21	62
Hematopoietic and lymphoid tissue	1732	21	8,406
Kidney	17	4	416
Colon/rectum	13	3	415
Liver	0	0	40
Lung	34	2	1,471
Meninges	0	0	29
Esophagus	0	0	114
Ovary	24	5	463
Pancreas	4	3	115
Pituitary	0	0	35
Placenta	0	0	9
Pleura	0	0	8
Prostate	1	1	88
Salivary gland	9	6	141
Skin	221	7	2,987
Small intestine	0	0	72
Soft tissue	3841	50	7,706
Stomach	2	1	357
Testis	52	9	558
Thymus	7	5	149
Thyroid	0	0	287
Upper aerodigestive tract	1	2	66
Urinary tract	0	0	28
Vagina	0	0	2
Vulva	0	0	5
Totals	6030	22	2,7306

conformation of the kinase. Mutations on codon 816 are resistant to imatinib and most KIT inhibitors that bind to the inactive form of the kinase.

Mutations of KIT in GIST

Two-thirds of GISTs exhibit mutations of KIT (insertions, deletions, missense mutations) in exon 11, which disrupt the normal juxtamembrane secondary structure that prevents the kinase activation loop to adopt an active conformation [28,43]. The deletions in this portion of the gene were associated with a shorter progression-free and overall survival (OS) before the imatinib era in comparison to the other exon 11 mutations [44–46].

Close to 10% of localized and metastatic GISTs have a mutation in the extracellular domain encoded by exon 9, most often in the form of a duplication of two amino acids (AY) in positions 902 and 903 [28]. These mutations mimic the conformational change occurring when the extracellular KIT receptor binds SCF [47]. Interestingly, this mutation occurs in GIST arising in the small and large intestine but is very uncommon in gastric GISTs.

In GIST, primary mutations, such as K642E, occurring in the ATP-binding region (encoded by exon 13), are uncommon [48]. Mutations in the activation loop encoded by exon 17 of the kinase are also uncommon in these tumors. As mentioned earlier, these mutations stabilize the active conformation of the kinase.

Multiple Secondary Mutations of KIT in Resistant GIST

Primary resistance is most often a consequence of an intrinsic resistance of the mutated protein (e.g., KIT D816V). Conversely, secondary resistance, occurring after a period of tumor control, often results from the emergence of resistant subclones. Interestingly, mutations in the activation loop or in the ATP-binding site are more frequent at the time of emergence of secondary resistance [28,30,49,50]. As discussed later, secondary resistance is occurring at a median of 30 months following the initiation of imatinib therapy in GIST patients in advanced stage [30,41–58] (Figure 6.1). This secondary resistance often occurs in the form of a multifocal clonal resistance, in different metastatic sites or in the same site [50,59]. The radiological presentation of a nodule within a mass illustrates this clonal evolution (Figure 6.2). The presence of secondary mutations and their topography on the protein influences the sensitivity to imatinib but also to second-line treatment with sunitinib [30,49,50].

Mutations of KIT in Melanoma, Thymic Carcinoma, and Germ Cell Tumors

In 5%–10% of melanoma, point mutations of KIT are observed in exons 11 and 13 and are similar to those observed in GIST [36–39]. There may be a higher frequency of report of mutations in exon 13 in melanoma as compared to GIST. The amplification of *KIT* has also been described [39]. In thymic carcinoma, mutations of exon 11 of KIT, as well as mutations of exon 13, have also been reported [40,122–125,136].

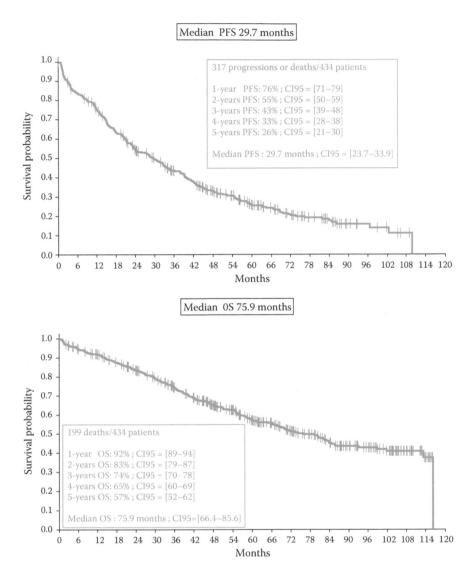

FIGURE 6.1   Updated progression-free and OS in the BFR14 series.

Mutations of KIT are observed in other histological subtypes of solid tumors, but the frequency reported is often low to very low (Table 6.1). In germ cell testicular cancers, these mutations are often observed in exon 17 and encode for a D816V mutation [136–139].

MUTATIONS OF KIT IN HEMATOLOGICAL MALIGNANCIES

Mutations of KIT are also observed in hematological malignancies, in particular, in systemic mastocytosis and AML with core binding factor gene alteration [10,31–35]. In these diseases also, most mutations occur also in the exon 17 portion of the gene,

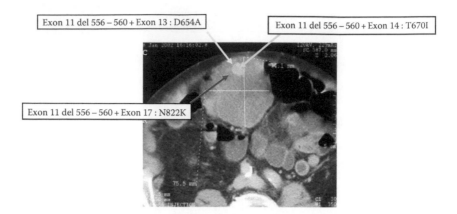

FIGURE 6.2 Multiclonal resistance. This occurs through the emergence of resistant clones equipped with different secondary mutations in a GIST patient resected at the time of progression.

in particular, on codon 816. These mutations may not always be the driver event but contribute to neoplastic progression in association with the fusion proteins [34,35].

ABNORMAL TRAFFICKING OF KIT RECEPTOR MUTANTS

The presence of KIT mutations induces an intracellular retention of the KIT receptor within the cell [60,61] (Figure 6.3). This has been observed in GIST cell lines, fresh clinical samples, as well as in NIH3T3 cells transfected with mutant forms of KIT [61–64]. In GIST, as well as in NIH3T3-infected cells, KIT mutated in exon 11 are expressed in an immature 125 kDa phosphorylated–activated form within the intracellular compartments of the Golgi and ER and with limited expression at the cell surface. This is not observed in cells expressing the wild-type (WT) form of KIT.

Importantly, imatinib-induced blockade of the activation of the immature form of KIT restores the expression of the mature form on the cell surface [61]. Similar observations have recently been reported with KIT D816V mutant cells treated with dasatinib [64].

The molecular pathways activated within the cells are different between WT *KIT* and mutated activated KIT [64]. Signaling pathways are also subtly different in cells expressing the exon 9 and exon 11 mutated KIT proteins and also among the different forms of the exon 11 mutations, associated with different miRNA expression profiles [65–69].

TYROSINE KINASE INHIBITORS OF KIT

The majority of the inhibitors of KIT used in the clinical setting, such as imatinib, nilotinib, and masitinib, exert inhibitory activities on receptors of the same family, that is, PDGFRA and CSF-1R. Other inhibitors, in particular, sunitinib, regorafenib, sorafenib, dovitinib, pazopanib, vatalanib, and motesanib, also block VEGFR2 and other RTKs.

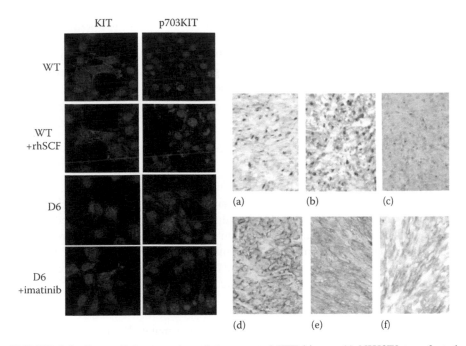

FIGURE 6.3 Intracellular retention of the mutated KIT kinase. (a) NIH3T3-transfected cells: Confocal microscopy analysis revealed that the KIT intracellular localization was different between cells transfected with the WT or the mutant D6 (*KIT* exon 11 del 554–560) forms: KIT staining (red) was diffused within cytoplasm and membranous in *KIT* WT cells, while it remained concentrated in the perinuclear region in *KIT*-mutated cells. Moreover, while the membrane *KIT* WT receptor needed rhSCF to be phosphorylated, mutants were activated in the intracellular compartment. Inhibition of KIT kinase activity of mutants led to receptor translocation to the membrane. (b) KIT immunohistochemical staining on GIST paraffin-embedded samples disclosed a predominant Golgi-like pattern in GISTs with homozygous KIT mutations (a, b, c) and membrane pattern in GISTs without mutations (d, e, f). A cytoplasmic staining was also present in most cases.

IMATINIB

Imatinib mesylate, a derivative of 2-phenylamino pyrimidine, is a small-molecule-selective TKI, given orally [11–14]. In vitro studies have shown that this drug binds and specifically inhibits the activity of Bcr–Abl, PDGF receptors, the WT and mutant KIT and MCSFR/CSF-1R [70]. Imatinib is a competitive antagonist of ATP binding that blocks transduction. At the molecular level, imatinib binds with high affinity to the conserved ATP-binding site in the tyrosine kinase domain of the kinases in their inactive form and blocks the ability to transfer phosphate groups from ATP to tyrosine residues on substrate proteins, thus blocking signaling.

SUNITINIB

Sunitinib inhibits multiple receptors for signaling pathways fundamental to tumor growth and survival, including PDGFR-α and PDGFR-β; KIT, RET, and CSF1R;

and FLT3 but also VEGFR-1, VEGFR-2, and VEGFR-3, in marked contrast with imatinib or nilotinib [71–74]. Although both sunitinib and imatinib bind within the ATP-binding domain of both KIT and PDGFRs, they are members of different chemical classes and have different binding characteristics and affinities. VEGFR kinases are essential for tumor-related angiogenesis, and this property is not shared by imatinib.

OTHER KIT INHIBITORS

Nilotinib

Nilotinib is a second-generation oral inhibitor of Bcr–Abl, designed to inhibit mutated activated tyrosine kinases resistant to imatinib, and also blocking KIT, PDGFRs, and MCSFR [75–77]. In vitro data in GIST882 cells show reduction of KIT autophosphorylation similar to imatinib, but nilotinib inhibits cell proliferation in imatinib-sensitive and imatinib-resistant GIST cell lines (GIST882, GIST430, and GIST48) more potently than imatinib [78]. This may be related to a preferential accumulation of nilotinib intracellular concentrations in GIST cell lines [76].

Masitinib

AB1010 is a protein–TKI that inhibits KIT receptor mutated in the juxtamembrane domain as well as WT receptor, PDGF receptor, and mutated FGFR3 [79]. At the cellular level, AB1010 inhibits *KIT* exon 11-dependent cell proliferation in the nanomolar range (IC_{50} 5 nM) and *KIT* WT-dependent cell proliferation in the 0.1 μM range [79]. Masitinib has been explored in phase II trials in first-line treatment, in GIST patient progressing after imatinib, and in GIST patients in progressing after both imatinib and sunitinib [80,81]. Two phase III trials are exploring this agent in first-line setting vs. imatinib and in second line vs. sunitinib.

Dasatinib

Dasatinib targets Abl, Src, and KIT, with IC50 < 1, 0.5, and 79 nM, respectively. Dasatinib inhibits mutated forms of KIT, with a specific activity on the D816V mutation known to be resistant to imatinib and other KIT inhibitors [82–85].

Ponatinib

Ponatinib is a novel TKI active on the T315I mutation of Bcr-Abl both in vitro and in the clinical setting [86,87]. This agent has also recently been reported to be active on WT *KIT* and mutated forms of KIT [88].

OTHER KINASE INHIBITORS TARGETING BOTH KIT AND VEGFR2

Regorafenib

Regorafenib is an oral kinase inhibitor that blocks the activity of multiple protein kinases, including those involved in the regulation of tumor angiogenesis (VEGFR-1, VEGFR-2, and VEGFR-3 and TIE2) and oncogenesis (KIT, RET, RAF-1, BRAF, BRAFV600E, PDGFR, and FGFR). It blocks VEGFR1, VEGFR2, VEGFR3, PDGFRβ, Kit, RET, and Raf-1 with IC50 of 13, 4.2, 46, 22, 7, 1.5, and

2.5 nM, respectively [89]. Its specific activity of the different KIT mutants is not precisely known.

Sorafenib

Sorafenib is a multikinase inhibitor against KIT, VEGFR, PDGFR, and RAF kinases. Sorafenib inhibits cells expressing *KIT* exon 11 mutants with an $IC_{50} < 100$ nmol/L, WT *KIT* with an IC_{50} close to 2.7 µM/L (similar to imatinib), and *KIT* exon 9 mutant kinase with an IC_{50} close to 1.8 µM/L, similar to imatinib. Sorafenib also inhibits the phosphorylation of KIT double mutants in which the second mutation occurred in the drug-/ATP-binding site of the receptor, including V560D and V654A or T670I (exons 11 and 13), while imatinib alone is ineffective. *KIT* exon 11 mutant kinases with a secondary mutation in the activation loop are all resistant to imatinib but are sensitive to sorafenib [90–92]. KIT D816V is also resistant to sorafenib.

Pazopanib

Pazopanib, a synthetic indazolpyrimidin, is a multitargeted TKI of VEGFR1, VEGFR2, VEGFR3, PDGFR, FGFR, KIT, and MCSFR, with IC_{50}s of 10, 30, 47, 84, 74, 140, and 146 nM, respectively [140]. Its activity on the different mutant forms of KIT has not been extensively reported yet. Pazopanib is registered for the treatment of advanced renal cell cancer and advanced soft tissue sarcoma failing doxorubicin [93]. Given its potent activity of KIT, this agent is currently being investigated in GIST progressing after imatinib and sunitinib.

Dovitinib

Dovitinib (TKI258, CHIR258) is a multitarget inhibitor for KIT, FLT3, FGFR1/3, VEGFR1/2/3, and PDGFRα/β with IC_{50}s of 2 nM, 1 nM, 8 nM/9nM and 10 nM/13 nM/8 nM, and 210 nM/27 nM, respectively [93,94]. Its activity on the different mutant forms of KIT has not been extensively reported yet. Dovitinib has been tested in the treatment of patients with advanced GIST in 2 phase II trials [95].

Motesanib

AMG706 is an orally bioavailable small-molecule multikinase inhibitor (KIT, PDGFR, VEGFR1–3, and RET) that exerts, like sunitinib, both strong antiangiogenic (VEGFR) and direct antitumor activity on activated tyrosine kinases on tumor cells [96]. This agent has been tested for the treatment of GIST failing imatinib [97].

Valatinib

PTK787/ZK222584 (PTK/ZK) is an inhibitor of the RTKs KIT, PDGFRs, VEGFR-1, and VEGFR-2 [98]. Initially developed for the treatment of advanced colorectal cancer in combination with chemotherapy, this agent has also been tested in the treatment of advanced GIST before its development being terminated [99].

TUMORS WITH MUTATIONS OF KIT

Different tumor types have been reported to express frequently or occasionally a mutated form of the KIT receptor. GISTs are the paradigmatic tumors of this category.

GIST

Clinical Presentation, Pathology, and Molecular Biology

GIST is the most frequent sarcoma of the gastrointestinal tract. It arises from pre-cursors of the ICCs, the pacemaker cells of the gastrointestinal tract [59]. The incidence of GIST ranges between 1 and 1.45/100,000 per year [100]. GISTs occur at a median age of 60, with rare pediatric forms. Primary GIST may range in size from less than 1 cm to larger than 30 cm. Although they can occur anywhere throughout the GI tract, GISTs predominantly originate from the stomach (60%) or small intestine (30%) and less commonly in the colon and rectum (5%) or the esophagus (1%).

MicroGIST

Very small GISTs discovered incidentally are common, with an incidence of up to 25% of the population for small lesions of a 3–9 mm size [101,102]. Their vast majority will not evolve toward an overt malignant behavior. MicroGIST and GIST are however equipped with the same sets of mutations, indicating that KIT mutation in this model is a very early event in the transformation process. Interestingly, while the mutated KIT protein is conveying the properties of a benign tumor in this model, it remains the key target for the treatment of its malignant counterpart.

Pathology and Molecular Biology

GISTs are characterized by the expression of CD34, KIT, and DOG1 in 70%, 95%, and >95% of the cases, respectively [28]. The gain-of-function KIT mutations in GIST were first reported in 1998 by Hirota [9]. Subsequently, activating mutations in PDGFRα, mutually exclusive of *KIT* mutations, were identified [9].

Approximately 12%–15% of GISTs have WT *KIT* or *PDGFRA*. Mutations on other genes, including NF1, BRAF, SDHA, B or C, K-Ras, and NRAS, have been described as possible initial mutational events in patients with these tumors. These activating mutations drive the aberrant behavior of GIST.

KIT-mutated GISTs represent more than 70% of GISTs, with *KIT* exon 11 muta-tions representing 60%–70%, exon 9 mutations 10%, and rare KIT mutations (on exon 13, 14, or 17) less than 2%.

Primary Treatment

Complete surgical resection, achieving negative margins whenever possible (R0 resection), is the standard approach for the initial management of primary local-ized GIST. Surgery must be performed en bloc, avoiding tumor rupture, with a margin of 1 cm around the tumor. Organ preservation (e.g., partial gastrectomy) is therefore possible in marked contrast with the more extensive standard surgical approach to GI carcinomas [59]. The risk of relapse following surgical resection may be estimated now using five parameters: (1) mitotic rate, (2) tumor size, (3) tumor site, (4) tumor rupture, and (5) the nature of the primary mutation [103]. The threshold level for high risk varies according to the prognostic classification.

Imatinib for the Treatment of GIST in Advanced Stage

Preceding the understanding of the role of KIT in the oncogenesis of these tumors and the introduction of imatinib, the prognosis of patients with advanced GISTs was very poor, with a median survival estimated between 12 and 18 months and a 5 year progression-free survival (PFS) and OS close to 5% [59]. In these patients, the introduction of imatinib has transformed the management of this previously untreatable neoplasm into a treatable entity and the paradigmatic model of targeted therapies in a solid tumor.

Imatinib provides response rates of between 50% and 70% in patients with advanced GIST, a median PFS between 20 and 30 months, and a median OS of approximately 5 years, with up to 25% of the patients alive at 9 years [52–58]. This represents at least a 300% increase in median OS and a likely >100% increase in 5 year and 10 year survival as compared to cytotoxic chemotherapy.

However, still 50% of patients experience disease progression within 30 months of starting therapy in advanced stage (Figure 6.1). Two phase III randomized trials compared two doses of imatinib, 400 g/day vs. 800 mg/day, in patients with advanced GIST, and these studies were subsequently merged in a meta-analysis [104]. In this total pooled series of 1640 patients with advanced GIST, there was a small but significant increase in median PFS in the high-dose group, without benefits in OS. *KIT* exon 9 mutations were the only predictive factor associated with significantly longer PFS and a higher objective response rate to high-dose imatinib [104]. No benefit was observed for the 800 mg/day dose for the other molecular subsets (exon 11 or WT) evaluated.

Based on these results, the National Comprehensive Cancer Network (NCCN) and the European Society of Medical Oncology (ESMO) guidelines have recommended initiating treatment in all patients with unresectable or metastatic GIST with imatinib 400 mg/day, with the exception of patients with GIST harboring *KIT* exon 9 mutations who should be given imatinib 800 mg/day [59]. In 2012, ESMO recommended the determination of the mutations as mandatory for routine clinical treatment. This is further justified by the fact that up to 20% of localized tumors of the stomach have a driver PDGFRA mutation, which is completely insensitive to imatinib.

In advanced stage, continuous KIT blockade should be maintained in the patients. The phase III BFR14 study investigated in a randomized setting the utility of maintenance imatinib treatment in advanced stage [54,58]. A randomized discontinuation design was performed after 1, 3, and then 5 years of treatment: at all these dates, interruption was demonstrated to be associated with a higher incidence of relapse. Interestingly, the median PFS of patients randomized to the interruption arm was significantly longer in those patients on therapy for 5 years (12.2 months) than in those on therapy for 1 (5.7 months) or 3 years (6.3 months) (Figure 6.4). It is therefore recommended to continue imatinib until progression or intolerance in the different clinical practice guidelines [59,105].

Imatinib in the Adjuvant and Neoadjuvant Setting in GIST

Following complete remission obtained by surgery on the primary tumor, it has been demonstrated that adjuvant administration of imatinib prevents relapse and

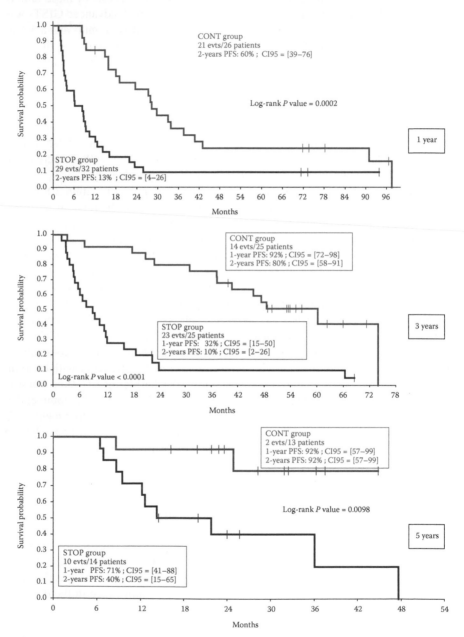

FIGURE 6.4   Updated PFS in the three groups of randomized patients in the BFR14 series: after 1, 3, and 5 years.

improves OS. Again, here the nature of the mutation guides the administration of an adjuvant treatment with imatinib [59].

The double-blind ACOSOG Z9001 multicenter phase III trial first demonstrated that patients who underwent complete surgical resection of the primary KIT+ GIST who were randomized to receive imatinib 400 mg/day (n=359) vs. placebo (n=354) for 1 year had a significantly lower rate of recurrence, after 1 year (HR 0.35; *P*=0.0001) [106]. Still, the recurrence rate increased sharply for patients after imatinib interruption suggesting that prolonged use of adjuvant imatinib beyond 1 year may be required [106].

Treatment with adjuvant imatinib therapy for 3 years was investigated in the SSGXVIII/AIO open-label, randomized, prospective, multicenter phase III trial: this trial compared 12 months with 36 months of adjuvant imatinib treatment following surgical resection of histologically confirmed KIT+GIST with a high risk of recurrence. RFS, the primary endpoint, was significantly longer in patients receiving adjuvant imatinib for 36 months compared with patients receiving imatinib for 12 months (HR 0.46; *P*<0.0001). Patients assigned to 36 months of imatinib also had significantly longer OS than the 12 month treatment group (HR 0.45; *P*=0.019) [107]. Again, however, the recurrence rate increased sharply for patients after imatinib interruption suggesting that a longer use of adjuvant imatinib may be required. Interestingly, the reintroduction of imatinib at the time of relapse induced again tumor control in the majority of patients, at a rate that was not significantly different between the two arms.

An important remaining question is whether adjuvant administration of imatinib influences the time to development of resistance to KIT inhibitors. The results of the largest randomized adjuvant phase III study of imatinib in intermediate- and high-risk patients performed by the EORTC in intergroup collaboration with the ISG, the FSG, and the AGITGC were reported at ASCO 2013. The primary endpoint was time to imatinib resistance, and no difference was observed between the two arms, even though a trend favoring adjuvant was observed for high-risk patients. As expected, PFS was significantly longer in the treated group. OS was not significantly different. These results point to the need of a longer duration of adjuvant imatinib and the need for careful selection of the patient candidate for adjuvant imatinib. They also confirm that adjuvant treatment does not induce the emergence of resistant clones.

To which extent KIT inhibition with imatinib *postpones* or *prevents* relapse remains an open question though.

The predictive value of molecular subtype for outcome after adjuvant therapy in ACOSOG Z9000 and Z9001 as well as SSGXVIII/AIO has also been reported for these two clinical trials [28,107]. The small number of patients in all subgroups but that of *KIT* exon 11 limits the power of this analysis. Overall, the HR achieved with adjuvant imatinib is similar in all smaller subgroups. Some of the molecular subgroups of GIST (PDGFRA D842V) may benefit less of not significantly from adjuvant imatinib.

Sunitinib as Second-Line TKI in GIST

The management of progression under imatinib 400 mg/day starts after having excluded false progressions (Figure 6.2) and evaluated the adherence and the compliance of the patient to the treatment. When confirmed, dose escalation of imatinib up to 800 mg/day is the recommended approach [50]. In a phase III trial, sunitinib, at 50 mg/day 4/6 weeks, significantly improved PFS over placebo [74]. In a phase II trial of continuous daily sunitinib at 37.5 mg/day, response and PFS were similar to that of the standard 4/6 weeks schedule [108]. No direct comparison of the two schedules has been performed in GIST.

The PFS of patients with *KIT* exon 9 mutations or WT *KIT* was found superior to that in a retrospective analysis of an early phase II trial [30]. No analysis of the pivotal trial was conducted to confirm this observation so far. This may be related to the frequent emergence of resistant subclones of GIST cells equipped with additional mutation of the KIT gene, encoding for a protein resistant to imatinib and sunitinib. This Darwinian selection of resistant clones seems to be more frequent in exon 11 mutated tumors.

Therapeutic Agents under Clinical Investigation

Several other agents have been explored in *KIT*-mutated GIST often without cross-resistance. We can distinguish here the agents with VEGFR2 inhibitory properties and other agents.

Regorafenib

As of May 2013, regorafenib is now approved for the treatment of GIST in several countries. In a phase II study, regorafenib yielded a 10 month median PFS in GIST patients progressing after imatinib and sunitinib [109]. A randomized, placebo-controlled, phase III trial (GRID) evaluated the efficacy and safety of regorafenib in 199 patients with metastatic and/or unresectable GIST progressing after failure of at least prior imatinib and sunitinib. Median PFS was 4.8 and 0.9 months in the regorafenib (n = 133) and placebo (n=66) groups, respectively (HR 0.27; $P<0.0001$). Median PFS for the 56 patients in the placebo group who crossed over to open-label regorafenib following progression was 5 months. The OS of the regorafenib and placebo groups were similar (HR 0.77; $P=0.19$). Similar benefits of regorafenib were observed in patients whose tumors with KIT mutations on exon 11 (HR 0.21) or exon 9 (HR 0.24) [110].

Sorafenib

Sorafenib has been explored in both retrospective analysis and prospective phase II studies, in patients with advanced GIST resistant to imatinib, sunitinib, and other agents. The results of these studies are very consistent with a median PFS in the range of 4–6 months and a response rate in the range of 10%–20% [111,112].

Dovitinib

At ESMO (2012), Kang et al. [95] reported on the efficacy and safety of dovitinib in 30 patients with advanced GIST (TKI) who had failed a minimum of both imatinib and sunitinib. Dovitinib was given orally at 500 mg qd for 5 consecutive days followed by a 2 day rest period [94]. There were no objective responses, but 19 (63%) had SD, and 5 (16%) PD as best response. Using EORTC PET criteria (at 4 weeks), 3 patients (10%) achieved a PR, 15 (50%) had SD, and 10 (33%) showed PD. Median PFS and OS were 3.6 and 6.2 months, respectively. PFS could be predicted by PET response (PD vs. no PD) at 4 weeks ($P=0.003$). Dovitinib has anti-tumor activity with manageable toxicities in this heavily pretreated cohort of GIST patients already exposed to KIT and VEGFR2 inhibitors [95]. The selective activity on KIT mutants is so far unknown.

Motesanib

In a multicenter single-arm phase 2 study of motesanib in 138 patients with advanced imatinib-resistant GISTs, response rates according to RECIST, PET, or Choi criteria [41] were 3%, 31%, and 38%, respectively, with durable SD ($\geq$22 weeks) in 30 of the 120 evaluable patients (25%) [97]. The activity of motesanib is in the range of that observed with sunitinib, but this agent was not further pursued. The selective activity on KIT mutants has not been precisely defined.

Valatinib

A phase II trial of valatinib 1250 mg/day once daily has been performed in patients failing imatinib (n = 26) or both imatinib and sunitinib (n = 19) [99]. A total of 18 patients (40%) had clinical benefit including 2 (4%) confirmed PR and 16 (36%) SDs (median duration, 12.5 months). Twelve (46.2%) out of the 26 patients who had received prior imatinib only achieved either PR or SD compared with 6 (31.6%, all SDs) out of the 19 patients who had received prior imatinib and sunitinib. The median time to progression was 5.8 months in the subset without prior sunitinib and 3.2 among those with prior imatinib and sunitinib. The activity of vatalanib is in the range of that observed with sunitinib, but again the selective activity on KIT mutants has not been precisely reported, and this agent is not being further developed.

The different TKIs blocking both KIT and VEGFR2 provide therefore very comparable results in second- or third-line patients. The results with pazopanib are pending. TKIs blocking KIT without VEGFR2 inhibitors have also been explored in this setting.

Nilotinib

A phase I study of AMN107 alone and in combination with imatinib has been performed in patients with imatinib-resistant GIST, 67% being also sunitinib resistant; 47% of the patients achieved SD lasting 2 to more than 6 months; 2 patients had PR [113]. A randomized phase III trial was subsequently performed comparing nilotinib vs. doctor's choice in the control arm (BSC alone or imatinib or sunitinib) [114]. The primary endpoint was PFS according to central radiological assessment. The study showed no significant difference between the two arms. However, the vast majority of patients received imatinib or sunitinib in the control arm, and a substantial proportion of patients were included with a reported intolerance to the previous treatment and without progression [141]. This may have impacted on the outcome of the study. Interestingly though, this work indicates that the maintenance of TKI blockade even at the time of resistance is of importance for these patients.

Masitinib

In a multicenter uncontrolled phase II study evaluating efficacy and safety of masitinib as a first-line treatment of advanced GIST, oral masitinib (7.5 mg/kg/day) was given until progression, refusal, or toxicity in 30 patients [115]. Median PFS was 41 months, with 74% survival at 4 years. Masitinib was explored in a second-line randomized phase II clinical trial in patients progressing after imatinib in a very small series of 44 patients randomized into masitinib (n=23) or sunitinib (n=21) [115,142]. Median PFS was 3.9 months for masitinib vs. 3.8 months for sunitinib. The 18 and 24 month OS rates for masitinib vs. sunitinib were 79% vs. 20%, respectively, possibly because of the imbalance in the crossover that was not possible for the sunitinib arm. A phase III study is scheduled.

Combination of Imatinib and mTOR or PI3K Inhibitors

In cell culture, the PI3K/mTOR pathway is activated in imatinib-resistant GIST cell lines, with a synergistic antitumor effect of the combination of imatinib and mTOR inhibitors or PI3K inhibitors [114]. A phase I/II clinical trial exploring the combination of imatinib and mTOR inhibitor everolimus was performed, showing significant drug/drug interaction with the combination of daily dosing and a recommended dose of imatinib 600 mg/day with 2.5 mg/day of everolimus. Two cohorts of patients in progression after imatinib or imatinib and sunitinib were included with a PFS of 17% and 39% at 4 months, then 0% and 14% progression-free at 12 months. Phase I combinations with PI3 kinase inhibitors BKM120 and BYL719 are ongoing. The simultaneous blockade of the KIT and mTOR pathways overcomes resistance to KIT inhibitors in a small group of patients with resistant GIST. Predictive biomarkers for response to the combination are needed and are currently investigated.

Dasatinib

A significant activity of dasatinib has been reported in GIST both in first-line setting and in second-line setting, but this activity is modest. Although pharmacodynamic markers have been identified, including Src phosphorylation [115,143] and PET imaging, its pattern of activity of KIT mutations resistant to other TKIs may deserve to be further investigated.

Ponatinib

Ponatinib has a broader spectrum of activity in mutated KIT proteins with resistance to other TKIs and may be worth exploring in clinical setting in resistant GIST and earlier.

Overall Results of KIT Inhibitors in GIST

There is a striking contrast between the activity of KIT inhibitors in the first-line setting, where median PFS is in the range of 20–30 months with imatinib, nilotinib, and in the small masitinib trial, and the results achieved with second or later lines with KIT inhibitors with or without VEGFR2 inhibitory properties, where PFS is in the range of 3–5 months only. Trials exploring agents in third-line setting report all median PFS in the range of 3–5 months. Only regorafenib was tested in a randomized trial vs. placebo and demonstrated a significant improvement in this setting. Other agents are currently being explored in later lines including pazopanib. With the exception of regorafenib, most agents provide slightly different results in the different KIT mutants.

Despite the short PFS achieved with these agents, long-term OS in patients failing imatinib is not infrequent, and it is interesting to note that, while the median

PFS of first-line GIST patients failing imatinib is 20–30 months, median OS of the same series extends beyond 58–74 months in the B2222 and BFR14 trials (Figure 6.1). Since most patients will experience long-term survival following imatinib resistance, it has been recently stressed in consensus conferences and clinical practice guidelines that continuous inhibition of KIT should be provided even in patients progressing on imatinib 400 mg/day [59,105]. Importantly, a trial performed in Korea is currently randomizing imatinib vs. no treatment in patients who have progressed under imatinib and have exhausted other options. This trial will provide important results.

New Strategies Needed to Avoid Resistance

Resistance occurs in the majority of patients with all KIT TKIs explored so far. Innovative strategies are therefore needed to prevent the emergence of this phenomenon. Surgical removal of metastasis, to reduce tumor cell mass and potentially resistant clone, could not be demonstrated to improve the risk of emergence of resistance, but randomized trials are still needed to address this question. Also, strategies to anticipate the emergence of resistant clones, through rapid rotation of noncrossresistant TKI agents, may be worth exploring (Figure 6.5).

More recently other solid tumors with KIT mutations have been identified. The results of KIT inhibitors are different, somewhat less favorable than with GIST, in these tumors.

MALIGNANT METASTATIC MELANOMA WITH **KIT** MUTATIONS

Melanomas arising from acral, mucosal, and chronically sun-damaged surfaces exhibit frequent KIT amplifications and mutations. These are reported in 21% of mucosal, 11% of acral, and 17% of chronically sun-damaged melanomas, although this may vary in different populations [33,39,116]. In phase 2 studies of single-agent

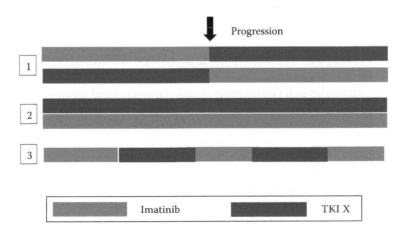

FIGURE 6.5 Possible strategies to improve PFS. Scenario 1: Each drug is given sequentially, the next drug being given at progression. Scenario 2: Combination treatment upfront. Scenario 3: Rotation of the treatments before the emergence of resistance.

imatinib in unselected patients (no alteration in KIT was needed for eligibility), imatinib was ineffective, with only one response among a total of 65 patients enrolled occurring in a patient with a point mutation in KIT (reviewed in 40).

Patients with melanoma with KIT mutations may have durable major responses with KIT inhibitors such as sorafenib, imatinib, sunitinib, nilotinib, and dasatinib [117–120]. In a phase II study, among 43 patients with melanoma with documented KIT mutations, 10 and 13 obtained a PR and an SD, respectively, with a 53% overall disease control rate, a median PFS of 3.5 months, and a median OS of 12 months [121]. Nine of the 10 responders had mutations in *KIT* exons 11 and 13. Amplifications of KIT or overexpression assessed by immunohistochemistry (IHC) has no predictive value for response.

Hence, despite similar KIT mutations with predictive value, metastatic melanoma has a much less favorable outcome than GIST patients with imatinib, with frequent primary and secondary resistance even in responding patients (median 9 months). The biological mechanisms underlying this differential pattern of response between GIST and MMM are unknown.

THYMIC CARCINOMAS

Thymomas and thymic carcinomas are rare malignant intrathoracic tumors characterized by a locoregional pattern of relapse for thymoma. Thymic carcinomas have a higher risk for metastatic relapse. Strobel et al. reported first on a response to imatinib in a metastatic thymic carcinoma with a KIT mutation [40]. The activity of sorafenib in other patients with thymic carcinoma and KIT mutations was subsequently reported in case reports [122–126].

Thymic carcinoma frequently expresses KIT, but KIT mutations are observed only in 7%–15% of the KIT-positive cases [124]. Schirosi et al. reported mutations involving exon 11 (four cases: V559A, L576P, Y553N, W557R), exon 9 (E490K), and exon 17 (D820E). Girard et al. reported on two thymic carcinomas with somatic KIT mutations (V560 del and H697Y) among seven tested, with specific sensitivity in cell viability assays, of the V560 del mutant to imatinib and sunitinib, while the H697Y mutant displayed greater sensitivity to sunitinib [123]. Buti et al. also reported on a single patient case with a massive response to imatinib in a thymic carcinoma with a codon 553 missense mutation of the KIT gene [126].

Overall, mutations in KIT are rare in thymic carcinoma and are most often occurring as point mutations within exon 11, more rarely 9, 13, 14, or 17, the latter being possibly more sensitive to sunitinib or sorafenib as already observed in GIST.

OTHER TUMOR TYPES

In other tumors, including mastocytosis, AML, or germ cell tumors, mutations of *KIT* have been extensively reported, mostly in exon 17 and encoding for proteins (e.g., D816V) often resistant to the majority of TKIs available, with the relative exception of dasatinib or PKC412 [84,127]. Rarer mutations on N822, in exon 8 or exon 11, may encode for sensitive protein to KIT inhibitors on these tumors [10].

EMPIRICAL USE OF KIT TYROSINE KINASE INHIBITORS

AGGRESSIVE FIBROMATOSIS

AF also known as desmoid tumors (AF/DT) are rare connective tissue tumors with a malignant locoregional behavior. Their hallmarks are the mutations of beta-catenin on exon 3 or the loss of the tumor suppressor gene APC [128]. When local treatments have failed, cytotoxic agents and hormonal treatment have been reported to induce tumor control in some patients, and only few prospective phase II trials have been reported in the literature. The antitumor activity of imatinib, used as a KIT inhibitor, in AF/DT was reported in three phase II trials.

The exact role of KIT and PDGFR modulation in imatinib activity is not precisely known; the overexpression of KIT may have been overestimated in this tumor due to technical artifacts. In a first series, a response rate of 17% and a 1 year PFS of 37% were reported [129]. In a second phase II trial including 40 patients treated with one year imatinib at the dose of 400 mg/day, PFS at 1 year was 71%. Imatinib induced prolonged disease stabilization in more than 2/3 of patients with AF/DT [130]. Interestingly, allelic variants or mutations in exon 10 of the KIT gene were observed in patients responding to imatinib [19,20].

The M541L allelic variant in particular is reported only in AF and systemic mastocytosis in the COSMIC database. However, these alterations are neither sufficient nor necessary for response to imatinib, and their significance remains unclear.

ADENOID CYSTIC CARCINOMAS

Adenoid cystic carcinomas are rare tumors with frequent overexpression of the KIT protein and rare mutations reported. Although occasional responses were observed in some patients [131], most patients could not achieve tumor control [132]. The molecular basis for response to imatinib in this disease is not known. Mutations of KIT are rare in these tumors [133,134].

CONCLUSION

The presence of activating mutations of KIT enables to identify efficiently sensitive tumor types, among GIST, melanoma, thymic carcinoma, cystic adenoid carcinoma, leukemia, and mastocytosis. Tumors with KIT mutations on exon 9 or exon 11 are generally responsive to TKIs. Mutations on exon 13, 14, or 17 often selected as resistance mutations under the therapeutic pressure have a variable sensitivity pattern to TKIs. These mutations are often heterogeneously distributed within the resistant tumor cell mass, representing thus a therapeutic challenge. These are the therapeutic challenges for KIT inhibitors. This is also the case for tumor types expressing a protein resistant to current TKIs, such as D816V in leukemia, mastocytosis, or germ cell tumors. Antibodies against KIT may represent a future alternative [135]. The prognostic and predictive values of allelic variants of *KIT* such as M541L as a predictive biomarker for response remain debated. Screening for these and other mutations is likely to be the most efficient strategy to identify novel nosological entities susceptible to tyrosine kinase inhibition in the future. KIT expression using IHC on tumor cells are neither necessary nor sufficient criteria to predict the efficacy of a KIT TKI in the clinical setting.

ACKNOWLEDGMENT

LYRIC project (INCA Grant 4664), Netsarc project (INCa Grant), RREPS project (INCA Grant), and euroSARC (FP7–278472)

REFERENCES

1. Blay JY, Lacombe D, Meunier F, and Stupp R. Personalised medicine in oncology: Questions for the next 20 years. *Lancet Oncol* 2012 May;13(5):448–449.
2. Blay JY, Le Cesne A, Alberti L, and Ray-Coquard I. Targeted cancer therapies. *Bull Cancer* 2005;92(2):E13–E18.
3. Soria JC, Blay JY, Spano JP, Pivot X, Coscas Y, and Khayat D. Added value of molecular targeted agents in oncology. *Ann Oncol* 2011;22:1703–1716.
4. Ashman LK. The biology of stem cell factor and its receptor c-kit. *Int J Biochem Cell Biol* 1999;31(10):1037–1051.
5. Furitsu T, Tsujimura T, Tono T et al. Identification of mutations in the coding sequence of the proto-oncogene c-kit in a human mast cell leukemia cell line causing ligand-independent activation of c-kit product. *J Clin Invest* 1993;92:1736–1744.
6. Vliagoftis H, Worobec AS, and Metcalf DD. The proto-oncogene c-kit and c-kit ligand in human disease. *J Allerg Clin Immunol* 1997;100:435–440.
7. Longley BJ, Reguera MJ, and Ma Y. Classes of c-kit activating mutations: Proposed mechanisms of action and implications for disease classification and therapy. *Leuk Res* 2001;25:571–576.
8. Lennartsson J, Jelacic T, Linnekin D, and Shivakrupa R. Normal and oncogenic forms of the receptor tyrosine kinase kit. *Stem Cells* 2005;23:16–43.
9. Hirota S, Isozaki K, Moriyama Y et al. Gain-of-function mutations of c-kit in human gastrointestinal stromal tumors. *Science* 1998;279:577–580.
10. Haenisch B, Nöthen MM, and Molderings GJ. Systemic mast cell activation disease: The role of molecular genetic alterations in pathogenesis, heritability and diagnostics. *Immunology* 2012;137:197–205.
11. Druker BJ, Tamura S, and Buchdunger E. Effects of a selective inhibitor of the Abl tyrosine kinase on the growth of Bcr-Abl positive cells. *Nat Med* 1996;2:561–566.
12. Buchdunger E, Cioffi CL, and Law N. Abl protein-tyrosine kinase inhibitor STI571 inhibits *in vitro* signal transduction mediated by c-kit and platelet-derived growth factor receptors. *J Pharmacol Exp Ther* 2000;295:139–145.
13. Savage DG and Antman KH. Imatinib mesylate—A new oral targeted therapy. *N Engl J Med* 2002;346:683–693.
14. Blay JY. A decade of tyrosine kinase inhibitor therapy: Historical and current perspectives on targeted therapy for GIST. *Cancer Treat Rev* 2011;37:373–384.
15. Ronnstrand L. Signal transduction via the stem cell factor receptor/c-kit. *Cell Mol Life Sci* 2004;61:2535–2548.
16. Ashman LK and Griffith R. Therapeutic targeting of c-KIT in cancer. *Expert Opin Invest Drugs* 2013; 22:103–115.
17. Hayashi S, Kunisada T, Ogawa M, Yamaguchi K, and Nishikawa S. Exon skipping by mutation of an authentic splice site of c-kit gene in W/W mouse. *Nucl Acids Res* 1991; 19:1267–1271.

18. Caruana G, Cambareri AC, and Ashman LK. Isoforms of c-KIT differ in activation of signalling pathways and transformation of NIH3T3 fibroblasts. *Oncogen* 1999;18:5573–5581.

19. Dufresne A, Bertucci F, Penel N et al. Identification of biological factors predictive of response to imatinib mesylate in aggressive fibromatosis. *Br J Cancer* 2010;103:482–485.

20. Kurtz JE, Asmane I, Voegeli AC, Neuville A, Dufresne A, Litique V, Chevreau C, and Bergerat JP. A V530I mutation in c-KIT exon 10 is associated to imatinib response in extra abdominal aggressive fibromatosis. *Sarcoma* 2010;458156.

21. Grabellus F, Worm K, Sheu SY, Siffert W, Schmid KW, and Bachmann HS. The prevalence of the c-kit exon 10 variant, M541L, in aggressive fibromatosis does not differ from the general population. *J Clin Pathol* 2011;64:1021–1024.

22. Molderings GJ, Brettner S, Homann J, and Afrin LB. Mast cell activation disease: A concise practical guide for diagnostic workup and therapeutic options. *J Hematol Oncol* 2011;4:10.

23. Akin C, Valent P, and Metcalfe DD. Mast cell activation syndrome: Proposed diagnostic criteria. *J Allergy Clin Immunol* 2010;126:1099–1104; Valent P, Akin C, Escribano L et al. Standards and standardization in mastocytosis: Consensus statements on diagnostics, treatment recommendations and response criteria. *Eur J Clin Invest* 2007;37:435–453.

24. Alvarez-Twose I, Gonzalez de Olano D, Sanchez-Munoz L et al. Clinical, biological, and molecular characteristics of clonal mast cell disorders presenting with systemic mast cell activation symptoms. *J Allergy Clin Immunol* 2010;125:1269–1278.

25. Hamilton MJ, Hornick JL, Akin C, Castells MC, and Greenberger NJ. Mast cell activation syndrome: A newly recognized disorder with systemic clinical manifestations. *J Allergy Clin Immunol* 2011;128:147–152.

26. Hermine O, Lortholary O, Leventhal PS et al. Case–control cohort study of patients' perceptions of disability in mastocytosis. *PLoS One* 2008;3:e2266.

27. Lanternier F, Cohen-Akenine A, Palmerini F et al. Phenotypic and genotypic characteristics of mastocytosis according to the age of onset. *PLoS One* 2008; 3:e1906.

28. Corless CL, Barnctt CM, and Heinrich MC. Gastrointestinal stromal tumours: Origin and molecular oncology. *Nat Rev Cancer* 2011;11:865–878.

29. Heinrich MC, Blanke CD, Druker BJ, and Corless CL. Inhibition of KIT tyrosine kinase activity: A novel molecular approach to the treatment of KIT-positive malignancies. *J Clin Oncol* 2002;20:1692–1703.

30. Heinrich MC, Maki RG, Corless CI. et al. Primary and secondary kinase genotypes correlate with the biological and clinical activity of sunitinib in imatinib-resistant gastrointestinal stromal tumor. *J Clin Oncol* 2008;26:5352–5359.

31. Malaise M, Steinbach D, and Corbacioglu S. Clinical implications of c-Kit mutations in acute myelogenous leukemia. *Curr Hematol Malig Rep* 2009;4:77–82.

32. Shen Y, Zhu YM, Fan X et al. Gene mutation patterns and their prognostic impact in a cohort of 1185 patients with acute myeloid leukemia. *Blood* 2011 November 17;118(20):5593–5603.

33. Nick HJ, Kim HG, Chang CW, Harris KW, Reddy V, and Klug CA. Distinct classes of c-Kit-activating mutations differ in their ability to promote RUNX1-ETO-associated acute myeloid leukemia. *Blood* 2012 February 9;119(6):1522–1531.

34. Park SH, Chi HS, Min SK, Park BG, Jang S, and Park CJ. Prognostic impact of c-KIT mutations in core binding factor acute myeloid leukemia. *Leuk Res* 2011;35:1376–1383.

35. Wang YY, Zhao LJ, Wu CF et al. C-KIT mutation cooperates with full-length AML1-ETO to induce acute myeloid leukemia in mice. *Proc Natl Acad Sci USA* 2011;108:2450–2455.

36. Curtin JA, Busam K, Pinkel D, and Bastian BC. Somatic activation of KIT in distinct subtypes of melanoma. *J Clin Oncol* 2006;24:4340–4346.

37. Kong Y, Si L, Zhu Y, Xu X, Corless CL, Flaherty KT, Li L, and Li H et al. Large-scale analysis of KIT aberrations in Chinese patients with melanoma. *Clin Cancer Res* 2011;17:1684–1691.

150   Targeted Therapies in Oncology

38. Eggermont AM and Melanoma RC. 2011. A new paradigm tumor for drug development. *Nat Rev Clin Oncol* 2012;9:74–76.
39. Romano E, Schwartz GK, Chapman PB, Wolchock JD, and Carvajal RD. Treatment implications of the emerging molecular classification system for melanoma. *Lancet Oncol* 2011;12:913–922.
40. Ströbel P, Hartmann M, Jakob A et al. Thymic carcinoma with overexpression of mutated KIT and the response to imatinib. *N Engl J Med* 2004;350:2625–2626.
41. Biermann K, Göke F, Nettersheim D et al. c-KIT is frequently mutated in bilateral germ cell tumours and down-regulated during progression from intratubular germ cell neoplasia to seminoma. *J Pathol* 2007;213:311–318.
42. Coffey J, Linger R, Pugh J et al. Somatic KIT mutations occur predominantly in seminoma germ cell tumors and are not predictive of bilateral disease: Report of 220 tumors and review of literature. *Genes Chromosome Cancer* 2008;47:34–42.
43. Mol CD, Dougan DR, Schneider TR et al. Structural basis for the autoinhibition and STI-571 inhibition of c-Kit tyrosine kinase. *J Biol Chem* 2004;279:31655–31663.
44. Wardelmann E, Losen I, Hans V et al. Deletion of Trp-557 and Lys-558 in the juxtamembrane domain of the c-kit protooncogene is associated with metastatic behavior of gastrointestinal stromal tumors. *Int J Cancer* 2003;106:887–895.
45. Martín J, Poveda A, Llombart-Bosch A et al. Deletions affecting codons 557–558 of the c-KIT gene indicate a poor prognosis in patients with completely resected gastrointestinal stromal tumors: A study by the Spanish Group for Sarcoma Research (GEIS). *J Clin Oncol* 2005;23:6190–6198.
46. Tzen CY and Mau BL. Analysis of CD117-negative gastrointestinal stromal tumors. *World J Gastroenterol* 2005;11:1052–1055.
47. Yuzawa S, Opatowsky Y, Zhang Z et al. Structural basis for activation of the receptor tyrosine kinase KIT by stem cell factor. *Cell* 2007;130:323–334.
48. Lasota J, Corless CL, Heinrich MC et al. Clinicopathologic profile of gastrointestinal stromal tumors (GISTs) with primary KIT exon 13 or exon 17 mutations: A multicenter study on 54 cases. *Mod Pathol* 2008;21:476–484.
49. Heinrich MC, Corless CL, Blanke CD et al. Molecular correlates of imatinib resistance in gastrointestinal stromal tumors. *J Clin Oncol* 2006;24:4764–4774.
50. Wardelmann E, Merkelbach-Bruse S, Pauls K, Thomas N, Schildhaus HU, Heinicke T, and Speidel N et al. Polyclonal evolution of multiple secondary KIT mutations in gastrointestinal stromal tumors under treatment with imatinib mesylate. *Clin Cancer Res* 2006;12:1743–1749.
51. Van Oosterom A, Judson I, Verwej J et al. Safety and efficacy of Imatinib (STI-571) in metastatic gastrointestinal stromal tumors: A phase I study. *Lancet* 2001;358: 1421–1423.
52. Demetri GD, von Mehren M, Blanke CD et al. Efficacy and safety of imatinib mesylate in advanced gastrointestinal stromal tumors. *N Engl J Med* 2002;347:472–480.
53. Verweij J, van Oosterom AT, Blay JY et al. Imatinib (Gleevec) an active agent for gastrointestinal stromal tumors (GIST), but not for other soft tissue sarcoma (STS) subtypes not characterized for KIT and PDGF-R expression, results of EORTC phase II studies. *Eur J Cancer* 2003;39:2006–2011.
54. Verweij J, Casali P, Zalcberg P et al. Improved progression free survival in gastrointestinal stromal tumors with high dose Imatinib. Results of a randomized phase III study of the EORTC, ISG and AGITG. *Lancet* 2004;364:1127–1134.
55. Blay JY, Le Cesne A, Ray-Coquard I et al. Prospective multicentric randomized phase III study of imatinib in patients with advanced gastrointestinal stromal tumors comparing interruption versus continuation of treatment beyond 1 year: The French Sarcoma Group. *J Clin Oncol* 2007;25:1107–1113.

56. Blanke CD, Rankin C, Demetri GD et al. Phase III randomized, intergroup trial assessing imatinib mesylate at two dose levels in patients with unresectable or metastatic gastrointestinal stromal tumors expressing the kit receptor tyrosine kinase: S0033. *J Clin Oncol* 2008;26:626–632.

57. Blanke CD, Demetri GD, von Mehren M et al. Long-term results from a randomized phase II trial of standard- versus higher-dose imatinib mesylate for patients with unresectable or metastatic gastrointestinal stromal tumors expressing KIT. *J Clin Oncol* 2008;26:620–625.

58. Le Cesne A, Ray-Coquard I, Bui BN et al. Discontinuation of imatinib in patients with advanced gastrointestinal stromal tumours after 3 years of treatment: An open-label multicentre randomised phase 3 trial. *Lancet Oncol* 2010;11:942–949.

59. ESMO/European Sarcoma Network Working Group. Gastrointestinal stromal tumors: ESMO Clinical Practice Guidelines for diagnosis, treatment and follow-up. *Ann Oncol* 2012;23(Suppl 7):vii49–vii55.

60. Xiang Z, Kreisel F, Cain J et al. Neoplasia driven by mutant c-kit is mediated by intracellular, not plasma membrane, receptor signaling. *Mol Cell Biol* 2007;27:267–282.

61. Tabone-Eglinger S, Subra F, El Sayadi H et al. KIT mutations induce intracellular retention and activation of an immature form of the KIT protein in gastrointestinal stromal tumors. *Clin Cancer Res* 2008;14:2285–2294.

62. Brahimi-Adouane S, Bachet JB, Tabone-Eglinger S et al. Effects of endoplasmic reticulum stressors on maturation and signaling of hemizygous and heterozygous wild-type and mutant forms of KIT. *Mol Oncol* 2012 Oct 30. doi:pii: S1574-7891(12)00106-8. 10.1016/j.molonc.2012.10.008. [Epub ahead of print] PubMed PMID: 23146721.

63. Bougherara H, Subra F, Crépin R, Tauc P, Auclair C, and Poul MA. The aberrant localization of oncogenic kit tyrosine kinase receptor mutants is reversed on specific inhibitory treatment. *Mol Cancer Res* 2009;7(9):1525–1533.

64. Bougherara H, Georgin-Lavialle S, Damaj G et al. Clinical implications. *Clin Lymphoma Myeloma Leuk* 2013;13:62–69.

65. Antonescu CR, Viale A, Sarran L et al. Gene expression in gastrointestinal stromal tumors is distinguished by KIT genotype and anatomic site. *Clin Cancer Res* 2004; 10:3282–3290.

66. Duensing A, Medeiros F, McConarty B et al. Mechanisms of oncogenic kit signal transduction in primary gastrointestinal stromal tumors (gists). *Oncogene* 2004;23: 3999–4006.

67. Chian R, Young S, Danilkovitch-Miagkova A et al. Phosphatidylinositol 3 kinase contributes to the transformation of hematopoietic cells by the d816v c-kit mutant. *Blood* 2001;98:1365–1373.

68. Ning ZQ, Li J, and Arceci RJ. Signal transducer and activator of transcription 3 activation is required for asp(816) mutant c-kit-mediated cytokine-independent survival and proliferation in human leukemia cells. *Blood* 2001;97:3559–3567.

69. Sun J, Pedersen M, and Ronnstrand L. The d816v mutation of c-kit circumvents a requirement for src family kinases in c-kit signal transduction. *J Biol Chem* 2009;284: 11039–11047.

70. Dewar AL, Cambareri AC, Zannettino AC et al. Macrophage colony-stimulating factor receptor c-fms is a novel target of imatinib. *Blood* 2005;105:3127–3132.

71. Mendel DB, Laird AD, X Xin et al. In vivo antitumor activity of SU11248, a novel tyrosine kinase inhibitor targeting vascular endothelial growth factor and platelet-derived growth factor receptors: Determination of a pharmacokinetic/pharmacodynamic relationship. *Clin Cancer Res* 2003;9:327–337.

72. Murray LJ, Abrams TJ, and Long KR et al. SU11248 inhibits tumor growth and CSF-1R-dependent osteolysis in an experimental breast cancer bone metastasis model. *Clin Exp Metastasis* 2003;20:757–766.

73. O'Farrell AM, Abrams TJ, and Yuen HA et al. SU11248 is a novel FLT3 tyrosine kinase inhibitor with potent activity in vitro and in vivo. *Blood* 2003;101:3597–3605.

74. Demetri GD, van Oosterom AT, Garrett CR et al. Efficacy and safety of sunitinib in patients with advanced gastrointestinal stromal tumour after failure of imatinib: A randomised controlled trial. *Lancet* 2006;368:1329–1338.

75. Weisberg E, Manley PW, Breitenstein W et al. Characterization of AMN107, a selective inhibitor of native and mutant Bcr-Abl. *Cancer Cell* 2005;7:129–141.

76. Prenen H, Guetens G, de Boeck G et al. Cellular uptake of the tyrosine kinase inhibitors imatinib and AMN107 in Gastrointestinal stromal tumor cell lines. *Pharmacology* 2006;77:11–16.

77. Blay JY, von Mehren M. Nilotinib: A novel, selective tyrosine kinase inhibitor. *Semin Oncol* 2011;38(Suppl 1):S3–S9.

78. Weisberg E, Wright RD, Jiang J et al. Effects of PKC412, nilotinib, and imatinib against GIST-associated PDGFRA mutants with differential imatinib sensitivity. *Gastroenterology* 2006;131:1734–1742.

79. Dubreuil P, Letard S, Ciufolini M et al. Masitinib (AB1010), a potent and selective tyrosine kinase inhibitor targeting KIT. *PLoS One* 30 September 2009;4(9):e7258.

80. Soria JC, Massard C, Magné N et al. Phase 1 dose-escalation study of oral tyrosine kinase inhibitor masitinib in advanced and/or metastatic solid cancers. *Eur J Cancer* 2009;45:2333–2341.

81. Le Cesne A, Blay JY, Bui BN et al. Phase II study of oral masitinib mesilate in imatinib-naïve patients with locally advanced or metastatic gastro-intestinal stromal tumour (GIST). *Eur J Cancer* 2010;46:1344–1351.

82. O'Hare T, Walters DK, Stoffregen EP et al. *In vitro* activity of Bcr-Abl inhibitors AMN107 and BMS-354825 against clinically relevant imatinib-resistant Abl kinase domain mutants. *Cancer Res* 2005;65:4500–4505.

83. Shah NP, Lee FY, Luo R, Jiang Y, Donker M, Akin C. Dasatinib (BMS-354825) inhibits KITD816V, an imatinib-resistant activating mutation that triggers neoplastic growth in most patients with systemic mastocytosis. *Blood* 2006;108:286–291.

84. Schittenhelm MM, Shiraga S, Schroeder A et al. Dasatinib (BMS-354825), a dual SRC/ABL kinase inhibitor, inhibits the kinase activity of wild-type, juxtamembrane, and activation loop mutant KIT isoforms associated with human malignancies. *Cancer Res* 2006;66:473–481.

85. Woodman SE, Trent JC, Stemke-Hale K. et al. Activity of dasatinib against L576P KIT mutant melanoma: Molecular, cellular, and clinical correlates. *Mol Cancer Ther* 2009;8:2079–2085.

86. O'Hare T, Shakespeare WC, Zhu X. et al. AP24534, a pan-BCR-ABL inhibitor for chronic myeloid leukemia, potently inhibits the T315I mutant and overcomes mutation-based resistance. *Cancer Cell* 2009;16:401–412.

87. Cortes JE, Kantarjian H, Shah NP et al. Ponatinib in refractory Philadelphia chromosome-positive leukemias. *N Engl J Med* 2012;367:2075–2088.

88. Lierman E, Smits S, Cools J, Dewaele B, Debiec-Rychter M, Vandenberghe P. Ponatinib is active against imatinib-resistant mutants of FIP1L1-PDGFRA and KIT, and against FGFR1-derived fusion kinases. *Leukemia* 2012;26:1693–1695.

89. Wilhelm SM, Dumas J, Adnane L et al. Regorafenib (BAY 73–4506): A new oral multikinase inhibitor of angiogenic, stromal and oncogenic receptor tyrosine kinases with potent preclinical antitumor activity. *Int J Cancer* 2011;129:245–255.

90. Guo T, Agaram NP, Wong GC et al. Sorafenib inhibits the imatinib-resistant KITT670I gatekeeper mutation in gastrointestinal stromal tumor. *Clin Cancer Res* 2007;13:4874–4881.

91. Guida T, Anaganti S, Provitera L et al. Sorafenib inhibits imatinib-resistant KIT and platelet-derived growth factor receptor beta gatekeeper mutants. *Clin Cancer Res* 2007;13: 3363–3369.

92. Heinrich MC, Marino-Enriquez A, Presnell A et al. Sorafenib inhibits many kinase mutations associated with drug-resistant gastrointestinal stromal tumors. *Mol Cancer Ther* 2012;11:1770–1780.
93. van der Graaf WT, Blay JY, Chawla SP et al. EORTC Soft Tissue and Bone Sarcoma Group; PALETTE study group. Pazopanib for metastatic soft-tissue sarcoma (PALETTE): A randomised, double-blind, placebo-controlled phase 3 trial. *Lancet* 2012;379:1879–1886; Trudel S, Li ZH, Wei E, Wiesmann M et al. CHIR-258, a novel, multitargeted tyrosine kinase inhibitor for the potential treatment of t(4;14) multiple myeloma. *Blood* 2005;105:2941–2948.
94. Sarker D, Molife R, Evans TR et al. A phase I pharmacokinetic and pharmacodynamic study of TKI258, an oral, multitargeted receptor tyrosine kinase inhibitor in patients with advanced solid tumors. *Clin Cancer Res* 2008;14:2075–2081.
95. Kang YK, Ryu MH, Lee JJ, Park I, Park JH, and Ryoo BY. Phase II study of dovitinib in first line metastatic or (non resectable primary) gastrointestinal stromal tumor (GIST) after progression on imatinib (IM) and sunitinib. *Proc ESMO* 2012 (abstract 3223).
96. Polverino A, Coxon A, Starnes C et al. AMG 706, an oral, multikinase inhibitor that selectively targets vascular endothelial growth factor, platelet-derived growth factor, and kit receptors, potently inhibits angiogenesis and induces regression in tumor xenografts. *Cancer Res* 2006;66:8715–8721.
97. Benjamin RS, Schöffski P, Hartmann JT et al. Efficacy and safety of motesanib, an oral inhibitor of VEGF, PDGF, and Kit receptors, in patients with imatinib-resistant gastrointestinal stromal tumors. *Cancer Chemother Pharmacol* 2011;68:69–77.
98. Wood JM, Bold G, Buchdunger E et al. PTK787/ZK 222584, a novel and potent inhibitor of vascular endothelial growth factor receptor tyrosine kinases, impairs vascular endothelial growth factor-induced responses and tumor growth after oral administration. *Cancer Res* 2000;60:2178–2189.
99. Joensuu H, De Braud F, Grignagni G et al. Vatalanib for metastatic gastrointestinal stromal tumour (GIST) resistant to imatinib: Final results of a phase II study. *Br J Cancer* 2011;104:1686–1690.
100. Cassier PA, Ducimetière F, Lurkin A et al. A prospective epidemiological study of new incident GISTs during two consecutive years in Rhone Alpes region: Incidence and molecular distribution of GIST in a European region. *Br J Cancer* 2010; 103:165–170.
101. Agaimy A, Dirnhofer S, Wünsch PH, Terracciano LM, Tornillo L, and Bihl MP. Multiple sporadic gastrointestinal stromal tumors (GISTs) of the proximal stomach are caused by different somatic KIT mutations suggesting a field effect. *Am J Surg Pathol* 2008;32:1553–1559.
102. Kawanowa K, Sakuma Y, Sakurai S et al. High incidence of microscopic gastrointestinal stromal tumors in the stomach. *Hum Pathol* 2006;37:1527–1535.
103. Reichardt P, Blay JY, Boukovinas I et al. Adjuvant therapy in primary GIST: State-of-the-art. *Ann Oncol* 2012;23:2776–2781.
104. Gastrointestinal Stromal Tumor Meta-Analysis Group (MetaGIST). Comparison of two doses of imatinib for the treatment of unresectable or metastatic gastrointestinal stromal tumors: A meta-analysis of 1,640 patients. *J Clin Oncol* 2010;28:1247–1253.
105. Demetri GD, von Mehren M, Antonescu CR et al. GIST. *J Natl Compr Canc Netw* 2010;8(Suppl 2):S1–S41.
106. DeMatteo RP, Ballman KV, Antonescu CR et al. Adjuvant imatinib mesylate after resection of localised, primary gastrointestinal stromal tumour: A randomised, double-blind, placebo-controlled trial. *Lancet* 2009;373:1097–1104.
107. Joensuu H, Eriksson M, Sundby Hall K et al. One vs three years of adjuvant imatinib for operable gastrointestinal stromal tumor: A randomized trial. *JAMA* 2012; 307:1265–1272.

108. George S, Blay JY, Casali PG et al. Clinical evaluation of continuous daily dosing of sunitinib malate in patients with advanced gastrointestinal stromal tumour after imatinib failure. *Eur J Cancer* 2009;45:1959–1968.

109. George S, Wang Q, Heinrich MC et al. Efficacy and safety of regorafenib in patients with metastatic and/or unresectable GI stromal tumor after failure of imatinib and sunitinib: A multicenter phase II trial. *J Clin Oncol* 2012;30:2401–2407.

110. Demetri GD, Reichardt P, Kang YK et al, GRID study investigators. Efficacy and safety of regorafenib for advanced gastrointestinal stromal tumours after failure of imatinib and sunitinib (GRID): An international, multicentre, randomised, placebo-controlled, phase 3 trial. *Lancet* 2013;381:295–302.

111. Montemurro M, Gelderblom H, Bitz U et al. Sorafenib as third- or fourth-line treatment of advanced gastrointestinal stromal tumour and pretreatment including both imatinib and sunitinib, and nilotinib: A retrospective analysis. *Eur J Cancer* 6 November 2012;doi:pii:S0959–S8049(12)00808–8. 10.1016/j.ejca.2012.10.009.

112. Park SH, Ryu MH, Ryoo BY et al. Sorafenib in patients with metastatic gastrointestinal stromal tumors who failed two or more prior tyrosine kinase inhibitors: A phase II study of Korean gastrointestinal stromal tumors study group. *Invest New Drugs* 2012;30:2377–2383.

113. Demetri GD, Casali PG, Blay JY et al. A phase I study of single-agent nilotinib or in combination with imatinib in patients with imatinib-resistant gastrointestinal stromal tumors. *Clin Cancer Res* 2009;15:5910–5916.

114. Schöffski P, Reichardt P, Blay JY et al. A phase I-II study of everolimus (RAD001) in combination with imatinib in patients with imatinib-resistant gastrointestinal stromal tumors. *Ann Oncol* 2010;21:1990–1998.

115. Montemurro M, Domont J, Blesius A et al. Dasatinib first-line treatment in gastrointestinal stromal tumors: A multicenter phase II trial of the SAKK (SAKK 56/07). *J Clin Oncol* 2012;30(suppl):abstr 10033.

116. Guo J, Si L, Kong Y et al. Phase II, open-label, single-arm trial of imatinib mesylate in patients with metastatic melanoma harboring c-Kit mutation or amplification. *J Clin Oncol* 2011;29:2904–2909.

117. Hodi FS, Friedlander P, Corless CL et al. Major response to imatinib mesylate in KIT-mutated melanoma. *J Clin Oncol* 2008;26:2046–2051.

118. Lutzky J, Bauer J, and Bastian BC. Dose-dependent, complete response to imatinib of a metastatic mucosal melanoma with a K642E KIT mutation. *Pigment Cell Melanoma Res* 2008;21:492–493.

119. Handolias D, Hamilton AL, Salemi R et al. Clinical responses observed with imatinib or sorafenib in melanoma patients expressing mutations in KIT. *Br J Cancer* 2010; 102:1219–1223.

120. Minor DR, Kashani-Sabet M, Garrido M, O'Day SJ, Hamid O, and Bastian BC. Sunitinib therapy for melanoma patients with KIT mutations. *Clin Cancer Res* 2012; 18:1457–1463.

121. Si L, Guo J. C-kit-mutated melanomas: The Chinese experience. *Curr Opin Oncol* 2013;25:160–165.

122. Giaccone G, Rajan A, Ruijter R, Smit E, van Groeningen C, and Hogendoorn PC. Imatinib mesylate in patients with WHO B3 thymomas and thymic carcinomas. *J Thorac Oncol* 2009;4:1270–1273.

123. Girard N, Shen R, Guo T et al. Comprehensive genomic analysis reveals clinically relevant molecular distinctions between thymic carcinomas and thymomas. *Clin Cancer Res* 2009;15:6790–6799.

124. Petrini I, Zucali PA, Lee HS, Pineda MA, Meltzer PS, Walter-Rodriguez B, Roncalli M et al. Expression and mutational status of c-kit in thymic epithelial tumors. *J Thorac Oncol* 2010;5:1447–1453.

125. Schirosi L, Nannini N, Nicoli D et al. Activating c-KIT mutations in a subset of thymic carcinoma and response to different c-KIT inhibitors. *Ann Oncol* 2012;23:2409–2414.
126. Buti S, Donini M, Sergio P et al. Impressive response with imatinib in a heavily pre-treated patient with metastatic c-KIT mutated thymic carcinoma. *J Clin Oncol* 2011; 29:e803–e805.
127. Gleixner KV, Mayerhofer M, Sonneck K et al. Synergistic growth-inhibitory effects of two tyrosine kinase inhibitors, dasatinib and PKC412, on neoplastic mast cells expressing the D816V-mutated oncogenic variant of KIT. *Haematologica* 2007;92:1451–1459.
128. Salas S, Dufresne A, Bui B, Blay JY et al. Prognostic factors influencing progression-free survival determined from a series of sporadic desmoid tumors: A wait-and-see policy according to tumor presentation. *J Clin Oncol* 201;29:3553–3558.
129. Heinrich MC, McArthur GA, Demetri GD et al. Clinical and molecular studies of the effect of imatinib on advanced aggressive fibromatosis (desmoid tumor). *J Clin Oncol* 2006;24:1195–1203.
130. Penel N, Le Cesne A, Bui BN et al. Imatinib for progressive and recurrent aggressive fibromatosis (desmoid tumors): An FNCLCC/French Sarcoma Group phase II trial with a long-term follow-up. *Ann Oncol* 2010; 22:452–457.
131. Faivre S, Raymond E, Casiraghi O, Temam S, and Berthaud P. Imatinib mesylate can induce objective response in progressing, highly expressing KIT adenoid cystic carcinoma of the salivary glands. *J Clin Oncol* 2005;23:6271–6273.
132. Pfeffer MR, Talmi Y, Catane R, Symon Z, Yosepovitch A, and Levitt M. A phase II study of Imatinib for advanced adenoid cystic carcinoma of head and neck salivary glands. *Oral Oncol* 2007;43:33–36.
133. Vila L, Liu H, Al-Quran SZ, Coco DP, Dong HJ, and Liu C. Identification of c-kit gene mutations in primary adenoid cystic carcinoma of the salivary gland. *Mod Pathol* 2009; 22:1296–1302.
134. Chau NG, Hotte SJ, Chen EX et al. A phase II study of sunitinib in recurrent and/or metastatic adenoid cystic carcinoma (ACC) of the salivary glands: Current progress and challenges in evaluating molecularly targeted agents in ACC. *Ann Oncol* 2012; 23:1562–1570.
135. Edris B, Willingham SB, Weiskopf K et al. Anti-KIT monoclonal antibody inhibits imatinib-resistant gastrointestinal stromal tumor growth. *Proc Natl Acad Sci USA*. 4 February 2013. [Epub ahead of print] PubMed PMID: 23382202.
136. Tian Q, Frierson HF Jr, Krystal GW, and Moskaluk CA. Activating c-kit gene mutations in human germ cell tumors. *Am J Pathol* 1999;154:1643–1647.
137. Kemmer K, Corless CL, Fletcher JA et al. KIT mutations are common in testicular seminomas. *Am J Pathol* 2004;164:305–313.
138. Rapley EA, Hockley S, Warren W et al. Somatic mutations of KIT in familial testicular germ cell tumours. *Br J Cancer* 2004;90:2397–2401.
139. Sihto H, Sarlomo-Rikala M, Tynninen O et al. KIT and platelet-derived growth factor receptor alpha tyrosine kinase gene mutations and KIT amplifications in human solid tumors. *J Clin Oncol* 2005;23:49–57.
140. Sloan B and Scheinfeld NS. Pazopanib, a VEGF receptor tyrosine kinase inhibitor for cancer therapy. *Curr Opin Investig Drugs* 2008;9:1324–1335.
141. Reichardt P, Blay JY, Gelderblom H et al. Phase III study of nilotinib versus best supportive care with or without a TKI in patients with gastrointestinal stromal tumors resistant to or intolerant of imatinib and sunitinib. *Ann Oncol* 2012;23:1680–1687.
142. Adenis A, Le Cesne A, Bui BN et al. Masitinib mesylate in imatinib-resistant advanced GIST: A randomized phase II trial. *J Clin Oncol* 30, 2012 (suppl; abstr 10007)
143. Trent JC, Wathen K, von Mehren M et al. A phase II study of dasatinib for patients with imatinib-resistant gastrointestinal stromal tumor (GIST). *J Clin Oncol* 2011;29(suppl): abstr 10006.

7 Targeting the Fibroblast Growth Factor Receptor Pathway in Human Cancer

Maria Vittoria Dieci
Institut Gustave Roussy

Fabrice Andre
Institut Gustave Roussy
Paris Sud University

CONTENTS

INTRODUCTION

The signaling pathway mediated by the fibroblast growth factor receptors (FGFRs) and their ligands fibroblast growth factors (FGFs) regulates key functions in human physiology. Alterations of FGF signaling have been linked to different human diseases including cancer. These observations suggested that this pathway may represent a potential target for anticancer therapies.

FGF/FGFR SIGNALING

The 18 members of the mammalian FGFs are secreted glycoproteins that are readily sequestered by heparan sulfate proteoglycans (HPSGs), localized both in the extracellular matrix and on cell surface. Once FGFs are released from the extracellular matrix by proteases, they become available to interact with FGFRs on the cell surface. The FGF–FGFR binding is stabilized through the formation of a ternary complex that involves cell surface HPSG [1]. FGF19, FGF21, and FGF23 have a lower affinity for heparin-like molecules. Indeed, they depend on the presence of Klotho proteins in their respective target tissues for the stabilization of ligand–receptor affinity [1].

To date, five FGFRs have been identified. FGFR1 to FGFR4 are highly conserved transmembrane tyrosine kinase receptors (FGFR1–4). They present an extracellular domain for ligand–receptor interaction and an intracellular domain containing a tyrosine kinase domain and a COOH-tail. The binding with ligands and HPSGs is mediated by two of the three immunoglobulin (Ig)-like fragments that constitute the receptor's extracellular domain (Ig-II and Ig-III) [1]. The last receptor, FGFRL1, lacks the tyrosine kinase domain and its function is still unclear [2].

The activation of FGFR is a consequence of FGF/FGFR binding, receptor dimerization, and phosphorylation of several tyrosine residues in the intracellular domain. FGFR then activates FGFR substrate 2 (FRS2) that triggers growth factor receptor-bound 2 (GRB2), leading to the activation of RAS and its downstream RAF/mitogen-activated protein kinase (MAPK) pathway. In a parallel way, GRB2 induces the activation of the PI3K/Akt-dependent signaling. Independently of FRS2, phospholipase Cγ (PLCγ) binds to a phosphotyrosine at the COOH-tail and hydrolyzes phosphatidylinositol-4,5-biphosphate (PIP2) to phosphoatidylinositol-3,4,5-triphosphate (PIP3) and diacylglycerol (DAG), thus activating protein kinase C (PKC), which reinforces the MAPK pathway activation [3].

Several regulatory mechanisms of FGF signaling have been proposed (ubiquitination, interaction between FGFR1 and the cell surface neural cell adhesion molecule, MAPK phosphatase 3, Sprouty proteins, and similar expression to FGF family members); however, the entire feedback network is not fully understood [3,4].

FGF/FGFR PATHWAY FUNCTIONS

The FGFR pathway activates various processes including proliferation (MAPK cascade), migration, antiapoptosis (PI3K/Akt cascade), and angiogenesis [3]. However, depending on the cellular context, FGF signaling has also been shown to induce growth arrest and cell differentiation. Various factors underlie this context-dependent signaling, including the spatial and temporal cell-type-specific expression of FGFs, FGFRs, adaptor molecules, and signal-transduction enhancers [5].

FGFRs/FGFs are key molecules during embryogenesis, regulating epithelial–mesenchymal communication and organogenesis. In adults, FGFR signaling orchestrates tissue homeostasis and is involved in tissue repair and inflammation [6]. Indeed, FGF1 and FGF2 have been shown to be potent proangiogenic factors by affecting angiogenesis both directly and indirectly through cross-talk and synergism with the vascular endothelial growth factor (VEGF) and platelet-derived growth factor (PDGF) pathways [7].

MECHANISMS FOR FGF/FGFR SIGNALING DYSREGULATION IN HUMAN CANCER

Two hundred and ten human cancers including breast, lung, colorectal, gastric, testis, ovarian, renal, melanoma, glioma, and acute lymphoblastic leukemia have been recently screened for somatic mutations in the coding exons and splice junctions of the 518 protein kinase genes. The sequencing yielded 921 base substitution somatic mutations, and the FGF pathway showed the highest enrichment for kinases containing non-synonymous mutations [8]. These observations strongly support a role for FGF signaling in cancer promotion. Genomic activating mutations in the FGF/FGFR cascade members are only one of the mechanisms by which the pathway may be dysregulated in human cancers. Other reported genomic mechanisms include chromosomal rearrangements and *FGFR* gene amplifications.

Moreover, aberrant FGF signaling may be the consequence of an increased FGF availability, deriving from either upregulated expression in cancer or stromal cells or enhanced release of FGFs from the extracellular matrix. At the same time, cancer cells may overexpress FGFRs. Interestingly, in physiological conditions, two different receptor isoforms can be generated by alternative splicing of the Ig-III fragment of FGFR1, FGFR2, and FGFR3. These splicing variants (Ig-IIIb and Ig-IIIc) differ in terms of ligand-binding specificity and are differentially expressed in the epithelia and in the mesenchyme. During malignancies, the balance between the tissue-specific expression of these two isoforms can be disrupted, and a switch between IIIb and IIIc splicing variants of FGFR1–3 may occur, broadening the range of FGFs that can stimulate tumor cells. The final result of increased FGF availability, FGFR overexpression, and imbalance in the physiologic expression patterns of receptor splicing variants is the generation and maintenance of autocrine/paracrine loops that sustain cancer growth [3,9].

Finally, an extensive cross-talk and synergism between FGFR signaling and other pathways promoting cancer cell proliferation, antiapoptosis, and angiogenesis has been described [3,9]. This is the prerequisite to interpret recent data describing FGF/FGFR signaling activation as an emergent mechanism of resistance to targeted endocrine and anti-angiogenic drugs.

In the following paragraphs, the role of FGF/FGFR pathways in specific human cancers will be discussed.

HEMATOLOGIC DISEASES

Chromosomal rearrangements involving the *FGFR* genes have been firstly detected in hematological malignancies.

Translocations or insertions at the 8p11 locus, involving *FGFR1*, characterize the 8p11 myeloproliferative syndrome (EMS), an aggressive and acute leukemic disease. The N-terminal portion of the fusion protein comprises a dimerization domain, and the C-terminal portion includes the FGFR1 tyrosine kinase domain. The most common translocation is t(8;13)(p11;q12), which generates a fusion gene with the N-terminal proportion of the proline-rich zinc finger motif of ZNF198. Fusion proteins are located in the cytosol, escape degradation or feedback attenuations, and are constitutively dimerized and activated [10]. Targeting FGFR1 with FGFR inhibitors results in reduced growth and apoptosis induction in cell lines harboring *FGFR1* gene rearrangements [11].

Another chromosomal translocation found in hematological diseases is t(4;14). It involves a chromosomal region including both *FGFR3* and the adjacent multiple myeloma SET domain (*MMSET*) and the Ig heavy chain promoter. The final result is an aberrant *FGFR3* and *MMSET* gene expression. This chromosomal alteration is found in about 15%–20% of multiple myeloma (MM) patients [12]. When the translocation is present, MM cells are strongly dependent from FGFR3 signaling both *in vitro* and *in vivo* [13]. Furthermore, this rearrangement is rarely identified in MM prodromal conditions, suggesting a role in driving a rapid evolution to MM.

BREAST CANCER

The amplification of 8p11–12, harboring *FGFR1*, occurs in 8%–10% of breast cancers, mainly in estrogen receptor (ER)-positive cases [14,15]. In a study including 880 unselected breast cancer samples, *FGFR1* amplification (8%) showed an independent poor prognostic value; however, when cases were dichotomized on the basis of ER status, *FGFR1* amplification maintained its prognostic role only for the ER-positive group [16]. In a retrospective evaluation, including 87 ER-positive breast cancer patients treated with tamoxifen, FGFR1 overexpression/amplification was found in 87.5% of highly proliferative cases (Ki67 $\geq$ 14%) and significantly correlated with a decreased metastasis-free survival [17]. *FGFR1*-amplified breast cancer cells are highly sensitive to anti-FGFR1 tyrosine kinase inhibitors (TKIs) [18]. Moreover, in cell line assays, FGFR1 overexpression/amplification was demonstrated to mediate resistance to 4-hydroxytamoxifen, and the effect was reverted by the inhibition of *FGFR1* by small interfering RNA (siRNA) [17].

In triple-negative (TN) breast cancer, *FGFR2* amplification confers sensitivity to PD173074 *in vitro* and can be detected in up to 4% of the cases [19].

As previously mentioned, sustained FGF signaling in human cancer may also be the consequence of paracrine and autocrine loops. As an illustration, an autocrine loop involving FGF2 with a potential carcinogenetic role has been described in basal-like TN breast cancer cells [20]. High expression of multiple FGFs has also been reported in breast cancer. FGF3 amplification occurs in 15%–20% of the cases and may correlate with invasiveness in node-negative breast cancer patients.

Moreover, a differential expression of FGF8 between breast cancer tissue and normal breast tissue has been reported, with FGF8 overexpression showing oncogenic activity in cell culture and mouse models. *In vivo*, a neutralizing antibody directed against FGF8 showed a potent antitumor effect [9].

GENITOURINARY CANCERS

Approximately 50% of bladder cancer cases present an activating mutation of *FGFR3*. The most frequent mutations lead to the introduction of an unpaired cysteine in the extracellular domain, resulting in constitutive receptor dimerization and activation [21]. The knockdown of mutated *FGFR3*, the use of anti-FGFR3 antibodies (R3Mab), or the use of small-molecule inhibitors (SU5402 and PD173074) reduced tumor growth in both bladder cancer cell cultures and mouse models [22–24]. In humans, *FGFR3* mutations are linked to low-grade, non-muscle-invasive tumors. However, within this favorable subset, *FGFR3* mutation is associated with higher recurrence rates [25]. The detection of *FGFR3* mutation on voided urine samples from patients with *FGFR3*-mutated low-grade bladder cancer has been identified as a potential tool to predict recurrences during surveillance [26].

With regards to prostate cancer, FGF/FGFR pathway activation seems to mainly occur through the establishment of autocrine and paracrine loops. Indeed, tumor stroma has been shown to overexpress many FGFs, and at the same time, FGFR1 expression by cancer cells is increased in poorly differentiated prostate cancers [9]. This interplay between stroma and cancer cells is able to promote cancer progression, angiogenesis, and epithelial to mesenchymal transition and could be disrupted *in vitro* by anti-FGF/FGFR agents. In humans, increased FGF8 expression in malignant prostate epithelium has been linked with tumor progression and poor outcome [27,28].

GYNECOLOGICAL CANCERS

FGFR2-activating mutations involving the extracellular domain (S252W, P253R) and, less frequently, the kinase domain (N549K, K659N) have been found in 12% of endometrial carcinomas. Endometrial cancer cell lines harboring *FGFR2* mutations showed high sensitivity to PD173074, an FGFR TKI [29].

FGF/FGFR abnormalities have been also found in ovarian cancer. As an illustration, amplification of FGF1 and FGF3 and overexpression of FGF2 have been described and correlated with a poorer prognosis [30]. Amplification of FGF1 is linked with microvessel density in ovarian cancer samples, supporting the proangiogenic role for this growth factor [30]. Notably, FGF2 and FGF7 may also be found in malignant ascites and in serum of ovarian cancer patients [9].

LUNG CANCER

FGFR1 amplification has been observed in approximately 20% of squamous non-small cell lung cancers (NSCLC). Squamous NSCLC harboring this alteration showed sensitivity to FGFR inhibition (PD173074) in *in vivo* assays [31]. Results of several studies have demonstrated the coexpression of specific FGFs, particularly

FGF2 and FGF9, along with FGFR1–2 in human lung cancers. FGF2 and FGFR1 were able to induce epithelial–mesenchymal transition in NSCLC cell lines, and this loop could be effectively targeted *in vitro* [32]. Even though conflicting results have emerged, some studies have found a correlation between FGF2 and FGFR1 high expression with poor prognosis in NSCLC patients [32].

FGF2 and FGF9 specifically bind the FGFR-IIIc variants of FGFR1 and FGFR2, which are expressed in gefitinib-resistant NSCLC cell lines [33]. Recently, EGFR inhibitors have been shown to induce transcriptional derepression of FGFR2 and FGFR3 expression in NSCLC cell lines, depicting a novel mechanism for acquired resistance to anti-EGFR agents [34].

FGF2 is supposed to impact oncogenesis also in small cell lung cancer (SCLC), since high FGF2 serum level results are associated with poorer prognosis [35]. In cell line studies, FGF2 was able to stimulate proliferation, inhibit apoptosis, and mediate chemoresistance; these effects were switched off by using PD173074 both *in vitro* and in xenograft models [36].

GASTROINTESTINAL CANCERS

Gastric cancer may harbor *FGFR2* amplification and/or mutation in ~10% of the cases, and this is most frequently observed in the poor-prognosis diffuse-type histotype. *FGFR2* amplified gastric cell lines are highly sensitive to FGFR2 inhibition [37].

FGF19 has been reported to be overexpressed in a subgroup of colorectal carcinomas. A monoclonal antibody that traps FGF19 blocked the growth and migration of colonic cancer cells that expressed FGF19 both *in vitro* and *in vivo* [3]. Moreover, clinical evidences in the advanced and neoadjuvant settings support the role of FGF2 in mediating resistance to bevacizumab-containing regimens [7].

HEPATOCELLULAR CARCINOMA

In a study evaluating 34 human hepatocellular carcinoma (HCC) samples, 82% of the cases showed upregulation of at least one FGF8 subfamily member (FGF8, 17 or 18) and/or one FGFR. The upregulation of FGF2, FGF8, FGF17, FGF18, and FGF19 has been shown to initiate growth stimulation, cell survival, and angiogenesis in an autocrine fashion in HCC [38,39]. A peculiar loop in HCC involves FGFR4, which is predominantly expressed in human hepatocytes, and its specific ligand FGF19, which relies on the high liver expression of Klotho β for receptor interaction [39]. In a recent study, the progeny of FGF19 transgenic mice, which have previously been shown to develop HCCs, bred with FGFR4 knockout mice, fails to develop liver tumors. Moreover, an anti-FGFR4 monoclonal antibody was able to contrast FGF1 and FGF19 binding to FGFR4 as well as FGFR4 tumorigenic functions both *in vitro* and *in vivo* [39].

OTHER CANCERS

Four FGFR4 missense substitutions at codons 535 and 550, involving the kinase domain, have been identified in rhabdomyosarcoma (7%–8% of the cases).

These alterations induced invasiveness, metastatic potential, and poor survival in rhabdomyosarcoma cell lines and murine models [40].

The role of FGF/FGFR pathway is under investigation also for many other cancer types. Some of the most recent results suggest that deregulated FGF/FGFR signaling may mediate resistance to cetuximab in squamous tumor cells and in glioblastoma patients treated with a vascular endothelial growth factor receptor (VEGFR) TKI and vemurafenib in BRAF V600E-mutated melanoma [41,42].

TARGETING FGF PATHWAY IN THE CLINIC

Many attempts have been made to develop agents that inhibit FGF/FGFR activity in human cancer. Those agents that have entered clinical trials are reported in Table 7.1.

TABLE 7.1
Anti-FGF/FGFR Compounds Currently under Clinical Evaluation

Drug	Ongoing Clinical Investigation
Multitargeted TKIs	
TKI258 (dovitinib)	Phase III (RCC)
BIBF1120 (nintedanib)	Phase III (NSCLC, ovarian)
E3810	Phase I (solid tumors)
E7080 (lenvatinib)	Phase III (thyroid)
BMS582664 (brivanib)	Phase III (HCC, CRC)
ENMD-2076	Phase II (breast, ovarian)
TSU 68 (orantinib)	Phase III (HCC)
AP24534 (ponatinib)	Phase II (ALL, CML)
Selective TKIs	
AZD4547	Phase II (breast, gastric)
BGJ398	Phase I (solid tumors)
LY2874455	Phase I (solid tumors)
Monoclonal antibodies	
MGFR1877S	Phase I (MM, solid tumors)
FGF traps	
HGS1036/FP-1039	Phase I (solid tumors)

TKIs, tyrosine-kinase inhibitors; FGFR, fibroblast growth factor receptor; FGF, fibroblast growth factor; RCC, renal cell carcinoma; NSCLC, non-small cell lung cancer; HCC, hepatocellular carcinoma; CRC, colorectal cancer; GIST; gastrointestinal stromal tumor; ALL, acute lymphoblastic leukemia; CML, chronic myeloid leukemia; MM, multiple myeloma.

SMALL-MOLECULE TYROSINE KINASE INHIBITORS

Anti-FGFR small-molecule TKIs target the ATP-binding site of the intracellular domain. Some of these drugs have entered the clinical phases of development and are discussed hereafter.

Nonselective FGFR TKIs

Nonselective FGFR TKIs are multitarget drugs that include FGFR family members in their spectrum of activity. They are often good VEGF inhibitors and they usually show a modest, although significant, bioactivity against FGFRs.

TKI258 (Dovitinib)

Dovitinib is a potent TKI, highly active against VEGFR-1, VEGFR-2, and VEGFR-3; platelet-derived growth factor receptor (PDGFR)-h; FGFR-1, FGFR-2, and FGFR-3; fetal liver tyrosine kinase receptor 3 (FLT-3); KIT; Ret; TrkA; and csf-1. Due to its peculiar activity profile, TKI258 demonstrated significant activity in a broad range of preclinical models [43]. Dovitinib induced apoptosis in FGFR-expressing mammary cells via inhibition of PI3K/Akt signaling pathway. Moreover, it specifically reduced proliferation and survival of cell lines with FGFR1 fusion genes associated with the 8p11 EMS [44]. Furthermore, dovitinib potently affected tumor growth of HCC xenograft models [45].

In a phase I trial including 35 patients with advanced solid tumors, the more frequently observed drug-related toxicities were gastrointestinal and fatigue, whereas cardiovascular events were seen in 5 patients. One partial response (PR) and two stable diseases (SDs) >6 months were observed [46].

A phase I/II dose-escalation study that enrolled 47 patients with advanced melanoma resistant or refractory to standard therapies reported SD in 12 patients as the best observed tumor response. The safety data were similar to those from the first phase I study. As for the results of the pharmacodynamics studies, treatment with dovitinib effectively inhibited VEGFR and FGFR [47].

Eighty-one human epidermal growth factor receptor 2 (HER2)-negative, previously treated metastatic breast cancer patients were included in a phase II study of dovitinib monotherapy. Among them, 68 had measurable disease and were included in the analysis of the first step of the study. The protocol predefined requirements for proceeding to step 2 (≥2 confirmed responses in one group) were not reached; however, encouraging efficacy results were reported for the FGFR-amplified/hormone receptor (HR)-positive subset of patients (25% of non-confirmed PR and/or SD ≥ 4 weeks). In addition, the investigators found that the coamplification of FGFR1 and FGF3 might represent a predictor for dovitinib sensitivity [48]. More information will derive from an ongoing phase II randomized trial of fulvestrant plus dovitinib versus placebo for postmenopausal HER2-negative/HR-positive advanced breast cancer patients (clinicaltrials.gov, NCT01528345).

Dovitinib has been tested in a phase II trial including 59 patients with metastatic renal cell carcinoma (RCC) who previously received a VEGFR-TKI and/or a mammalian target of rapamycin (mTOR) inhibitor or other therapies. PRs were observed in 3.4% of the patients, whereas SD $\geq$ 2 months and SD $\geq$ 4 months were reported at a rate of 49.2% and 27.1%, respectively. Median progression-free survival (PFS) was 5.5 months and median overall survival (OS) was 11.8 months. The most common grade 3 adverse events (AEs) were nausea/vomiting, fatigue, diarrhea, and hypertension; grade 4 hypertriglyceridemia occurred in 8.5% of patients [49]. An ongoing phase III trial is comparing dovitinib versus sorafenib as a third-line treatment (clinicaltrials.gov, NCT01223027).

Finally, other phase I/II trials for many other cancer types are ongoing (clinicaltrials.gov, accessed June 2012). In particular, following promising preclinical findings, phase II studies are currently testing dovitinib in GIST patients resistant to imatinib and sunitinib (clinicaltrials.gov; NCT01478373, NCT01440959).

BIBF1120 (Nintedanib)

Another multitarget TKI, BIBF1120, shows the highest activity against VEGFR1 to VEGFR3 and FGFR2 [50]. BIBF1120 inhibited MAPK and Akt signaling pathways in three cell types involved in angiogenesis (endothelial cells, pericytes, and smooth muscle cells), resulting in inhibition of cell proliferation and apoptosis. In human tumor xenograft models, BIBF 1120 was highly active at well-tolerated doses, reducing vessel density and vessel integrity after 5 days and inducing profound growth inhibition [50].

A phase I dose-escalating study including 61 patients with advanced cancers reported gastrointestinal symptoms as the main drug-related AEs. The dose limiting toxicities (DLTs) were reversible hepatic enzyme elevations. Interestingly, one complete response in RCC and two PRs in RCC and colorectal cancer (CRC) were observed [51]. Encouraging efficacy results were also derived from other phase I and phase II trials evaluating BIBF1120 either as monotherapy or in combination with chemotherapy for NSCLC [52–55].

These findings have lead to the design of phase III trials testing BIBF 1120 in NSCLC in combination with docetaxel or pemetrexed (clinicaltrials.gov; NCT00805194, NCT00806819).

BIBF1120 has also been studied as maintenance treatment for relapsed ovarian cancer. Eighty-three patients achieving a response to chemotherapy and at high risk of further recurrence were treated with either BIBF1120 or placebo in a phase II study. A tendency to a better PFS with BIBF1120 was reported (p=0.06) [56]. This potential for BIBF1120 in the treatment of ovarian cancer is under investigation in a phase III trial (clinicaltrials.gov; NCT01015118).

E3810

E3810 potently inhibits VEGFRs and FGFRs (mainly FGFR1 and FGFR2) [57]. A phase I trial is ongoing, testing this compound in advanced solid tumor patients. Among the 17 patients who were included in the dose-escalation phase, 3 SDs beyond one year were reported. Common AEs included hypertension and proteinuria. The DLT was glomerular thrombotic microangiopathy. A dose-expansion phase is including breast cancer patients with FGFR1 amplification and patients with tumors sensitive to anti-angiogenic therapy failing a prior anti-angiogenic regimen [58].

E7080 (Lenvatinib)

E7080 is an orally available multi-TKI, mainly active against VEGFR1, VEGFR2, and VEGFR3 but also FGFR1, PDGFRα, and PDGFRβ. Phase I studies demonstrated hypertension and proteinuria as DLTs, these being common side effects of VEGFR-targeted therapies [59]. Encouraging results from phase I/II studies, mainly for melanoma, HCC, and thyroid cancer patients, prompted further evaluation of this drug [60–62].

BMS582664 (Brivanib)

Like E7080, brivanib is more potent against VEGFRs than FGFRs. In the phase I study, brivanib monotherapy resulted in 3% of PR and 35% of SD. Frequently occurring treatment-related toxic effects were nausea, diarrhea, fatigue, dizziness, hypertension, headache, and anorexia. VEGF inhibition class effects observed with brivanib included hypertension (33.8%), proteinuria (14.7%), hemorrhage (11.8%), thrombosis-related events (4.4%), and reversible posterior leukoencephalopathy (1.5%) [63]. Due to the findings of phase I and phase II studies [64,65], brivanib is under evaluation for the treatment of CRC in combination with cetuximab and is being compared to sorafenib as first-line therapy for HCC (clinicaltrials.gov; NCT00858871, NCT00640471).

Other nonselective anti-FGFR TKIs have entered clinical phases of development such as ENMD-2076 [66] and TSU-68 (orantinib) [67]; however, they only show a marginal activity against FGFR.

Selective Anti-FGFR TKIs

Recently, second-generation selective anti-FGFR TKIs have been developed. The potential advantage is that they do not present VEGF-related toxicity profiles. However, their initial development has been complicated by an emerging class-specific toxicity. Indeed, FGF23 is involved in phosphate homeostasis, and in preclinical models, these compounds have caused hyperphosphatemia-mediated tissue calcification due to the blockade of FGF23 signaling [3]. Three selective FGFR TKIs have entered the clinical phases of evaluation.

AZD4547

Potent nanomolar IC50 values were obtained when AZD4547 was examined against recombinant FGFR kinases, whereas activity versus VEGFR2 was approximately 120-fold lower. In preclinical assays, it showed anticancer activity against tumor cell lines and xenograft models harboring FGFR alterations [68]. This prompted the design of early phase clinical trials testing the compound in cancer patients presenting FGFR1 and/or FGFR2 polysomy or amplification (clinicaltrials.gov; NCT00979134, NCT01202591, NCT01457846).

BGJ398

BGJ398, selectively inhibiting FGFR1–3, showed significant antitumor activity in RT112 bladder cancer xenograft models overexpressing wild-type FGFR3 [69].

In the context of an ongoing phase I trial, 26 patients (including 10 patients with FGFR1-amplified breast cancer and 3 patients with FGFR1-amplified squamous NSCLC) have been treated so far. AEs were generally grades 1–2 (diarrhea, fatigue, and nausea). Hyperphosphatemia was observed, with increasing frequency at higher doses of BGJ398, and could be managed with phosphate binders and diuretics. One lung cancer patient with an *FGFR1* amplification achieved a 33% reduction in target lesions [70].

LY287445

LY2874455 is a pan-FGFR inhibitor targeting FGFR1 to FGFR4. This drug was able to reduce the proliferation of cancer cells with a significantly increased FGFR signaling activity especially those with elevated FGF or FGFR levels such as gastric cancer, bladder cancer, MM, and NSCLC cell lines. Moreover, LY2874455 inhibited the growth of tumor xenografts derived from gastric and MM cell lines carrying a highly amplified FGFR2 and an overexpressed FGFR3 due to a chromosomal translocation, respectively. Furthermore, LY2874455 did not show VEGFR2-mediated toxicities at efficacious doses [71]. A phase I trial is currently enrolling advanced breast cancer patients (clinicaltrials.gov, NCT01212107).

MONOCLONAL ANTIBODIES AND FGF-LIGAND TRAPS

Other attempts to target FGFR pathway are represented by anti-FGFR monoclonal antibodies and FGF-ligand traps.

Due to a severe side effect in mouse models (anorexia), an antibody targeting FGFR1-IIIc did not enter the clinical phases of development. To the opposite, MGFR1877S, an anti-FGFR3 antibody, is currently under clinical investigation (clinicaltrials.gov, NCT01363024 and NCT01122875).

The ligand-trap FP-1039 sequesters FGFs, so that they are no longer available for FGFR binding. In *in vivo* studies, it inhibited FGF2- and VEGF-induced neovascularization and tumor growth [72]. Phase I studies testing this drug are ongoing (clinicaltrials.gov, NCT00687505).

CONCLUSIONS

In summary, several FGF signaling aberrations have been described in many cancer types, with preclinical assays often confirming their carcinogenetic role, thereby highlighting this pathway as a potential therapeutic target. The role played by FGFR signaling in tumor angiogenesis and in mediating resistance to other targeted agents further reinforces the rationale for developing anti-FGFR agents for cancer treatment. Various anti-FGFR drugs with different mechanisms of action and FGFR selectivity have already reached the clinical phases of development. The results of these ongoing trials and further research will help in defining the role of these new potential effective drugs in human cancer treatment and to allocate them to the correct settings for each specific disease.

REFERENCES

1. Beenken A, Mohammadi M. The FGF family: Biology, pathophysiology and therapy. *Nat Rev Drug Discov* 2009;8:235–253.
2. Trueb B. Biology of FGFRL1, the fifth fibroblast growth factor receptor. *Cell Mol Life Sci* 2011;68:951–964.
3. Turner N, Grose R. Fibroblast growth factor signaling: From development to cancer. *Nat Rev Cancer* 2010;10:116–129.
4. Thien CB, Langdon WY. Cbl: Many adaptations to regulate protein tyrosine kinases. *Nat Rev Mol Cell Biol* 2001;2:294–307.
5. Dailey L, Ambrosetti D, Mansukhani A, Basilico C. Mechanisms underlying differential responses to FGF signaling. *Cytokine Growth Factor Rev* 2005;16:233–247.
6. Powers CJ, McLeskey SW, Wellstein A. Fibroblast growth factors, their receptors and signaling. *Endocr Relat Cancer* 2000;7:165–197.
7. Lieu C, Heymach J, Overman M, Tran H, Kopetz S. Beyond VEGF: Inhibition of the fibroblast growth factor pathway and antiangiogenesis. *Clin Cancer Res* 2011;17:6130–6139.
8. Greenman C, Stephens P, Smith R, Dalgliesh GL, Hunter C, Bignell G et al. Patterns of somatic mutation in human cancer genomes. *Nature* 2007;446:153–158.
9. Wesche J, Haglund K, Haugsten EM. Fibroblast growth factors and their receptors in cancer. *Biochem J* 2011;437:199–213.
10. Jackson CC, Medeiros LJ, Miranda RN. 8p11 myeloproliferative syndrome: A review. *Hum Pathol* 2010;41:461–476.
11. Chase A, Grand FH, Cross NC. Activity of TKI258 against primary cells and cell lines with FGFR1 fusion genes associated with the 8p11 myeloproliferative syndrome. *Blood* 2007;110:3729–3734.
12. Chesi M, Nardini E, Brents LA, Schröck E, Ried T, Kuehl WM et al. Frequent translocation t(4;14) (p16.3;q32.3) in multiple myeloma is associated with increased expression and activating mutations of fibroblast growth factor receptor 3. *Nat Genet* 1997;16:260–264.
13. Qing J, Du X, Chen Y, Chan P, Li H, Wu P et al. Antibody-based targeting of FGFR3 in bladder carcinoma and t(4;14)-positive multiple myeloma in mice. *J Clin Invest* 2009;119:1216–1229.
14. Courjal F, Cuny M, Simony-Lafontaine J, Louason G, Speiser P, Zeillinger R et al. Mapping of DNA amplifications at 15 chromosomal localizations in 1875 breast tumors: definition of phenotypic groups. *Cancer Res* 1997;57:4360–4367.
15. Andre F, Job B, Dessen P, Tordai A, Michiels S, Liedtke C et al. Molecular characterization of breast cancer with high-resolution oligonucleotide comparative genomic hybridization array. *Clin Cancer Res* 2009;15:441–451.
16. Elbauomy ES, Green AR, Lambros MB, Turner NC, Grainge MJ, Powe D et al. FGFR1 amplification in breast carcinomas: A chromogenic in situ hybridisation analysis. *Breast Cancer Res* 2007;9:R23.
17. Turner N, Pearson A, Sharpe R, Lambros M, Geyer F, Lopez-Garcia MA et al. FGFR1 amplification drives endocrine therapy resistance and is a therapeutic target in breast cancer. *Cancer Res* 2010;70:2085–2094.
18. Reis-Filho JS, Simpson PT, Turner NC, Lambros MB, Jones C, Mackay A et al. FGFR1 emerges as a potential therapeutic target for lobular breast carcinomas. *Clin Cancer Res* 2006;12: 6652–6662.
19. Turner N, Lambros MB, Horlings HM, Pearson A, Sharpe R, Natrajan R et al. Integrative molecular profiling of triple negative breast cancers identifies amplicon drivers and potential therapeutic targets. *Oncogene* 2010;29:2013–2023.

20. Sharpe R, Pearson A, Herrera-Abreu MT, Johnson D, Mackay A, Welti JC, Natrajan R, Reynolds AR, Reis-Filho JS, Ashworth A, Turner NC. FGFR signaling promotes the growth of triple-negative and basal-like breast cancer cell lines both in vitro and in vivo. *Clin Cancer Res* 2011;17(16):5275–5286.

21. van Rhijn BW, vanTilborg AA, Lurkin I, Bonaventure J, deVries A, Thiery JP et al. Novel fibroblast growth factor receptor 3 (FGFR3) mutations in bladder cancer previously identified in non-lethal skeletal disorders. *Eur J Hum Genet* 2002;10:819–824.

22. Lamont FR, Tomlinson DC, Cooper PA, Shnyder SD, Chester JD, Knowles MA et al. Small molecule FGF receptor inhibitors block FGFR-dependent urothelial carcinoma growth in vitro and in vivo. *Br J Cancer* 2011;104:75–82.

23. Tomlinson DC, Hurst CD, Knowles MA. Knock down by shRNA identifies S249C mutant FGFR3 as a potential therapeutic target in bladder cancer. *Oncogene* 2007;26:5889–5899.

24. Martínez-Torrecuadrada J, Cifuentes G, López-Serra P, Saenz P, Martínez A, Casal JI. Targeting the extra cellular domain of fibro blast growth factor receptor3 with human single-chain Fv anti bodies inhibits bladder carcinoma cell line proliferation. *Clin Cancer Res* 2005;11:6280–6290.

25. Hernández S, López-Knowles E, Lloreta J, Kogevinas M, Amorós A, Tardón A et al. Prospective study of FGFR3 mutations as a prognostic factor in nonmuscle invasive urothelial bladder carcinomas. *J Clin Oncol* 2006;24:3664–3671.

26. Zuiverloon TC, Tjin SS, Busstra M, Bangma CH, Boevé ER, Zwarthoff EC. Optimization of non muscle invasive bladder cancer recurrence detection using a urine based FGFR3 mutation assay. *J Urol* 2011;186:707–712.

27. Acevedo VD, Gangula RD, Freeman KW, Li R, Zhang Y, Wang F et al. Inducible FGFR-1 activation leads to irreversible prostate adenocarcinoma and an epithelial-to mesenchymal transition. *Cancer Cell* 2007; 12:559–571.

28. Feng S, Shao LJ, Yu W, Gavine PR, Ittmann MM. Targeting fibroblast growth factor receptor signaling inhibits prostate cancer progression. *Clin Cancer Res* 2012; 18:3880–3888 [Epub ahead of print].

29. Dutt A, Salvesen HB, Chen TH, Ramos AH, Onofrio RC, Hatton C et al. Drug-sensitive FGFR2 mutations in endometrial carcinoma. *Proc Natl Acad Sci USA* 2008;105:8713–8717.

30. Birrer MJ, Johnson ME, Hao K, Wong KK, Park DC, Bell A et al. Whole genome oligonucleotide-based array comparative genomic hybridization analysis identified fibroblast growth factor 1 as a prognostic marker for advanced-stage serous ovarian adenocarcinomas. *J Clin Oncol* 2007;25:2281–2287.

31. Weiss J, Sos ML, Seidel D, Peifer M, Zander T, Heuckmann JM et al. Frequent and focal FGFR1 amplification associates with therapeutically tractable FGFR1 dependency in squamous cell lung cancer. *Sci Trans Med* 2010;2:62ra93.

32. Semrad TJ, Mack PC. Fibroblast growth factor signaling in non-small-cell lung cancer. *Clin Lung Cancer* 2012;13:90–95.

33. Marek L, Ware KE, Fritzsche A, Hercule P, Helton WR, Smith JE et al. Fibroblast growth factor (FGF) and FGF receptor-mediated autocrine signaling in non-small-cell lung cancer cells. *Mol Pharmacol* 2009;75:196–207.

34. Ware KE, Marshall ME, Heasley LR, Marek L, Hinz TK, Hercule P et al. Rapidly acquired resistance to EGFR tyrosine kinase inhibitors in NSCLC cell lines through de-repression of FGFR2 and FGFR3 expression. *PLoS One* 2010;5:e14117.

35. Ruotsalainen T, Joensuu H, Mattson K, Salven P. High pretreatment serum concentration of basic fibroblast growth factor is a predictor of poor prognosis in small cell lung cancer. *Cancer Epidemiol Biomarkers Prev* 2002;11:1492–1495.

36. Pardo OE, Wellbrock C, Khanzada UK, Aubert M, Arozarena I, Davidson S et al. FGF-2 protects small cell lung cancer cells from apoptosis through a complex involving PKCepsilon, B-Raf and S6K2. *EMBO J* 2006;25:3078–3088.

37. Kunii K, Davis L, Gorenstein J, Hatch H, Yashiro M, DiBacco A et al. FGFR2-amplified gastric cancer cell lines require FGFR2 and Erbb3 signaling for growth and survival. *Cancer Res* 2008;68:2340–2348.

38. Brooks N, Kilgour E, Smith PD. Molecular pathways: Fibroblast growth factor signaling: a new therapeutic opportunity in cancer. *Clin Cancer Res* 2012;18:1855–1862.

39. French DM, Lin BC, Wang M, Adams C, Shek T, Hötzel K et al. Targeting FGFR4 inhibits hepatocellular carcinoma in preclinical mouse models. *PLoS One* 2012;7(5):e36713.

40. Taylor JG, Cheuk AT, Tsang PS, Chung JY, Song YK, Desai K et al. Identification of FGFR4-activating mutations in human rhabdomyosarcomas that promote metastasis in xenotransplanted models. *J Clin Invest* 2009;119:3395–3407.

41. Oliveras-Ferraros C, Cufí S, Queralt B, Vazquez-Martin A, Martin-Castillo B, deLlorens R et al. Cross-suppression of EGFR ligands amphiregulin and epiregulin and de-repression of FGFR3 signalling contribute to cetuximab resistance in wild-type KRAS tumour cells. *Br J Cancer* 2012;106:1406–1414.

42. Yadav V, Zhang X, Liu J, Estrem S, Li S, Gong XQ et al. Reactivation of mitogen-activated protein kinase(MAPK) pathway by FGF receptor3(FGFR3)/ras mediates resistance to vemurafenib in human BRAF V600E mutant melanoma. *J Biol Chem* 2012; 287:28087–28098. [Epub ahead of print.]

43. Lee SH, Lopes de MD, Vora J, Harris A, Ye H, Nordahl L et al. In vivo target modulation and biological activity of CHIR-258, a multitargeted growth factor receptor kinase inhibitor, in colon cancer models. *Clin Cancer Res* 2005;11:3633–3641.

44. Trudel S, Li ZH, Wei E, Wiesmann M, Chang H, Chen C et al. CHIR-258, a novel, multitargeted tyrosine kinase inhibitor for the potential treatment oft(4;14) multiple myeloma. *Blood* 2005;105:2941–2948.

45. Huynh H, Chow PK, Tai WM, Choo SP, Chung AY, Ong HS et al. Dovitinib demonstrates anti tumor and anti metastatic activities in xenograft models of hepatocellular carcinoma. *J Hepatol* 2012;56:595–601.

46. Sarker D, Molife R, Evans TR, Hardie M, Marriott C, Butzberger-Zimmerli P et al. A phase I pharmacokinetic and pharmacodynamic study of TKI258, an oral, multitargeted receptor tyrosine kinase inhibitor in patients with advanced solid tumors. *Clin Cancer Res* 2008;14:2075–2081.

47. Kim KB, Chesney J, Robinson D, Gardner H, Shi MM, Kirkwood JM. Phase I/II and pharmacodynamic study of dovitinib (TKI258), an inhibitor of fibroblast growth factor receptors and VEGF receptors, in patients with advanced melanoma. *Clin Cancer Res* 2011;17:7451–7461.

48. Andre F, Bachelot D, Campone M, Dalenc F, Perez-Garcia JM, Hurvitz SA et al. A multicenter, open-label phase II trial of dovitinib, an FGFR1 inhibitor, in FGFR1 amplified and non-amplified metastatic breast cancer. Data presented at the *2011 American Society of Clinical oncology Annual Meeting. J Clin Oncol* 2011; 29(suppl):Abstract 508.

49. Angevin E, Grunwald V, Ravaud A, Castellano DE, Lin CC, Gschwend JE et al. A phase II study of dovitinib (TKI258), an FGFR- and VEGFR-inhibitor, in patients with advanced or metastatic renal cell cancer (mRCC). Data presented at *the 2011 American Society of Clinical oncology Annual Meeting. J Clin Oncol* 2011; 29(suppl):Abstract 4551.

50. Hilberg F, Roth GJ, Krssak M, Kautschitsch S, Sommergruber W, Tontsch-Grunt U et al. BIBF 1120: Triple angiokinase inhibitor with sustained receptor blockade and good antitumor efficacy. *Cancer Res* 2008;68:4774–4782.

51. Mross K, StefanicM, Gmehling D, Frost A, Baas F, Unger C et al. Phase I study of the angiogenesis inhibitor BIBF 1120 in patients with advanced solid tumors. *Clin Cancer Res* 2010;16:311–319.
52. Okamoto I, Kaneda H, Satoh T, Okamoto W, Miyazaki M, Morinaga R et al. Phase I safety, pharmacokinetic, and biomarker study of BIBF 1120, an oral triple tyrosine kinase inhibitor in patients with advanced solid tumors. *Mol Cancer Ther* 2010;9:2825–2833.
53. Doebele RC, Conkling P, Traynor AM, Otterson GA, Zhao Y, Wind S et al. A phase I, open-label dose-escalation study of continuous treatment with BIBF 1120 in combination with paclitaxel and carboplatin as first-line treatment in patients with advanced non-small-cell lung cancer. *Ann Oncol* 2012;23:2094–2102.
54. Ellis PM, Kaiser R, Zhao Y, Stopfer P, Gyorffy S, Hanna N. Phase I open-label study of continuous treatment with BIBF 1120, a triple angiokinase inhibitor, and pemetrexed in pretreated non-small cell lung cancer patients. *Clin Cancer Res* 2010;16:2881–2889.
55. Reck M, Kaiser R, Eschbach C, Stefanic M, Love J, Gatzemeier U et al. A phase II double-blind study to investigate efficacy and safety of two doses of the triple angio kinase inhibitor BIBF 1120 in patients with relapsed advanced non-small-cell lung cancer. *Ann Oncol* 2011;22:1374–1381.
56. Ledermann JA, Hackshaw A, Kaye S, Jayson G, Gabra H, McNeish I et al. Randomized phase II placebo-controlled trial of maintenance therapy using the oral triple angiokinase inhibitor BIBF 1120 after chemotherapy for relapsed ovarian cancer. *J Clin Oncol* 2011;29:3798–3804.
57. Bello E, Colella G, Scarlato V, Oliva P, Berndt A, Valbusa G et al. E-3810 is a potent dual inhibitor of VEGFR and FGFR that exerts antitumor activity in multiple preclinical models. *Cancer Res* 2011;71:1396–1405.
58. Soria JC, Dienstmann R, de Braud F, Cereda R, Bahleda R, Hollebecque A et al. First-in-man study of E-3810, a novel VEGFR and FGFR inhibitor, in patients with advanced solid tumors. *Ann Oncol* 2012;23 (Suppl 1): i15–i25, Abstract L2.5.
59. Yamada K, Yamamoto N, Yamada Y, Nokihara H, Fujiwara Y, Hirata T et al. Phase I dose-escalation study and biomarker analysis of E7080 in patients with advanced solid tumors. *Cancer Res* 2011;17:2528–2537.
60. Hong DS, Boss DS, Glen H, Mink J, Ren M, Andresen C et al. Assessment of clinical activity of E7080, a multitargeted kinase inhibitor, in patients with advanced melanoma treated in two phase I trials. *J Clin Oncol* 2011;29(Suppl):Abstract 8527.
61. Schlumberger M, Jarzab B, Cabanillas ME, Robinson B, Pacini F, Ball DW et al. A phase II trial of the multitargeted kinase inhibitor lenvatinib (E7080) in advanced medullary thyroid cancer (MTC). *J Clin Oncol* 30, 2012(Suppl):Abstract 5591.
62. Okita K, Kumada H, Ikeda K, Kudo M, Kawazoe S, Osaki Y et al. Phase I/II study of E7080 (lenvatinib), a multitargeted tyrosine kinase inhibitor, in patients (pts) with advanced hepatocellular carcinoma (HCC): Initial assessment of response rate. *J Clin Oncol* 30, 2012(Suppl 4):Abstract 320.
63. Jonker DJ, Rosen LS, Sawyer MB, deBraud F, Wilding G, Sweeney CJ et al. A phase I study to determine the safety, pharmacokinetics and pharmacodynamics of a dual VEGFR and FGFR inhibitor, brivanib, in patients with advanced or metastatic solid tumors. *Ann Oncol* 2011;22:1413–1419.
64. Garrett CR, Siu LL, El-Khoueiry A, Buter J, Rocha-Lima CM, Marshall J et al. Phase I dose-escalation study to determine the safety, pharmacokinetics and pharmacodynamics of brivanib alaninate in combination with full-dose cetuximab in patients with advanced gastrointestinal malignancies who have failed prior therapy. *Br J Cancer* 2011;105:44–52.
65. Finn RS, Kang YK, Mulcahy M, Polite BN, Lim HY, Walters I et al. Phase II, open-label study of brivanib as second-line therapy in patients with advanced hepatocellular carcinoma. *Clin Cancer Res* 2012;18:2090–2098.

66. Fletcher GC, Brokx RD, Denny TA, Hembrough TA, Plum SM, Fogler WE et al. ENMD-2076 is an orally active kinase inhibitor with anti angiogenic and anti proliferative mechanisms of action. *Mol Cancer Ther* 2011;10:126–137.

67. Laird AD, Vajkoczy P, Shawver LK, Thurnher A, Liang C, Mohammadi M et al. SU6668 is a potent antiangiogenic and antitumor agent that induces regression of established tumors. *Cancer Res* 2000;60:4152–4160.

68. Gavine PR, Mooney L, Kilgour E, Thomas AP, Al-Kadhimi K, Beck S et al. AZD4547: An orally bioavailable, potent, and selective inhibitor of the fibroblast growth factor receptor tyrosine kinase family. *Cancer Res* 2012;72:2045–2056.

69. Guagnano V, Furet P, Spanka C, Bordas V, LeDouget M, Stamm C et al. Discovery of 3-(2,6-dichloro-3,5-dimethoxy-phenyl)-1-{6-[4-(4-ethyl-piperazin-1-yl)-phenylamino]-pyrimidin-4-yl}-1-methyl-urea (NVP-BGJ398), a potent and selective inhibitor of the fibroblast growth factor receptor family of receptor tyrosine kinase. *J Med Chem* 2011;54:7066–7083.

70. Wolf J, LoRusso PM, Camidge RD, Perez JM, Tabernero J, Hidalgo M et al. A phase I dose escalation study of NVP-BGJ398, a selective pan FGFR inhibitor in genetically preselected advanced solid tumors. Data presented at the *Annual Meeting of the American Association for Cancer Research* 2012; March 31 to April 4; Chicago, IL. Philadelphia, PA: AACR; 2012. Abstract LB-122.

71. Zhao G, Li WY, Chen D, Henry JR, Li HY, Chen Z et al. A novel, selective inhibitor of fibroblast growth factor receptors that shows a potent broad spectrum of antitumor activity in several tumor xenograft models. *Mol Cancer Ther* 2011;10:2200–2210.

72. Long L, Tom Brennan, Jim Zanghi, Palencia S, Cheung R, Aguirre M et al. Antitumor efficacy of FP-1039, a soluble FGF receptor 1:Fc conjugate, as a single agent or in combination with anticancer drugs. Data presented at the *Annual Meeting of the American Association for Cancer Research* 2009; April 18–22; Denver, CO. Philadelphia, PA: AACR; 2009. Abstract 2789.

8 Anaplastic Lymphoma Kinase

Aparna Rao
Peter MacCallum Cancer Centre

Benjamin Solomon
Peter MacCallum Cancer Centre

CONTENTS

INTRODUCTION

Anaplastic lymphoma kinase (ALK) was originally identified in 1994 as a tyrosine kinase activated by a chromosomal translocation in an uncommon T cell lymphoma called anaplastic large-cell lymphoma (ALCL) [1]. Following its subsequent identification in a subset of non-small cell lung cancers (NSCLCs) in 2007 [2,3], ALK has emerged as a readily identifiable and therapeutically tractable molecular target in cancer [4]. Activation of ALK, which occurs primarily through gene rearrangements and point mutations, is found in a spectrum of diseases including ALCL [1], NSCLC [2,3], inflammatory myofibroblastic tumors (IMTs) [5], and neuroblastoma [6]. A variety of approaches to target ALK are in development, the most advanced of which is the ALK tyrosine kinase inhibitor crizotinib.

BIOLOGY OF ALK

The *ALK* gene on chromosome 2p23 encodes a 1620 amino acid tyrosine kinase [7,8], which is a member of the insulin receptor superfamily and shares the most identity with the leukocyte tyrosine kinase and ROS1 [9]. ALK has three structural domains, an extracellular ligand-binding domain, a transmembrane region, and an intracellular tyrosine kinase domain. In *Drosophila melanogaster*, the ligand Jelly belly (Jeb) has been shown to bind and activate the ortholog for ALK [10]. While there are two proposed ALK ligands in humans, pleiotrophin and midkine, a definitive homolog of Jeb remains to be identified [11].

The physiological function of ALK in mammals is incompletely understood. In mice, expression of ALK is prominent in the brain and the nervous system of embryos [12] and may contribute to behavioral control in adult mice [13]. In human adults, ALK is expressed at low levels within the central nervous system (CNS) [14] and in the small intestine and testis [1].

The downstream effectors of ALK include the Ras/MAPK/ERK, PI3K/AKT, and JAK3/STAT3 pathways. These pathways play important and likely overlapping roles in cell survival and proliferation [15]. Different oncogenic abnormalities of the *ALK* gene may result in differential activation of these pathways in different cellular contexts.

ALK was first identified in 1994 as a tyrosine-phosphorylated protein component of a fusion protein with nucleophosmin (NPM1), which arose as a result of a translocation between chromosomes 2 and 5 (2;5)(p23;q35) in ALCL [1,16]. Since that time, other fusion genes have been identified in ALCL including *TFG-ALK*, *ATIC-ALK*, and *CLTC-ALK* [17] (Table 8.1). Furthermore, a number of fusion proteins have been identified in other tumors, such as IMTs, NSCLC, esophageal cancer, and renal cancer [7].

In 2007, a novel fusion gene *EML4-ALK* was identified in NSCLC [2], which arose from an inversion on the short arm of chromosome 2 (inv (2) (p21p23)). This fusion gene encoded for a protein made up of the amino-terminal portion of EML4 and the intracellular tyrosine kinase domain-containing portion of ALK. This fusion gene was simultaneously and independently identified in NSCLC cell lines using a phosphoproteomic approach [3]. *EML4-ALK* was demonstrated to transform cells both *in vitro* and *in vivo* [2]. Subsequently, it was demonstrated that the expression of *EML4-ALK* in the lungs of transgenic mice resulted in the induction of adenocarcinoma [18,19] confirming the oncogenic role of ALK.

ALK AND MALIGNANCY

In addition to gene rearrangements resulting in fusion proteins containing the ALK tyrosine kinase, other oncogenic abnormalities have been identified in cancer including point mutations in the *ALK* kinase domain and *ALK* gene amplification. The most common of these abnormalities are shown in Figure 8.1 and summarized in Table 8.1, with further information regarding the clinical and pathologic correlates being detailed in the following sections.

TABLE 8.1
ALK as an Oncogene

Tumor Type	Pathogenic Abnormality	Frequency
Anaplastic large-cell lymphoma	Translocation resulting in fusion genes: *NPM1-ALK* [1]; rarer partners *TFG-ALK, ATIC-ALK,* and *CLTC-ALK* [21].	50%–75% [1]
Non-small cell lung cancer	Translocation resulting in fusion genes: *EML4-ALK* [2]; rarer fusion partners *KIF5B-ALK* [24], *TFG-ALK* [3], and *KLC1-ALK* [25]	3%–6% [7]
Inflammatory myofibroblastic tumors	Translocation resulting in fusion genes of *ALK* with *TPM3, TPM4, CLTC, ATIC, CARS, RANB2, SEC31l1,* and *PPFIBP1* [49–52]	50% [5]
Neuroblastoma	Germline mutations of tyrosine kinase domain, e.g., R1275 mutation [6]	>90% in some pedigrees of hereditary neuroblastoma [6]
	Sporadic mutations of tyrosine kinase domain: R1275, F1174, F1245, and K1062M [59–61]	8% in sporadic neuroblastoma [62]
	Rarely gene amplification [65]	
Rare abnormalities		
Breast cancer	Translocation resulting in *EML4-ALK* fusion gene [66]	Very rarely, observed in cases only
Colorectal cancer	Translocations resulting in fusion genes: *EML4-ALK* [66] and *C2orff44-ALK* [72]	
Renal medullary carcinoma	Translocation resulting in fusion gene *VCL-ALK* [71]	
Diffuse large B cell lymphoma	Translocation resulting in fusion genes: *NPM-ALK* [67], *CLTC-ALK* [68], *SEC31a-ALK* [69], and *SQSTM1-ALK* [70]	
Anaplastic thyroid cancer	Missense mutation of tyrosine kinase domain [73]	
Inflammatory breast cancer	Gene amplification [74]	
Rhabdomyosarcoma	Frequent copy number gain of *ALK* [75].	

ANAPLASTIC LARGE-CELL LYMPHOMA

ALCL is a rare lymphoma in adults but is more common in the pediatric population. The first identified *ALK* fusion protein in ALCL was the NPM1-ALK fusion protein [1,16] with the t (2;5)(p23;q35) translocation occurring in 50%–75% of ALCL. The nucleophosmin (NPM1) portion drives aberrant expression, in this case within the nucleus, and mediates dimerization and subsequent autoactivation of the ALK kinase [20]. Other less frequent translocations have been identified including t (1;2), t (2;3), inv (2), and t (2;17) [21], which result in the fusion of *ALK* with other genes, as outlined in Table 8.1.

ALK rearrangement-positive ALCL more commonly occurs in younger patients and in males (a ratio of 6.5:1 for females) [22]. In ALCL, ALK positivity (as defined

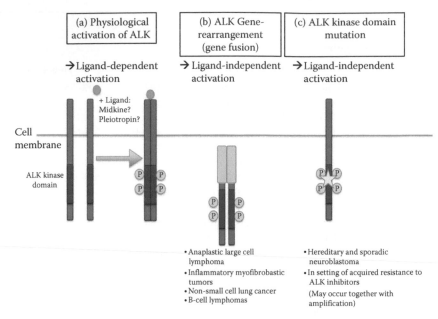

| (a) Physiological activation of ALK | (b) ALK Gene-rearrangement (gene fusion) | (c) ALK kinase domain mutation |

→ Ligand-dependent activation   → Ligand-independent activation   → Ligand-independent activation

+ Ligand: Midkine? Pleiotropin?

Cell membrane

ALK kinase domain

• Anaplastic large cell lymphoma
• Inflammatory myofibrobastic tumors
• Non-small cell lung cancer
• B-cell lymphomas

• Hereditary and sporadic neuroblastoma
• In setting of acquired resistance to ALK inhibitors
(May occur together with amplification)

FIGURE 8.1 Physiological and common mechanism of ALK dysregulation in human cancers. (a) Physiological activation of ALK occurs through binding of membrane-bound ALK with its putative ligands midkine or pleiotropin, which results in homodimerization and activation of the ALK kinase by transautophosphorylation. (b) ALK gene rearrangements result in a fusion protein that is aberrantly expressed and subject to ligand-independent dimerization and constitutive activation of the ALK. (c) Mutations in the ALK kinase domain result in constitutive activation of the ALK kinase activity. ALK gene copy number changes have been reported, but the pathological significance of these remains uncertain. See text for details. (Modified from La Madrid, A.M. et al., *Target. Oncol.* 7, 199, 2012.)

by positive immunostaining) is associated with a favorable prognosis, with a 5 year survival of 79.8% for *ALK*-positive disease, compared with 32.9% for *ALK*-negative disease [23].

Non-Small Cell Lung Cancer

ALK rearrangements are present in up to 3%–5% of NSCLC [7]. The most common 5′ partner is *EML4* as previously described [2]; rarer fusion partners include *KIF5B* [24], *TFG* [3], and *KLC1* [25,26]. *ALK*-rearranged tumors are typically adenocarcinomas and have been associated with characteristic morphological features, such as mucinous cribriform or solid signet-ring histology [27,28], and commonly express both thyroid transcription factor-1 (TTF1) and p63. In general, *ALK* rearrangements typically occur independently of *EGFR* or *KRAS* mutations [29–32] although uncommon exceptions to this rule have been reported.

ALK rearrangements in NSCLC can be detected by several methods including fluorescence *in situ* hybridization (FISH), reverse transcriptase polymerase chain reaction (RT PCR), or immunohistochemistry, each with advantages and limitations [33,34]. FISH was used to identify patients in clinical trials with crizotinib and was recently approved as a companion diagnostic by the US Food and Drug Administration (FDA) and in many respects represents the gold standard for the detection of *ALK* rearrangements. The FISH assay involves labeling of the 5' and 3' ends of the ALK gene with fluorescent probes, with rearrangements resulting in a break-apart appearance, regardless of the ALK fusion partner or the *EML4-ALK* variant [33]. A high sensitivity and specificity is seen when cutoffs of >15% of cells and >/4 fields are examined [35,36]. RT PCR is specific and can define both the fusion partner and the variant and can be applied to limited tissue samples; however, the variants or fusion partners that can be detected are limited by the available primers [7,33]. Finally, immunohistochemistry is a readily available technique, which may offer a sensitivity comparable to FISH but may have limited specificity [36]. Ultimately, the technique utilized in each clinical situation will be dependent on available resources and expertise, as well as the suitability of tissue.

In terms of clinical features, *ALK* rearrangement-positive NSCLC is associated with a younger age of onset, with one study demonstrating a median age of 54 years compared with 64 in the *ALK*-negative population [37]. Patients with *ALK* rearrangements are more likely to be light or never-smokers and have adenocarcinoma histology [4,38–40], highlighting the overlapping clinical and pathologic features with other NSCLC subtypes, such as those harboring an EGFR mutation. There are exceptions to this stereotypical phenotype; in particular, *EML4-ALK* has been detected in smokers in some studies [41] and in rare patients with squamous cell carcinoma.

The prognostic implications of *ALK* rearrangement in NSCLC have been explored retrospectively. In early stage disease, post-resection studies have provided conflicting reports of improved and worsened survival in ALK-positive patients [26,29,42]. In the advanced disease setting, ALK positivity seems to be associated with an improved prognosis particularly in the context of treatment with ALK inhibitors [43]. Some studies have demonstrated improved response rates and progression-free survival than that seen in wild-type patients with pemetrexed treatment [44], although more modest results have been seen in other series [45]. Perhaps more clear is the poor response of ALK-positive patients to EGFR tyrosine kinase inhibitor therapy [38,46,47].

INFLAMMATORY MYOFIBROBLASTIC TUMORS

IMTs are rare soft tissue tumors that predominantly affect children and young adults and most frequently arise in the lung, abdomen, and retroperitoneum [48]. *ALK* rearrangements in IMTs were first described in 1999 and are thought to occur in approximately 50% of IMTs [5], with some studies indicating that this occurs more frequently in children and young adults than in older patients. In IMTs, several chromosomal rearrangements that result in a fusion protein have been identified including the fusion of *ALK* with *TPM3, TPM4, CLTC, ATIC, CARS, RANB2, SEC31l1,* and *PPFIBP1* [49–52]. In IMTs, ALK positivity has been demonstrated with conventional immunohistochemistry techniques. However, more sensitive methods such as immunohistochemistry with an intercalated antibody-enhanced polymer method [53] and FISH [54] are emerging as important techniques.

There are conflicting studies regarding the prognostic significance of ALK expression in IMTs. Diffuse cytoplasmic expression of ALK has been correlated with a younger age and increased risk of local recurrence rather than distant failure [55]. Although ALK-positive IMTs have been correlated with a favorable outcome [56] more recently, nuclear membrane and perinuclear staining of ALK associated with an epithelioid morphology has been correlated with a more aggressive phenotype of IMTs, with large intra-abdominal tumors associated with potentially fatal rapid local recurrence [57].

NEUROBLASTOMA

Neuroblastoma, an embryonal tumor of the autonomic nervous system, is the most common malignancy diagnosed within the 1st year of age and is a leading cause of childhood cancer death [58]. In contrast to the gene rearrangements described in ALCL, NSCLC, and IMTs, oncogenic activation of *ALK* in neuroblastoma is predominantly through germ line or sporadic mutations of the tyrosine kinase domain of *ALK*. In pedigrees of families with high rates of neuroblastoma, mutations of *ALK* have been identified in almost all (>90%) pedigrees, with the most frequent germ line mutation being the R1275 mutation, which occurs in up to 50% of all tumors with an *ALK* mutation [6]. Common sporadic mutations include R1275, F1174, F1245, and K1062M [59–61]. Through systematic re-sequencing of 1600 cases of sporadic neuroblastoma, it was demonstrated that *ALK* is mutated in 8% of tumor samples [62]. Of note, the mutations in *ALK* have varying transforming ability, with each mutant affecting downstream signaling differently and subtle structural differences resulting in different sensitivities to ALK inhibitors [63,64]. Another infrequently observed abnormality of *ALK* in neuroblastoma is that of amplification, the clinical relevance of which is yet to be determined [65].

OTHER TUMORS

Oncogenic abnormalities in *ALK* have been reported in small numbers in other tumor types. The *EML4-ALK* fusion gene has been detected in rare cases of breast and colorectal cancers [66]. In addition to ALCL, a T cell neoplasm, a number of pathogenic fusion genes have been identified in ALK-positive diffuse large B cell lymphoma, including *NPM-ALK* [67], *CLTC-ALK* [68], *SEC31a-ALK* [69], and *SQSTM1-ALK* [70]. More novel ALK fusion genes include *VCL-ALK* in renal medullary carcinoma [71] and *C2orff44-ALK* in colorectal cancer [72]. Analogous to those seen in neuroblastoma, missense mutations have been reported in anaplastic thyroid cancer [73]. *ALK* gene amplification has been observed in inflammatory breast cancer [74], as well as in rhabdomyosarcoma, where frequent copy number gain of *ALK* is associated with an increased level of ALK protein and clinically associated with poor survival and the occurrence of metastases [75].

ALK INHIBITORS

Treatment of preclinical models of *ALK*-rearranged ALCL and NSCLC with ALK inhibitors resulted in growth inhibition and apoptosis *in vitro* and reduction in tumor size *in vivo* [2,18,33,74,76,77]. The most studied tyrosine kinase inhibitor of ALK is crizotinib; however, novel, more potent inhibitors are in varying stages of preclinical and clinical development, as summarized in Table 8.2.

CRIZOTINIB

Crizotinib (PF 02341066, Pfizer) was originally developed as an oral small-molecule tyrosine kinase inhibitor of mesenchymal–epithelial transition growth factor (c-MET) [78] but is also an inhibitor of ALK and ROS1 [79]. Preclinically, crizotinib has been shown to inhibit ALK phosphorylation and signal transduction, resulting in G1–S-phase cell-cycle arrest and apoptosis through induction of BIM, in cell lines of *NPM-ALK*-positive ALCL [77], as well as *EML4-ALK*-positive NSCLC [76].

In 2007, coincident with the identification of *EML4-ALK* in NSCLC, a phase 1 trial of crizotinib was underway to investigate the safety, pharmacokinetics, and antitumor activity of this agent with a plan to explore activity in patients with MET amplification [4]. Two patients with *EML4-ALK*-positive NSCLC were treated with crizotinib during the dose escalation, with an excellent symptomatic improvement, leading to an expanded molecular cohort of patients with *EML4-ALK*-positive NSCLC being treated with the MTD of 250 mg BD. This enriched NSCLC cohort included 149 patients, 143 of whom were evaluable for response in a recent update [80].

TABLE 8.2
ALK Tyrosine Kinase Inhibitors in Development

Drug	Manufacturer	Stage of Investigation	Activity against ALK Kinase Domain Mutations
Crizotinib (PF02341066)	Pfizer	Phases II and III for NSCLC, Phases I and II for other tumor types	
LDK378	Novartis	Phase 1 trial	
CH5424802	Chugai Pharmaceuticals	Phase 1 trial	L1196M, C1156Y, and F1174L secondary mutations
AP-26113	Ariad Pharmaceuticals	Phase 1 trial	L1196M, S1206R, and G1269S mutations
X-276/396	Xcovery	Phase 1 trial	L1196M ALK secondary mutations
ASP3026	Astellas	Phase 1 trial	
CEP-37440	Cephalon	Preclinical	
NMS-E628	Nerviano medical	Preclinical	
TAE684	Novartis	Not a clinical candidate	L1196M and F1174L ALK secondary mutations

The objective response rate was 60.8%, which essentially was independent of age, sex, performance status, or line of therapy. The overall survival data are not yet mature; however, the median progression-free survival was 9.7 months and estimated overall survival at 12 months was 74.8%.

The subsequent single-arm Phase II study of crizotinib (PROFILE 1005) also demonstrated an objective response rate of 53% in the first 439 evaluable patients [81]. Of note, the patient-reported outcome data demonstrated significant improvements in pain, dyspnea, cough, and fatigue after 6 weeks of therapy [82]. On the basis of these promising phase I and phase II trial results, in August 2011, the FDA granted accelerated approval of crizotinib and a companion diagnostic FISH test, for the use in patients with ALK-positive lung cancer. This approval is conditional on the results of the two Phase III studies that are currently being conducted, which compare crizotinib with standard chemotherapy, that is, PROFILE 1014 (a first-line study comparing crizotinib with platinum/pemetrexed doublet, NCT 01154140) and PROFILE 1007 (second-line and beyond study comparing crizotinib with either docetaxel or pemetrexed, NCT00932893). The preliminary results from the first 347 patients treated on PROFILE 1007 were recently presented [83]. Crizotinib had a superior progression-free survival when compared with docetaxel or pemetrexed chemotherapy (median 7.7 versus 3.0 months, HR 0.49, $p < 0.0001$) and also a significantly improved overall response rate of 65% versus 20%. Both PROFILE 1007 and PROFILE 1014 have a primary end point of progression-free survival, as crossover to crizotinib after progression on chemotherapy is possible, making it difficult to formally assess the impact of crizotinib on overall survival.

Crizotinib is generally well tolerated, and the common toxicities observed in the Phase 1 study are listed in Table 8.3, the most frequent being visual changes, nausea and vomiting, diarrhea, and peripheral edema [80]. Of note, the visual changes usually occur during light adaptation and are characterized by light trails, flashes, or persistence of images at the edge of the visual field. Uncommon but major or severe adverse events include transaminitis, neutropenia, and pneumonitis [80]. Other unusual and less common toxicities include renal cysts, asymptomatic bradycardia [80], and hypogonadism [84].

Beyond its use in ALK-positive NSCLC, there is emerging evidence for the activity of crizotinib in other ALK-driven tumors. The aforementioned Phase 1 trial included two patients with IMTs [85], one of whom carried the *ALK-RANBP2* rearrangement and had an initial 53% reduction in disease burden and, following resection of new lesions, had a complete remission for 25 months. The ALK-negative patient in that study did not achieve a response.

More recently, the Children's Oncology Group Consortium reported initial results of a Phase I dose escalation trial and pharmacokinetic trial in children with solid tumors or ALCL [86]. In this study, seven out of eight (88%) of the children with ALCL achieved a complete response. Furthermore, two patients with neuroblastoma have had a complete response, and one patient with an IMT has had a partial response. Thus, there is emerging evidence that crizotinib can be effectively used in a range of ALK-driven tumors, beyond the subset of NSCLC patients with ALK gene rearrangements.

TABLE 8.3
Common Adverse Events Attributed to Crizotinib

Common Treatment-Related Adverse Events	Proportion of Patients with All Grades (%)	Proportion of Patient with Grade 3 or 4 (%)
Any adverse event	96.6	24.2
Vision disorder	64.4	0
Nausea	56.4	0.7
Diarrhea	49.7	0
Vomiting	38.9	0.7
Peripheral edema	29.5	0
Constipation	27.5	0.7
Decreased appetite	16.1	0
Fatigue	16.1	1.3
ALT increased	12.1	4.0
Rash	11.4	0
Dysgeusia	10.7	0
AST increased	10.1	3.4

Source: Camidge, D.R. et al., *Lancet Oncol.*, 13, 1011, 2012.

MECHANISMS OF RESISTANCE TO CRIZOTINIB AND OTHER ALK INHIBITORS

As has been seen with other targeted therapies, the utility of crizotinib in ALK-positive cancer is limited by the development of acquired resistance. Despite dramatic initial responses to crizotinib, disease progression develops after a median progression-free survival of approximately 10 months. Although data are available from relatively small series, several mechanisms underlying such resistance have emerged including multiple mechanisms that may occur simultaneously in the same patient. Thus far, the major mechanisms of resistance appear to include genetic alteration of *ALK* itself (through secondary mutations or copy number gain) and activation of other oncogenic kinases that restore downstream signaling pathways [33,87,88].

Mutations of the kinase domain of *ALK* represent one mechanism of acquired resistance. Indeed, the initial publication of the Phase I trial of crizotinib [4] was accompanied by details of a case report of an NSCLC patient demonstrating acquired resistance to crizotinib with two separate mutations of the kinase domain, L1196M and C1156Y [89]. Analogous to the T790M mutation in *EGFR*-mutant NSCLC [90] or the T315I substitution in *BCR-ABL*, the aforementioned L1196M is a gatekeeper mutation in the *ALK* kinase domain, which interferes with affinity to crizotinib. However, unlike *EGFR*-mutant NSCLC where T790M is the predominant secondary mutation, a number of other mutations have also been described including L1152R, G1269A, S1206Y, G1202R, and 1151Tins [87,88,91]. In a patient with a *RANBP2-ALK*-positive IMT [92], an F1174L mutation was described (which interestingly is also a frequent mutation identified in neuroblastoma). These mutations have been discovered both through modeling of resistance in cell lines *in vitro* [93] and in studies of patients who were biopsied after progression while being treated with crizotinib [87,88], with the rate of mutations of the kinase domain in these biopsy studies ranging from 22% to 36%. Another demonstrated mechanism of crizotinib resistance is gene amplification, which was seen in 1 of 18 [87] and 2 of 14 [88] patients biopsied at progression while being treated with crizotinib. Preclinical data thus far show that the identified mutations vary in their sensitivity to both crizotinib and novel ALK inhibitors [87,94,95]. This variable response, combined with the intra- and interpatient heterogeneity of mutations detected, poses a significant challenge when considering the development of second-line agents to be used in the setting of crizotinib resistance.

Activations of alternate oncogenic signaling pathways may also be a cause of resistance. For example, a recent study [91] demonstrated that activation of the EGFR signaling pathway can contribute to ALK inhibitor resistance. In one of the previously described biopsy studies [88], 3 of 11 patients had either an *EGFR* or *KRAS* mutation following treatment with crizotinib. Amplification of *KIT* may also have a role, having been demonstrated in 2 of 18 patients post crizotinib [87]. In light of this, combination treatment may prove to be a legitimate therapeutic approach to the treatment of crizotinib-resistant patients, as is being explored in an ongoing Phase I trial of crizotinib and PF 299804, an irreversible HER2 inhibitor (NCT01121575).

Finally, one clinical pattern of resistance for patients on crizotinib is that of progression within the CNS [96]. This CNS progression may in part be due to relative underexposure of the drug in cerebrospinal fluid (CSF). While there is limited evidence regarding this, in one patient where CSF and serum levels of crizotinib were measured [97], the CSF levels were <0.3% of those in the blood. Thus, resection or radiotherapy to areas of progression within the CNS, particularly in the context of stable extracranial disease, may be an appropriate strategy. Further studies are required with regard to formulation of novel agents or approaches that result in ALK inhibitors effectively crossing the blood–brain barrier, which may reduce the rates of CNS progression.

OTHER ALK INHIBITORS

Unlike crizotinib, which was originally developed as an inhibitor of c-MET, LDK378 is a potent inhibitor of ALK that does not inhibit c-MET. Preclinical models have been used to confirm the activity of LDK378 in ALK-positive tumor models, including those that demonstrate crizotinib resistance [98], suggesting that LDK378 might be used in both crizotinib-naive and crizotinib-resistant patients. A first-in-man Phase 1 trial of LDK378 is currently under way, and in a preliminary report, a response rate of 81% (21/26) was seen in ALK-positive crizotinib-refractory NSCLC patients treated at ≥400 mg [99]. The most frequent adverse events were nausea, vomiting, and diarrhea. The study is still ongoing in dose escalation, but early results suggest that this may be a promising ALK inhibitor for both previously treated and crizotinib-naive patients.

Recently, another first-in-man Phase 1 trial of a novel ALK inhibitor, CH5424802, was reported [100]. Thus far, a total of 24 crizotinib-naive patients have been treated, with all patients, at all dose levels, demonstrating tumor regression. The main toxicity observed was myalgia, with hypophosphatemia, hypermagnesemia, neutropenia, and increased blood CPK being rarer toxicities. This study is also ongoing, with a Phase II component being planned. There are a number of other potential ALK inhibitors under investigation, as detailed in Table 8.2.

Hsp90 Inhibitors: Another Approach of Targeting ALK

Heat shock protein 90 (Hsp90) inhibitors are another class of agents that may have activity in ALK-positive tumors. ALK fusion proteins serve as client proteins for the chaperone protein Hsp90 in preclinical models [93,101]. Hsp90 inhibitors have been shown to reduce the levels of ALK protein and have antitumor activity in ALK-driven preclinical models. Two Hsp90 inhibitors, retaspimycin (IPI-504) [102] and ganetespib (STA-9090) [103], have been shown in early phase clinical trials to have efficacy in ALK-positive NSCLC patients, who were predominantly crizotinib naive. Further studies are required to determine if this class of agents may be useful in patients who have acquired resistance to crizotinib and whether they should be administered alone or potentially in combination with ALK inhibitors.

FUTURE CHALLENGES

The emergence of ALK as a new therapeutic target in NSCLC and beyond has been one of the success stories of modern oncology. Particularly spectacular has been the short timeline from the identification of *ALK* gene rearrangements in NSCLC (2007) to FDA approval of crizotinib for this indication (2011). However, there are a number of challenges that scientists, clinicians, and patients alike will face in the years to come. Understanding the optimal methods for testing and the most cost-effective screening strategies to identify patients with ALK-driven tumors represent initial challenges. Elucidating mechanisms of acquired resistance to ALK inhibitors and developing therapeutic strategies that may overcome these will be paramount to achieving long-term disease control in patients harboring ALK-driven malignancies.

REFERENCES

1. Morris SW, Kirstein MN, Valentine MB, Dittmer KG, Shapiro DN, Saltman DL et al. Fusion of a kinase gene, ALK, to a nucleolar protein gene, NPM, in non-Hodgkin's lymphoma. *Science*. 1994;263(5151):1281–1284. Epub 1994/03/04.
2. Soda M, Choi YL, Enomoto M, Takada S, Yamashita Y, Ishikawa S et al. Identification of the transforming EML4-ALK fusion gene in non-small-cell lung cancer. *Nature*. 2007;448(7153):561–566. Epub 2007/07/13.
3. Rikova K, Guo A, Zeng Q, Possemato A, Yu J, Haack H et al. Global survey of phosphotyrosine signaling identifies oncogenic kinases in lung cancer. *Cell*. 2007;131(6):1190–1203. Epub 2007/12/18.
4. Kwak EL, Bang YJ, Camidge DR, Shaw AT, Solomon B, Maki RG et al. Anaplastic lymphoma kinase inhibition in non-small-cell lung cancer. *The New England Journal of Medicine*. 2010;363(18):1693–1703. Epub 2010/10/29.

5. Griffin CA, Hawkins AL, Dvorak C, Henkle C, Ellingham T, Perlman EJ. Recurrent involvement of 2p23 in inflammatory myofibroblastic tumors. *Cancer Research*. 1999;59(12):2776–2780. Epub 1999/06/26.

6. Mosse YP, Laudenslager M, Longo L, Cole KA, Wood A, Attiyeh EF et al. Identification of ALK as a major familial neuroblastoma predisposition gene. *Nature*. 2008;455(7215):930–935. Epub 2008/08/30.

7. Mano H. ALKoma: A cancer subtype with a shared target. *Cancer Discovery*. 2012;2(6):495–502. Epub 2012/05/23.

8. Iwahara T, Fujimoto J, Wen D, Cupples R, Bucay N, Arakawa T et al. Molecular characterization of ALK, a receptor tyrosine kinase expressed specifically in the nervous system. *Oncogene*. 1997;14(4):439–449. Epub 1997/01/30.

9. Morris SW, Naeve C, Mathew P, James PL, Kirstein MN, Cui X et al. ALK, the chromosome 2 gene locus altered by the t(2;5) in non-Hodgkin's lymphoma, encodes a novel neural receptor tyrosine kinase that is highly related to leukocyte tyrosine kinase (LTK). *Oncogene*. 1997;14(18):2175–2188. Epub 1997/05/08.

10. Lee HH, Norris A, Weiss JB, Frasch M. Jelly belly protein activates the receptor tyrosine kinase Alk to specify visceral muscle pioneers. *Nature*. 2003;425(6957):507–512. Epub 2003/10/03.

11. Schonherr C, Hallberg B, Palmer R. Anaplastic lymphoma kinase in human cancer. *Critical Reviews in Oncogenesis*. 2012;17(2):123–143. Epub 2012/04/05.

12. Vernersson E, Khoo NK, Henriksson ML, Roos G, Palmer RH, Hallberg B. Characterization of the expression of the ALK receptor tyrosine kinase in mice. *Gene Expression Patterns*. 2006;6(5):448–461. Epub 2006/02/07.

13. Lasek AW, Lim J, Kliethermes CL, Berger KH, Joslyn G, Brush G et al. An evolutionary conserved role for anaplastic lymphoma kinase in behavioral responses to ethanol. *PLoS One*. 2011;6(7):e22636. Epub 2011/07/30.

14. Pulford K, Lamant L, Morris SW, Butler LH, Wood KM, Stroud D et al. Detection of anaplastic lymphoma kinase (ALK) and nucleolar protein nucleophosmin (NPM)-ALK proteins in normal and neoplastic cells with the monoclonal antibody ALK1. *Blood*. 1997;89(4):1394–1404. Epub 1997/02/15.

15. Shaw AT, Solomon B. Targeting anaplastic lymphoma kinase in lung cancer. *Clinical Cancer Research*. 2011;17(8):2081–2086. Epub 2011/02/04.

16. Shiota M, Fujimoto J, Semba T, Satoh H, Yamamoto T, Mori S. Hyperphosphorylation of a novel 80 kDa protein-tyrosine kinase similar to Ltk in a human Ki-1 lymphoma cell line, AMS3. *Oncogene*. 1994;9(6):1567–1574. Epub 1994/06/01.

17. Drexler HG, Gignac SM, von Wasielewski R, Werner M, Dirks WG. Pathobiology of NPM-ALK and variant fusion genes in anaplastic large cell lymphoma and other lymphomas. *Leukemia*. 2000;14(9):1533–1559. Epub 2000/09/20.

18. Soda M, Takada S, Takeuchi K, Choi YL, Enomoto M, Ueno T et al. A mouse model for EML4-ALK-positive lung cancer. *Proceedings of the National Academy of Sciences of the United States of America*. 2008;105(50):19893–19897. Epub 2008/12/10.

19. Chen Z, Sasaki T, Tan X, Carretero J, Shimamura T, Li D et al. Inhibition of ALK, PI3K/MEK, and HSP90 in murine lung adenocarcinoma induced by EML4-ALK fusion oncogene. *Cancer Research*. 2010;70(23):9827–9836. Epub 2010/10/19.

20. Pulford K, Lamant L, Espinos E, Jiang Q, Xue L, Turturro F et al. The emerging normal and disease-related roles of anaplastic lymphoma kinase. *Cellular and Molecular Life Sciences*. 2004;61(23):2939–2953. Epub 2004/12/08.

21. Passoni L, Gambacorti-Passerini C. ALK a novel lymphoma-associated tumor antigen for vaccination strategies. *Leukemia & Lymphoma*. 2003;44(10):1675–1681. Epub 2003/12/25.

22. Falini B, Pileri S, Zinzani PL, Carbone A, Zagonel V, Wolf-Peeters C et al. ALK + lymphoma: Clinico-pathological findings and outcome. *Blood*. 1999;93(8):2697–2706. Epub 1999/04/09.

23. Shiota M, Nakamura S, Ichinohasama R, Abe M, Akagi T, Takeshita M et al. Anaplastic large cell lymphomas expressing the novel chimeric protein p80NPM/ALK: A distinct clinicopathologic entity. *Blood*. 1995;86(5):1954–1960. Epub 1995/09/01.

24. Takeuchi K, Choi YL, Togashi Y, Soda M, Hatano S, Inamura K et al. KIF5B-ALK, a novel fusion oncokinase identified by an immunohistochemistry-based diagnostic system for ALK-positive lung cancer. *Clinical Cancer Research: An Official Journal of the American Association for Cancer Research*. 2009;15(9):3143–3149. Epub 2009/04/23.

25. Togashi Y, Soda M, Sakata S, Sugawara E, Hatano S, Asaka R et al. KLC1-ALK: A novel fusion in lung cancer identified using a formalin-fixed paraffin-embedded tissue only. *PLoS One*. 2012;7(2):e31323. Epub 2012/02/22.

26. Solomon B, Shaw AT. Are anaplastic lymphoma kinase gene rearrangements in non-small cell lung cancer prognostic, predictive, or both? *Journal of Thoracic Oncology*. 2012;7(1):5–7. Epub 2011/12/17.

27. Rodig SJ, Mino-Kenudson M, Dacic S, Yeap BY, Shaw A, Barletta JA et al. Unique clinicopathologic features characterize ALK-rearranged lung adenocarcinoma in the western population. *Clinical Cancer Research: An Official Journal of the American Association for Cancer Research*. 2009;15(16):5216–5223. Epub 2009/08/13.

28. Yoshida A, Tsuta K, Watanabe S, Sekine I, Fukayama M, Tsuda H et al. Frequent ALK rearrangement and TTF-1/p63 co-expression in lung adenocarcinoma with signet-ring cell component. *Lung Cancer*. 2011;72(3):309–315. Epub 2010/11/03.

29. Zhang X, Zhang S, Yang X, Yang J, Zhou Q, Yin L et al. Fusion of EML4 and ALK is associated with development of lung adenocarcinomas lacking EGFR and KRAS mutations and is correlated with ALK expression. *Molecular Cancer*. 2010;9:188. Epub 2010/07/14.

30. Inamura K, Takeuchi K, Togashi Y, Hatano S, Ninomiya H, Motoi N et al. EML4-ALK lung cancers are characterized by rare other mutations, a TTF-1 cell lineage, an acinar histology, and young onset. *Modern Pathology: An Official Journal of the United States and Canadian Academy of Pathology, Inc.* 2009;22(4):508–515. Epub 2009/02/24.

31. Boland JM, Erdogan S, Vasmatzis G, Yang P, Tillmans LS, Johnson MR et al. Anaplastic lymphoma kinase immunoreactivity correlates with ALK gene rearrangement and transcriptional up-regulation in non-small cell lung carcinomas. *Human Pathology*. 2009;40(8):1152–1158. Epub 2009/04/24.

32. Takahashi T, Sonobe M, Kobayashi M, Yoshizawa A, Menju T, Nakayama E et al. Clinicopathologic features of non-small-cell lung cancer with EML4-ALK fusion gene. *Annals of Surgical Oncology*. 2010;17(3):889–897. Epub 2010/02/26.

33. Sasaki T, Janne PA. New strategies for treatment of ALK-rearranged non-small cell lung cancers. *Clinical Cancer Research*. 2011;17(23):7213–7218. Epub 2011/10/20.

34. Shaw AT, Solomon B, Kenudson MM. Crizotinib and testing for ALK. *Journal of the National Comprehensive Cancer Network*. 2011;9(12):1335–1341. Epub 2011/12/14.

35. Camidge DR, Kono SA, Flacco A, Tan AC, Doebele RC, Zhou Q et al. Optimizing the detection of lung cancer patients harboring anaplastic lymphoma kinase (ALK) gene rearrangements potentially suitable for ALK inhibitor treatment. *Clinical Cancer Research: An Official Journal of the American Association for Cancer Research*. 2010;16(22):5581–5590. Epub 2010/11/11.

36. Mino-Kenudson M, Chirieac LR, Law K, Hornick JL, Lindeman N, Mark EJ et al. A novel, highly sensitive antibody allows for the routine detection of ALK-rearranged lung adenocarcinomas by standard immunohistochemistry. *Clinical Cancer Research: An Official Journal of the American Association for Cancer Research*. 2010;16(5):1561–1571. Epub 2010/02/25.

37. Shaw AT, Yeap B, Costa DB, Solomon BJ, Kwak EL, Nguyen AT et al. Prognostic versus predictive value of EML4-ALK translocation in metastatic non-small cell lung cancer. *ASCO Meeting Abstracts*. 2010;28(15_suppl):7606.

38. Shaw AT, Yeap BY, Mino-Kenudson M, Digumarthy SR, Costa DB, Heist RS et al. Clinical features and outcome of patients with non-small-cell lung cancer who harbor EML4-ALK. *Journal of Clinical Oncology*. 2009;27(26):4247–4253. Epub 2009/08/12.

39. Wong DW, Leung EL, So KK, Tam IY, Sihoe AD, Cheng LC et al. The EML4-ALK fusion gene is involved in various histologic types of lung cancers from nonsmokers with wild-type EGFR and KRAS. *Cancer*. 2009;115(8):1723–1733. Epub 2009/01/27.

40. Paik JH, Choe G, Kim H, Choe JY, Lee HJ, Lee CT et al. Screening of anaplastic lymphoma kinase rearrangement by immunohistochemistry in non-small cell lung cancer: Correlation with fluorescence in situ hybridization. *Journal of Thoracic Oncology*. 2011;6(3):466–472. Epub 2011/01/25.

41. Shinmura K, Kageyama S, Tao H, Bunai T, Suzuki M, Kamo T et al. EML4-ALK fusion transcripts, but no NPM-, TPM3-, CLTC-, ATIC-, or TFG-ALK fusion transcripts, in non-small cell lung carcinomas. *Lung Cancer*. 2008;61(2):163–169. Epub 2008/02/05.

42. Yang P, Kulig K, Boland JM, Erickson-Johnson MR, Oliveira AM, Wampfler J et al. Worse disease-free survival in never-smokers with ALK + lung adenocarcinoma. *Journal of Thoracic Oncology*. 2012;7(1):90–97. Epub 2011/12/03.

43. Shaw AT, Yeap BY, Solomon BJ, Riely GJ, Gainor J, Engelman JA et al. Effect of crizotinib on overall survival in patients with advanced non-small-cell lung cancer harbouring ALK gene rearrangement: A retrospective analysis. *The Lancet Oncology*. 2011;12(11):1004–1012. Epub 2011/09/22.

44. Camidge DR, Kono SA, Lu X, Okuyama S, Baron AE, Oton AB et al. Anaplastic lymphoma kinase gene rearrangements in non-small cell lung cancer are associated with prolonged progression-free survival on pemetrexed. *Journal of Thoracic Oncology*. 2011;6(4):774–780. Epub 2011/02/22.

45. Shaw AT, Varghese AM, Solomon BJ, Costa DB, Novello S, Mino-Kenudson M et al. Pemetrexed-based chemotherapy in patients with advanced, ALK-positive non-small cell lung cancer. *Annals of Oncology*. 2012;24:59–66. Epub 2012/08/14.

46. Lee JK, Park HS, Kim DW, Kulig K, Kim TM, Lee SH et al. Comparative analyses of overall survival in patients with anaplastic lymphoma kinase-positive and matched wild-type advanced nonsmall cell lung cancer. *Cancer*. 2012;118(14):3579–3586. Epub 2011/11/17.

47. Kim HR, Shim HS, Chung JH, Lee YJ, Hong YK, Rha SY et al. Distinct clinical features and outcomes in never-smokers with nonsmall cell lung cancer who harbor EGFR or KRAS mutations or ALK rearrangement. *Cancer*. 2012;118(3):729–739. Epub 2011/07/02.

48. Tothova Z, Wagner AJ. Anaplastic lymphoma kinase-directed therapy in inflammatory myofibroblastic tumors. *Current Opinion in Oncology*. 2012;24(4):409–413. Epub 2012/06/06.

49. Lawrence B, Perez-Atayde A, Hibbard MK, Rubin BP, Dal Cin P, Pinkus JL et al. TPM3-ALK and TPM4-ALK oncogenes in inflammatory myofibroblastic tumors. *The American Journal of Pathology*. 2000;157(2):377–384. Epub 2000/08/10.

50. Bridge JA, Kanamori M, Ma Z, Pickering D, Hill DA, Lydiatt W et al. Fusion of the ALK gene to the clathrin heavy chain gene, CLTC, in inflammatory myofibroblastic tumor. *The American Journal of Pathology*. 2001;159(2):411–415. Epub 2001/08/04.

51. Panagopoulos I, Nilsson T, Domanski HA, Isaksson M, Lindblom P, Mertens F et al. Fusion of the SEC31L1 and ALK genes in an inflammatory myofibroblastic tumor. *International Journal of Cancer*. 2006;118(5):1181–1186. Epub 2005/09/15.

52. Ma Z, Hill DA, Collins MH, Morris SW, Sumegi J, Zhou M et al. Fusion of ALK to the Ran-binding protein 2 (RANBP2) gene in inflammatory myofibroblastic tumor. *Genes Chromosomes Cancer*. 2003;37(1):98–105. Epub 2003/03/28.

53. Takeuchi K, Soda M, Togashi Y, Sugawara E, Hatano S, Asaka R et al. Pulmonary inflammatory myofibroblastic tumor expressing a novel fusion, PPFIBP1-ALK: Reappraisal of anti-ALK immunohistochemistry as a tool for novel ALK fusion identification. *Clinical Cancer Research.* 2011;17(10):3341–3348. Epub 2011/03/25.

54. Siminovich MH, Galluzzo Mutti ML, Lopez JM, Lubieniecki FJ, MT GdD. Inflammatory myofibroblastic tumor of the lung in children: Anaplastic lymphoma kinase (alk) expression and clinico-pathological correlation. *Pediatric and Developmental Pathology.* 2012. Epub 2012/01/28.

55. Coffin CM, Hornick JL, Fletcher CD. Inflammatory myofibroblastic tumor: Comparison of clinicopathologic, histologic, and immunohistochemical features including ALK expression in atypical and aggressive cases. *The American Journal of Surgical Pathology.* 2007;31(4):509–520. Epub 2007/04/07.

56. Chan JK, Cheuk W, Shimizu M. Anaplastic lymphoma kinase expression in inflammatory pseudotumors. *The American Journal of Surgical Pathology.* 2001;25(6):761–768. Epub 2001/06/08.

57. Marino-Enriquez A, Wang WL, Roy A, Lopez-Terrada D, Lazar AJ, Fletcher CD et al. Epithelioid inflammatory myofibroblastic sarcoma: An aggressive intra-abdominal variant of inflammatory myofibroblastic tumor with nuclear membrane or perinuclear ALK. *The American Journal of Surgical Pathology.* 2011;35(1):135–144. Epub 2010/12/18.

58. Carpenter EL, Mosse YP. Targeting ALK in neuroblastoma-preclinical and clinical advancements. *Nature Reviews. Clinical Oncology.* 2012;9(7):391–399. Epub 2012/05/16.

59. Chen Y, Takita J, Choi YL, Kato M, Ohira M, Sanada M et al. Oncogenic mutations of ALK kinase in neuroblastoma. *Nature.* 2008;455(7215):971–974. Epub 2008/10/17.

60. George RE, Sanda T, Hanna M, Frohling S, Luther W, 2nd, Zhang J et al. Activating mutations in ALK provide a therapeutic target in neuroblastoma. *Nature.* 2008;455(7215):975–978. Epub 2008/10/17.

61. Janoueix-Lerosey I, Lequin D, Brugieres L, Ribeiro A, de Pontual L, Combaret V et al. Somatic and germline activating mutations of the ALK kinase receptor in neuroblastoma. *Nature.* 2008;455(7215):967–970. Epub 2008/10/17.

62. Weiser D, Laudenslager M, Rappaport E, Carpenter E, Attiyeh EF, Diskin S et al. Stratification of patients with neuroblastoma for targeted ALK inhibitor therapy. *ASCO Meeting Abstracts.* 2011;29(15_suppl):9514.

63. Bresler SC, Wood AC, Haglund EA, Courtright J, Belcastro LT, Plegaria JS et al. Differential inhibitor sensitivity of anaplastic lymphoma kinase variants found in neuroblastoma. *Science Translational Medicine.* 2011;3(108):108ra14. Epub 2011/11/11.

64. Schonherr C, Ruuth K, Yamazaki Y, Eriksson T, Christensen J, Palmer RH et al. Activating ALK mutations found in neuroblastoma are inhibited by Crizotinib and NVP-TAE684. *The Biochemical Journal.* 2011;440(3):405–413. Epub 2011/08/16.

65. George RE, Attiyeh EF, Li S, Moreau LA, Neuberg D, Li C et al. Genome-wide analysis of neuroblastomas using high-density single nucleotide polymorphism arrays. *PLoS One.* 2007;2(2):e255. Epub 2007/03/01.

66. Lin E, Li L, Guan Y, Soriano R, Rivers CS, Mohan S et al. Exon array profiling detects EML4-ALK fusion in breast, colorectal, and non-small cell lung cancers. *Molecular Cancer Research.* 2009;7(9):1466–1476. Epub 2009/09/10.

67. Onciu M, Behm FG, Downing JR, Shurtleff SA, Raimondi SC, Ma Z et al. ALK-positive plasmablastic B-cell lymphoma with expression of the NPM-ALK fusion transcript: Report of 2 cases. *Blood.* 2003;102(7):2642–2644. Epub 2003/06/21.

68. Gascoyne RD, Lamant L, Martin-Subero JI, Lestou VS, Harris NL, Muller-Hermelink HK et al. ALK-positive diffuse large B-cell lymphoma is associated with Clathrin-ALK rearrangements: report of 6 cases. *Blood.* 2003;102(7):2568–2573. Epub 2003/05/24.

69. Van Roosbroeck K, Cools J, Dierickx D, Thomas J, Vandenberghe P, Stul M et al. ALK-positive large B-cell lymphomas with cryptic SEC31A-ALK and NPM1-ALK fusions. *Haematologica*. 2010;95(3):509–513. Epub 2010/03/09.

70. Takeuchi K, Soda M, Togashi Y, Ota Y, Sekiguchi Y, Hatano S et al. Identification of a novel fusion, SQSTM1-ALK, in ALK-positive large B-cell lymphoma. *Haematologica*. 2011;96(3):464–467. Epub 2010/12/08.

71. Debelenko LV, Raimondi SC, Daw N, Shivakumar BR, Huang D, Nelson M et al. Renal cell carcinoma with novel VCL-ALK fusion: New representative of ALK-associated tumor spectrum. *Modern Pathology: An Official Journal of the United States and Canadian Academy of Pathology, Inc.* 2011;24(3):430–442. Epub 2010/11/16.

72. Lipson D, Capelletti M, Yelensky R, Otto G, Parker A, Jarosz M et al. Identification of new ALK and RET gene fusions from colorectal and lung cancer biopsies. *Nature Medicine*. 2012;18(3):382–384. Epub 2012/02/14.

73. Murugan AK, Xing M. Anaplastic thyroid cancers harbor novel oncogenic mutations of the ALK gene. *Cancer Research*. 2011;71(13):4403–4411. Epub 2011/05/21.

74. Tuma RS. ALK gene amplified in most inflammatory breast cancers. *Journal of the National Cancer Institute*. 2012;104(2):87–88.

75. van Gaal JC, Flucke UE, Roeffen MH, de Bont ES, Sleijfer S, Mavinkurve-Groothuis AM et al. Anaplastic lymphoma kinase aberrations in rhabdomyosarcoma: Clinical and prognostic implications. *Journal of Clinical Oncology*. 2012;30(3):308–315. Epub 2011/12/21.

76. Tanizaki J, Okamoto I, Takezawa K, Sakai K, Azuma K, Kuwata K et al. Combined effect of ALK and MEK inhibitors in EML4-ALK-positive non-small-cell lung cancer cells. *British Journal of Cancer*. 2012;106(4):763–767. Epub 2012/01/14.

77. Christensen JG, Zou HY, Arango ME, Li Q, Lee JH, McDonnell SR et al. Cytoreductive antitumor activity of PF-2341066, a novel inhibitor of anaplastic lymphoma kinase and c-Met, in experimental models of anaplastic large-cell lymphoma. *Molecular Cancer Therapeutics*. 2007;6(12 Pt 1):3314–3322. Epub 2007/12/20.

78. Zou HY, Li Q, Lee JH, Arango ME, McDonnell SR, Yamazaki S et al. An orally available small-molecule inhibitor of c-Met, PF-2341066, exhibits cytoreductive antitumor efficacy through antiproliferative and antiangiogenic mechanisms. *Cancer Research*. 2007;67(9):4408–4417. Epub 2007/05/08.

79. Bergethon K, Shaw AT, Ignatius Ou SH, Katayama R, Lovly CM, McDonald NT et al. ROS1 rearrangements define a unique molecular class of lung cancers. *Journal of Clinical Oncology*. 2012;30(8):863–870. Epub 2012/01/05.

80. Camidge DR, Bang YJ, Kwak EL, Iafrate AJ, Varella-Garcia M, Fox SB et al. Activity and safety of crizotinib in patients with ALK-positive non-small-cell lung cancer: Updated results from a phase 1 study. *The Lancet Oncology*. 2012;13:1011–1019. Epub 2012/09/08.

81. Kim D-W, Ahn M-J, Shi Y, De Pas TM, Yang P-C, Riely GJ et al. Results of a global phase II study with crizotinib in advanced ALK-positive non-small cell lung cancer (NSCLC). *ASCO Meeting Abstracts*. 2012;30(15_suppl):7533.

82. Blackhall FH, Peterson JA, Wilner K, Hirsch V, Shaw AT, Dong-Wan K et al. PROFILE 1005: Preliminary patient-reported outcomes (PROS) from an ongoing phase 2 study of crizotinib (PF-02341066) in anaplastic lymphoma kinase (ALK)-positive advanced non-small cell lung cancer. *Journal of Thoracic Oncology*. 2011;6(suppl 6):S413–S414.

83. Shaw AT, Kim DW, Nakagawa K, Seto T, Crinò L, Ahn M et al. Phase III study of crizotinib vs pemetrexed or docetaxel chemotherapy in patients with advanced ALK-positive NSCLC (PROFILE 1007). *Annals of Oncology*. 2012;23(suppl 9):ixe211.

84. Weickhardt AJ, Rothman MS, Salian-Mehta S, Kiseljak-Vassiliades K, Oton AB, Doebele RC et al. Rapid-onset hypogonadism secondary to crizotinib use in men with metastatic nonsmall cell lung cancer. *Cancer*. 2012;118:5302–5309. Epub 2012/04/11.

85. Butrynski JE, D'Adamo DR, Hornick JL, Dal Cin P, Antonescu CR, Jhanwar SC et al. Crizotinib in ALK-rearranged inflammatory myofibroblastic tumor. *The New England Journal of Medicine*. 2010;363(18):1727–1733. Epub 2010/10/29.

86. Mosse YP, Balis FM, Lim MS, Laliberte J, Voss SD, Fox E et al. Efficacy of crizotinib in children with relapsed/refractory ALK-driven tumors including anaplastic large cell lymphoma and neuroblastoma: A Children's Oncology Group phase I consortium study. *ASCO Meeting Abstracts*. 2012;30(15_suppl):9500.

87. Katayama R, Shaw AT, Khan TM, Mino-Kenudson M, Solomon BJ, Halmos B et al. Mechanisms of acquired crizotinib resistance in ALK-rearranged lung cancers. *Science Translational Medicine*. 2012;4(120):120ra17. Epub 2012/01/27.

88. Doebele RC, Pilling AB, Aisner DL, Kutateladze TG, Le AT, Weickhardt AJ et al. Mechanisms of resistance to crizotinib in patients with alk gene rearranged non-small cell lung cancer. *Clinical Cancer Research: An Official Journal of the American Association for Cancer Research*. 2012;18(5):1472–1482. Epub 2012/01/12.

89. Choi YL, Soda M, Yamashita Y, Ueno T, Takashima J, Nakajima T et al. EML4-ALK mutations in lung cancer that confer resistance to ALK inhibitors. *The New England Journal of Medicine*. 2010;363(18):1734–1739. Epub 2010/10/29.

90. Pao W, Miller VA, Politi KA, Riely GJ, Somwar R, Zakowski MF et al. Acquired resistance of lung adenocarcinomas to gefitinib or erlotinib is associated with a second mutation in the EGFR kinase domain. *PLoS Medicine*. 2005;2(3):e73. Epub 2005/03/02.

91. Sasaki T, Koivunen J, Ogino A, Yanagita M, Nikiforow S, Zheng W et al. A novel ALK secondary mutation and EGFR signaling cause resistance to ALK kinase inhibitors. *Cancer Research*. 2011;71(18):6051–6060. Epub 2011/07/28.

92. Sasaki T, Okuda K, Zheng W, Butrynski J, Capelletti M, Wang L et al. The neuroblastoma associated F1174L ALK mutation causes resistance to an ALK kinase inhibitor in ALK-translocated cancers. *Cancer Research*. 2010;70(24):10038–10043. Epub 2010/10/30.

93. Katayama R, Khan TM, Benes C, Lifshits E, Ebi H, Rivera VM et al. Therapeutic strategies to overcome crizotinib resistance in non-small cell lung cancers harboring the fusion oncogene EML4-ALK. *Proceedings of the National Academy of Sciences of the United States of America*. 2011;108(18):7535–7540. Epub 2011/04/20.

94. Zhang S, Wang F, Keats J, Zhu X, Ning Y, Wardwell SD et al. Crizotinib-resistant mutants of EML4-ALK identified through an accelerated mutagenesis screen. *Chemical Biology & Drug Design*. 2011;78(6):999–1005. Epub 2011/11/01.

95. Heuckmann JM, Holzel M, Sos ML, Heynck S, Balke-Want H, Koker M et al. ALK mutations conferring differential resistance to structurally diverse ALK inhibitors. *Clinical Cancer Research*. 2011;17(23):7394–7401. Epub 2011/09/29.

96. Camidge DR, Doebele RC. Treating ALK-positive lung cancer—Early successes and future challenges. *Nature Reviews Clinical Oncology*. 2012;9(5):268–277. Epub 2012/04/05.

97. Costa DB, Kobayashi S, Pandya SS, Yeo WL, Shen Z, Tan W et al. CSF concentration of the anaplastic lymphoma kinase inhibitor crizotinib. *Journal of Clinical Oncology*. 2011;29(15):e443–e445. Epub 2011/03/23.

98. Li N, Michellys P-Y, Kim S, Pferdekamper AC, Li J, Kasibhatla S et al. Abstract B232: Activity of a potent and selective phase I ALK inhibitor LDK378 in naive and crizotinib-resistant preclinical tumor models. *Molecular Cancer Therapeutics*. 2011;10(1 suppl):B232.

99. Mehra R, Camidge DR, Sharma S, Felip E, Tan DS-W, Vansteenkiste JF et al. First-in-human phase I study of the ALK inhibitor LDK378 in advanced solid tumors. *ASCO Meeting Abstracts*. 2012;30(15_suppl):3007.

100. Kiura K, Seto T, Yamamoto N, Nishio M, Nakagawa K, Tamura T. A first-in-human phase I/II study of ALK inhibitor CH5424802 in patients with ALK-positive NSCLC. *ASCO Meeting Abstracts*. 2012;30(15_suppl):7602.

101. Normant E, Paez G, West KA, Lim AR, Slocum KL, Tunkey C et al. The Hsp90 inhibitor IPI-504 rapidly lowers EML4-ALK levels and induces tumor regression in ALK-driven NSCLC models. *Oncogene*. 2011;30(22):2581–2586. Epub 2011/01/25.
102. Sequist LV, Gettinger S, Senzer NN, Martins RG, Janne PA, Lilenbaum R et al. Activity of IPI-504, a novel heat-shock protein 90 inhibitor, in patients with molecularly defined non-small-cell lung cancer. *Journal of Clinical Oncology*. 2010;28(33):4953–4960. Epub 2010/10/14.
103. Wong K. An open-label phase II study of the Hsp90 inhibitor ganetespib (STA-9090) as monotherapy in patients with advanced non-small cell lung cancer (NSCLC). *Journal of Clinical Oncology* 2011;29:(suppl; abstr 7500). 2011.
104. La Marid AM, Campbell N, Smith S, Cohn SL, Salgia R. Targeting ALK: A promising strategy for the treatment of non-small cell lung cancer, non-Hodgkin's lymphoma, and neuroblastoma. *Targeted Oncology* 2012;7:199–210.

9 MET Inhibitors

Apoorva Chawla
University of Chicago

Ravi Salgia
University of Chicago

Victoria M. Villaflor
University of Chicago

CONTENTS

INTRODUCTION

Cancer therapeutics has seen the rapid growth and development of targeted therapy. As the molecular pathways in each cancer subtype have been better elucidated, personalized medicine has revolutionized the field of oncology. Targets such as epidermal growth factor receptor (EGFR) have not only seen directed therapies but also attempts at the development of pharmacologic drugs to target resistance.[1–3] Since its discovery in the 1980s, MET and its associated ligand hepatocyte growth factor/scatter factor (HGF/SF) have become attractive targets in several types of cancer.[4–6] MET overexpression correlates with poor prognosis in several solid tumors,[7] and activation of the MET pathway plays a primary role in cancer cell survival, growth, and migration.[8–10] Over the past three decades, the signal transduction pathways and cross-talk involving the oncogene MET have been elucidated. Target-based therapeutic development has led to pharmacologic drugs in the form of MET inhibitors, which include small-molecule inhibitors (SMIs) and monoclonal antibodies (mAbs). These SMIs and mAbs are being studied in tumors with MET overexpression, including head and neck cancers, breast cancer, esophageal cancer, gastric cancer, lung cancer, renal cancer, and hepatocellular cancer, among others. This chapter reviews the biology of MET in normal and cancer cells, MET inhibitors in development and clinical trials, and the therapeutic implications of MET inhibition.

MET STRUCTURE, BIOLOGY, AND SIGNALING IN NORMAL CELLS

MET was discovered in 1984 and subsequently found to be a receptor tyrosine kinase (RTK) located at 7q21–q31.[4,11] It is composed of a 50 kDa alpha chain and 140 kDa transmembrane beta chain, linked by a disulfide bond. The beta chain is frequently divided into seven domains, including the SEMA domain, PSI domain, four IPT repeats, transmembrane domain, juxtamembrane (JM) domain, tyrosine kinase (TK), and carboxyterminal tail.[12,13] The JM domain contains two key phosphorylation sites, S985 and Y1003. Phosphorylation at S985 negatively regulates kinase activity.[14] Phosphorylation at Y1003 recruits c-CBL, which targets MET for internalization and degradation through MET ubiquitination.[15–17] The TK domain consists of several tyrosine phosphorylation sites: Y1230, Y1234, and Y1235 are involved in autophosphorylation[18]; Y1313 directs activation of PI3K and recruitment of p85[19]; and Y1349 and Y1356 are docking sites for SRC-homology-2 domain (SH2), phosphotyrosine binding (PTB), and MET binding domain (MBD)-containing proteins[20,21] (Figure 9.1). These phosphorylation sites are potential sites of pharmacologic drug targeting as they regulate internalization, catalytic activity, docking of substrates that subsequently activate key signal transducers, and, in the case of c-CBL, targeting MET degradation.

The sole ligand for MET is HGF/SF. This molecule is secreted by mesenchymal cells, particularly fibroblasts and smooth muscle cells,[22–24] but can also be secreted by tumor cells.[5] In normal cells, HGF-induced MET activation is under tight regulation by paracrine ligand delivery. Among the genes upregulated by HGF are those encoding proteases required for HGF and MET processing, as well as MET,

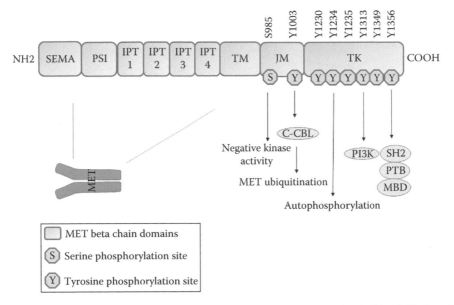

FIGURE 9.1 MET structure and beta chain domains; SEMA (semaphorin-like); PSI (found in plexins, semaphorins, and integrins); IPT (found in Ig-like regions, plexins, and transcription factors); TM (transmembrane); JM (juxtamembrane); TK (intracellular tyrosine kinase); S (serine); Y (tyrosine), PI3K (phosphatidylinositol-3 kinase); SH2 (Src homology-2); PTB (phosphotyrosine binding); and MBD-containing proteins.

creating the potential for overexpression through persistent ligand stimulation.[25] MET TK is activated when HGF/SF ligand binds to the SEMA domain of MET at the plasma membrane.[26–28] Upon binding of the HGF/SF ligand to MET, MET dimerization, autophosphorylation, and activation of TK catalytic activity occur (Figure 9.2). The cytoplasmic TK domain of MET has several key serine and tyrosine phosphorylation sites. Tyrosine phosphorylation of JM, TK, and tail domains respectively regulate internalization, catalytic activity, and docking of substrates to MET's docking site.[21,29,30] GRB2-associated-binding protein 1 (GAB1), growth factor receptor-bound protein 2 (GRB2), phospholipase C (PLC), and SRC are among the proteins recruited to MET's bidentate docking site.[31,32] These proteins, in turn, activate signal transducers such as PI3K, STAT, ERK1, ERK2, and FAK. The net effect is the activation of two major downstream pathways, including the RAS–RAF–MAPKK–ERK pathway as well as the PI3K–AKT–mTOR–NF-kB pathway.[29,33] The RAS-MAPK and PI3K–AKT pathways, in turn, direct gene expression and cell cycle progression through nuclear migration. Cytoplasmic signaling mediated by PI3K–AKT and the GTPases RAC-1 or cell division control protein 42 (CDC42) affect cell survival and modulate cytoskeletal changes. RAP-1 and RAC1–CDC42 pathways control cell migration and adhesion, mainly through their effects on integrins and cadherins.[34]

MET has been shown to cross-talk with various signaling pathways (Figure 9.3). Cross-signaling of the MET–vascular endothelial growth factor receptor (VEGFR),[35,36]

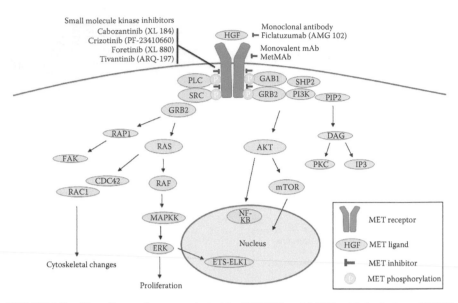

FIGURE 9.2 Signaling pathways activated by HGF/SF and MET, with inclusion of HGF/ MET inhibitors in clinical trial. HGF/SF binds to MET to trigger dimerization and activation of MET at the plasma membrane. The phosphorylation (P) sites of MET are indicated and more fully depicted in Figure 9.1. Cytoplasmic effector molecules, including growth factor receptor-bound protein 2 (GRB2), GRB2-associated binding protein (GAB1), phospholipase C (PLC), and SRC, are recruited to the docking site. GAB1 bound to MET attracts further docking proteins, including SRC homology 2 domain-containing phosphatase 2 (SHP2), PI3K, and others, which activate downstream signal transduction cascades. Two such pathways include the RAS–MAPK and PI3K–AKT, which reach the nucleus to affect gene expression and cell cycle progression. The pathway mediated by RAC1-cell division control protein 42 (CDC42) elicits cytoskeletal changes. Also depicted are HGF/MET inhibitors in clinical trial. These include the monoclonal antibody (mAb) against HGF (ficlatuzumab), the monovalent mAb against MET (MetMAb, or Onartuzumab), and the small kinase inhibitors cabozantinib (XL 184), crizotinib (PF-23410660), foretinib (XL 880), and tivantinib (ARQ-197). Abbreviations: HGF, hepatocyte growth factor; mAb, monoclonal antibody; PLC, phospholipase C; GRB2, growth factor receptor-bound protein 2; RAP1, rhoptry-associated protein 1; FAK, focal adhesion kinase; CDC42, cell division control protein 42; RAC-1; Ras-related C3 botulinum toxin substrate 1; MAPKK, mitogen-activated protein kinase kinase; ERK, extracellular signal-regulated kinase; GAB1, GRB2-associated binding protein; SHP2, SRC homology 2 domain-containing phosphatase 2; PI3K, phosphatidylinositol-3-kinase; AKT, acutely transforming retrovirus AKT8 in rodent T-cell lymphoma; NF-kB, nuclear factor kappa B; mTOR, mammalian target of rapamycin; PIP2, phosphatidylinositol 4,5-bisphosphate; DAG, diacylglycerol; PKC, protein kinase C; IP3, inositol triphosphate; ETS-ELK1, E26-AMV virus oncogene cellular homolog-1.

MET–EGFR,[3,37] and MET–WNT pathways[38–40] has emerged in the past years. Interaction between MET and EGFR/HER family receptors has implications in lung and breast cancer therapeutics and is discussed later. Cross-talk between MET and K-RAS has been described in lung carcinoma cell lines with much preclinical and clinical interest.

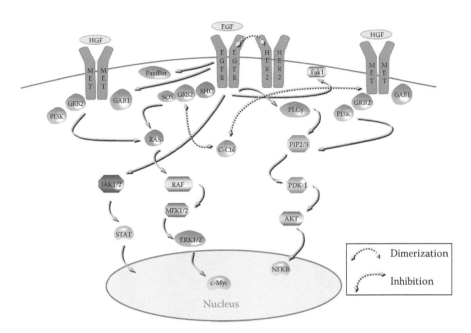

FIGURE 9.3 Cross-talk between the EGFR (ErbB-1; Her-1 in humans) and MET pathways. Multiple mechanisms allow for interaction between MET and the ERB-receptor family, of which a few are shown here. EGFR is the cell surface receptor for members of the epidermal growth factor family of extracellular protein ligands. EGFR dimerization is shown, which stimulates its intrinsic intracellular protein-tyrosine kinase activity. Autophosphorylation of EGFR elicits downstream activation and signaling of several key proteins, including RAS, ERK, PI3K/AKT, and JAK/STAT. The MET signaling pathway cooperates with the EGFR pathway by converging upon and activating the RAS–RAF–MEK–ERK signaling cascade as well as the PI3K–AKT–NF-kB cascade. C-CBL can affect MET degradation through MET ubiquitination. Abbreviations: HGF, hepatocyte growth factor; EGF, epidermal growth factor; EGFR, epidermal growth factor receptor; Her-2, human epidermal growth factor receptor 2; GAB1, GRB2-associated binding protein; GRB2, growth factor receptor-bound protein 2; FAK1, focal adhesion kinase-1; SOS, Son of sevenless; MEK, mitogen-activated protein kinase; ERK, extracellular signal-regulated kinase; c-Myc, Avian myelocytomatosis virus oncogene cellular homolog; PLC, phospholipase C; PIP2, phosphatidylinositol 3,4-bisphosphate; PIP3, phosphatidylinositol 3,4,5-trisphosphate; PDK1, 3-phosphoinositide-dependent protein kinase-1; AKT, acutely transforming retrovirus AKT8 in rodent T-cell lymphoma; NF-kB, nuclear factor kappa B; JAK, Janus-family tyrosine kinase; STAT, signal transducer and activator of transcription.

MET IN CANCER CELLS

Discovered in 1984 as a fusion partner with translocated-promoter region (TPR),[4] MET was found to be a potent oncogene in the early 1990s,[41] as cells from the mouse embryonic 3T3 fibroblast cell lines that co-expressed MET and HGF metastasized in an animal model.[42] The regulation of HGF/SF and MET signaling typically observed in normal cells can become deranged in cancer cells at multiple levels. Mechanisms of MET activation include (a) binding to its ligand HGF,

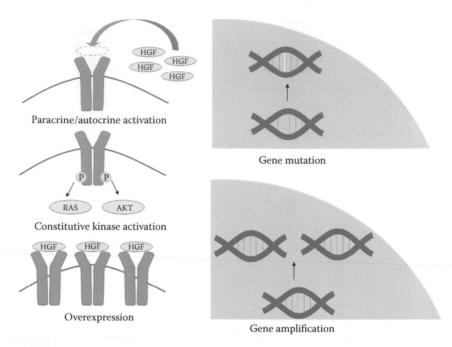

FIGURE 9.4 Common mechanisms of MET activation include binding to ligand HGF, with associated paracrine/autocrine activation via HGF; constitutive kinase activation (which can occur through activating mutations in the sema domain and JM domain); MET receptor overexpression; MET gene mutation; or MET gene amplification.

with associated paracrine/autocrine activation via HGF; (b) activating mutations, including those causing constitutive kinase activity, as seen in the sema domain and JM domain of the MET gene; (c) MET gene overexpression/amplification; and (d) decreased degradation (Figure 9.4). With respect to ligand-dependent activation, HGF can become upregulated through increased HGF originating from tumor cells and stromal cells.[9] MET can also become activated through a ligand-independent manner, including activating MET mutations, overexpression and constitutive ligand-independent dimerization, truncation, translocation, rearrangement, hypoxic activation, transactivation, or loss of inhibitory regulators.[43–46] Genetic abnormalities and activating point mutations of the MET gene are seen in sporadic and inherited human renal carcinomas, hepatocellular carcinomas, and several other cancer types.[5,6] The majority of these mutations are at the kinase domain and parallel the activating mutations seen in other RTKs, such as EGFR, RET, and KIT. Proof of principle has been shown as mutated MET in mouse models has caused a variety of tumors including sarcoma, lymphoma, and carcinoma, and basal-like breast carcinomas. Finally, amplification of MET is seen in certain human gastric and colorectal carcinomas[47–49] and is further discussed later when reviewing the role of MET in GI malignancies. MET degradation occurs through the E3 ubiquitin ligase c-CBL. Investigators have shown that c-CBL is decreased via loss of heterozygosity and can sometimes be mutated in lung cancer.[50] The microenvironment has also been shown to play a critical role in tumorigenesis, as hypoxic areas of tumors have been shown to overexpress MET.[51] Hypoxic activation leads to transcription of the MET proto-oncogene, higher MET levels, and amplification of HGF signaling. Upon inhibition of MET expression, hypoxia-induced invasive growth was prevented.[51] The diversity of cellular responses seen with MET activation confirms its role as a key mediator and its cooperation with other signaling pathways. Interplay between MET with EGFR, ERBB2, or insulin-like growth factor 1 receptor (IGF1R) has been described in several systems[52,53] and has emerged as a mechanism for cancer spread and resistance to therapy. These are briefly discussed in specific tumor types, as applicable, in the following text.

Hepatocyte growth factor receptor (HGFR) is the protein product of the MET gene and directs the oncogenic processes of cell proliferation, survival, invasion, motility, and metastases. The biology and mechanism for HGF-mediated mitogenesis and motogenesis have been described and involve phosphatidylinositol-3 kinase, among other proteins, which when inhibited leads to reduced chemotaxis.[54] In addition, paxillin, which is overexpressed in non-small-cell lung cancer (NSCLC), shows increased phosphorylation in the presence of activating HGFR mutations (T1010I and R988C).[55] The earlier protein and target have significant implications in cytoskeletal function and metastatic potential.

MET IN RENAL CELL CANCER

MET kinase mutations were first identified in hereditary papillary renal cell carcinoma (HPRCC).[6] The genetic defect underlying HPRCC is MET; mutations in MET have also been identified in a subset of patients with sporadic type 1 papillary renal cell cancer (RCC). Involvement of HGF/c-MET in papillary RCC oncogenesis is supported by the frequently seen trisomy of chromosome 7 in sporadic type 1 papillary RCC. In biopsy samples, MET has been shown to be frequently gained and occasionally mutated (13%) through trisomy 7, gain of 7q31, or activating mutations in the TK domain of the c-MET gene at 7q31, in sporadic papillary RCCs.[56] In addition, an early-onset HPRCC phenotype has been described, which involves metastasis progression.[57] Drugs targeting the c-MET pathway through antagonism of ligand interaction, inhibition of TK catalytic activity, or blockade of receptor–effector interactions may bear fruition in this early-onset metastatic phenotype.[58] Recent screening has also detected c-MET as a requirement for survival in Von Hippel–Lindau (VHL)-defective renal cancer cells, leading to an interest in targeting c-MET in clear cell kidney cancer.[59] hTid-1, a heat shock protein chaperone and the human counterpart of the Drosophila tumor suppressor gene *lethal (2) tumorous imaginal discs*, has been described as a modulator of c-MET receptor signaling in renal cell carcinomas and represents another target for inhibition.[60] Clinical trials targeting the MET pathway with single agents (i.e., XL 880 monotherapy) as well as dual inhibition with VEGF-R inhibitors (i.e., ARQ 197 with pazopanib, ARQ 197 with sorafenib) are in early phase I–II trials in patients with HPRCC and sporadic (nonhereditary) papillary kidney cancer (Table 9.1).

TABLE 9.1

HGF and MET Inhibitors in Phase II and III Clinical Evaluation

Drug Name	Mechanism/Target	Company	Type of Tumor/Phase of Study
AMG 102 (Rilotumumab)	Antibody/human HGF	Amgen	Castrate-resistant prostate cancer—phase II with mitoxantrone and prednisone
			Colorectal cancer—phase II with panitumumab
			Gastric or esophagogastric cancer—phase IB/II with ECX (epirubicin, cisplatin, capecitabine)
			Gastroesophageal adenocarcinoma—phase II with FOLFOX
			Lung (NSCLC)—phase I/II with erlotinib
			Malignant glioma—phase II
			Malignant glioma—phase I/II with bevacizumab
			Renal cell—phase II
			Small-cell lung cancer—phase IB/II with platinum-based chemotherapy
			Ovarian cancer—phase II
MetMAb (Onartuzumab)	Monovalent antibody/ Human MET	Genentech	Breast—phase II with paclitaxel
			Colorectal cancer—phase II with FOLFOX/bevacizumab
			Gastroesophageal cancer—phase II with mFOLFOX6
			Glioblastoma—with bevacizumab
			Lung (NSCLC)—phase II with erlotinib
			Lung (non-squamous NSCLC)—phase II with bevacizumab, platinum, paclitaxel, pemetrexed
			Lung (squamous NSCLC)—phase II with paclitaxel, platinum
			Lung (NSCLC)—phase III with erlotinib
ARQ-197 (Tivantinib)	Selective kinase inhibitor, non-ATP competitive/met	ArQule	Breast cancer—phase II
			Colorectal cancer—phase I/II with irinotecan and cetuximab
			Gastric cancer—phase II as monotherapy (completed)
			Gastroesophageal cancer—phase I/II with FOLFOX
			Germ cell tumors—phase II
			Hepatocellular cancer—phase II (completed)
			Kidney cancer—phase II with erlotinib
			Lung (NSCLC)—phase II with erlotinib

Drug	Mechanism	Company	Indications
XL 184 (Cabozantinib)	Broad-spectrum kinase inhibitor, ATP competitive/met, VEGFR1–3, Ret, Kit, Flt-3, Tie-2	Exelixis	Lung (non-squamous NSCLC)—phase III with erlotinib Microphthalmia transcription factor associated (MiT) tumors—phase II (completed) Myeloma—phase II Pancreatic adenocarcinoma—phase II compared to gemcitabine (completed) Prostate cancer—phase II Advanced solid malignancy—phase II Breast cancer (hormone receptor positive)—phase II Castrate-resistant prostate cancer—phase II Castrate-resistant prostate cancer—phase III vs. prednisone Castrate-resistant prostate cancer—phase III vs. mitoxantrone Glioblastoma—phase II Lung (NSCLC)—phase II Lung (NSCLC)—phase II with erlotinib Medullary thyroid cancer—phase III Pancreatic neuroendocrine/carcinoid tumors—phase II Prostate cancer (androgen dependent)—phase II with androgen ablation Urothelial cancer—phase II
PF-2341066 (Crizotinib)	Broad spectrum kinase inhibitor, ATP competitive/met, Alk, ROS-1	Pfizer	Lung (NSCLC)—phase II with erlotinib Lung (ALK positive)—phase II Lung (ALK-positive NSCLC)—phase III vs. platinum+pemetrexed
XL 880 (Foretinib)	Broad-spectrum kinase inhibitor, ATP competitive/met, Ron, VEGFR1–3, PDGFR, Kit, Flt-3, Tie-2	Exelixis	Breast cancer—phase I/II with lapatinib Breast cancer, recurrent/metastatic—phase II Gastric cancer—phase II (completed) Head and neck squamous cell cancer—phase II Lung (NSCLC)—phase II with erlotinib Papillary renal cell carcinoma—phase II

Note: NSCLC, non-small-cell lung cancer. Full clinical trial listing can be found at the U.S. National Institutes of Health registry of Clinical Trials (see the ClinicalTrials.gov website).

MET IN HEAD AND NECK CANCER

MET has been shown to be functionally important in head and neck squamous cell cancer (HNSCC) through overexpression, increased gene copy number, and mutation.

Interestingly, somatic activating mutations of the MET oncogene are selected for, during the metastases of human head and neck cancers, as cells expressing mutant MET likely undergo clonal expansion during HNSCC progression, suggesting that MET is a critical oncogene controlling the progression of primary cancer to metastases.[61] In vitro and in vivo models have confirmed that MET inhibition in HNSCC can abrogate MET functions, such as proliferation, migration/motility, and angiogenesis.[62,63] Though EGFR is overexpressed in up to 90% of tumor cells, EGFR inhibition in HNSCC has yielded only modest response rates in clinical practice,[64,65] leading to studies of dual blockade of c-MET with EGFR[66] due to the known cross-talk between the two pathways. One such study has shown that EGFR ligand, TGF-alpha, can induce the activation of the c-MET pathway in HNSCC.[66] Early data are promising in the preclinical models evaluating MET inhibitors in combination with cisplatin or EGFR inhibitors.[63]

MET IN LUNG CANCER

MET alterations can occur through receptor mutations, overexpression, genomic amplification, or alternative splicing. MET gene mutations are seen in a variety of tumor subtypes, particularly NSCLC with adenocarcinoma histology, but are also described in neuroendocrine subtypes, including small-cell lung cancer (SCLC). These MET receptor mutations are typically seen in the extracellular sema and JM domains. The sema domain is needed for receptor dimerization and activation.[67] Certain JM domain mutations (R988C, T1010I, alternative spliced JM-deleting variant) are oncogenic activating variants with enhanced oncogenic signaling, cell motility, and migration. There have also been reports of exon skipping with exon 14 of MET and gain of function.[68] In SCLC, JM domain mutations (S1040P, T992I, and R970C) have been characterized.[55] Both somatic and germline variants of MET have been reported in thoracic malignancies. Though the presence of these mutations has been defined in lung cancer, detailed understanding of their functional and biologic significance remains to be determined.

MET receptor is overexpressed in SCLC and NSCLC. MET is particularly over-expressed in NSCLC of the non-squamous subtype. In protein studies of human lung cancer tissue, 67% of adenocarcinomas, 60% of carcinoids, 57% of large-cell carcinomas, 57% of squamous cell carcinomas, and 25% of SCLC strongly express MET.[69] PAX5, a nuclear transcription factor required for B-cell development, seems to be an important regulator of c-MET transcriptional control in SCLC. Kanteti et al. have noted that PAX5 protein expression is strongly expressed in SCLC, whereas PAX8 is expressed in NSCLC.[70] The active form of MET (phospho-c-MET) and PAX5 have been shown to localize to the same intranuclear compartment in HGF-treated SCLC cells and interact together. PAX5 is frequently coexpressed with MET in intermediate-grade and high-grade neuroendocrine tumors including atypical carcinoids, SCLCs, and large-cell neuroendocrine tumors. This may have significant therapeutic translational potential, as PAX5 knockdown SCLC lines, in conjunction with topoisomerase I inhibitor (SN38) and c-MET inhibitor (SU11274), have maximally decreased the viability of SCLC cell lines.[70]

Clinically, the role of MET in the development of EGFR TK inhibitor (TKI) resistance has been an active area of research. In an in vitro model, Engelman et al. showed that MET amplification causes gefitinib resistance through ERBB3 (Her-3)-dependent activation of PI3K.[3] Cells with MET amplification may undergo a kinase switch when exposed to EGFR blockade and subsequently rely on MET to maintain activation of AKT in the presence of EGFR-TKIs.[71] In some preclinical models, resistance appears to be overcome by combined dual inhibition of EGFR and MET, as shown in lung, pancreatic, and breast tumor xenografts. These results provide a rationale for ongoing clinical studies of MET inhibitor, alone, and in combination with EGFR-TKI in NSCLC. Several such studies are in progress (Table 9.1).

MET in Esophageal, Gastric, and GI Cancers

In certain human gastric and colorectal carcinomas, as well as in other tumors, amplification of MET on chromosome 7q31 is seen. MET is overexpressed in esophageal adenocarcinoma (EA) compared to normal esophageal squamous epithelium and Barrett's esophagus columnar epithelium without dysplasia. Met-dependent loss of Cbl protein in MET-amplified gastric cancer cell lines represents a recently described mechanism contributing to signal dysregulation.[72] Graziano et al. recently investigated whether prognosis of patients with high-risk gastric cancer may depend on MET copy number gain or an activating truncation mutation within the deoxyadenosine tract element in the promoter region of the MET ligand HGF. It was shown that increasing MET gene copy number in stages II and III gastric adenocarcinoma correlates with the risk of recurrence and decreased survival.[73] Although MET amplification in gastroesophageal cancers was uncommon and observed in only 2% of their cohort, Lennerz et al. confirmed that an increase in MET gene copy number was associated with higher presenting tumor grade and stage, and shorter median survival.[74]

Investigators have analyzed the effects of a c-MET-specific SMI (PHA665752) on MET-overexpressing EA cell lines. PHA665752 was shown to inhibit constitutive and HGF-induced phosphorylation of c-MET. However, c-MET inhibition with PHA665752 induced apoptosis and inhibited motility and invasion only in cells in which PI3K/AKT signaling was stimulated by HGF.[75] This suggests that factors other than MET receptor overexpression, such as c-MET-dependent PI3K/AKT signaling, may predict a tumor's response to MET inhibition.

Parallel to EGFR-TKI resistance in lung cancer, MET activation mediates resistance to lapatinib inhibition of HER2-amplified gastric cancer cells[76] and is a novel mechanism that may decrease sustained efficacy of HER2-targeted agents in gastric cancer cells. MET is also frequently overexpressed in colon cancers with high metastatic tendency. Concomitant downregulation of miR-1 and increase in MACC1 has been shown to contribute to MET overexpression and to the metastatic behavior of colon cancer cells.[77] The Wnt pathway has been implicated in controlling MET expression in colorectal cancer, and cross-talk between the two pathways has been described.[38] MET signaling, however, can lead to increased transformation of colon epithelial cells independent of Wnt signaling and in this way can play an essential role in the onset and progression of colorectal cancer.[78]

Despite previously described mechanisms of EGFR resistance and sensitivity, the involved pathways are indeed multifactorial. In the case of metastatic colorectal cancer, resistance to anti-EGFR therapy is likely based on more than K-RAS mutation. Recently, the cross talk of IGF1R and c-MET pathways with respect to resistance to cetuximab is being elucidated and may likely allow for improved understanding and ultimately rational targeting.[79] As well, there can be synergism of MET and RON, especially in gastroesophageal junction carcinoma.[80]

MET IN BREAST CANCER

With the development and approval of trastuzumab (Herceptin), a humanized mAb directed against Her-2, patient survival in breast cancer has been prolonged. Despite these successes, resistance to trastuzumab therapy has been described and is a barrier to effective treatment of Her-2 (+) breast cancer. Investigators have reported resistance to single-agent trastuzumab as 66%–88% and 20%–50% for combination therapy.[81,82] MET receptor has been shown to be aberrantly expressed in breast cancer and is an independent predictor of poor prognosis. This is of particular importance as MET and Her-2 synergize in promoting cellular invasion. MET is felt to contribute to trastuzumab resistance, as attenuation of MET activity leads to sensitization to trastuzumab treatment. MET activation protects cells from the growth inhibitory effects of trastuzumab through sustained AKT activation and by preventing trastuzumab-mediated p27 induction.[83] In addition, MET is also involved in IGF-IR-mediated trastuzumab resistance, as MET is required for several IGF-IR-driven cellular responses.[52] Interestingly, laboratory studies have shown that Her-2 overexpressing breast cancers react to trastuzumab treatment with rapid upregulation of MET, thereby promoting their own resistance. Blocking of MET, in breast cancer preclinical models, through RNA interference-mediated depletion or SMIs, has been shown to improve response to trastuzumab.[83]

CANCER THERAPEUTICS

With our improved understanding of the structure and function of c-MET, its downstream signaling, and its associated receptor–ligand interactions, the past decade has seen much progress in the development of MET-HGF/SF inhibitors in cancer therapeutics. MET inhibitors can be subdivided into MET antagonists (which include MET/HGF mAbs) and MET small-molecule/kinase inhibitors (Figure 9.2).

MET ANTAGONISTS

HGF/MET pathway antagonists are directed against ligand–receptor binding, or related cell surface events such as receptor clustering, and include (a) truncated HGF splice variants and isoforms, (b) HGF forms that resist proteolytic activation, (c) truncated soluble forms of MET ectodomain, and (d) neutralizing mAbs against HGF or MET.

NK1 is the shortest splice variant of HGF/SF. Despite agonist activity in vivo,[84] it can be converted to a receptor antagonist by mutations such as Tyr124 and Asn127.[85] Typically with partial agonist and antagonist activity in vivo, NK-2 can become mutated at the Cys214 position, yielding a variant with receptor antagonist activity.[86] NK-4 has been described as having MET antagonist activity, along with broad anti-angiogenic activity.[87]

MONOCLONAL ANTIBODIES AGAINST MET/HGF

AMG 102 (Rilotumumab)

AMG 102, or rilotumumab (AMGEN), is a humanized mAb that blocks HGF/SF binding to MET by binding to the SPH domain.[88] AMG 102 enhances temozolomide or docetaxel effectiveness in U-87 MG cells and xenograft models.[89] AMG 102 has been studied in advanced solid tumors, gastric and esophagogastric junction adenocarcinoma, renal cell carcinoma, and glioblastoma multiforme, as discussed later.

Rosen et al., in a phase IB study, reviewed overall safety and toxicity profile of AMG 102 when combined with bevacizumab or motesanib in advanced solid tumors.[90] In this study, patients with treatment-refractory advanced solid tumors were enrolled into four cohorts (3, 10, or 20 mg/kg AMG 102 plus 10 mg/kg bevacizumab intravenously every 2 weeks, or 3 mg/kg AMG 102 intravenously every 2 weeks plus 75 mg motesanib orally once daily). The number of patients who received AMG 102 plus motesanib was insufficient to adequately assess safety, though the combination of AMG 102 with bevacizumab (n = 12) seemed to have acceptable toxicity. Enrollment in the motesanib cohort was suspended due to reports of cholecystitis in other motesanib studies. Treatment-emergent adverse events among patients receiving AMG 102 plus bevacizumab were generally mild and included fatigue (75%), nausea (58%), constipation (42%), and peripheral edema (42%). Bevacizumab did not seem to affect AMG 102 pharmacokinetics. Of 10 evaluable patients, 8 had reductions in tumor dimensions. Stable disease at ≥ 8, ≥ 16, and ≥ 24 weeks occurred in 9, 7, and 4 patients, respectively. Progression-free survival (PFS) ranged from 7.9 to 121.9 weeks.[90]

In another study, overall survival (OS) benefit with the addition of AMG 102 to ECX (epirubicin, cisplatin, and capecitabine) in patients with unresectable locally advanced or metastatic gastric or esophagogastric junction adenocarcinoma was recently reported at the 2012 annual ASCO meeting.[91] In this double-blind, placebo-controlled, phase II trial of 121 patients with gastric/esophagogastric junction cancer, rilotumumab (7.5 or 15 mg/kg) + ECX showed trends for improved OS and PFS compared to ECX alone through exposure–response analysis using pharmacokinetic, biomarker, efficacy, and safety data.[91]

On the other hand, a phase II study of AMG 102 in patients with metastatic renal cell carcinoma showed safety, but it was unclear if the agent was growth inhibitory in the studied population.[92] Recently reported results from a Phase II trial of AMG102 in patients with recurrent glioblastoma multiforme also showed that while AMG 102 was generally well tolerated at doses of 10 and 20 mg/kg once every 2 weeks, there did not seem to be single-agent antitumor activity in this heavily pretreated population.[93] Finally, AMG 102 with erlotinib in patients with recurrent or progressive advanced stage NSCLC is in progress as a phase I/II study (NCT01233687).

MetMAb (Onartuzumab, OA-5D5)

MetMAb, also known as onartuzumab, is a single-armed humanized mAb developed by Genentech that binds the SEMA domain of MET.[94] It was designed as a monovalent antibody to avoid any agonist activity that can occur when a bivalent antibody binds two MET molecules. By competing for the binding of HGF to MET, MetMAb acts like a classic receptor antagonist. MetMAb blocks ligand-induced MET dimerization and prevents activation of MET's kinase domain.

Preclinical studies confirmed MetMAb as a potent anti-c-Met inhibitor. In one such preclinical study, MetMAb was shown to inhibit glioblastoma growth in vivo. Specifically, U87 tumor growth (c-Met and SF/HGF positive) was inhibited >95% with OA-5D5 treatment. In contrast, G55 tumors, which are not SF/HGF driven, did not respond to OA-5D5.[94] MetMAb has also been shown to inhibit orthotopic pancreatic tumor growth and improve survival.[95] Subsequent studies suggested a role for its use in combination with EGFR and/or VEGF inhibitors. These studies have shown that a triple combination of MetMAb with an EGFR and VEGF inhibitor had more robust antitumor effects than any two agents alone.

Salgia et al. reported on a phase I, open-label, dose-escalation study of MetMAb at the 20th Annual AACR-NCI-EORTC International Conference, and MetMAb was reported to be safe and well tolerated as a single agent at doses up to 30 mg/kg. A phase IB dose-escalation study established the safety and tolerability of MetMAb in locally advanced or metastatic solid tumors.[96] Interestingly, one response in the phase I trial of MetMAb consisted of a durable complete response obtained in a patient with chemo-refractory metastatic gastric cancer, with the biology underlying the response involving high MET gene polysomy and evidence for an autocrine production of HGF, the growth factor ligand of Met.[97]

Dual inhibition of c-MET and EGFR in NSCLC was recently studied in a randomized, double-blind, phase II study. This study compared MetMAb with erlotinib vs. placebo with erlotinib as the second-/third-line therapy in advanced NSCLC. MetMAb with erlotinib resulted in improved PFS and OS, with OS benefit noted in the arm with MET FISH $\geq$ 5 copies as well as FISH ($-$)/IHC (2+/3+) arm (HR = 0.37, median 12.6 months vs. 4.6 months, p = 0.002).[98]

Ficlatuzumab

Ficlatuzumab (AV-299), previously SCH 900105, was developed by AVEO and is an anti-HGF IgG1 mAb currently in phase II development. Prior phase I studies indicated a satisfactory tolerability profile with the EGFR inhibitors and no dose-limiting toxicities up to the highest dose tested (20 mg/kg).[99] An ongoing phase II trial of ficlatuzumab with gefitinib as first-line therapy for wild-type and mutant EGFR NSCLC is still pending.

DN-30 and 11E1

The MET antibody DN-30 causes MET activation and ectodomain shedding through ADAM10.[100] Conversion into a monovalent form eradicated agonist activity and subsequently produced an antagonist.[101] A MET antibody with antagonist activity in bivalent form, 11E1, has also been described. Its detailed mechanism remains to be elucidated, but is felt to differ from MetMAb and DN-30.

MET KINASE INHIBITORS

Parallel efforts in the structural analysis of MET kinase have led to the extensive development of MET kinase inhibitors for cancer therapy. Three major classes of inhibitors have emerged that differ in binding mode, activity on MET kinase mutants, and enzyme specificity. The first grouping, including compounds such as crizotinib, bind at the ATP-binding pocket. They are competitive inhibitors of ATP binding, with the majority having preferential binding to the inactive conformation of the enzyme. Type II inhibitors, in addition to occupying the ATP-binding pocket, encompass a second pocket that is formed when the side chain of Asp 1222 points away from the ATP-binding pocket. The less common type III inhibitors occupy the ATP-binding pocket while extending into a hydrophobic cavity formed by the displacement of an alpha-C helix. However, it is clear that not all of the MET kinase inhibitors cleanly fit into one of the earlier categories. In addition, even small modifications can dramatically alter potency and specificity. For example, the type I inhibitor PF-02341066 has strong activity against anaplastic lymphoma kinase (ALK) and has shown activity in patients with NSCLC and EML4-ALK fusions. BMS-777607 has potent activity against MET, RON, and AXL. XL880 inhibits MET, AXL, VEGFR2, and PDGFR-beta.

ARQ-197 (Tivantinib)

ARQ-197, also known as tivantinib, is an oral, non-ATP-dependent selective MET inhibitor developed by ArQule in partnership with Daiichi-Sankyo. Its mechanism involves inhibition of MET autophosphorylation, with selectivity for the unphosphorylated form of MET. Interestingly, when biochemically assessed on a panel of 230 kinases, only c-MET was inhibited to moderate to high extent. Due to its rapid metabolism by CYP2C19 and moderate metabolism by CYP3A4, ARQ-197 dosing has been modified based on classification as a poor or extensive metabolizer.

In preclinical experiments, ARQ197 has inhibited HGF-stimulated and constitutive c-Met phosphorylation in multiple human cancer cell lines and decreased phosphorylation of downstream effectors, including AKT, MAPK, and STAT-3. ARQ-197 has been studied in NSCLC, hepatocellular, and pancreatic carcinomas.

Perhaps the most compelling data have been seen in locally advanced or metastatic NSCLC. ARQ 197–209, a randomized, placebo-controlled phase II clinical trial of erlotinib + ARQ 197 in previously treated EGFR inhibitor-naive patients was found to be superior to erlotinib + placebo.[102] In this study, 167 patients were randomized to erlotinib (E) + ARQ-197 (A) (n = 84) or erlotinib (E) + placebo (P) (n = 83). PFS was prolonged with E + A (HR 0.81 [95% CI 0.57, 1.15]; p = 0.23), with more dramatic results in patients with non-squamous histology, EGFR WT status, and KRAS mutations.[102] A subsequent phase III trial with this drug combination was initiated and was powered to detect improvement in median OS in the E + A arm over E alone. In a recent press release, Daiichi-ArQule announced that the trial failed to meet its primary endpoint. However, further biomarkers need to be assessed and a potential biomarker-driven trial needs to be performed.

In other clinical trials, monotherapy with ARQ-197 inhibited the growth of hepatocellular and pancreatic carcinomas, as well as tumors driven by microphthalmia-associated transcription factor.[103] In a recent multicenter randomized phase II trial, ARQ-197 was tested for efficacy and safety for the second-line treatment of advanced hepatocellular carcinoma. Patients with advanced hepatocellular carcinoma and Child–Pugh A cirrhosis who had progressed on, or were unable to tolerate, first-line systemic therapy were eligible. Patients were randomly assigned to receive tivantinib 360 mg twice daily, or placebo, until disease progression. Of note, the tivantinib dose was amended to 240 mg twice daily because of high incidence of grade 3 or worse neutropenia. The study met its primary endpoint of time to progression, according to independent radiologic review in the intention to treat population [(1.6 months for patients treated with tivantinib [95% CI 1.4–2.8] versus 1.4 months for patients receiving placebo [95% CI 1.4–1.5]); hazard ratio 0.64, 90% CI 0.43–0.94, p=0.04]. At the time of analysis, 46 patients (65%) in the tivantinib group and 26 patients (72%) in the placebo group had progressive disease. In subgroup analysis, tumor samples were assessed for MET expression with immunohistochemistry, with high expression regarded as $\geq 2+$ in $\geq 50\%$ of tumor cells. For MET-high tumors, median time to progression was longer for patients on tivantinib than for those receiving placebo [(2.7 months [95% CI 1.4–8.5] for 22 MET-high patients on tivantinib versus 1.4 months [95% CI 1.4–1.6] for 15 MET-high patients on placebo); hazard ratio 0.43, 95% CI 0.19–0.97, p=0.03].[104] While requiring completion of phase III data, ARQ-197 may hold promise for the second-line treatment for advanced hepatocellular carcinoma, particularly for patients with MET-high tumors.

XL 184 (Cabozantinib)

Cabozantinib predominantly targets MET and VEGFR2, but also has an inhibitory activity against RET, KIT, AXL, and FLT3. Mechanistically, cabozantinib has been shown to inhibit endothelial cell tubule formation, cellular migration and invasion, and tumor cell proliferation, as well as with MET/VEGFR2 phosphorylation in vivo.[105]

In an experimental model of metastasis, treatment with cabozantinib did not show any increase in lung tumor burden, which has been observed with other VEGF signaling inhibitors that do not target the MET pathway.[105] The earlier point suggests that cabozantinib may hold promise in inhibiting tumor angiogenesis and metastasis in cancers with dysregulated MET and VEGFR signaling.

In a phase II randomized discontinuation trial (RDT) of nine different types of solid tumors, XL 184 showed substantial activity in several advanced solid tumors including breast cancer, NSCLC, liver cancer, and melanoma. Ovarian cancer and hepatocellular cancer also displayed notable responses to XL 184 in similar phase II RDTs.[106]

In addition, in a phase II study in metastatic castrate-resistant prostate cancer with up to one prior chemotherapy, cabozantinib resulted in tumor response, partial or complete resolution of lesions on bone scan, and symptom relief.[107]

A phase Ib/II study of XL184 with and without erlotinib in patients with NSCLC was recently presented. Dual treatment resulted in substantial decrease in pMET and pERK, without major drug–drug interactions. Overall, there was encouraging clinical activity of XL184 with erlotinib in a largely erlotinib pretreated population, including patients with EGFR T790M mutation and MET amplification. This suggests that XL184 may resensitize cells resistant to the EGFR inhibitors gefitinib and erlotinib.

Cabozantinib has been shown to be active in medullary thyroid cancer (MTC), likely through its targeting of multiple pathways of importance in MTC, including MET, VEGFR2, and RET.[108] In one such study, 17 patients with MTC were treated with XL184 and demonstrated a >50% response rate and a 100% disease control rate. Of the patients with MTC, nine were previously treated with TKIs. A subsequent global phase III pivotal study of cabozantinib vs. placebo in MTC was recently reported and met its primary objective of improved PFS (11.2 vs. 4.0 months, p<0.0001), which led to cabozantinib's recent approval for metastatic MTC.[109]

Crizotinib (PF-2341066)

While largely thought of, and approved, as an inhibitor of EML4-ALK fusion protein in NSCLC, crizotinib was initially developed as an ATP-competitive, small-molecule MET inhibitor by Pfizer. Initial preclinical studies showed that crizotinib potently inhibited HGF-stimulated endothelial cell survival or invasion and serum-stimulated tubulogenesis in vitro, thereby decreasing c-Met phosphorylation.[110] In mouse xenografts of human NCI-H441 NSCLC cells, tumor volume decreased by over 40% after 38 days of PF-2341066 treatment. Similarly, in gastric carcinoma, renal cell, glioblastoma, and prostate cancer xenografts, tumor volume decreased by 53%–97%. Additional studies demonstrated that PF-2341066-treated gastric carcinoma cells had decreased phosphorylation of MET, AKT, ERK, and STAT-5.[110]

In MET-amplified lung cancer cell lines, MET signaling inhibition by crizotinib has been shown to induce apoptosis along with the inhibition of AKT and extracellular signal-regulated kinase phosphorylation.[111] Rapid durable clinical responses with crizotinib in NSCLC patients with de novo MET amplification and without ALK rearrangement have been described. Similar results have been described in MET-amplified recurrent glioblastoma multiforme.[112] It is certainly possible that crizotinib will not only be utilized as an ALK and ROS-1 inhibitor but also in a subset of MET-activated tumors.

XL 880 (Foretinib)

XL 880 (also called foretinib, EXEL-2880, or GSK 1363089) is an orally available multi-target MET inhibitor that targets the HGF family as well as VEGF RTK families, including VEGFR-2. In preclinical models, XL 880 has shown inhibitory activity against Flt-3, KIT, PDGFR-beta, and Tie2 RTKs, though in vivo, potent inhibition has not been demonstrated.

Thus far, three phase I studies have been completed, describing safety and bio-availability.[113] Different administration schedules have been analyzed, either on a 5 day on/9 day off schedule, or as a fixed daily dose. Reversible increases in hepatic transaminases and pancreatic lipase were seen. Hypertension was seen in over a quarter of patients, but was grade 3 in only 5% and was manageable with medication. In the study that utilized a 5 day on/9 day off schedule (n=41), four had confirmed partial response (>30% tumor shrinkage by RECIST criteria), four had minor responses (RECIST response >20% and <30%), and seven patients had stable disease. The longest response was over 54 months.[114]

Two phase II studies have been completed in patients with head and neck cancer and gastric cancer. There is currently a randomized phase I/II trial looking at side effects of erlotinib with or without the MET/VEGFR2 inhibitor foretinib.

OTHER AGENTS IN EARLY CLINICAL TRIALS

Several other agents are undergoing early phase and preclinical testing. Some of these include the multikinase inhibitor MGCD265 that targets MET, VEGF, Tie-2, and RON RTKs, and HPK-56 that inhibits KIT, PDGF, and MET kinase. In addition, a new generation of highly selective MET inhibitors, including SAR125844 (Sanofi), PF-04217903 (Pfizer), JNJ-38877605 (Johnson and Johnson), and SGX 523 (SGX Pharmaceuticals, Inc), are currently undergoing phase I testing.

SUMMARY AND FUTURE DIRECTIONS

Cancer therapeutics seems to be entering a new era, as traditional cytotoxic systemic chemotherapy is being supplemented with targeted drugs, which relies on specific pathways upregulated in malignancy. One such oncogenic pathway, MET, plays a primary role in cancer cell survival, growth, and migration, through its activation of two major downstream pathways, including the RAS–RAF–MAPKK–ERK pathway as well as the PI3K–AKT–mTOR–NF-kB pathway. As such, MET has become an attractive target in several types of cancer, including lung cancer, esophageal and gastric cancer, head and neck cancer, breast cancer, and renal cancer, among others. mAbs against MET/HGF (i.e., rilotumumab, onartuzumab, and ficlatuzumab), as well as MET kinase inhibitors (i.e., tivantinib, cabozantinib, crizotinib, and foretinib), have shown substantial promise in clinical trials. As we continue to understand more about MET amplification, mutation, and overexpression, future studies will likely analyze the subset of patients most likely to benefit from MET inhibition therapy. These predictors of response will likely occur through advancement of diagnostic and predictive biomarkers.[115] In addition, the role of MET inhibition as a single agent or in combination with currently approved pharmacotherapies will need to be elucidated and better defined. As seen earlier, tumor cells appear to undergo a kinase switch when exposed to certain targeted agents such as erlotinib, providing a possible rationale for combination therapy. Mechanisms of resistance to MET inhibitors, whether primary or acquired, will also need to be explored. Future directions will help us better define whether these agents are best used as first-line or second-line therapy. Additionally, whether these agents should be used with or without cytotoxic chemotherapy, or other targeted agents, remains to be determined.

ABBREVIATIONS

ALK   anaplastic lymphoma kinas
CDC42 cell division control protein 42
EA   esophageal adenocarcinoma
EGFR   epidermal growth factor receptor

GAB1   GRB2-associated protein 1
GRB2   growth factor receptor-bound protein 2
HGF   hepatocyte growth factor
HGFR   hepatocyte growth factor receptor
HNSCC   head and neck squamous cell cancer
HPRCC   hereditary renal cell carcinoma
IGF1R   insulin-like growth factor 1 receptor
JM   juxtamembrane
mAbs   monoclonal antibodies
MBD   MET binding domain
MTC   medullary thyroid cancer
NSCLC   non-small-cell lung cancer
OS   overall survival
PFS   progression-free survival
PI3K   phosphatidylinositol-3 kinase
PLC   phospholipase C
PTB   phosphotyrosine binding
RDT   randomized discontinuation trial
RTK   receptor tyrosine kinase
SCLC   small-cell lung cancer
SF   scatter factor
SH2   SRC-homology domain
SMIs   small-molecule inhibitors
TK   tyrosine kinase
TKI   tyrosine kinase inhibitor
TPR   translocated-promoter region
VEGFR   vascular endothelial growth factor receptor
VHL   Von Hippel–Lindau

REFERENCES

1. Puri N, Salgia R. Synergism of EGFR and c-Met pathways, cross-talk and inhibition, in non-small cell lung cancer. *Journal of Carcinogenesis.* 2008;7:9.
2. Tang Z, Du R, Jiang S et al. Dual MET-EGFR combinatorial inhibition against T790M-EGFR-mediated erlotinib-resistant lung cancer. *British Journal of Cancer.* 2008;99(6):911–922.
3. Engelman JA, Zejnullahu K, Mitsudomi T et al. MET amplification leads to gefitinib resistance in lung cancer by activating ERBB3 signaling. *Science.* 2007;316(5827):1039–1043.
4. Cooper CS, Park M, Blair DG et al. Molecular cloning of a new transforming gene from a chemically transformed human cell line. *Nature.* 1984;311(5981):29–33.
5. Ma PC, Tretiakova MS, MacKinnon AC et al. Expression and mutational analysis of MET in human solid cancers. *Genes, Chromosomes and Cancer.* 2008;47(12):1025–1037.
6. Schmidt L, Duh FM, Chen F et al. Germline and somatic mutations in the tyrosine kinase domain of the MET proto-oncogene in papillary renal carcinomas. *Nature Genetics.* 1997;16(1):68–73.
7. Raghav KP, Wang W, Liu S et al. cMET and phospho-cMET protein levels in breast cancers and survival outcomes. *Clinical Cancer Research.* 2012;18(8):2269–2277.

8. Comoglio PM, Boccaccio C. Scatter factors and invasive growth. *Seminars in Cancer Biology.* 2001;11(2):153–165.
9. Jiang W, Hiscox S, Matsumoto K et al. Hepatocyte growth factor/scatter factor, its molecular, cellular and clinical implications in cancer. *Critical Reviews in Oncology/ Hematology.* 1999;29(3):209–248.
10. Tretiakova M, Salama AK, Karrison T et al. MET and phosphorylated MET as potential biomarkers in lung cancer. *Journal of Environmental Pathology, Toxicology and Oncology.* 2011;30(4):341–354.
11. Dean M, Park M, Le Beau MM et al. The human met oncogene is related to the tyrosine kinase oncogenes. *Nature.* 1985;318(6044):385–388.
12. Maestrini E, Tamagnone L, Longati P et al. A family of transmembrane proteins with homology to the MET-hepatocyte growth factor receptor. *Proceedings of the National Academy of Sciences of the United States of America.* 1996;93(2):674–678.
13. Sattler M, Salgia R. c-Met and hepatocyte growth factor: Potential as novel targets in cancer therapy. *Current Oncology Reports.* 2007;9(2):102–108.
14. Gandino L, Longati P, Medico E et al. Phosphorylation of serine 985 negatively regulates the hepatocyte growth factor receptor kinase. *The Journal of Biological Chemistry.* 1994;269(3):1815–1820.
15. Abella JV, Peschard P, Naujokas MA et al. Met/hepatocyte growth factor receptor ubiquitination suppresses transformation and is required for Hrs phosphorylation. *Molecular and Cellular Biology.* 2005;25(21):9632–9645.
16. Soubeyran P, Kowanetz K, Szymkiewicz I et al. Cbl-CIN85-endophilin complex mediates ligand-induced downregulation of EGF receptors. *Nature.* 2002;416(6877):183–187.
17. Petrelli A, Gilestro GF, Lanzardo S et al. The endophilin-CIN85-Cbl complex mediates ligand-dependent downregulation of c-Met. *Nature.* 2002;416(6877):187–190.
18. Rodrigues GA, Park M. Autophosphorylation modulates the kinase activity and oncogenic potential of the Met receptor tyrosine kinase. *Oncogene.* 1994;9(7):2019–2027.
19. Fournier TM, Kamikura D, Teng K et al. Branching tubulogenesis but not scatter of madin-darby canine kidney cells requires a functional Grb2 binding site in the Met receptor tyrosine kinase. *The Journal of Biological Chemistry.* 1996;271(36):22211–22217.
20. Furge KA, Zhang YW, Vande Woude GF. Met receptor tyrosine kinase: enhanced signaling through adapter proteins. *Oncogene.* 2000;19(49):5582–5589.
21. Ponzetto C, Bardelli A, Zhen Z et al. A multifunctional docking site mediates signaling and transformation by the hepatocyte growth factor/scatter factor receptor family. *Cell.* 1994;77(2):261–271.
22. Sonnenberg E, Meyer D, Weidner KM et al. Scatter factor/hepatocyte growth factor and its receptor, the c-met tyrosine kinase, can mediate a signal exchange between mesenchyme and epithelia during mouse development. *The Journal of Cell Biology.* 1993;123(1):223–235.
23. Naldini L, Weidner KM, Vigna E et al. Scatter factor and hepatocyte growth factor are indistinguishable ligands for the MET receptor. *The EMBO Journal.* 1991;10(10):2867–2878.
24. Kim ES, Salgia R. MET pathway as a therapeutic target. *Journal of Thoracic Oncology.* 2009;4(4):444–447.
25. Cecchi F, Rabe DC, Bottaro DP. Targeting the HGF/Met signalling pathway in cancer. *European Journal of Cancer.* 2010;46(7):1260–1270.
26. Hammond DE, Urbe S, Vande Woude GF et al. Down-regulation of MET, the receptor for hepatocyte growth factor. *Oncogene.* 2001;20(22):2761–2770.
27. Peruzzi B, Bottaro DP. Targeting the c-Met signaling pathway in cancer. *Clinical Cancer Research.* 2006;12(12):3657–3660.
28. Teis D, Huber LA. The odd couple: signal transduction and endocytosis. *Cellular and Molecular Life Sciences.* 2003;60(10):2020–2033.

29. Birchmeier C, Birchmeier W, Gherardi E et al. Met, metastasis, motility and more. *Nature Reviews Molecular Cell Biology.* 2003;4(12):915–925.

30. Weidner KM, Di Cesare S, Sachs M et al. Interaction between Gab1 and the c-Met receptor tyrosine kinase is responsible for epithelial morphogenesis. *Nature.* 1996;384(6605):173–176.

31. Zhang YW, Vande Woude GF. HGF/SF-met signaling in the control of branching morphogenesis and invasion. *Journal of Cellular Biochemistry.* 2003;88(2):408–417.

32. Corso S, Comoglio PM, Giordano S. Cancer therapy: Can the challenge be MET? *Trends in Molecular Medicine.* 2005;11(6):284–292.

33. Lai AZ, Abella JV, Park M. Crosstalk in Met receptor oncogenesis. *Trends in Cell Biology.* 2009;19(10):542–551.

34. Gherardi E, Birchmeier W, Birchmeier C et al. Targeting MET in cancer: Rationale and progress. *Nature Reviews Cancer.* 2012;12(2):89–103.

35. Zhang YW, Su Y, Volpert OV et al. Hepatocyte growth factor/scatter factor mediates angiogenesis through positive VEGF and negative thrombospondin 1 regulation. *Proceedings of the National Academy of Sciences of the United States of America.* 2003;100(22):12718–12723.

36. Sulpice E, Ding S, Muscatelli-Groux B et al. Cross-talk between the VEGF-A and HGF signalling pathways in endothelial cells. *Biology of the Cell/under the Auspices of the European Cell Biology Organization.* 2009;101(9):525–539.

37. Turke AB, Zejnullahu K, Wu YL et al. Preexistence and clonal selection of MET amplification in EGFR mutant NSCLC. *Cancer Cell.* 2010;17(1):77–88.

38. Boon EM, van der Neut R, van de Wetering M et al. Wnt signaling regulates expression of the receptor tyrosine kinase met in colorectal cancer. *Cancer Research.* 2002;62(18):5126–5128.

39. Liu Y, Chattopadhyay N, Qin S et al. Coordinate integrin and c-Met signaling regulate Wnt gene expression during epithelial morphogenesis. *Development.* 2009; 136(5):843–853.

40. Monga SP, Mars WM, Pediaditakis P et al. Hepatocyte growth factor induces Wnt-independent nuclear translocation of beta-catenin after Met-beta-catenin dissociation in hepatocytes. *Cancer Research.* 2002;62(7):2064–2071.

41. Rong S, Bodescot M, Blair D et al. Tumorigenicity of the met proto-oncogene and the gene for hepatocyte growth factor. *Molecular and Cellular Biology.* 1992;12(11):5152–5158.

42. Rong S, Segal S, Anver M et al. Invasiveness and metastasis of NIH 3T3 cells induced by Met-hepatocyte growth factor/scatter factor autocrine stimulation. *Proceedings of the National Academy of Sciences of the United States of America.* 1994;91(11):4731–4735.

43. Follenzi A, Bakovic S, Gual P et al. Cross-talk between the proto-oncogenes Met and Ron. *Oncogene.* 2000;19(27):3041–3049.

44. Park M, Dean M, Cooper CS et al. Mechanism of met oncogene activation. *Cell.* 1986;45(6):895–904.

45. Prat M, Crepaldi T, Gandino L et al. C-terminal truncated forms of Met, the hepatocyte growth factor receptor. *Molecular and Cellular Biology.* 1991;11(12):5954–5962.

46. Wallenius V, Hisaoka M, Helou K et al. Overexpression of the hepatocyte growth factor (HGF) receptor (Met) and presence of a truncated and activated intracellular HGF receptor fragment in locally aggressive/malignant human musculoskeletal tumors. *The American Journal of Pathology.* 2000;156(3):821–829.

47. Houldsworth J, Cordon-Cardo C, Ladanyi M et al. Gene amplification in gastric and esophageal adenocarcinomas. *Cancer Research.* 1990;50(19):6417–6422.

48. Kuniyasu H, Yasui W, Kitadai Y et al. Frequent amplification of the c-met gene in scirrhous type stomach cancer. *Biochemical and Biophysical Research Communications.* 1992;189(1):227–232.

49. Rege-Cambrin G, Scaravaglio P, Carozzi F et al. Karyotypic analysis of gastric carcinoma cell lines carrying an amplified c-met oncogene. *Cancer Genetics and Cytogenetics.* 1992;64(2):170–173.

50. Tan YH, Krishnaswamy S, Nandi S et al. CBL is frequently altered in lung cancers: its relationship to mutations in MET and EGFR tyrosine kinases. *PloS One.* 2010;5(1):e8972.

51. Pennacchietti S, Michieli P, Galluzzo M et al. Hypoxia promotes invasive growth by transcriptional activation of the met protooncogene. *Cancer Cell.* 2003;3(4):347–361.

52. Bauer TW, Somcio RJ, Fan F et al. Regulatory role of c-Met in insulin-like growth factor-I receptor-mediated migration and invasion of human pancreatic carcinoma cells. *Molecular Cancer Therapeutics.* 2006;5(7):1676–1682.

53. Khoury H, Naujokas MA, Zuo D et al. HGF converts ErbB2/Neu epithelial morphogenesis to cell invasion. *Molecular Biology of the Cell.* 2005;16(2):550–561.

54. Derman MP, Cunha MJ, Barros EJ et al. HGF-mediated chemotaxis and tubulogenesis require activation of the phosphatidylinositol 3-kinase. *The American Journal of Physiology.* 1995;268(6 Pt 2):F1211–F1217.

55. Ma PC, Kijima T, Maulik G et al. c-MET mutational analysis in small cell lung cancer: novel juxtamembrane domain mutations regulating cytoskeletal functions. *Cancer Research.* 2003;63(19):6272–6281.

56. Allory Y, Culine S, de la Taille A. Kidney cancer pathology in the new context of targeted therapy. *Pathobiology: Journal of Immunopathology, Molecular and Cellular Biology.* 2011;78(2):90–98.

57. Schmidt LS, Nickerson ML, Angeloni D et al. Early onset hereditary papillary renal carcinoma: Germline missense mutations in the tyrosine kinase domain of the met proto-oncogene. *The Journal of Urology.* 2004;172(4 Pt 1):1256–1261.

58. Bellon SF, Kaplan-Lefko P, Yang Y et al. c-Met inhibitors with novel binding mode show activity against several hereditary papillary renal cell carcinoma-related mutations. *The Journal of Biological Chemistry.* 2008;283(5):2675–2683.

59. Bommi-Reddy A, Almeciga I, Sawyer J et al. Kinase requirements in human cells: III. Altered kinase requirements in VHL-/- cancer cells detected in a pilot synthetic lethal screen. *Proceedings of the National Academy of Sciences of the United States of America.* 2008;105(43):16484–16489.

60. Copeland E, Balgobin S, Lee CM et al. hTID-1 defines a novel regulator of c-Met Receptor signaling in renal cell carcinomas. *Oncogene.* 2011;30(19):2252–2263.

61. Di Renzo MF, Olivero M, Martone T et al. Somatic mutations of the MET oncogene are selected during metastatic spread of human HNSC carcinomas. *Oncogene.* 2000;19(12):1547–1555.

62. Li Y, Zhang S, Tang Z et al. Silencing of c-Met by RNA interference inhibits the survival, proliferation, and invasion of nasopharyngeal carcinoma cells. *Tumour Biology: The Journal of the International Society for Oncodevelopmental Biology and Medicine.* 2011;32(6):1217–1224.

63. Seiwert TY, Jagadeeswaran R, Faoro L et al. The MET receptor tyrosine kinase is a potential novel therapeutic target for head and neck squamous cell carcinoma. *Cancer Research.* 2009;69(7):3021–3031.

64. Vermorken JB, Trigo J, Hitt R et al. Open-label, uncontrolled, multicenter phase II study to evaluate the efficacy and toxicity of cetuximab as a single agent in patients with recurrent and/or metastatic squamous cell carcinoma of the head and neck who failed to respond to platinum-based therapy. *Journal of Clinical Oncology.* 2007;25(16):2171–2177.

65. Grandis JR, Tweardy DJ. Elevated levels of transforming growth factor alpha and epidermal growth factor receptor messenger RNA are early markers of carcinogenesis in head and neck cancer. *Cancer Research.* 1993;53(15):3579–3584.

66. Xu H, Stabile LP, Gubish CT et al. Dual blockade of EGFR and c-Met abrogates redundant signaling and proliferation in head and neck carcinoma cells. *Clinical Cancer Research*. 2011;17(13):4425–4438.
67. Kong-Beltran M, Stamos J, Wickramasinghe D. The Sema domain of Met is necessary for receptor dimerization and activation. *Cancer Cell*. 2004;6(1):75–84.
68. Seo JS, Ju YS, Lee WC et al. The transcriptional landscape and mutational profile of lung adenocarcinoma. *Genome Research*. 2012;22(11):2109–2119.
69. Ma PC, Jagadeeswaran R, Jagadeesh S et al. Functional expression and mutations of c-Met and its therapeutic inhibition with SU11274 and small interfering RNA in non-small cell lung cancer. *Cancer Research*. 2005;65(4):1479–1488.
70. Kanteti R, Nallasura V, Loganathan S et al. PAX5 is expressed in small-cell lung cancer and positively regulates c-Met transcription. *Laboratory Investigation; A Journal of Technical Methods and Pathology*. 2009;89(3):301–314.
71. Pao W, Chmielecki J. Rational, biologically based treatment of EGFR-mutant non-small-cell lung cancer. *Nature Reviews Cancer*. 2010;10(11):760–774.
72. Lai AZ, Durrant M, Zuo D et al. Met kinase-dependent loss of the E3 ligase Cbl in gastric cancer. *The Journal of Biological Chemistry*. 2012;287(11):8048–8059.
73. Graziano F, Galluccio N, Lorenzini P et al. Genetic activation of the MET pathway and prognosis of patients with high-risk, radically resected gastric cancer. *Journal of Clinical Oncology*. 2011;29(36):4789–4795.
74. Lennerz JK, Kwak EL, Ackerman A et al. MET amplification identifies a small and aggressive subgroup of esophagogastric adenocarcinoma with evidence of responsiveness to crizotinib. *Journal of Clinical Oncology*. 2011;29(36):4803–4810.
75. Watson GA, Zhang X, Stang MT et al. Inhibition of c-Met as a therapeutic strategy for esophageal adenocarcinoma. *Neoplasia*. 2006;8(11):949–955.
76. Chen CT, Kim H, Liska D et al. MET activation mediates resistance to lapatinib inhibition of HER2-amplified gastric cancer cells. *Molecular Cancer Therapeutics*. 2012;11(3):660–669.
77. Migliore C, Martin V, Leoni VP et al. MiR-1 downregulation cooperates with MACC1 in promoting MET overexpression in human colon cancer. *Clinical Cancer Research*. 2012;18(3):737–747.
78. Boon EM, Kovarikova M, Derksen PW et al. MET signalling in primary colon epithelial cells leads to increased transformation irrespective of aberrant Wnt signalling. *British Journal of Cancer*. 2005;92(6):1078–1083.
79. Inno A, Di Salvatore M, Cenci T et al. Is there a role for IGF1R and c-MET pathways in resistance to cetuximab in metastatic colorectal cancer? *Clinical Colorectal Cancer*. 2011;10(4):325–332.
80. Catenacci DV, Cervantes G, Yala S et al. RON (MST1R) is a novel prognostic marker and therapeutic target for gastroesophageal adenocarcinoma. *Cancer Biology and Therapy*. 2011;12(1):9–46.
81. Nahta R, Esteva FJ. Trastuzumab: Triumphs and tribulations. *Oncogene*. 2007;26(25):3637–3643.
82. Valabrega G, Montemurro F, Aglietta M. Trastuzumab: Mechanism of action, resistance and future perspectives in HER2-overexpressing breast cancer. *Annals of Oncology*. 2007;18(6):977–984.
83. Shattuck DL, Miller JK, Carraway KL, 3rd et al. Met receptor contributes to trastuzumab resistance of Her2-overexpressing breast cancer cells. *Cancer Research*. 2008;68(5):1471–1477.
84. Jakubczak JL, LaRochelle WJ, Merlino G. NK1, a natural splice variant of hepatocyte growth factor/scatter factor, is a partial agonist in vivo. *Molecular and Cellular Biology*. 1998;18(3):1275–1283.

85. Youles M, Holmes O, Petoukhov MV et al. Engineering the NK1 fragment of hepatocyte growth factor/scatter factor as a MET receptor antagonist. *Journal of Molecular Biology.* 2008;377(3):616–622.

86. Tolbert WD, Daugherty-Holtrop J, Gherardi E et al. Structural basis for agonism and antagonism of hepatocyte growth factor. *Proceedings of the National Academy of Sciences of the United States of America.* 2010;107(30):13264–13269.

87. Date K, Matsumoto K, Shimura H et al. HGF/NK4 is a specific antagonist for pleiotrophic actions of hepatocyte growth factor. *FEBS Letters.* 1997;420(1):1–6.

88. Giordano S. Rilotumumab, a mAb against human hepatocyte growth factor for the treatment of cancer. *Current Opinion in Molecular Therapeutics.* 2009;11(4):448–455.

89. Jun HT, Sun J, Rex K et al. AMG 102, a fully human anti-hepatocyte growth factor/ scatter factor neutralizing antibody, enhances the efficacy of temozolomide or docetaxel in U-87 MG cells and xenografts. *Clinical Cancer Research.* 2007;13(22 Pt 1): 6735–6742.

90. Rosen PJ, Sweeney CJ, Park DJ et al. A phase Ib study of AMG 102 in combination with bevacizumab or motesanib in patients with advanced solid tumors. *Clinical Cancer Research.* 2010;16(9):2677–2687.

91. Zhu M, Tang R, Doshi S et al. Exposure-response (E-R) analysis of rilotumumab (R, AMG 102) plus epirubicin/cisplatin/capecitabine (ECX) in patients (pts) with locally advanced or metastatic gastric or esophagogastric junction (G/EGJ) cancer. *Journal of Clinical Oncology.* 2012;30(suppl):abstr 2535.

92. Schoffski P, Garcia JA, Stadler WM et al. A phase II study of the efficacy and safety of AMG 102 in patients with metastatic renal cell carcinoma. *BJU International.* 2011;108(5):679–686.

93. Wen PY, Schiff D, Cloughesy TF et al. A phase II study evaluating the efficacy and safety of AMG 102 (rilotumumab) in patients with recurrent glioblastoma. *Neuro-Oncology.* 2011;13(4):437–446.

94. Martens T, Schmidt NO, Eckerich C et al. A novel one-armed anti-c-Met antibody inhibits glioblastoma growth in vivo. *Clinical Cancer Research.* 2006;12(20 Pt 1):6144–6152.

95. Jin H, Yang R, Zheng Z et al. MetMAb, the one-armed 5D5 anti-c-Met antibody, inhibits orthotopic pancreatic tumor growth and improves survival. *Cancer Research.* 2008;68(11):4360–4368.

96. Moss RA, Bothos JG, Filvaroff E et al. Phase Ib dose-escalation study of MetMAb, a monovalent antagonist antibody to the receptor MET, in combination with bevacizumab in patients with locally advanced or metastatic solid tumors. *Journal of Clinical Oncology.* 2010;28(suppl):abstr e13050.

97. Catenacci DV, Henderson L, Xiao SY et al. Durable complete response of metastatic gastric cancer with anti-Met therapy followed by resistance at recurrence. *Cancer Discovery.* 2011;1(7):573–579.

98. Spigel DR, Ervin TJ, Ramlau R et al. Final efficacy results from OAM4558g, a randomized phase II study evaluating MetMAb or placebo in combination with erlotinib in advanced NSCLC. *Journal of Clinical Oncology.* 2011;29:(suppl);abstr 7505.

99. Tan E, Park K, Lim WT et al. Phase 1b study of ficlatuzumab (AV-299), an anti-hepatocyte growth factor monoclonal antibody, in combination with gefitinib in Asian patients with NSCLC, in poster presented at the *2010 ASCO Annual Meeting 2010*, Chicago, IL.

100. Schelter F, Kobuch J, Moss ML et al. A disintegrin and metalloproteinase-10 (ADAM-10) mediates DN30 antibody-induced shedding of the met surface receptor. *The Journal of Biological Chemistry.* 2010;285(34):26335–26340.

101. Pacchiana G, Chiriaco C, Stella MC et al. Monovalency unleashes the full therapeutic potential of the DN-30 anti-Met antibody. *The Journal of Biological Chemistry.* 2010;285(46):36149–36157.

102. Schiller JH, Akerley WL, Brugger W et al. Results from ARQ 197–209: A global randomized placebo-controlled phase II clinical trial of erlotinib plus ARQ 197 versus erlotinib plus placebo in previously treated EGFR inhibitor-naive patients with locally advanced or metastatic non-small cell lung cancer (NSCLC). *Journal of Clinical Oncology.* 28:18s, 2010 (suppl; abstr LBA7502).

103. Wagner AJ, Goldberg JM, Dubois SG et al. Tivantinib (ARQ 197), a selective inhibitor of MET, in patients with microphthalmia transcription factor-associated tumors: Results of a multicenter phase 2 trial. *Cancer.* 2012;118(23):5894–5902.

104. Santoro A, Rimassa L, Borbath I et al. Tivantinib for second-line treatment of advanced hepatocellular carcinoma: A randomised, placebo-controlled phase 2 study. *The Lancet Oncology.* 2013;14(1):55–63.

105. Yakes FM, Chen J, Tan J et al. Cabozantinib (XL184), a novel MET and VEGFR2 inhibitor, simultaneously suppresses metastasis, angiogenesis, and tumor growth. *Molecular Cancer Therapeutics.* 2011;10(12):2298–2308.

106. Cohn AL, Kelley RK, Yang TS et al. Activity of cabozantinib (XL184) in hepatocellular carcinoma patients (pts): Results from a phase II randomized discontinuation trial (RDT). *Journal of Clinical Oncology* 2012;30(suppl 4): abstr 261.

107. Hussain M, Smith MR, Sweeney C et al. Cabozantinib (XL184) in metastatic castration-resistant prostate cancer (mCRPC): Results from a phase II randomized discontinuation trial. *Journal of Clinical Oncology* 2011;29(suppl):abstr 4516.

108. Kurzrock R, Sherman SI, Ball DW et al. Activity of XL184 (Cabozantinib), an oral tyrosine kinase inhibitor, in patients with medullary thyroid cancer. *Journal of Clinical Oncology.* 2011;29(19):2660–2666.

109. Schoffski P, Elisei R, Müller S et al. An international, double-blind, randomized, placebo-controlled phase III trial (EXAM) of cabozantinib (XL184) in medullary thyroid carcinoma (MTC) patients (pts) with documented RECIST progression at baseline. *Journal of Clinical Oncology* 2012;30(suppl):abstr 5508.

110. Zou HY, Li Q, Lee JH et al. An orally available small-molecule inhibitor of c-Met, PF-2341066, exhibits cytoreductive antitumor efficacy through antiproliferative and antiangiogenic mechanisms. *Cancer Research.* 2007;67(9):4408–4417.

111. Tanizaki J, Okamoto I, Okamoto K et al. MET tyrosine kinase inhibitor crizotinib (PF-02341066) shows differential antitumor effects in non-small cell lung cancer according to MET alterations. *Journal of Thoracic Oncology.* 2011;6(10):1624–1631.

112. Chi AS, Batchelor TT, Kwak EL et al. Rapid radiographic and clinical improvement after treatment of a MET-amplified recurrent glioblastoma with a mesenchymal-epithelial transition inhibitor. *Journal of Clinical Oncology.* 2012;30(3):e30–e33.

113. Eder JP, Shapiro GI, Appleman LJ et al. A phase I study of foretinib, a multi-targeted inhibitor of c-Met and vascular endothelial growth factor receptor 2. *Clinical Cancer Research.* 2010;16(13):3507–3516.

114. Eder JP, Heath E, Appleman L et al. Phase I experience with c-MET inhibitor XL880 administered orally to patients (pts) with solid tumors. *Journal of Clinical Oncology, 2007 ASCO Annual Meeting Proceedings Part I* 2007;25(18S) (June 20 Supplement):3526.

115. Abidoye O, Murukurthy N, Salgia R. Review of clinic trials: Agents targeting c-Met. *Reviews on Recent Clinical Trials.* 2007;2(2):143–147.

10 Targeting Stem Cells

Marcello Maugeri-Saccà
Regina Elena National Cancer Institute

Ruggero De Maria
Regina Elena National Cancer Institute

CONTENTS

INTRODUCTION

The heterogenic nature of tumors has been noted since the earliest pathological examinations. This heterogeneity is traditionally explained by coexisting distinct tumorigenic and mutant clones arising from random genetic and epigenetic events. According to this belief, cells undergoing these changes gain a survival advantage over other inhabitants of the tumor and a greater plasticity in enduring and adapting to environmental perturbations (stochastic or clonal evolution model).[1] Accumulating evidence suggests that tumorigenic ability is not a trait that all cancer cells share, but it is confined to an uncommon and phenotypically distinct population possessing two peculiar properties: capacity for self-renewal and ability to differentiate into multiple lineages.[2–6] Such properties are characteristics of adult stem cells that enable them to fulfill physiological needs and to thwart conditions requiring an accelerated cellular turnover. Through self-renewal, stem cells divide without depleting the undifferentiated pool, while providing a progeny that lost "stemness" properties to undertake a stepwise differentiation. The existence of a subset of cancer cells resembling normal stem cells, referred to as cancer stem cells (CSCs), allowed to predict a "stem-cell-centric" model of cancer. This model of the origin of cancer helped to envision an adult stem cell as the target of oncogenic hits and to postulate the existence of a stringent cellular hierarchy also in tumors. According to this "hierarchical model," a tumor possesses a pyramidal organization where the entire tumor population descends from a common ancestor represented by a CSC residing at the apex of the pyramid.[7] In this scenario, the intrinsic plasticity of the founder, which retains the functional properties of its normal counterpart, explains tumor heterogeneity. Although the two models of the origin of cancer are seemingly contradictory, both theories have evolved partially losing their exclusive nature. The convergence of the clonal evolution and hierarchical models derived from a more profound characterization of the actual tumor-propagating population and a better definition of the role of microenvironmental stimuli on tumor cells. While the CSC model originally stated that only stem-like cells can propagate the tumor, recent evidence shows that multiple tumor-initiating clones, represented by both CSCs and their proximal offspring, can coexist and account for the different temporal patterns of tumor formation upon serial transplantation into the murine background.[8] Therefore, this type of biological behavior is probably due to the clonal evolution of distinct CSC clones. Secondly, the possibility of reprogramming differentiated cells into pluripotent cells through the forced expression of four embryonic stem cell-specific transcription factors indicated that the "stemness" state is not a static condition and that the differentiation program is not unidirectional.[9] Although this groundbreaking evidence was perceived as a major advancement for regenerative medicine, it also triggered the same effect in experimental oncology. For instance, investigations revealed that both paracrine-acting pathways and some adverse conditions existing within the tumor microenvironment, such as hypoxia and low pH, instruct cancer cells to gain stem-like traits.[10,11] Even though it is unlikely that exogenous influences generate the whole CSC pool, these stimuli are involved in the process of maintaining and enriching CSCs, highlighting the fact that the retention/acquisition of stem-like features is a dynamic process. The CSC theory has therefore been refined by introducing microenvironmental variables, adding a further feature of the Darwinian evolutionary principles on which the clonal evolution model was shaped (Figure 10.1). The mechanisms driving the CSC–microenvironment interactions also assumed a bidirectional nature with the ability of CSCs to participate in generating blood vessels, a property interpreted as an attempt to render the microenvironment a tumor-promoting site.[12,13] In this chapter, we discuss recent advances in CSC biology that translate into innovative therapeutic opportunities, spanning from the development of anti-CSC compounds to generating innovative animal models for optimal preclinical testing of established and investigational anticancer agents. Finally, we discuss the exploitation of CSC-related parameters in the clinical setting.

DEVELOPMENT OF CSC-FOCUSED ANTICANCER AGENTS

Even though it is still unclear whether pharmacological strategies directed against the CSC compartment lead to improving patient long-term outcomes, much effort toward identifying CSC-restricted pathways valuable for pharmacological inhibition has been done. The first wave of preclinical studies took advantage of the expanded knowledge on molecular mechanisms governing normal stem cell fate, relying on the assumption that stem cell-dedicated pathways may also be active in CSCs. This conceptual approach sparked researchers to focus on the developmental

Clonal evolution model
random genetic events/
hostile microenvironmental conditions

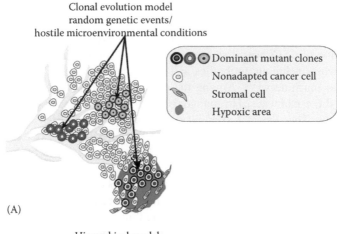

Dominant mutant clones
Nonadapted cancer cell
Stromal cell
Hypoxic area

(A)

Hierarchical model
The architecture of the tumor pyramid

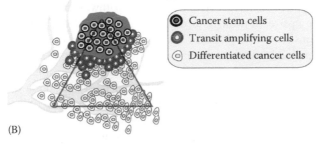

Cancer stem cells
Transit amplifying cells
Differentiated cancer cells

(B)

Clonal-Hierarchical model
The heterogeneity at the apex of the pyramid

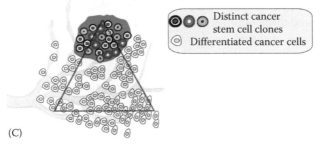

Distinct cancer
stem cell clones
Differentiated cancer cells

(C)

FIGURE 10.1 The "clonal evolution model" (panel A) postulates that dominant mutant clones arise from random genetic events and acquire a greater plasticity to adapt hostile conditions. According to the "hierarchical model" (panel B), tumors possess a pyramidal organization with CSCs at the apex of the pyramid. The combined "clonal evolution–hierarchical model" (panel C) suggests the coexistence of different CSC clones with distinct biological properties.

signals involved in the self-renewal program and the maintenance of the undifferentiated state, including Hedgehog (Hh), Notch, and Wnt pathways, as potential key regulators of many biological properties of CSCs. In the preclinical setting a preferential distribution of effectors of the aforementioned signals was observed in the CSC compartment compared to differentiated progeny.[14] In addition, a selective depletion of CSCs was documented in diverse tumor models adopting different approaches including antibodies and molecules acting at various levels of the intracellular machinery.[15–17] Among the pharmacological strategies developed for inhibiting these pathways, Hh antagonists are under advanced stages of clinical investigations. The steroidal alkaloid cyclopamine was the first molecule discovered to possess anti-Hh activity,[18] while additional Hh inhibitors endowed with more favorable pharmacological properties have been identified by high-throughput screening of small-molecule libraries.[19] By using this approach, a number of antagonists acting upstream the Hh cascade have been identified, and subsequent efforts have been carried out in order to characterize alternative strategies for pathway inhibition. Such investigations culminated into a number of clinical trials with different compounds (Table 10.1). Hh inhibition displayed encouraging antitumor activity against a niche of tumors, such as medulloblastoma and basal cell carcinoma, displaying the constitutive activation of the pathway produced by mutational events involving upstream positive or negative regulators.[20,21] Therefore, this clinical activity is consistent with targeting oncogene-addicted cells. Nevertheless, clinical trials designed to investigate the activity of GDC-0449 in metastatic colorectal and ovarian cancers, tumors characterized by a functional rather than constitutive activation of the pathway, failed to meet the primary endpoint.[22,23] A further aspect proposed for developing Hh antagonists is the co-targeting of interconnected signals triggering the Hh pathway in a noncanonical manner, such as the PI3K/AKT axis and TGF-β pathway.[24,25] Although this approach seemed effective in preclinical models, such combinations can be difficult to evaluate in the clinical setting until evidence of either single-agent activity or synergism with established anticancer regimens is proven. The developmental Notch pathway is a juxtacrine signaling activated through cell-to-cell contacts.[26] This interaction produces a dual enzymatic cleavage of the engaged receptor that generates the Notch intracellular domain. This fragment moves to the nucleus and interacts with other effectors for assembling the transcriptional complex. The abrogation of Notch activity through gamma-secretase inhibitors (GSIs) or anti-receptor antibodies demonstrated a significant activity against glioblastoma and mammary CSCs.[27–29] Moreover, it has been shown that in breast cancer Notch interacts with established and targetable oncogenic pathways such as the estrogen receptor[30] and Erb-b family members,[28] thus opening the path for associating molecular-targeted agents. For instance, evidence that Notch becomes engaged when hormonal signals are pharmacologically inhibited has been translated into clinical trials aimed at assessing whether the addition of GSIs to endocrine therapy enhances the activity of current antihormone manipulations. The pharmacological interference with the Notch pathway has been explored also in colon CSCs in which the association of irinotecan with an anti-delta-like ligand 4 led to a reduced frequency of KRAS-mutant CSCs.[31] This finding contained potential clinical implications given that tumors harboring KRAS

TABLE 10.1

Clinical Trials with Smoothened Inhibitors

Drug	Tumor (Phase)	Therapy
GDC-0449	Basal cell carcinoma (approved)	Single agent
(Vismodegib)	Medulloblastoma (II)	Single agent, temozolomide
	Pancreatic cancer (II)	Gemcitabine and nab-paclitaxel, gemcitabine, erlotinib and gemcitabine, sirolimus
	Ovarian cancer (II)	Single agent
	Colorectal cancer (II)	FOLFOX or FOLFIRI plus bevacizumab
	Small cell lung cancer (II)	Cisplatin and etoposide
	Glioblastoma multiforme (II)	Single agent
	Sarcoma (II)	RO4929097 (GSI)
	Multiple myeloma (I)	RO4929097 (GSI)
	Breast cancer (I)	Single agent
BMS-833923	Small cell lung cancer (I)	Carboplatin and etoposide
	Basal cell carcinoma and basal cell nevoid Syndrome (I)	Single agent
	Chronic myeloid leukemia (I/II)	Dasatinib
	Gastric, gastroesophageal or esophageal adenocarcinomas (I)	Cisplatin and capecitabine
	Multiple myeloma (I)	Single agent, lenalidomide and dexamethasone, bortezomib
IPI-926	Pancreatic cancer (I/II)	Gemcitabine, FOLFIRINOX
(Saridegib)	Myelofibrosis (II)	Single agent
	Chondrosarcoma (II)	Single agent
	Head and neck cancer (I)	Cetuximab
PF-04449913	Acute myeloid leukemia and high-risk myelody splastic syndrome (I)	Cytarabine, decitabine, and daunorubicin
	Solid tumors (I)	Single agent
LDE-225	Basal cell carcinoma (II)	Single agent
	Small cell lung cancer (I)	Cisplatin and etoposide
	Pancreatic adenocarcinoma (I/II)	Gemcitabine, FOLFIRINOX
	Pediatric solid tumors (I)	Single agent
	Myeloid leukemia (I)	Nilotinib
	Advanced solid tumors (I)	PI3K inhibitor BKM120
LEQ-506	Advanced solid tumors (I)	Single agent

mutations are insensitive to anti-EGFR therapies. When considering the potential of anti-Notch strategies, however, it is worth noting that molecular mechanisms driving pathway activation have not yet been fully elucidated. In addition, in the context of the Notch family, some receptors seem to exert tumor-suppressive properties. This picture is further complicated by the tumor-dependent activity of Notch paralogs.[32,33] This observation calls for investigating anti-Notch therapies in more depth since the activity of GSIs could be hampered by the concomitant abrogation of negative pathway regulators. Although the exploitation of anti-delta-like ligand

4 has been proposed to overcome this drawback, preclinical investigations revealed considerable toxicity consisting in the onset of vascular tumors and liver histopathological alterations.[34] An overview of clinical trials with GSIs is provided in Tables 10.2 and 10.3. Wnt is the third pathway traditionally associated with stem cell maintenance. The on/off state of canonical Wnt signaling is mainly regulated at the level of β-catenin, a cytoplasmic protein that is usually maintained at low concentration by a destruction complex. Upon ligand–receptor interaction the inhibitory effects of the destruction complex are relieved enabling β-catenin to translocate to the nucleus and to recruit a set of proteins to form a transcriptional complex.[35] Even

TABLE 10.2
Clinical Trials with GSIs

Drug	Tumor (Phase)	Therapy
MK-0752	Breast cancer (no specified, neoadjuvant therapy)	Tamoxifen or letrozole
	Breast cancer (I/II)	Docetaxel
	Pancreatic cancer (I/II)	Gemcitabine
	Ovarian cancer, fallopian tube cancer, primary peritoneal cancer, colorectal cancer (I)	Dalotuzumab (IGFR1 inhibitor)
	CNS malignancies (I)	Single agent
	Leukemia/lymphoma	Single agent
	Advanced solid tumors	Ridaforolimus (mTOR inhibitor)
RO4929097	Breast cancer (I/II)	Exemestane
	Breast cancer (II)	Single agent
	Breast cancer (I, neoadjuvant therapy)	Letrozole
	Breast cancer (I)	GDC-0449 (smoothened inhibitor)
	Triple-negative breast cancer (I, neoadjuvant therapy)	Paclitaxel and carboplatin
	Brain metastases (I/II)	Radiotherapy
	Colorectal cancer (II)	FOLFOX plus bevacizumab
	Colorectal cancer (II)	Single agent
	Colorectal cancer (I)	Cetuximab
	Non-small cell lung cancer (II)	Single agent
	Non-small cell lung cancer (I)	Erlotinib
	Sarcoma (I/II)	GDC-0449 (smoothened inhibitor)
	Prostate cancer (II)	Bicalutamide
	Pancreatic cancer (I, neoadjuvant therapy)	Single agent
	Pancreatic cancer (II)	Single agent
	Glioblastoma (II)	Single agent
	Glioblastoma (I)	Radiotherapy and temozolomide
	Glioblastoma (I/II)	Bevacizumab
	Multiple myeloma(II)	Melphalan
	Melanoma (II)	Single agent
	Melanoma (I)	Cisplatin, vinblastine, and temozolomide
	Advanced solid tumors (I)	Cediranib
	Childhood cancers (I)	Dexamethasone

TABLE 10.3

Completed Clinical Trials with GSIs

Drug	Trial Combination (Phase, Tumor)	Number of Patients	Schedule	MTD/DLTs	Antitumor Activity	Notes
MK-0752[66]	Single agent (I, advanced solid tumors)	103	Continuous daily dosing (schedule A, n=21) or 3 days on/4 days off (schedule B, n=17) or once per week (schedule C, n=65)	Schedule A: 450 and 600 mg exceeded the MTD/nausea, vomiting, diarrhea Schedule B: 450 mg once daily/fatigue Schedule C: 3200 mg/ diarrhea and fatigue	1CR (anaplastic astrocytoma/schedule C) 1 SD>1 year (glioblastoma multiforme/schedule C) 11 SD>4 cycles (10 gliomas/10 in schedule C and 1 in schedule B)	Effective modulation of Notch genes in hair follicles No evidence of activity in extracranial tumors
MK-0752[67]	Single agent (I, children with CNS malignancies)	23	3 days on/4 days off of a 28-day cycle	260 mg/m^2 once daily/ increased transaminases	2 SD>3 cycles	Notch pathway expressed and active (nuclear expression of HES1 and HES5)

(continued)

TABLE 10.3 (continued)
Completed Clinical Trials with GSIs

Drug	Trial Combination (Phase, Tumor)	Number of Patients	Schedule	MTD/DLTs	Antitumor Activity	Notes
RO4929097[68]	Single agent (I, advanced solid tumors)	110	3 days on/4 days off for 2 weeks followed by a week of rest (schedule A, n=58) or days 1–7 of a 3-week cycle (schedule B, n=47) or continuous daily dosing for a 3-week cycle (schedule C, n=5; expanded cohort)	Schedule A: MTD not defined (dose escalation continued to 270 mg) Schedule B: MTD not defined (dose escalation continued to 135 mg)	1 PR (colorectal adenocarcinoma/ schedule B) 1 mixed response-stable disease (sarcoma/ schedule B) 1 nearly CR (melanoma, schedule B) 34 SD>4 cycles (16 in schedule A, 18 in schedule B)	SD more common in melanoma, sarcoma, and ovarian carcinoma Dose escalation (schedules A and B) halted for PK evidence of CYP3A4 autoinduction
RO4929097[69]	Single agent (II, pretreated metastatic colorectal cancer)	37	20 mg daily, 3 days on/4 days off of a 28-day cycle		0 CR/PR 6 SD mPFS 1.8 months OS 6.0 months	No drug-related G3–4 toxicities G1–2 toxicities mainly gastrointestinal

Abbreviations: MTD, maximum tolerated dose; DLTs, dose-limiting toxicities; CR, complete response; PR, partial response; SD, stable disease; HES1 and HES5, hairy enhancer of split-1 and split-5.

though the tumor-promoting ability of this pathway was elucidated since the "adenoma to carcinoma sequence," Wnt continues to be an orphan pathway, given that its modulation has been achieved mainly indirectly, and specific molecular-targeted agents are at very early stage of clinical development. Moreover, the impact of Wnt signal on the biological properties of CSCs remains largely unexplored and confined to colon cancer. In this model, increased Wnt activity identifies colon CSCs, while myofibroblast-derived factors activate the pathway conferring stem-like traits to cancer cells.[36] More recently, elevated nuclear β-catenin content has been associated with resistance to PI3K and AKT inhibitors in patient-derived primary cultures and deriving xenografts.[37] Overall, when considering the therapeutic applications of molecular-targeted agents inhibiting self-renewal pathways and, more in general, putative anti-CSC compounds, some bottlenecks are encountered and should be overcome before embarking in clinical trials. Among these is the difficulty in isolating pure CSC populations, a degree of interlaboratory variability in the isolation and characterization procedures, and optimal methods for measuring CSC-based endpoints.

ALTERNATIVE STRATEGIES FOR CSC TARGETING

It is known that different cells possess a distinct spectrum of resistance to endogenous and environmental stress. When the ability to survive stressful conditions, such as the exposition to chemotherapeutics, has been explored within the context of the hierarchical organization of adult tissues, a greater resistance was observed in the stem cell compartment compared to more differentiated cells.[38] This distinct pattern of response is correlated with the need for protecting cellular precursors deputed to reestablish the damaged tissue. The first clinical implication emerging from the characterization of CSCs isolated from patient specimens was that standard chemotherapeutic agents are rather ineffective against this cellular subset.[39] Therefore, a further key functional property appeared to be common to normal and malignant stem cells. Although the development of chemo-potentiating strategies has been pursued since the beginning of oncological research, such attempts failed in clinical investigations. However, both the development of a renewed pipeline of chemotherapy-enhancing agents and the possibility to test such compounds in the actual tumorigenic population isolated from each patient tumor instead of commercial cell lines allowed to better define the biological context for blocking chemoresistance-associated mechanisms. The most relevant of these is the system deputed to protect the integrity of the genome. The DNA damage response (DDR), the network ensuring the repair of genetic lesions, is composed by a large set of proteins belonging to different but interconnected pathways that can be grouped into cell cycle checkpoints, DNA damage repair pathways, and apoptotic signals.[40] While these pathways physiologically avoid that nonlethal mutations are amplified through the transmission to the offspring, in cancer cells these signals are improperly activated and exploited for constraining harmful insults. The biological framework for the hyperproficient activation of these protective signals in cancer cells is probably the need for counteracting oncogene-induced senescence and apoptosis.[41] In fact, the development of a fully malignant phenotype requires the evolution of a compensatory response to endogenous stresses, such as those correlated with rapid replicative kinetics. To a similar extent, these molecular circuits are used to limit chemotherapy-induced death. The first event of the molecular cascade is the activation of cell cycle checkpoints deputed to halt the cell cycle when a DNA damage is sensed. This activity permits the recruitment of DNA repair pathways and subsequently of the apoptotic machinery if the repair activity cannot be successfully carried out or the damage exceeds repair ability. The checkpoint kinases 1 and 2 (Chk1 and Chk2) are central components of the DDR. While Chk2 is generally accepted to be an amplifier, Chk1 exerts a wider spectrum of activity spanning from cell cycle checkpoints (intra-S-phase checkpoint, G2-M checkpoint, mitotic spindle checkpoint) to the homologous recombination, the Fanconi anemia/BRCA pathway, and the apoptotic response.[42] Evidence that CSCs activate the DDR network more rapidly than the differentiated counterparts stemmed from experiments conducted with CSCs isolated form primary brain tumors. Investigators reported that the CSC pool survived ionizing radiations through a prompt activation of Chk1 and Chk2, as opposed to the non-CSC population.[43] A further report indirectly linked an increased basal activation of the DDR machinery to chemo-radioresistance of glioblastoma stem cells.[44] Likewise, the activation of Chk1 was the most precocious molecular event detected in lung CSCs exposed to chemotherapy.[45] In this experimental setting, the pharmacological abrogation of Chk1 restored chemosensitivity, while a similar outcome was observed in colon CSCs.[46] Given this multifaceted involvement of Chk1 and Chk2 into the DDR, many Chk1 or dual Chk1/Chk2 inhibitors have been developed and entered early phases of clinical development (Table 10.4), although safety issues emerged with some of these compounds.[47] The interference with the apoptotic machinery and the use of differentiation-inducing agents are further pharmacological strategies proposed for increasing chemotherapy efficacy against CSCs. In different epithelial cancers interleukin-4 (IL-4) produces an amplification of anti-apoptotic mediators,[48] a mechanism that seems to be maintained also by CSCs.[49] Consistent with this, the abrogation of the IL-4 signal with either a neutralizing antibody or a mutant form of IL-4 reverted the chemotherapy-resistant phenotype of CSCs.[50] When considering compounds capable of inducing differentiation, the attention turns to retinoic acid, a molecule used for treating patients with hematological malignancies and investigated also in solid tumors. Retinoic acid efficiently differentiates glioblastoma stem cells in a process accompanied by the downregulation of Notch components.[51] Furthermore, the identification of differentiation-inducing agents is taking advantage of the growing body of knowledge on the differentiation path of normal stem cells. Bone morphogenetic protein 4 (BMP4) promotes the differentiation of normal colonic stem cells, a phenomenon recapitulated in the malignant counterpart in which the BMP4-inducted differentiation is associated with chemosensitization.[52] Finally, molecules inhibiting adenosine triphosphate (ATP)-binding cassette transporters (ABC transporters) have been proposed as potential anti-CSC drugs, based on the observations that ABC pumps are highly expressed in adult stem cells and CSCs. Nevertheless, both preclinical observations showing that chemoresistance of CSCs is probably independent from multidrug resistance proteins[53] and clinical evidence demonstrating

TABLE 10.4

Clinical Development of Chk1 Inhibitors

Drug	Trial Combination (Phase, Tumor)	DLTs	Future Development
AZD7762[47,70]	AZD7762 + irinotecan (I, AST)	Cardiotoxicity, diarrhea, decreased appetite, dehydration, increased alanine aminotransferase, febrile neutropenia	Program stopped
	AZD7762 + gemcitabine (I, AST)	Cardiotoxicity, neutropenia, vomiting, and nausea	
PF00477736[71]	PF00477736 + gemcitabine (I, AST)	Thrombocytopenia, sudden death, mucositis, elevated lipase	Program stopped
SCH900776[72]	SCH900776 + gemcitabine (I, AST)	Cardiotoxicity, thrombocytopenia	Unknown (no active trials)
LY2603618[73]	LY2603618 + pemetrexed (I, AST)	Diarrhea, infusion-related reaction, thrombocytopenia, fatigue	Phase I/II (NSCLC) in combination with cisplatin and pemetrexed Phase I/II (pancreatic cancer) in combination with gemcitabine

Abbreviations: DLTs, dose-limiting toxicities; AST, advanced solid tumors; NSCLC, non-small cell lung cancer.

an overall ineffectiveness of first- and second-generation ABC inhibitors are hindering the development of this class of anticancer agents.[54]

CSC-BASED ANIMAL MODELS

It is estimated that ~95% of compounds with documented anticancer activity in the preclinical setting fail during clinical development. Although multiple factors concur in determining this high attrition rate for anticancer drugs, the unreliability of current animal models represents a critical hurdle. The screening of new molecules has been traditionally conducted across the NCI 60 panel. However, it is known that commercial cell lines fail to recreate a tumor resembling the human disease since genetic/epigenetic changes occur as an adaptive response to nonphysiological environmental conditions. Commercial cell lines are broadly used for generating subcutaneous xenografts. One the one hand, this model allows to explore candidate predictive biomarkers in the target tissue, avoids the need for imaging techniques for monitoring tumor response, and further permits pharmacokinetic, pharmacodynamic, and safety evaluations.[55] On the other hand, subcutaneous xenografts lack appropriate microenvironmental stimuli and fail to recapitulate the natural history of human tumors due to the limited rate of metastasis generation. Although part of these major criticisms has been addressed with the development of orthotopic models, consisting in the implantation of tumor cells into the anatomical site of origin, the exploitation of commercial cell lines remains a critical barrier for the development of novel anticancer agents. To overcome these drawbacks, investigators explored patient-derived tumor xenografts, consisting in the ectopic or orthotopic implantation of fresh surgical tissues.[56] These xenografts preserve the histological architecture of the parental tumor, contain functional human stromal components, and have been used for evaluating the concordance between outcomes produced by an anticancer treatment in mice and humans and for testing investigational compounds.[57,58] Potential limitations of this model consist in requiring fresh tumors, the poor take rate of some tumors, the amount of time required, the definition of the optimal recipient strains, and an experimental algorithm requiring a large number of animals. The discovery of tumorigenic CSCs fueled an alternative way for obtaining tumor in mice that retain the biological characteristics of each individual patient tumor.[59] The delivery of spheroids, which are enriched for CSCs, has been found to recapitulate the parental tumor in mice at the histological level. Moreover, our unpublished data suggest that CSC-generated xenografts possess and maintain the proteomic profile of the tumor of origin and continue to reproduce the original tumor after long-term culture. Therefore, CSCs represent a virtually unlimited source of biological materials and allow to investigate both innovative anticancer agents and predictive biomarkers within the context of the tumor hierarchy. Even more importantly, the onset of liver metastasis has been observed upon the orthotopic injection of colon CSCs, but not in subcutaneous models, a finding that further highlights the biological relevance of maintaining appropriate environmental conditions.[59] In conclusion, setting up reliable animal models is of utmost importance for optimally delineating the spectrum of antitumor activities of novel molecular-targeted agents. To do this, a direct comparison of primary tumor fragment-derived and CSC-derived xenografts should be performed in order to determine the reliability of the two systems in terms of rate of tumor formation, metastasis generation, and maintenance of the original molecular portraits. A further key step toward optimal preclinical testing of anticancer agents is to model in animals both human tumors and patient-related factors for testing new classes of anticancer agents, such as microenvironment-acting compounds or agents targeting immune checkpoints.

CSC CONCEPT APPLIED TO TRANSLATIONAL ONCOLOGY

The growing body of knowledge on CSC biology has fostered clinical investigations aimed at assessing the prognostic or predictive value of CSC-related endpoints. By comparing gene-expression profiles of tumorigenic breast cancer cells and normal breast epithelium, investigators developed a prognostic signature predicting clinical outcomes of breast cancer patients.[60] This set of 186 differentially expressed genes, named "invasiveness" gene signature (IGS), correlated with metastasis-free survival and overall survival. Notably, the prognostic value of the IGS was conserved across different tumor types (medulloblastoma, lung cancer, and prostate cancer). Moreover, none of the 186 genes overlapped with other established molecular predictors, and only six genes were shared with the wound-response signature. Similarly, a microarray signature profile dominated by an embryonic stem cell expression pattern seemed to identify a subset of prostate cancer patients with poor survival outcome.[61] In addition, the potential usefulness of this approach has been further confirmed with the identification of a leukemia stem cell–specific signature.[62] The prognostic utility of CSC-associated parameters has also been explored in a cohort of glioblastoma patients treated with surgical resection followed by chemoradiotherapy.[63] The in vitro generation of CSCs and the expression of CSC markers correlated with overall and progression-free survival. In this patient cohort the coexpression of CD133 and Ki67 was associated with very poor clinical outcomes. Finally, the analysis of 25 germline polymorphisms in a panel of genes previously associated with colon CSCs revealed that LGR5, CD44, and ALDH1A1 polymorphisms identify a subset of high-risk stage II and stage III colon cancer patients with a significant shorter time to tumor recurrence.[64] The concept that CSCs are equipped with a multifaceted defensive machinery against chemicals provided a ready background for exploring the correlation between CSC-related parameters and effectiveness of current chemotherapeutic protocols. For instance, pre- and post neoadjuvant chemotherapy analysis of stem cell-associated parameters revealed an increase in the percentage of cells possessing stem cell markers and in the mammosphere formation efficiency following chemotherapy.[65] This suggested that while chemotherapy is effective against the bulk of tumor cells, the small fraction of CSCs survives unaltered current treatment protocols. Although evidence indicates that the measurement of CSC-related endpoints could add a further level of accuracy to current predictors, the small cohort of patients examined and the retrospective nature of these studies impose further evaluation to delineate the clinical applicability of stemness-related molecular endpoints. Moreover, how to measure the CSC pool still remains a controversial issue. Pre- and post therapy sphere-forming efficiency could determine CSC content, thus allowing to evaluate whether a given therapy successfully kills tumor-initiating cells. However, this approach is technically challenging and requires laboratories with a strong expertise in stem cell manipulation. The evaluation of putative CSC markers is less difficult and can be carried out also on circulating tumor cells, thus avoiding the need for collecting tissue samples. However, current CSC markers seem not to be restricted to the target population, and at least in some tumor types, both positive and negative cells meet the operative criteria to be defined CSCs.

CONCLUSIONS AND FUTURE DIRECTIONS

The discovery of CSCs has been the focus of an intense debate in the scientific research community. The existence of a cellular hierarchy in tumors brought into question decades of experimental research relying on the Darwinian evolutionary principles applied to neoplastic diseases. However, subsequent evidence allows to postulate a combined clonal evolution–hierarchical model, in which also external cues play a fundamental role in the maintenance and generation of cancer cells with stem-like biological properties, while in the meantime the apex of the pyramid is progressively losing its homogenous architecture. The functional characterization of CSCs exploited the elucidation of molecular mechanisms governing the homeostasis of healthy tissues. Based on the assumption that CSCs share the molecular machinery governing the fate of adult stem cells, a first wave of preclinical research has been conducted to determine whether also CSCs mainly rely on dedicated signal transduction pathways. This allowed to elucidate the existence of an asymmetry in the distribution of self-renewal pathway components, with a preferential distribution of these molecular effectors at the top of the tumor pyramid, and a preferential activity of self-renewal pathway inhibitors against CSCs. Nevertheless, early clinical investigations conducted with compounds inhibiting these pathways produced contradictory results. For instance, the activity of Hh antagonists appears to be until now confined to oncogene-addicted tumors, and clear evidence of anti-CSC activity is still lacking in the clinical setting due to the difficulty in exploring the CSC pool. Similar considerations can be applied to Notch inhibitors. While recent clinical trials provided some initial hints of antitumor activity,[66-69] whether this is ascribable to the targeting of the tumorigenic population is yet to be explored. In such a scenario, a better delineation of the modalities of pathway activation in each tumor and the development of inhibitors acting downstream the intracellular cascade are required. To a similar extent, whether or not pharmacological strategies developed for potentiating the cytotoxic effects of chemotherapy, such as Chk1 inhibitors,[47,70-73] or for reverting chemoresistance improve patients' outcomes remains to be addressed. Moreover, the development of compounds directed against CSCs might be burdened by off-target effects on normal stem cells. This potential effect should be considered and ideally assessed, before moving these agents to clinical investigations. The definition of the target population permits a more careful preclinical evaluation of investigational anticancer agents and avoids common artifacts coming from the use of commercial cancer cell lines. Nowadays, the generation of CSC-based tumor xenografts is considered the gold standard for recapitulating the human disease in mice. In this scenario, the orthotopic transplantation of CSCs in the appropriate murine background allows to recapitulate the various phases of the human disease in animals and to test new compounds in a close simulation of each clinical setting. However, the heterogeneity existing at the apex of the tumor pyramid should be taken into account, and a deeper characterization of distinct CSC clones is required to precisely dissect the antitumor properties of investigational agents. Finally, growing evidence suggests that innovative endpoints consisting in CSC-based molecular parameters could identify tumors characterized by an aggressive biological behavior. To this end, a more in-depth examination is required in order to define whether the integration of these molecular parameters into current predictors improves their accuracy. To sum up, the identification and characterization of the tumor-propagating population has added a further level of complexity to the pathobiology of tumors. Although many nodes remain to be solved, the examination and inhibition of signal transduction pathways linked to

CSC biology, the possibility to exploit CSCs for recreating the parental tumor in mice, and the examination of molecular endpoints correlated with CSCs in the clinical setting are expected to optimize the path from discovery to the clinic of innovative anticancer strategies.

ACKNOWLEDGMENT

The authors thank Giuseppe Loreto and Tania Merlino for technical assistance.

REFERENCES

1. Nowell PC. The clonal evolution of tumor cell populations. *Science* 1976;194:23–28.
2. Bonnet D, Dick JE. Human acute myeloid leukemia is organized as a hierarchy that originates from a primitive hematopoietic cell. *Nat Med* 1997;3:730–737.
3. Al-Hajj M, Wicha MS, Benito-Hernandez A et al. Prospective identification of tumorigenic breast cancer cells. *Proc Natl Acad Sci USA* 2003;100:3983–3988.
4. Eramo A, Lotti F, Sette G et al. Identification and expansion of the tumorigenic lung cancer stem cell population. *Cell Death Differ* 2008;15:504–514.
5. Ricci-Vitiani L, Lombardi DG, Pilozzi E et al. Identification and expansion of human colon-cancer-initiating cells. *Nature* 2007;445:111–115.
6. Todaro M, Iovino F, Eterno V et al. Tumorigenic and metastatic activity of human thyroid cancer stem cells. *Cancer Res* 2010;70:8874–8885.
7. Magee JA, Piskounova E, Morrison SJ. Cancer stem cells: Impact, heterogeneity, and uncertainty. *Cancer Cell* 2012;21:283–296.
8. Dieter SM, Ball CR, Hoffmann CM et al. Distinct types of tumor-initiating cells form human colon cancer tumors and metastases. *Cell Stem Cell* 2011;9:357–365.
9. Takahashi K, Yamanaka S. Induction of pluripotent stem cells from mouse embryonic and adult fibroblast cultures by defined factors. *Cell* 2006;126:663–676.
10. Li Z, Bao S, Wu Q et al. Hypoxia-inducible factors regulate tumorigenic capacity of glioma stem cells. *Cancer Cell* 2009;15:501–513.
11. Hjelmeland AB, Wu Q, Heddleston JM et al. Acidic stress promotes a glioma stem cell phenotype. *Cell Death Differ* 2011;18:829–840.
12. Ricci-Vitiani L, Pallini R, Biffoni M et al. Tumour vascularization via endothelial differentiation of glioblastoma stem-like cells. *Nature* 9;468:824–828.
13. Wang R, Chadalavada K, Wilshire J et al. Glioblastoma stem-like cells give rise to tumour endothelium. *Nature* 2010;468:829–833.
14. Peacock CD, Wang Q, Gesell GS et al. Hedgehog signaling maintains a tumor stem cell compartment in multiple myeloma. *Proc Natl Acad Sci USA* 2007;104:4048–4053.
15. Lauth M, Bergstrom A, Shimokawa T, Toftgard R. Inhibition of GLI-mediated transcription and tumor cell growth by small-molecule antagonists. *Proc Natl Acad Sci USA* 2007;104:8455–8460.
16. Hoey T, Yen WC, Axelrod F et al. DLL4 blockade inhibits tumor growth and reduces tumor-initiating cell frequency. *Cell Stem Cell* 2009;5:168–177.
17. Bar EE, Chaudhry A, Lin A et al. Cyclopamine-mediated hedgehog pathway inhibition depletes stem-like cancer cells in glioblastoma. *Stem Cells* 2007;25:2524–2533.
18. Chen JK, Taipale J, Cooper MK, Beachy PA. Inhibition of Hedgehog signaling by direct binding of cyclopamine to Smoothened. *Genes Dev* 2002;16:2743–2748.
19. Frank-Kamenetsky M, Zhang XM, Bottega S et al. Small-molecule modulators of Hedgehog signaling: Identification and characterization of smoothened agonists and antagonists. *J Biol* 2002;1:10.

20. Von Hoff DD, LoRusso PM, Rudin CM et al. Inhibition of the hedgehog pathway in advanced basal-cell carcinoma. *N Engl J Med* 2009;361:1164–1172.

21. Rudin CM, Hann CL, Laterra J et al. Treatment of medulloblastoma with hedgehog pathway inhibitor GDC-0449. *N Engl J Med* 2009;361:1173–1178.

22. Berlin J BJ, Hart LL, Firdaus I et al. A phase 2, randomized, double-blind, placebo-controlled study of hedgehog pathway inhibitor (HPI) GDC-0449 in patients with previously untreated metastatic colorectal cancer. *Ann Oncol* 2010;21(Suppl 8):Abstract LBA21.

23. Kaye SB FL, Holloway R, Horowitz N et al. A phase 2, randomized, placebo-controlled study of Hedgehog (Hh) pathway inhibitor GDC-0449 as maintenance therapy in patients with ovarian cancer in 2nd or 3rd complete remission. *Ann Oncol* 2010; 21(Suppl 8):Abstract LBA25.

24. Riobo NA, Lu K, Ai X et al. Phosphoinositide 3-kinase and Akt are essential for Sonic Hedgehog signaling. *Proc Natl Acad Sci USA* 2006;103:4505–4510.

25. Dennler S, Andre J, Alexaki I et al. Induction of sonic hedgehog mediators by transforming growth factor-beta: Smad3-dependent activation of Gli2 and Gli1 expression in vitro and in vivo. *Cancer Res* 2007;67:6981–6986.

26. Koch U, Radtke F. Notch and cancer: A double-edged sword. *Cell Mol Life Sci* 2007;64:2746–2762.

27. Farnie G, Clarke RB, Spence K et al. Novel cell culture technique for primary ductal carcinoma in situ: Role of Notch and epidermal growth factor receptor signaling pathways. *J Natl Cancer Inst* 2007;99:616–627.

28. Magnifico A, Albano L, Campaner S et al. Tumor-initiating cells of HER2-positive carcinoma cell lines express the highest oncoprotein levels and are sensitive to trastuzumab. *Clin Cancer Res* 2009;15:2010–2021.

29. Wang J, Wakeman TP, Lathia JD et al. Notch promotes radioresistance of glioma stem cells. *Stem Cells* 2010;28:17–28.

30. Rizzo P, Miao H, D'Souza G et al. Cross-talk between notch and the estrogen receptor in breast cancer suggests novel therapeutic approaches. *Cancer Res* 2008;68:5226–5235.

31. Fischer M, Yen WC, Kapoun AM et al. Anti-DLL4 inhibits growth and reduces tumor-initiating cell frequency in colorectal tumors with oncogenic KRAS mutations. *Cancer Res* 2011;71:1520–1525.

32. Parr C, Watkins G, Jiang WG. The possible correlation of Notch-1 and Notch-2 with clinical outcome and tumour clinicopathological parameters in human breast cancer. *Int J Mol Med* 2004;14:779–786.

33. Graziani I, Eliasz S, De Marco MA et al. Opposite effects of Notch-1 and Notch-2 on mesothelioma cell survival under hypoxia are exerted through the Akt pathway. *Cancer Res* 2008;68:9678–9685.

34. Li JL, Jubb AM, Harris AL. Targeting DLL4 in tumors shows preclinical activity but potentially significant toxicity. *Future Oncol* 2010;6:1099–1103.

35. Moon RT, Bowerman B, Boutros M, Perrimon N. The promise and perils of Wnt signaling through beta-catenin. *Science* 2002;296:1644–1646.

36. Vermeulen L, De Sousa EMF, van der Heijden M et al. Wnt activity defines colon cancer stem cells and is regulated by the microenvironment. *Nat Cell Biol* 2010;12:468–476.

37. Tenbaum SP, Ordonez-Moran P, Puig I et al. Beta-catenin confers resistance to PI3K and AKT inhibitors and subverts FOXO3a to promote metastasis in colon cancer. *Nat Med* 2012;18:892–901. doi: 10.1038/nm.2772. [Epub ahead of print].

38. Blanpain C, Mohrin M, Sotiropoulou PA, Passegue E. DNA-damage response in tissue-specific and cancer stem cells. *Cell Stem Cell* 2011 7;8:16–29.

39. Maugeri-Sacca M, Vigneri P, De Maria R. Cancer stem cells and chemosensitivity. *Clin Cancer Res* 2011;17:4942–4947.

40. Hoeijmakers JH. Genome maintenance mechanisms for preventing cancer. *Nature* 2001;411:366–374.
41. Larsson LG. Oncogene- and tumor suppressor gene-mediated suppression of cellular senescence. *Semin Cancer Biol* 2011;21:367–376.
42. Dai Y, Grant S. New insights into checkpoint kinase 1 in the DNA damage response signaling network. *Clin Cancer Res* 2010;16:376–383.
43. Bao S, Wu Q, McLendon RE et al. Glioma stem cells promote radioresistance by preferential activation of the DNA damage response. *Nature* 2006;444:756–760.
44. Ropolo M, Daga A, Griffero F et al. Comparative analysis of DNA repair in stem and nonstem glioma cell cultures. *Mol Cancer Res* 2009;7:383–392.
45. Bartucci M, Svensson S, Romania P et al. Therapeutic targeting of Chk1 in NSCLC stem cells during chemotherapy. *Cell Death Differ* 2012;19:768–778.
46. Gallmeier E, Hermann PC, Mueller MT et al. Inhibition of ataxia telangiectasia- and Rad3-related function abrogates the in vitro and in vivo tumorigenicity of human colon cancer cells through depletion of the CD133(+) tumor-initiating cell fraction. *Stem Cells* 2011;29:418–429.
47. Sausville EA, Barker PN, Agbo F et al. Phase I dose-escalation study of AZD7762 in combination with gemcitabine (gem) in patients (pts) with advanced solid tumors. *J Clin Oncol* 2011;29(Suppl 15):Abstract 3058.
48. Todaro M, Lombardo Y, Francipane MG et al. Apoptosis resistance in epithelial tumors is mediated by tumor-cell-derived interleukin-4. *Cell Death Differ* 2008;15:762–772.
49. Todaro M, Alea MP, Di Stefano AB et al. Colon cancer stem cells dictate tumor growth and resist cell death by production of interleukin-4. *Cell Stem Cell* 2007;1:389–402.
50. Francipane MG, Alea MP, Lombardo Y et al. Crucial role of interleukin 4 in the survival of colon cancer stem cells. *Cancer Res* 2008;68:4022–4025.
51. Ying M, Wang S, Sang Y et al. Regulation of glioblastoma stem cells by retinoic acid: Role for Notch pathway inhibition. *Oncogene* 2011;30:3454–3467.
52. Lombardo Y, Scopelliti A, Cammareri P et al. Bone morphogenetic protein 4 induces differentiation of colorectal cancer stem cells and increases their response to chemotherapy in mice. *Gastroenterology* 2011;140:297–309.
53. Eramo A, Ricci-Vitiani L, Zeuner A et al. Chemotherapy resistance of glioblastoma stem cells. *Cell Death Differ* 2006;13:1238–1241.
54. Wu CP, Calcagno AM, Ambudkar SV. Reversal of ABC drug transporter-mediated multidrug resistance in cancer cells: Evaluation of current strategies. *Curr Mol Pharmacol* 2008;1:93–105.
55. Firestone B. The challenge of selecting the 'right' in vivo oncology pharmacology model. *Curr Opin Pharmacol* 2010;10:391–396.
56. Tentler JJ, Tan AC, Weekes CD et al. Patient-derived tumour xenografts as models for oncology drug development. *Nat Rev Clin Oncol* 2012;9:338–350.
57. Garrido-Laguna I, Uson M, Rajeshkumar NV et al. Tumor engraftment in nude mice and enrichment in stroma-related gene pathways predict poor survival and resistance to gemcitabine in patients with pancreatic cancer. *Clin Cancer Res* 2011;17:5793–5800.
58. Ma CX, Cai S, Li S et al. Targeting Chk1 in p53-deficient triple-negative breast cancer is therapeutically beneficial in human-in-mouse tumor models. *J Clin Invest* 2012;122:1541–1552.
59. Baiocchi M, Biffoni M, Ricci-Vitiani L, Pilozzi E, De Maria R. New models for cancer research: Human cancer stem cell xenografts. *Curr Opin Pharmacol* 2010;10:380–384.
60. Liu R, Wang X, Chen GY et al. The prognostic role of a gene signature from tumorigenic breast-cancer cells. *N Engl J Med* 2007;356:217–226.
61. Markert EK, Mizuno H, Vazquez A, Levine AJ. Molecular classification of prostate cancer using curated expression signatures. *Proc Natl Acad Sci USA* 2011;108:21276–21281.

62. Gentles AJ, Plevritis SK, Majeti R, Alizadeh AA. Association of a leukemic stem cell gene expression signature with clinical outcomes in acute myeloid leukemia. *JAMA* 2010;304:2706–2715.
63. Pallini R, Ricci-Vitiani L, Banna GL et al. Cancer stem cell analysis and clinical outcome in patients with glioblastoma multiforme. *Clin Cancer Res* 2008;14:8205–8212.
64. Gerger A, Zhang W, Yang D et al. Common cancer stem cell gene variants predict colon cancer recurrence. *Clin Cancer Res* 2011;17:6934–6943.
65. Li X, Lewis MT, Huang J, Gutierrez C, Osborne CK, Wu MF et al. Intrinsic resistance of tumorigenic breast cancer cells to chemotherapy. *J Natl Cancer Inst* 2008;100:672–679.
66. Krop I, Demuth T, Guthrie T et al. Phase I pharmacologic and pharmacodynamic study of the gamma secretase (Notch) inhibitor MK-0752 in adult patients with advanced solid tumors. *J Clin Oncol* 2012;30:2307–2313.
67. Fouladi M, Stewart CF, Olson J et al. Phase I trial of MK-0752 in children with refractory CNS malignancies: A pediatric brain tumor consortium study. *J Clin Oncol* 2011;29:3529–3534.
68. Tolcher AW, Messersmith WA, Mikulski SM et al. Phase I study of RO4929097, a gamma secretase inhibitor of Notch signaling, in patients with refractory metastatic or locally advanced solid tumors. *J Clin Oncol* 2012; 30:2348–2353.
69. Strosberg JR, Yeatman T, Weber J et al. A phase II study of RO4929097 in metastatic colorectal cancer. *Eur J Cancer* 2012;48:997–1003.
70. Ho AL, Bendell JC, Cleary JM et al. Phase I, open-label, dose-escalation study of AZD7762 in combination with irinotecan (irino) in patients (pts) with advanced solid tumors. [abstract 3033]. *J Clin Oncol* 2011;29(Suppl 15):3033.
71. Brega N, McArthur GA, Britten SG et al. Phase I clinical trial of gemcitabine (GEM) in combination with PF-00477736 (PF-736), a selective inhibitor of CHK1 kinase. [abstract 3062]. *J Clin Oncol* 2010;28 (Suppl 15): 3062.
72. Daud A, Springett GM, Mendelson DS et al. A phase I dose-escalation study of SCH 900776, a selective inhibitor of checkpoint kinase 1 (CHK1), in combination with gemcitabine (Gem) in subjects with advanced solid tumors. [abstract]. *J Clin Oncol* 2010;28(Suppl 15):3064.
73. Weiss GJ, Donehower RC, Iyengar T et al. Phase I dose-escalation study to examine the safety and tolerability of LY2603618, a checkpoint 1 kinase inhibitor, administered 1 day after pemetrexed 500 mg/m(2) every 21 days in patients with cancer. *Invest New Drugs* 2012;31:136–144. [Epub ahead of print].

11 The Cancer Super-Chaperone Hsp90

Its Posttranslational Regulation and Drug Targeting

Annerleim Walton-Diaz
National Cancer Institute

Sahar Khan
National Cancer Institute

Jane B. Trepel
National Cancer Institute

Mehdi Mollapour
National Cancer Institute

Len Neckers
National Cancer Institute

CONTENTS

BACKGROUND AND BIOLOGY OF HSP90

During the past decade, much has been learned about the nature and function of heat shock protein 90 (Hsp90), especially concerning its association with several molecules and pathways important in cancer. Hsp90 is an abundant (2%–5% of total cellular protein) molecular chaperone whose homeostatic functions include stabilization and modulation of a number of proteins (clients) that comprise various cell signaling nodes, and fostering cellular responses to environmental stress.[1-3] The chaperone has been high jacked by and represents a nononcogene addiction of cancer cells, where its expression is further elevated above that of untransformed cells.[4] Hsp90 is found in all kingdoms except *Archaea*.[5] In humans, as in other eukaryotes, there are two Hsp90 isoforms: stress-inducible Hsp90α and constitutively expressed Hsp90β.[6] These isoforms, although highly homologous, do not fully complement each other. Hsp90β knockout is embryologically lethal, while mice lacking Hsp90α are viable but sterile.[7] Eukaryotes also express organelle specific Hsp90 paralogs: Glucose-regulated protein 94 (Grp94), also known as Hsp90B1, is found in the endoplasmic reticulum, where it participates in folding proteins destined for secretion.[8,9] Hsp75, also known as TNF receptor-associated protein 1 (TRAP1), is a mitochondrial paralog that provides protection from proteotoxic stress and may impact mitochondrial metabolism.[10,11] Hsp90 is a member of the ATPase/kinase GHKL (DNA gyrase, Hsp90, histidine kinase, MutL) superfamily—a small group of proteins that are characterized by a unique ATP binding cleft.[2,12] The N-terminal domain of the chaperone contains an ATP-binding site, which is also the target for Hsp90 inhibitors now in clinical trial. The middle (M) domain has binding sites for clients and co-chaperones, and the C-terminal domain contains a dimerization motif and binding sites for other co-chaperones. Connecting the N- and M-domains are a number of charged amino acids. This unstructured region is referred to as the "charged linker" and plays an important role in Hsp90 chaperone function.[13-15]

Hsp90 is a dynamic protein that undergoes a conformational cycle determined in part by ATP binding/hydrolysis and co-chaperone binding (see Figure 11.1). However, the Hsp90-directed chaperone cycle is complex and its regulation is also impacted by numerous posttranslational modifications (PTMs) to Hsp90 and the various co-chaperones. Clinically evaluated Hsp90 inhibitors disrupt the chaperone cycle by occupying the ATP binding pocket. Co-chaperones interact with distinct Hsp90 conformational states (see Figure 11.2). Presumably, these interactions lower the energy barrier between certain conformations, thus providing directionality to the Hsp90 cycle.[16,17] Further, certain co-chaperones, such as Hop and Cdc37, assist in the delivery of distinct sets of client proteins (steroid hormone receptors and kinases, respectively) to the Hsp90 chaperone machine. The complex and highly regulated conformational dynamics allow Hsp90 to bind, chaperone, and release client proteins. During this process, the conformation and activity/stability of the client protein are altered.[16-20] As stated earlier, Hsp90 inhibitors currently in clinical trial replace ATP in the N-domain nucleotide-binding pocket, thereby preventing the chaperone cycle from progressing. As a result, Hsp90-dependent client proteins are ubiquitinated and degraded in the proteasome, in a process involving Hsp70 and several chaperone-interacting E3 ubiquitin ligases.[4,12,21]

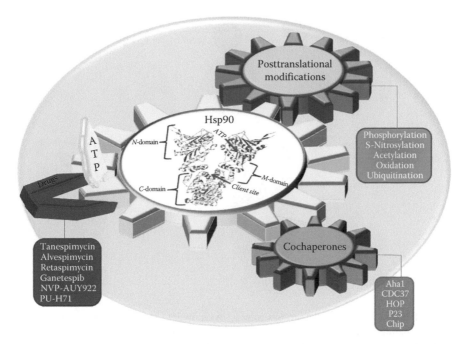

FIGURE 11.1 Hsp90 chaperone machine is comprised of dimeric Hsp90 protein that interacts with various cochaperones to promote client protein folding. This process depends on the binding and hydrolysis of ATP and is further modulated in cells by numerous posttranslational modifications to Hsp90 that help coordinate cochaperone binding. Hsp90 inhibitors displace ATP from its binding site in Hsp90 and block the chaperone cycle.

POSTTRANSLATIONAL MODIFICATIONS OF HSP90

In eukaryotes, numerous PTMs contribute to the regulation of the Hsp90 chaperone cycle (see Figure 11.1).[22] These PTMs seem likely to be an evolutionarily acquired characteristic since bacterial Hsp90 lacks any known PTM. Further, the extent of Hsp90 PTM is greater in metazoans compared to single cell eukaryotes, suggesting that increased use of PTMs provides the possibility for more complex regulation of Hsp90 activity as its client repertoire has increased during evolution. For a detailed description of Hsp90 PTM sites, the interested reader is directed to two curated websites: PhosphoSitePlus (www.phosphosite.org/protein) and PhosphoPep (www.phosphopep.org/index.php). In the following sections, we will briefly discuss several recently reported Hsp90 PTMs.

PHOSPHORYLATION

Phosphorylation of Hsp90 was first described in the 1980s.[23] More recently, Muller et al. reported that C-terminal phosphorylation of Hsp90 determines co-chaperone binding. These authors showed that phosphorylation of Hsp90 and Hsp70 prevents binding of CHIP (a co-chaperone with ubiquitin ligase activity), while simultaneously enhancing the binding of the co-chaperone p60[HOP]. Since both co-chaperones

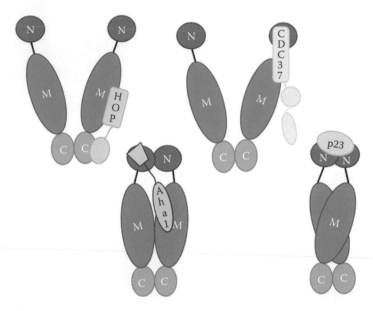

FIGURE 11.2 Various cochaperones interact with distinct Hsp90 conformations and have unique binding modes. These cochaperones deliver client proteins to Hsp90 and regulate Hsp90-mediated ATP hydrolysis by stabilizing distinct Hsp90 conformational states.

compete for the same binding site on Hsp90 but have opposing activities (CHIP promotes client degradation while p60[HOP] is involved in client folding), these findings demonstrate how specific phosphorylation events determine whether an Hsp90-dependent client is more likely to be degraded or properly folded.[24] Further, the authors show that cancer cells are characterized by excessive phosphorylation of Hsp90 in this region and this is coincident with increased binding of p60[HOP] at the expense of CHIP, suggesting that this PTM could be targeted in certain malignancies.

CK2 is a ubiquitous Ser/Thr kinase whose activity depends on Hsp90 function.[25–27] CK2 phosphorylates two serine residues, Ser-231 and Ser-263, in the charged linker of Hsp90α.[28] Equivalent residues in Hsp90β (Ser-226 and Ser-255) are also phosphorylated in untransformed cells but not in leukemic cells.[29] The leukemogenic tyrosine kinases, Bcr-Abl, FLT3/D835Y, and Tel-PDGFRβ, all suppress constitutive phosphorylation of Hsp90β at these sites, and this leads to inhibition of apoptosome function. This is achieved by stabilization of a strong interaction between Hsp90β and apoptotic peptidase activating factor 1 (Apaf-1), which prevents cytochrome c-induced Apaf-1 oligomerization and caspase-9 recruitment. Stabilization of the Hsp90β–apoptosome interaction by suppression of Ser-226 and Ser-255 phosphorylation may contribute to chemoresistance in leukemias.[29]

CK2 also phosphorylates a conserved threonine residue (Thr-22) in the N-domain of yeast Hsp90 both *in vitro* and *in vivo*. Thr-22 is the only threonine residue in the N-domain targeted by CK2. We recently showed that ATP binding to the Hsp90 N-domain is necessary for CK2-mediated phosphorylation of Thr-22, suggesting that this PTM participates in the ATP-driven chaperone cycle.[30,31] In support of this hypothesis, we found that mutation of this residue significantly reduced Hsp90 interaction with Aha1, a co-chaperone that upregulates the rate of ATP hydrolysis and chaperone activity. As expected from these data, mutation of Thr-22 affected Hsp90-dependent chaperoning of kinase (v-Src, Mpk1/Slt2, Raf-1, HER2/ErbB2, and CDK4) and nonkinase (heat shock factor 1, cystic fibrosis transmembrane conductance regulator protein, and glucocorticoid receptor) clients.[30,31] In addition, Thr-22 phosphorylation status also affects Hsp90 inhibitor sensitivity.[31]

Other phosphorylations of Hsp90 also directly impact the interaction of Aha1, consistent with recent structural data, suggesting that interaction of this co-chaperone with Hsp90 is necessary to lower the energy barrier of a critical conformational step in the chaperone cycle.[32] Thus, cSrc-dependent phosphorylation of Y301 in Hsp90β leads to decreased Aha1 interaction,[33,34] while phosphorylation of Hsp90α Y313 has been shown to dramatically enhance Hsp90 binding to Aha1.[35] More recently, interaction of another co-chaperone, CDC37, was also shown to be regulated by Hsp90 phosphorylation.[35] Taken together, this growing body of data suggests that eukaryotic cells utilize a diverse set of phosphorylation events to regulate co-chaperone interactions with Hsp90.

Nitrosylation/Oxidation

Hsp90 also undergoes S-nitrosylation. Nitric oxide promotes S-nitrosylation of Hsp90 Cys-597 in endothelial cells and this inhibits Hsp90 chaperone activity.[36] Since endothelial nitric oxide synthase (eNOS) is an Hsp90 client, S-nitrosylation provides a way to regulate NO production that relies on direct feedback inhibition of Hsp90 chaperone activity.[36–38] Oxidative stress has also been shown to cause PTM of Hsp90. Tubocapsenolide, a novel withanolide, increases reactive oxygen species (ROS), decreases glutathione levels, and causes direct thiol oxidation of Hsp90.[39] Likewise, 4-hydroxy-2-nonenal targets Hsp90 Cys-572 and inhibits its ability to chaperone clients.[40]

Acetylation

Acetylation is a reversible PTM that adds acetyl groups to proteins, usually on lysine residues. Histones are a major target for acetylation, and historically acetylating and deacetylating enzymes were termed histone acetylases (HATs) and histone deacetylases (HDACs), respectively. However, these enzymes are now known to be capable of modifying numerous nonhistone proteins, including Hsp90. Hsp90 acetylation in response to HDAC inhibitors (HDACi) was first reported by Yu and colleagues. These investigators showed that the HDACi depsipeptide (romidepsin) increased steady-state acetylation of Hsp90 while simultaneously destabilizing Hsp90 interaction with several client proteins, including ErbB2, Raf-1, and mutant p53.[41] Others have shown that additional HDACi also cause Hsp90 hyperacetylation.[42] p300 and HDAC6 promote acetylation and deacetylation of Hsp90, respectively.[43–46] Acetylated Hsp90 levels are increased in HDAC6-deficient mouse embryonic fibroblasts and glucocorticoid receptor function in these cells is compromised.[47] Androgen receptor, an Hsp90 client, is also downregulated upon HDAC6 inhibition.[48] Reduction in *HDAC6* expression also promotes destabilization of another Hsp90 client protein, the hypoxia-inducible transcription factor HIF-1α.[49] HDAC6 and HDAC10 have shown regulation of Hsp90-mediated VEGF receptor.[50] Although the impact of HDAC6 on Hsp90 acetylation has been extensively studied, other HDACs also are able to deacetylate the chaperone. HDAC1 has been reported to deacetylate Hsp90 in the nucleus of human breast cancer cells,[51] and both HDAC1 and HDAC10 inhibit the productive Hsp90 chaperoning of VEGF receptor proteins.[50]

Treating SKBr3 breast cancer cells with the pan-HDACi trichostatin A (TSA) caused hyperacetylation of Hsp90α at lysine 294.[52] Interestingly, K294 acetylation can be detected even in the absence of HDACi, suggesting that a pool of Hsp90α may be constitutively acetylated on this lysine residue.[52] K294Q or K294A Hsp90 mutants (acetylated lysine mimics) displayed reduced interaction with numerous client proteins (ErbB2, p60$^{v\text{-}Src}$, mutant p53, androgen receptor, Raf-1, HIF1α), and they failed to associate with the co-chaperones Aha1, CHIP, and FKBP52. Conversely, the nonacetylable mutant K294R displayed an equivalent or stronger interaction with these co-chaperone and client proteins compared to wild-type Hsp90.[52] Treating human embryonic kidney 293 cells (HEK293) with the pan-HDACi panobinostat (LBH589) led to the identification of 7 additional acetylated lysine residues in Hsp90. Mutation of these lysine residues to glutamine affected the binding of Hsp90α to several co-chaperones, including CHIP, Hsp70, and p23, inhibited ATP binding, and inhibited Hsp90 chaperoning of Raf-1.[53] Taken together, these data suggest that reversible acetylation of Hsp90 at multiple sites is a dynamic, tightly regulated process impacting Hsp90 function.

CLIENT-DEPENDENT REGULATION OF HSP90 PTMs: A NOVEL APPROACH TO THERAPY?

Hsp90 is frequently modified, and its activity impacted, by its own clients. An illustrative example is the tyrosine kinase Wee1. Wee1 is involved in the regulation of the G2/M cell cycle checkpoint and is an Hsp90 client. Wee1 phosphorylates Hsp90 on a conserved tyrosine residue (Y38 on Hsp90α) in the N-domain. Phosphorylation of Hsp90 at this site increases its ability to chaperone several cancer-related kinases including HER2/ErbB2, Src, C-Raf, Cdk4, and Wee1 itself. These data suggest that Wee1 inhibitors might potentiate or synergize with Hsp90 inhibitors. In support of this hypothesis, we recently reported that inhibition of Wee1 sensitizes prostate and cervical cancer cells to Hsp90 inhibitors and causes activation of the intrinsic apoptotic pathway. Dual Wee1 and Hsp90 inhibition in prostate cancer causes downregulation of Wee1 and Survivin, a suppressor of apoptosis.[54] Combined inhibition of Wee1 and Hsp90, using drug concentrations that individually were ineffective *in vivo*, caused significant inhibition of tumor growth and led to prolonged survival. These data suggest a novel strategy to enhance the efficacy of Hsp90 inhibitors by combining Hsp90 inhibitors with inhibitors of certain Hsp90 clients that themselves modify Hsp90.

TARGETING HSP90: IMPLICATIONS AND
BEST CLINICAL OUTCOMES

The concept of targeting Hsp90 for cancer therapy was initially viewed with some skepticism because its high expression in nontransformed cells suggested the significant possibility of generating unwanted toxicity. This concern has proven not to be relevant, however, for reasons that are still the subject of intense investigation. Surprisingly, Hsp90 inhibitors *in vivo* tend to concentrate and persist in tumors while being more rapidly cleared from blood and normal tissues.[4] Thus, perhaps even more relevant than with most drugs, Hsp90 inhibitor dose and schedule of administration are important. Careful consideration of these parameters, together with an appreciation of the specific role of Hsp90 relevant to the cancer in question, will be key to designing the most informative clinical trials going forward.

Although the first Hsp90 inhibitors to be identified, the natural products geldanamycin and radicicol, proved too toxic for clinical use, these agents served as invaluable chemical tools for probing the biology of Hsp90 and validating this molecular chaperone as a therapeutic target. These compounds also provided the foundation for development of future clinically well-tolerated drugs. Of these, the first drug to progress to clinical trials was the geldanamycin derivative tanespimycin (17-allylamino-17-demethoxygeldanamycin, 17-AAG). This drug demonstrated clinical activity (as defined by RECIST criteria) in HER2/ErbB2-positive, trastuzumab-resistant breast cancer patients.[55]

Other examples of first-generation Hsp90 inhibitors that have been clinically evaluated include a second geldanamycin derivative, alvespimycin (17-dimethylaminoethylamino-17-demethoxygeldanamycin, 17-DMAG), in castrate-refractory prostate cancer, chondrosarcoma, and renal cancer,[56] and retaspimycin (IPI-504, a soluble, stable hydroquinone form of 17-AAG), which remains in clinical development.[57] The trailblazing proof-of-concept work with geldanamycin analogues stimulated the race to discover synthetic small molecule Hsp90 inhibitors that would overcome some or all of the limitations of this class and would provide the ability to use doses and schedules capable of insuring sufficiently sustained client depletion while sparing liver toxicity, and a large number of synthetic Hsp90 inhibitors are now in clinical development (see Figure 11.3 and Table 11.1; as of this writing, 9 drugs are being evaluated in a total of 44 clinical trials).

As more is learned about the role of Hsp90 in modulating signaling networks in cancer (and normal) cells, and about the sensitivity of various client proteins to Hsp90 inhibition (and the importance of these sensitive clients for tumor survival), we will be better able to predict the patient population most likely to benefit from Hsp90 inhibition, either as a single treatment strategy or in combination with other therapies. As of this writing, several selection criteria already seem apparent and will be briefly discussed (see Figure 11.4). These include (1) targeting cancers that depend on highly sensitive Hsp90 clients (e.g., HER2/ErbB2-positive breast cancer, ALK-positive non-small cell lung cancer); (2) targeting cancers that are characterized by constitutive proteotoxic stress (e.g., multiple myeloma and K-Ras-driven tumors); and (3) employing Hsp90 inhibitors to prevent or combat tumor escape from molecularly targeted therapy (e.g., escape from tyrosine kinase inhibitors).

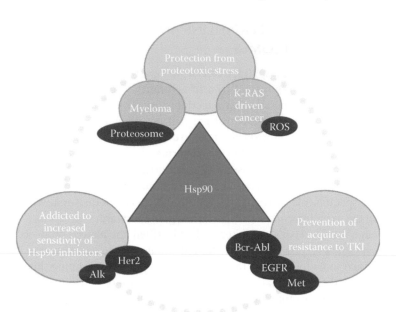

FIGURE 11.3 Available preclinical and clinical data suggest that Hsp90 inhibitors are likely to be especially effective in targeting cancers that are (a) driven by proteins that are highly dependent on Hsp90 for stability/activity (e.g., HER2 and ALK), (b) highly susceptible to proteotoxic stress and thus critically dependent on maintaining maximally efficient protein homeostasis (e.g., multiple myeloma and KRAS-driven cancers), or (c) initially responsive to tyrosine kinase inhibitors targeting Hsp90-dependent kinases (e.g., cancers driven by BCR-ABL, mutated EGFR, and MET). In the later case, combination of Hsp90 inhibitor and TKI is expected to reduce the frequency of TKI resistance.

TARGETING SENSITIVE CLIENTS THAT ARE ALSO TUMOR DRIVERS

HER2/ErbB2 is one of the most sensitive clients of Hsp90. In breast cancer, the role of HER2 as an important driver oncoprotein has been well established in the literature.[58] In 2011, Scaltriti et al. assessed the antitumor activity of retaspimycin in trastuzumab-resistant HER2 + breast cancer cells. They tested trastuzumab, retaspimycin, and a combination of both agents *in vitro* and in xenograft models. Retaspimycin was able to reduce total levels of HER2 equally in trastuzumab-sensitive and trastuzumab-resistant cells. The Hsp90 inhibitor was also able to inhibit tumor growth in xenografts when used as a single agent or in combination with trastuzumab.[59]

As mentioned earlier, the closely related Hsp90 inhibitor tanespimycin has shown clinical activity in phase I and II trials in HER2 +, trastuzumab-refractory breast cancer. RECIST responses were seen with a weekly schedule of 450 mg/m². The overall response rate was 22% and the clinical benefit rate (complete response + partial response + stable disease) was 59%.[60,61]

Another ongoing trial is the ENCHANT trial, evaluating the Hsp90 inhibitor ganetespib (STA-9090) in breast cancer. This is a phase II trial for evaluating ganetespib as frontline treatment for HER2 + and triple-negative metastatic breast

TABLE 11.1

Hsp90 Inhibitors Currently in Clinical Trial (as of February, 2013)

AT13387	I	Refractory solid tumors
(Astex pharma)	I, II	Single agent or with abiraterone
	I, II	With or without crizotinib in NSCLC
	II	With or without imatinib in GIST
AUY922	I	Advanced solid malignancies
(Novartis)	I, II	Undesignated
	II	Undesignated
	I	With BYL719 (PI3K inhibitor) in advanced/metastatic gastric cancer
	I, II	With erlotinib (NSCLC)
	II	Refractory GIST
	II	Refractory metastatic pancreatic cancer
	II	Myelofibrosis
	II	NSCLC with EGFR mutations
	Ib	With LDK378 in ALK-rearranged NSCLC
	II	GIST
	II	NSCLC after two lines of prior chemotherapy
	II	Advanced ALK + NSCLC
	I	With cetuximab in metastatic KRAS mutant metastatic colorectal cancer
Ganetespib	II	Small cell lung cancer (SCLC)
(Synta pharma)	II	NSCLC
	II	Prostate cancer after docetaxel
	II	Metastatic pancreatic cancer (2nd or 3rd line)
	II	Metastatic ocular melanoma
	II	With fulvestrant in hormone receptor-positive breast cancer
	II	Unresectable melanoma (stage III or IV)
	I	Advance hepatocellular carcinoma
	II	ALK-positive NSCLC
	I	With or without bortezomib in relapsed/refractory
	I	Multiple myeloma
	II	Refractory solid tumors
	I	Metastatic HER2 + or triple-negative breast cancer
	II/III	With capecitabine and radiation in rectal cancer
	I	With docetaxel in advanced NSCLC
	I, II	With docetaxel in solid tumors
	I, II	With crizotinib in ALK + lung cancers
		With pemetrexed–cisplatin in malignant pleural mesothelioma
SNX-5422	I	Refractory solid tumors
(Esanex)	I	Hematologic cancers
PU-H71	I	Advanced malignancies
(Samus	I	Solid tumors/low-grade non-Hodgkin's lymphoma not responding to treatment
therapeutics)	0	PET imaging of tumors
XL-888	I	With vemurafenib in unresectable BRAF-mutated stage III/IV melanoma

(continued)

TABLE 11.1 (continued)
Hsp90 Inhibitors Currently in Clinical Trial (as of February, 2013)

DS-2248 (Daiichi sankyo)	I	Advanced solid tumors
Debio 0932 (Debiopharm)	I	With standard care in NSCLC
IPI-504 (Infinity pharma)	I, II	With everolimus in KRAS mutant NSCLC

Source: Information was obtained from www.cancer.gov/clinicaltrials
Drug, trial phase, and indication are shown.

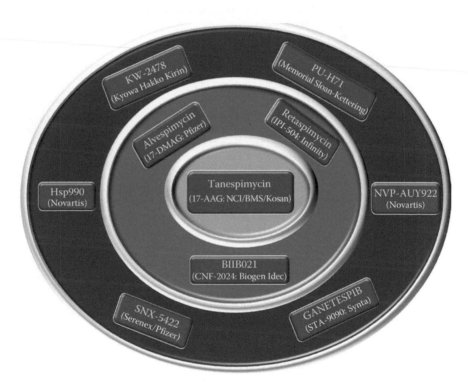

FIGURE 11.4 A natural benzoquinone ansamycin derivative, tanespimycin (17-AAG), was the first-in-human Hsp90 inhibitor. Other benzoquinone ansamycin derivatives (alvespimycin, 17-DMAG; retaspimycin, IPI-504) and numerous second generation synthetic inhibitors have been or are being evaluated in cancer patients.

cancer.[62] This study is of much interest since it evaluates the use of Hsp90 inhibitors in patients naive to other lines of therapy.

There have been promising studies assessing the activity of ganetespib in non-small cell lung cancer (NSCLC) patients whose tumors harbor ALK fusion proteins and who have progressed on other lines of therapy. In these studies, ganetespib showed response rates of 50%.[63] Recently, Proia et al. also evaluated the activity of ganetespib alone and in combination with crizotinib, in crizotinib-sensitive and crizotinib-resistant cancers harboring ALK fusions, and in cells expressing amplified ALK or ROS1 translocations. They reported that single-agent ganetespib displayed antitumor activity. Furthermore, there was strong synergy between this Hsp90 inhibitor and the ALK inhibitor crizotinib.[63]

Recently, at the European Society for Medical Oncology (ESMO) Meeting in 2012, preliminary results were presented for a phase II trial in patients with ALK-rearranged (ALK +) or EGFR-mutated lung cancer who had progressed following at least one line of chemotherapy and who were treated with the Hsp90 inhibitor NVP-AUY922. In this study, 61% of the patients had received three or more lines of treatment. Up to April 2012, 121 patients were treated with 70 mg/m^2 NVP-AUY922 once weekly. Of these, 29% of ALK + and 20% of EGFR-mutated patients had partial responses. Four of the 6 ALK + responders were naïve to crizotinib. The median progression-free survival rate at 18 weeks was 42% in ALK + and 34% in EGFR-mutated patients.[64]

Ganetespib was also studied by Kau et al. who reported a phase I and pharmacokinetic study of multiple schedules of ganetespib in combination with docetaxel for patients with advanced solid tumors. This combination was well tolerated at doses of 75 mg/m^2 for docetaxel and 150 mg/m^2 for ganetespib. As of this writing, a randomized phase 2b/3 study with a regimen including docetaxel on day 1 and ganetespib on days 1 and 15 is ongoing for advanced lung cancer.[65,66]

Hsp90 and Proteotoxic Stress

In some cancers, there is a delicate balance between proteotoxic stress and cancer cell survival. For example, the proteasome machinery is used to maximum capacity in highly secretory multiple myeloma cells and the proteasome is a validated molecular target in this cancer.[67] Hsp90 inhibitors (which redirect many Hsp90-dependent clients to the proteasome) have been shown to synergize with proteasome inhibitors in multiple myeloma and other cancers.[68] A phase 1/2 trial was undertaken to evaluate combination of the Hsp90 inhibitor tanespimycin and the proteasome inhibitor bortezomib. Among evaluable patients, 3% had a complete response and 12% had a partial response. The objective response rate was 27%. Of note, the highest response rates were observed in patients naïve to bortezonib.[69,70] Unfortunately, the development of tanespimycin was discontinued, due in part to patent issues (www.myelomabeacon.com/news/2010//tanespymicin-development-halted). However, given this promising activity, additional Hsp90 inhibitors are being evaluated in combination with proteasome inhibitors in multiple myeloma.[71] For example, a current phase I study is comparing ganetespib alone versus ganetespib plus bortezomib in patients with relapsed and/or refractory multiple myeloma. Although results are not available as of this writing (http://clinicaltrials.gov/ct2/show/NCT01485835?term=ganetespib&rank=2), Hsp90 inhibitors are likely to be efficacious in such a setting because they interfere with the machinery, already running at maximum capacity, used by myeloma cells to maintain cellular homeostasis.

K-Ras is mutated in 25% of NSCLC and is recognized as an important oncogenic driver. Patients whose cancers harbor this mutation respond poorly to existing therapies. Hes et al. recently published a study evaluating ganetespib in patients with K-Ras mutations. They observed single-agent activity and even better outcomes when ganetespib was combined with MEK or PI3K/mTOR inhibitors. Of interest, these investigators reported that ganetespib sensitized mutant K-Ras cells to standard of care therapies.[72]

Mutant K-Ras-driven tumor cells depend on optimal function of the cellular stress response machinery necessary to cope with constitutively elevated ROS. Moderate ROS levels are needed by K-Ras-driven tumor cells to regulate important signal transduction pathways on which they depend for proliferation.[73] However, excessive oxidative stress can overwhelm the stress response machinery, damaging proteins and leading to cell death. For this reason, K-Ras-driven tumors rely on an active chaperone network and on mTOR to maintain sufficient levels of reduced glutathione needed to modulate oxidative stress. In this context, Hsp90 inhibitors help to collapse this safety net, and, when combined with mTOR inhibition, this strategy provides a novel therapeutic approach to attack such cancers.[74] A phase 1b/2 clinical trial evaluating the safety and efficacy of retaspimycin plus the mTOR inhibitor everolimus in patients with K-Ras mutant NSCLC is ongoing (http:/www.infi.com/product-candidates-pipeline-IPI-504.asp). In this case, as with proteasome inhibitor combination in multiple myeloma, Hsp90 inhibition is not aimed at inactivating a specific tumor driver, but at compromising the cancer cell's ability to cope with persistent environmental stress.

Hsp90 Inhibitors and TKIs

Chronic myeloid leukemia (CML) is a hematologic disorder characterized by a translocation between chromosomes 9 and 22.[75] This produces the constitutively active chimeric oncogenic tyrosine kinase BCR-ABL. Tyrosine kinase inhibitors (TKIs), such as imatinib mesylate (Gleevec), have been an important tool for treatment of these malignancies since BCR-ABL is necessary to maintain their deregulated growth.[76] Although responses to Gleevec are dramatic, this TKI is not able to completely eradicate BCR-ABL + tumor cells, and resistance eventually develops. BCR-ABL kinase domain mutations account for up to 90% of secondary resistance mechanisms in CML.[77] Among the strategies explored to combat this resistance is the use of Hsp90 inhibitors, since Hsp90 is known to chaperone and promote the stability of BCR-ABL.[78] Investigators have shown that both Gleevec-sensitive and Gleevec-resistant BCR-ABL retain dependence on Hsp90 and sensitivity to Hsp90 inhibitors.[76] Peng et al. evaluated the combination of retaspimycin and Gleevec in mice with leukemia harboring Gleevec-resistant BCR-ABL. These investigators reported that this combination was more effective than either drug alone and was able to significantly prolong survival in mice.[79] These studies provide evidence that Hsp90 inhibitors might abrogate or significantly delay escape of certain kinase-driven cancers from TKIs.

Hsp90 inhibition has also been studied in relation to tyrosine kinase KIT-driven gastrointestinal stromal tumors (GIST). Investigators at Memorial Sloan–Kettering Cancer Center reported a phase 2 trial using the Hsp90 inhibitor BIIB021 in which they observed a metabolic response. This was assessed by fluorodeoxyglucose positron emission tomography (FDG-PET). The study included 23 patients with

GIST refractory to Gleevec and sunitinib (Sutent). The investigators reported a partial response in three patients treated with a dose of 600 mg biweekly and in two patients treated with a dose of 400 mg three times a week, with an overall response rate of 22%.[80]

CONCLUDING REMARKS

As described in this chapter, ongoing efforts are being made to better understand the structure and functional biology of Hsp90 in cancer and in normal cells, as well as to identify sensitive tumor-driving clients and novel approaches to sensitize cancer cells to Hsp90 inhibitors. We continue to learn about additional PTMs of Hsp90 that affect not only the chaperone itself but its interaction with numerous client proteins and affect its sensitivity to Hsp90 inhibitors. However, one should not lose sight of the fact that Hsp90 is also highly expressed in normal cells where it contributes toward maintaining protein homeostasis. This needs to be considered in trial design so as to take advantage of the beneficial, if not completely understood, property of current clinically evaluated Hsp90 inhibitors to persist preferentially in tumors and not in normal tissues. Further, predicting those cancers most likely to respond to Hsp90 inhibition is a work in progress. It is likely that initial success will be best achieved by using these inhibitors to treat cancers that are addicted to particular amplified, mutated, or translocated driver oncogenes that are themselves highly dependent Hsp90 clients, such as HER2/ErrbB2 and ALK. Use of Hsp90 inhibitors to interfere with cancer cells' ability to cope with persistent proteotoxic or other environmental stresses is likely to represent an additional paradigm, as is their use to combat development of TKI resistance or escape. Going forward, realization of the full therapeutic potential of inhibiting Hsp90 will certainly also benefit from a more complete genetic profiling of tumors.

REFERENCES

1. Wandinger SK, Richter K, Buchner J. The Hsp90 chaperone machinery. *J Biol Chem* 2008;283(27):18473–18477.
2. Picard D. Heat-shock protein 90, a chaperone for folding and regulation. *Cell Mol Life Sci* 2002;59(10):1640–1648.
3. Taipale M, Jarosz DF, Lindquist S. HSP90 at the hub of protein homeostasis: emerging mechanistic insights. *Nat Rev Mol Cell Biol* 2010;11(7):515–528.
4. Trepel J, Mollapour M, Giaccone G et al. Targeting the dynamic HSP90 complex in cancer. *Nat Rev Cancer* 2010;10(8):537–549.
5. Large AT, Goldberg MD, Lund PA. Chaperones and protein folding in the archaea. *Biochem Soc Trans* 2009;37(Pt 1):46–51.
6. Grad I, Cederroth CR, Walicki J et al. The molecular chaperone Hsp90alpha is required for meiotic progression of spermatocytes beyond pachytene in the mouse. *PLoS One* 2010;5(12):e15770.
7. Voss AK, Thomas T, Gruss P. Mice lacking HSP90beta fail to develop a placental labyrinth. *Development* 2000;127(1):1–11.
8. Dollins DE, Warren JJ, Immormino RM et al. Structures of GRP94-nucleotide complexes reveal mechanistic differences between the hsp90 chaperones. *Mol Cell* 2007;28(1):41–56.

9. Frey S, Leskovar A, Reinstein J et al. The ATPase cycle of the endoplasmic chaperone Grp94. *J Biol Chem* 2007;282(49):35612–32620.

10. Felts SJ, Owen BA, Nguyen P et al. The hsp90-related protein TRAP1 is a mitochondrial protein with distinct functional properties. *J Biol Chem* 2000;275(5):3305–3312.

11. Leskovar A, Wegele H, Werbeck ND et al. The ATPase cycle of the mitochondrial Hsp90 analog Trap1. *J Biol Chem* 2008;283(17):11677–11688.

12. Pearl LH, Prodromou C. Structure and mechanism of the Hsp90 molecular chaperone machinery. *Annu Rev Biochem* 2006;75:271–294.

13. Tsutsumi S, Mollapour M, Prodromou C et al. Charged linker sequence modulates eukaryotic heat shock protein 90 (Hsp90) chaperone activity. *Proc Natl Acad Sci USA* 2012;109(8):2937–2942.

14. Tsutsumi S, Mollapour M, Graf C et al. Hsp90 charged-linker truncation reverses the functional consequences of weakened hydrophobic contacts in the N domain. *Nat Struct Mol Biol* 2009;16(11):1141–1147.

15. Hainzl O, Lapina MC, Buchner J et al. The charged linker region is an important regulator of Hsp90 function. *J Biol Chem* 2009;284(34):22559–22567.

16. Hessling M, Richter K, Buchner J. Dissection of the ATP-induced conformational cycle of the molecular chaperone Hsp90. *Nat Struct Mol Biol* 2009;16(3):287–293.

17. Mickler M, Hessling M, Ratzke C et al. The large conformational changes of Hsp90 are only weakly coupled to ATP hydrolysis. *Nat Struct Mol Biol* 2009;16(3):281–286.

18. Vaughan CK, Gohlke U, Sobott F et al. Structure of an Hsp90-Cdc37-Cdk4 complex. *Mol Cell* 2006;23(5):697–707.

19. McLaughlin SH, Ventouras LA, Lobbezoo B et al. Independent ATPase activity of Hsp90 subunits creates a flexible assembly platform. *J Mol Biol* 2004;344(3):813–826.

20. Shiau AK, Harris SF, Southworth DR et al. Structural Analysis of E. coli hsp90 reveals dramatic nucleotide-dependent conformational rearrangements. *Cell* 2006; 127(2):329–340.

21. Neckers L. Using natural product inhibitors to validate Hsp90 as a molecular target in cancer. *Curr Top Med Chem* 2006;6(11):1163–1171.

22. Mollapour M, Neckers L. Post-translational modifications of Hsp90 and their contributions to chaperone regulation. *Biochim Biophys Acta* 2012;1823(3):648–655.

23. Dougherty JJ, Puri RK, Toft DO. Phosphorylation in vivo of chicken oviduct progesterone receptor. *J Biol Chem* 1982;257(23):14226–14230.

24. Muller P, Ruckova E, Halada P et al. C-terminal phosphorylation of Hsp70 and Hsp90 regulates alternate binding to co-chaperones CHIP and HOP to determine cellular protein folding/degradation balances. *Oncogene* 2013;32(25)3001–3110.

25. Ruzzene M, Di Maira G, Tosoni K et al. Assessment of CK2 constitutive activity in cancer cells. *Methods Enzymol* 2010;484:495–514.

26. Miyata Y. Protein kinase CK2 in health and disease: CK2: The kinase controlling the Hsp90 chaperone machinery. *Cell Mol Life Sci* 2009;66(11–12):1840–1849.

27. Dougherty JJ, Rabideau DA, Iannotti AM et al. Identification of the 90 kDa substrate of rat liver type II casein kinase with the heat shock protein which binds steroid receptors. *Biochim Biophys Acta* 1987;927(1):74–80.

28. Lees-Miller SP, Anderson CW. Two human 90-kDa heat shock proteins are phosphorylated in vivo at conserved serines that are phosphorylated in vitro by casein kinase II. *J Biol Chem* 1989;264(5):2431–2437.

29. Kurokawa M, Zhao C, Reya T et al. Inhibition of apoptosome formation by suppression of Hsp90beta phosphorylation in tyrosine kinase-induced leukemias. *Mol Cell Biol* 2008;28(17):5494–5506.

30. Mollapour M, Tsutsumi S, Kim YS et al. Casein kinase 2 phosphorylation of Hsp90 threonine 22 modulates chaperone function and drug sensitivity. *Oncotarget* 2011;2(5):407–417.

31. Mollapour M, Tsutsumi S, Truman AW et al. Threonine 22 phosphorylation attenuates Hsp90 interaction with cochaperones and affects its chaperone activity. *Mol Cell* 2011;41(6):672–681.

32. Retzlaff M, Hagn F, Mitschke L et al. Asymmetric activation of the hsp90 dimer by its cochaperone aha1. *Mol Cell* 2010;37(3):344–354.

33. Desjardins F, Delisle C, Gratton JP. Modulation of the Cochaperone AHA1 Regulates Heat-Shock Protein 90 and Endothelial NO Synthase Activation by Vascular Endothelial Growth Factor. *Arterioscler Thromb Vasc Biol* 2012;32(10):2484–2492.

34. Duval M, Le Boeuf F, Huot J et al. Src-mediated phosphorylation of Hsp90 in response to vascular endothelial growth factor (VEGF) is required for VEGF receptor-2 signaling to endothelial NO synthase. *Mol Biol Cell* 2007;18(11):4659–4668.

35. Xu W, Mollapour M, Prodromou C et al. Dynamic tyrosine phosphorylation modulates cycling of the HSP90-P50(CDC37)-AHA1 chaperone machine. *Mol Cell* 2012;47(3):434–443.

36. Martinez-Ruiz A, Villanueva L, Gonzalez de Orduna C et al. S-nitrosylation of Hsp90 promotes the inhibition of its ATPase and endothelial nitric oxide synthase regulatory activities. *Proc Natl Acad Sci USA* 2005;102(24):8525–8530.

37. Retzlaff M, Stahl M, Eberl HC et al. Hsp90 is regulated by a switch point in the C-terminal domain. *EMBO Rep* 2009;10(10):1147–1153.

38. Garcia-Cardena G, Fan R, Shah V et al. Dynamic activation of endothelial nitric oxide synthase by Hsp90. *Nature* 1998;392(6678):821–824.

39. Chen WY, Chang FR, Huang ZY et al. Tubocapsenolide A, a novel withanolide, inhibits proliferation and induces apoptosis in MDA-MB-231 cells by thiol oxidation of heat shock proteins. *J Biol Chem* 2008;283(25):17184–17193.

40. Carbone DL, Doorn JA, Kiebler Z et al. Modification of heat shock protein 90 by 4-hydroxynonenal in a rat model of chronic alcoholic liver disease. *J Pharmacol Exp Ther* 2005;315(1):8–15.

41. Yu X, Guo ZS, Marcu MG et al. Modulation of p53, ErbB1, ErbB2, and Raf-1 expression in lung cancer cells by depsipeptide FR901228. *J Natl Cancer Inst* 2002;94(7):504–513.

42. Nimmanapalli R, Fuino L, Bali P et al. Histone deacetylase inhibitor LAQ824 both lowers expression and promotes proteasomal degradation of Bcr-Abl and induces apoptosis of imatinib mesylate-sensitive or -refractory chronic myelogenous leukemia-blast crisis cells. *Cancer Res* 2003;63(16):5126–5135.

43. Bali P, Pranpat M, Bradner J et al. Inhibition of histone deacetylase 6 acetylates and disrupts the chaperone function of heat shock protein 90: A novel basis for antileukemia activity of histone deacetylase inhibitors. *J Biol Chem* 2005;280(29):26729–26734.

44. Kovacs JJ, Murphy PJ, Gaillard S et al. HDAC6 regulates Hsp90 acetylation and chaperone-dependent activation of glucocorticoid receptor. *Mol Cell* 2005;18(5):601–607.

45. Kekatpure VD, Dannenberg AJ, Subbaramaiah K. HDAC6 modulates Hsp90 chaperone activity and regulates activation of aryl hydrocarbon receptor signaling. *J Biol Chem* 2009;284(12):7436–7445.

46. Murphy PJ, Morishima Y, Kovacs JJ et al. Regulation of the dynamics of hsp90 action on the glucocorticoid receptor by acetylation/deacetylation of the chaperone. *J Biol Chem* 2005;280(40):33792–33799.

47. Zhang Y, Kwon S, Yamaguchi T et al. Mice lacking histone deacetylase 6 have hyperacetylated tubulin but are viable and develop normally. *Mol Cell Biol* 2008;28(5):1688–1701.

48. Ai J, Wang Y, Dar JA et al. HDAC6 regulates androgen receptor hypersensitivity and nuclear localization via modulating Hsp90 acetylation in castration-resistant prostate cancer. *Mol Endocrinol* 2009;23(12):1963–1972.

49. Zhang Q, Denlinger DL. Molecular characterization of heat shock protein 90, 70 and 70 cognate cDNAs and their expression patterns during thermal stress and pupal diapause in the corn earworm. *J Insect Physiol* 2010;56(2):138–150.

50. Park JH, Kim SH, Choi MC et al. Class II histone deacetylases play pivotal roles in heat shock protein 90-mediated proteasomal degradation of vascular endothelial growth factor receptors. *Biochem Biophys Res Commun* 2008;368(2):318–322.
51. Zhou Q, Agoston AT, Atadja P et al. Inhibition of histone deacetylases promotes ubiquitin-dependent proteasomal degradation of DNA methyltransferase 1 in human breast cancer cells. *Mol Cancer Res* 2008;6(5):873–883.
52. Scroggins BT, Robzyk K, Wang D et al. An acetylation site in the middle domain of Hsp90 regulates chaperone function. *Mol Cell* 2007;25(1):151–159.
53. Yang Y, Rao R, Shen J et al. Role of acetylation and extracellular location of heat shock protein 90alpha in tumor cell invasion. *Cancer Res* 2008;68(12):4833–4842.
54. Iwai A, Bourboulia D, Mollapour M et al. Combined inhibition of Wee1 and Hsp90 activates intrinsic apoptosis in cancer cells. *Cell Cycle* 2012;11(19):3649–3655.
55. Modi S, Sugarman S, Stopeck A et al. Phase II trial of the Hsp90 inhibitor tanespimycin (Tan) + trastuzumab (T) in patients (pts) with HER2-positive metastatic breast cancer (MBC) [abstract]. *J Clin Oncol* 2008;26(15S):1027.
56. Pacey S, Wilson RH, Walton M et al. A phase I study of the heat shock protein 90 inhibitor alvespimycin (17-DMAG) given intravenously to patients with advanced solid tumors. *Clin Cancer Res* 2011;17(6):1561–1570.
57. Sequist LV, Gettinger S, Senzer NN et al. Activity of IPI-504, a novel heat-shock protein 90 inhibitor, in patients with molecularly defined non-small-cell lung cancer. *J Clin Oncol* 2010;28(33):4953–4960.
58. Loi S, de Azambuja E, Pugliano L et al. HER2-overexpressing breast cancer: Time for the cure with less chemotherapy? *Curr Opin Oncol* 2011;23(6):547–558.
59. Scaltriti M, Serra V, Normant E et al. Antitumor activity of the Hsp90 inhibitor IPI-504 in HER2-positive trastuzumab-resistant breast cancer. *Mol Cancer Ther* 2011;10(5):817–824.
60. Modi S, Stopeck A, Linden H et al. HSP90 inhibition is effective in breast cancer: A phase II trial of tanespimycin (17-AAG) plus trastuzumab in patients with HER2-positive metastatic breast cancer progressing on trastuzumab. *Clin Cancer Res* 2011;17(15):5132–5139.
61. Modi S, Stopeck AT, Gordon MS et al. Combination of trastuzumab and tanespimycin (17-AAG, KOS-953) is safe and active in trastuzumab-refractory HER-2 overexpressing breast cancer: A phase I dose-escalation study. *J Clin Oncol* 2007;25(34):5410–5417.
62. Cameron D, Mano MS, Vukovic V et al. The ENCHANT trial: An open label multi-center phase 2 window of opportunity study evaluating ganetespib (STA-9090) mono-therapy in women with previously untreated metastatic HER2 positive or triple negative breast cancer (TNBC). *European Society for Medical Oncology*, Vienna, Austria. 2012; Abstract 347P.
63. Proia DA, Acquaviva J, Jiang Q et al. Preclinical activity of the Hsp90 inhibitor, ganetespib, in ALK- and ROS1-driven cancers. *J Clin Oncol* 2012;30:3090.
64. Felip E, Carcereny E, Barlesi F et al. Phase II activity of the HSP90 inhibitor AUY922 in patients with ALK-rearranged (ALK +) or EGFR-mutated advanced non-small cell lung cancer (NSCLC). *European Society for Medical Oncology*, Vienna, Austria. 2012; Abstract 4380.
65. Kauh JS, Owonikoko TK, El-Rayes BF et al. A phase I and pharmacokinetic study of multiple schedules of ganetespib (STA-9090), a heat shock protein 90 inhibitor, in combination with docetaxel for subjects with advanced solid tumor malignancies. *J Clin Oncol* 2012;30:3094.
66. Ramalingam SS, Zaric B, Goss G et al. A randomized IIB/III study of ganetespib (STA-9090) in combination with docetaxel versus docetaxel alone as second line therapy in patients with stage IIIB or IV NSCLC. *European Society for Medical Oncology*, Vienna, Austria. 2012; Abstract 1248P-PR.

67. Lawasut P, Chauhan D, Laubach J et al. New proteasome inhibitors in myeloma. *Curr Hematol Malig Rep* 2012;7(4):258–266.
68. Mimnaugh EG, Xu W, Vos M et al. Simultaneous inhibition of hsp 90 and the proteasome promotes protein ubiquitination, causes endoplasmic reticulum-derived cytosolic vacuolization, and enhances antitumor activity. *Mol Cancer Ther* 2004;3(5):551–566.
69. Richardson PG, Chanan-Khan AA, Lonial S et al. Tanespimycin and bortezomib combination treatment in patients with relapsed or relapsed and refractory multiple myeloma: results of a phase 1/2 study. *Br J Haematol* 2011;153(6):729–740.
70. Richardson PG, Mitsiades CS, Laubach JP et al. Inhibition of heat shock protein 90 (HSP90) as a therapeutic strategy for the treatment of myeloma and other cancers. *Br J Haematol* 2011;152(4):367–379.
71. Ri M, Iida S, Nakashima T et al. Bortezomib-resistant myeloma cell lines: A role for mutated PSMB5 in preventing the accumulation of unfolded proteins and fatal ER stress. *Leukemia*. 2010;24(8):1506–1512.
72. Acquaviva J, Smith DL, Sang J et al. Targeting KRAS mutant non-small cell lung cancer with the Hsp90 inhibitor ganetespib. *Mol Cancer Ther* 2012;11(12): 2633–2643.
73. Xu W, Trepel J, Neckers L. Ras, ROS and proteotoxic stress: A delicate balance. *Cancer Cell* 2011;20(3):281–282.
74. De Raedt T, Walton Z, Yecies JL et al. Exploiting cancer cell vulnerabilities to develop a combination therapy for ras-driven tumors. *Cancer Cell* 2011;20(3):400–413.
75. Bartram CR, de Klein A, Hagemeijer A et al. Translocation of c-abl oncogene correlates with the presence of a Philadelphia chromosome in chronic myelocytic leukaemia. *Nature* 1983;306(5940):277–280.
76. Gorre ME, Ellwood-Yen K, Chiosis G et al. BCR-ABL point mutants isolated from patients with imatinib mesylate-resistant chronic myeloid leukemia remain sensitive to inhibitors of the BCR ABL chaperone heat shock protein 90. *Blood* 2002;100(8):3041–3044.
77. Weisberg E, Griffin JD. Mechanism of resistance to the ABL tyrosine kinase inhibitor STI571 in BCR/ABL-transformed hematopoietic cell lines. *Blood* 2000;95(11):3498–3505.
78. Gorre ME, Mohammed M, Ellwood K et al. Clinical resistance to STI-571 cancer therapy caused by BCR-ABL gene mutation or amplification. *Science* 2001;293(5531):876–880.
79. Peng C, Brain J, Hu Y et al. Inhibition of heat shock protein 90 prolongs survival of mice with BCR-ABL-T315I-induced leukemia and suppresses leukemic stem cells. *Blood* 2007;110(2):678–685.
80. Dickson MA, Okuno SH, Keohan ML et al. Phase II study of the HSP90-inhibitor BIIB021 in gastrointestinal stromal tumors. *Ann Oncol* 2013;24(1):252–257.

12 Targeting Apoptosis Pathways

Pamela M. Holland
Amgen, Inc.

David Reese
Amgen, Inc.

Jeffrey Wiezorek
Amgen, Inc.

CONTENTS

INTRODUCTION

In higher organisms, apoptosis induction originates through ligand engagement and receptor activation outside the cell or from stress-induced signals within the cell. Both of these pathways, termed the extrinsic and intrinsic pathways, respectively, converge on common cell death effector machinery comprised of a series of cysteine proteases called caspases. Caspases are the key effector components of apoptosis and cleave their substrates after aspartate residues. Once activated, they cleave substrate proteins within the cell, leading to the morphological changes associated with apoptosis. Adaptor proteins act as scaffolds that organize signaling complexes and also recruit pro- and anti-apoptotic regulatory proteins that provide critical control points and influence caspase activation. These core components are represented in both the extrinsic and intrinsic pathway machinery and will be discussed further in the relevant sections. The increased understanding of control points in apoptotic cell death pathways has yielded fundamental insights into basic biology and also aided in the development of rational apoptosis-inducing therapies.

EXTRINSIC PATHWAY

Engagement of the death domain (DD)-containing receptors within the tumor necrosis factor receptor (TNFR) superfamily by their cognate ligands initiates the extrinsic pathway. Of the 19 ligands that make up the TNF cytokine superfamily, three members, TNF (TNFSF2), Fas ligand (FasL, TNFSF6), and Apo2L/TRAIL (TNFSF10), have been most thoroughly evaluated as apoptosis-inducing cancer therapeutics.[1]

Strategies for extrinsic pathway activation for cancer therapy have focused on recombinant ligands that express only the extracellular domain or agonistic monoclonal antibodies that bind the receptors and trigger apoptosis. More recently, additional strategies are being employed, largely designed to enhance receptor clustering and downstream signaling.

TNF, FasL, and Apo2L/TRAIL are all type II transmembrane proteins and exist as both soluble and membrane-bound forms. Both forms assemble as noncovalent trimers and engage their cognate receptors, thereby generating stoichiometrically defined trimer complexes with threefold symmetry.[2] Increasing evidence has suggested that optimal signal transduction occurs when the receptors are clustered and aggregated into lipid rafts.[3] TNF, FasL, and Apo2L/TRAIL are all expressed on a variety of immune cells, including activated T cells and NK cells, and function endogenously to modulate innate as well as adaptive immunity.

Ligand-induced receptor oligomerization results in assembly of the cell death-inducing signaling complex (DISC), made up of the receptor, the adaptor protein FADD, and a regulatory protein. DISC formation facilitates activation of caspases 8 and 10, which subsequently activate the effector caspases 3, 6, and 7. These "executioner" caspases cleave intracellular substrates that mediate apoptotic cell death[4] (Figure 12.1).

The extrinsic pathway is negatively regulated at the level of the DISC as well as the downstream executioner caspases. The protein c-FLIP resides in the DISC and bears structural similarity to caspase 8 but lacks enzymatic activity, acting in a dominant negative fashion.[4] XIAP is another negative regulator, which can directly bind and sequester caspase 3.[5]

Although the principal signaling event through DD-containing receptors is apoptosis induction in susceptible cells, activation of NFkB and MAP kinase can also occur through the formation of secondary signaling complexes via recruitment of other adaptor proteins.[4,6,7] Signaling through these alternative pathways can result in pro-survival responses, including cell proliferation, migration, differentiation, and metastasis.[8] How these paradoxical cellular outcomes are regulated is an area of active investigation. For example, recent findings indicate that receptor internalization and endosomal trafficking may play a role in selectively transmitting

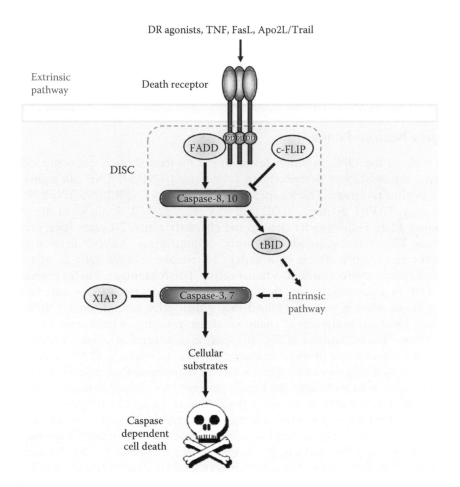

FIGURE 12.1   The extrinsic signaling pathway. The extrinsic pathway is triggered upon binding of death receptor agonists to the pro-apoptotic DD-containing receptors on the surface of a target cell, resulting in formation of the DISC. DISC formation involves recruitment of the adaptor protein FADD to the receptor via the DD and the inactive pro-caspases 8 and 10. This facilitates activation and self-processing of caspases 8 and 10, leading to their release into the cytoplasm, where they activate effector caspases 3 and 7. In some cells, active caspase 8 cleaves the pro-apoptotic BCL-2 family member BID. Truncated BID (tBID) then translocates to the mitochondria and triggers activation of the intrinsic pathway (Figure 12.3). The intrinsic pathway converges on caspases 3 and 7. c-FLIP is a negative regulator in the DISC, which bears structural similarity to caspase 8 but lacks enzymatic activity and can displace caspase 8 in the DISC. The ratio of caspase 8 to c-FLIP in the DISC is an important determinant of response to death receptor engagement. Once activated, caspases 3 and 7 cleave intracellular substrates that contribute to the morphological hallmarks of apoptosis, resulting in cell death. XIAP is another negative regulator of the extrinsic pathway and functions downstream of the DISC to bind and sequester active caspase 3, thereby inhibiting its activity.

the signals that lead to either cell survival or cell death.[9] Increased understanding of the mechanisms by which diverse biological effects are determined following death receptor agonism will be important in providing translational advances in the design of death receptor agonist therapies. As discussed in the following sections, emerging knowledge around the multifaceted signaling downstream of TNF, FasL, and Apo2L/TRAIL has resulted in a rethinking of the best way to harness these pathways for cancer therapy.

TUMOR NECROSIS FACTOR

As early as the 1960s, a serum factor from LPS-treated mice that could induce tumor regression was described and later termed TNF.[10,11] TNF can signal via two distinct receptors, TNFR1 (p55/TNFRSF1A) and TNFR2 (p75/TNFRSF1B), but only TNFR1 contains a DD and can promote cell death when agonized (Figure 12.2). Following its cloning and characterization 20 years later, recombinant TNF was evaluated extensively in preclinical studies, demonstrating immunomodulatory effects on a variety of immune effector cells as well as a direct cytotoxic effect on human tumor cells.[12] These findings led to the evaluation of TNF as a potential cancer therapeutic agent in humans. Efforts were largely abandoned when it was determined that systemically administered TNF could induce signs and symptoms of endotoxic shock, resulting in little or no therapeutic index.[13] The current use of TNF in cancer is in directed infusions, which avoid systemic toxicity and provide antitumor activity. Tasonermin (TNF alpha-1a) is approved by the European Medicines Agency for isolated limb perfusion (ILP) in combination with melphalan for locally advanced soft tissue sarcoma to prevent or delay limb amputation. In this setting, TNF is thought to trigger necrosis of endothelial cells and pericytes, leading to destruction of tumor vasculature and increased tumor uptake of melphalan.[14] TNF-based ILP achieves a response rate of approximately 75% and a limb salvage rate of approximately 85%.[15,16] Activity has also been demonstrated in other tumor types, including in-transit melanoma[17] and other types of skin cancer.[18]

Although named for its antitumor properties, TNF has been implicated in a wide spectrum of other diseases and is also implicated in tumor promotion. Expression of TNF in the tumor microenvironment is associated with inflammation-induced cancer, and mice lacking TNF are resistant to TPA–DMBA-induced skin carcinogenesis.[19,20] Moreover, several tumor cell types constitutively express TNF, including ovarian cancer, breast cancer, and others.[19] These findings suggest that blocking TNF activity may have a therapeutic effect in some settings, and studies aimed to address this are currently ongoing.[21]

FAS LIGAND

Another well-studied member of the TNF superfamily is FasL/CD95L (TNFSF6). The Fas/CD95 (TNFRSF6) receptor mediates apoptosis when triggered by its cognate ligand FasL or agonistic anti-Fas antibodies (Figure 12.1). The FasL/Fas system plays a critical role in the clonal deletion of T cells in the periphery, downregulation

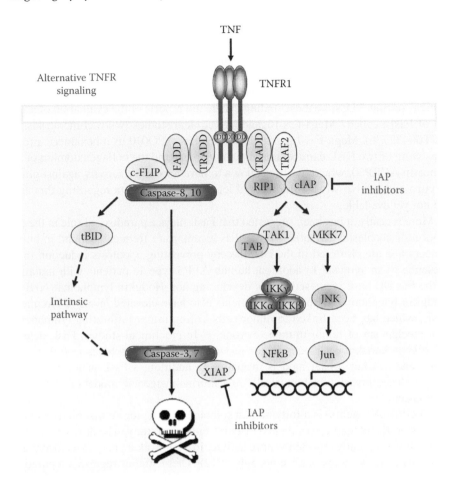

FIGURE 12.2 Alternative TNFR1 signaling pathways. TNFR1 recruits the adaptor protein TRADD via the DD. TRADD acts as a platform adaptor and allows the assembly of multiple signaling complexes through secondary adaptors. TRADD can bind to FADD to form the DISC and activate the extrinsic pathway as in Figure 12.1. A second signaling complex involves the kinase RIP1 that links receptor stimulation to the activation of NFkB through the canonical pathway. The presence of cIAP1 and cIAP2 regulates RIP1 and NFkB activity. Loss of cIAP1 and cIAP2 causes constitutive recruitment of RIP1, which forms a cytoplasmic complex with FADD and caspase 8, followed by induction of apoptosis. A third complex involves the adaptor protein TRAF2, which couples receptor engagement to activation of JNK. Ubiquitin linkages are not depicted in this diagram.

of immune responses, and cytotoxic T lymphocyte (CTL)-mediated cytotoxicity. Mice that harbor mutations in FasL that either decrease its expression or render it incapable of binding the Fas receptor develop lymphoproliferation, leading to lymphadenopathy and splenomegaly.[22] Autoimmune lymphoproliferative syndrome (ALPS) is a similar syndrome that has been described in humans, where patients display lymphadenopathy and splenomegaly due to impaired lymphocyte apoptosis.[23,24]

Collectively, these studies establish a role for Fas/FasL as a potent inducer of apoptosis in immune regulation.

The induction of apoptosis through the Fas receptor can also occur in tumor cells in vitro and in vivo. However, administration of anti-Fas agonistic antibodies to mice was shown to be highly hepatotoxic, thereby limiting its potential use in a clinical setting.[25] Despite these findings, there are reports of the evaluation of a variant of FasL, called "Mega-Fas-Ligand," in clinical studies (www.clinicaltrials.gov, NCT00437736). Mega-Fas-Ligand, also known as APO010, is a hexameric protein consisting of two FasL extracellular domain trimers and the collagen domain of adiponectin ACRP30, which has been shown to have antitumor activity against glioma in vitro and in vivo when administered locally.[26] Further data regarding this agent are not yet available.

More recently, it has been suggested that FasL plays a paradoxical role in the promotion of neoplasia.[7] Mutations in the Fas receptor are frequently found in human cancers and are clustered in the DD, thereby preventing apoptosis induction in the presence of an agonist.[7] In addition, human ALPS type 1a patients with mutations in the Fas DD have increased risk of developing non-Hodgkin lymphoma (NHL) or Hodgkin lymphoma.[7] Many cancer patients also have elevated levels of circulating FasL, which has been linked to tumor cells killing tumor-infiltrating lymphocytes as a mechanism of tumor immune evasion.[7,27] In preclinical studies, FasL deletion or shRNA knockdown blocks tumor growth in vitro and in hepatocellular carcinoma and ovarian cancer models in vivo.[28] In addition, a FasL-neutralizing antibody reduced invasion of tumor cells in a murine syngeneic model of intracranial glioblastoma.[29]

APG101 (Apogenix) is a fully human soluble Fas receptor Fc that binds and neutralizes FasL and has been evaluated in a first-in-human study in healthy volunteers.[30] APG101 was recently reported to have activity in a controlled phase II recurrent glioblastoma trial (www.apogenix.com, July 2012). These studies represent a paradigm shift in our thinking about strategies of targeting death receptors and the role of Fas/FasL in oncogenesis, and the results of additional clinical studies aimed at blocking FasL activity to treat cancer will be of significant interest.

Apo2L/TRAIL and Agonistic Death Receptor Antibodies

Given the initial toxicity associated with the administration of TNF and FasL agonists, TNF related apoptosis-inducing ligand (Apo2L/TRAIL, TNFSF10) emerged as the most promising death ligand with potential clinical application. This was due in large part to early observations, indicating that Apo2L/TRAIL could preferentially kill transformed or virally infected cells over normal cells.[31,32] Unlike TNF and FasL, Apo2L/TRAIL binds two distinct DD-containing receptors, DR4/TRAIL-R1 (TNFRSF10A) and DR5/TRAIL-R2 (TNFRSF10B), in addition to binding decoy receptors.[4]

Extensive preclinical experiments evaluating the antitumor effects of Apo2L/TRAIL have been performed. Apo2L/TRAIL as well as agonist antibodies targeting either DR4 or DR5 have shown activity in vitro and in vivo against a wide range of tumor types, including lung, colon, pancreatic, NHL, multiple myeloma, glioma, and breast cancer.[31,33] Combinations of Apo2L/TRAIL receptor agonists with conventional chemotherapeutics and multiple targeted agents also yielded promising preclinical results, warranting the evaluation of these agents in a clinical setting.[33]

Several agents for agonizing Apo2L/TRAIL death receptors have been evaluated in the clinic[34] (Table 12.1). Dulanermin is an optimized, zinc-coordinated, homotrimeric recombinant protein consisting of amino acids 114–281 of the endogenous polypeptide and is the only agonist that engages both Apo2L/TRAIL death receptors. Conatumumab, drozitumab, tigatuzumab, and lexatumumab are all monoclonal agonist antibodies selectively targeting DR5, whereas mapatumumab is a fully human agonist antibody against DR4.

Phase 1 trials have demonstrated these agents were tolerable as monotherapy.[34] Concerns regarding fulminant hepatotoxicity as seen with FasL have not been substantiated. No consistent dose-limiting toxicities have been identified. Single-agent antitumor activity, however, has been modest with only a few durable partial responses reported across different tumor histologies including chondrosarcoma,[35] follicular lymphoma,[36] and non-small cell lung cancer.[37–41] Increases in circulating cell death markers after treatment have suggested that there was pharmacodynamic activity but have not been useful as predictive markers of response, perhaps due to the small number of clinical responses observed.[42]

Death receptor agonists have also been combined with chemotherapy and other targeted agents in phase 1b/2 clinical trials. Preclinically these combinations enhance the antitumor activity of the class through cross talk of the intrinsic and extrinsic pathways. These combinations have been tolerable and did not seem to significantly further sensitize normal cells to apoptosis. The efficacy results of these studies, however, have not convincingly demonstrated meaningful clinical benefit to date, and no agent has progressed to phase 3 trials. Results are still awaited for studies of mapatumumab and tigatuzumab in hepatocellular carcinoma in combination with sorafenib and tigatuzumab with protein-bound paclitaxel (Abraxane) in triple-negative breast cancer. Clearly, novel approaches are needed to translate the promise of targeting death receptors to clinically meaningful activity.

NEW APPROACHES TO TARGET THE EXTRINSIC PATHWAY

Although phase 1/1b studies using Apo2L/TRAIL agonists provided encouraging preliminary results, findings from randomized phase 2 studies failed to demonstrate significant clinical benefit. For agonist antibodies, one possible reason may be attributed to the cross-linking requirement for effective receptor engagement and clustering. For example, conatumumab is dependent on cross-linking for activity in vitro and in vivo.[43] In vivo, cross-linking is mediated by Fcγ receptors (FcγR) expressed on the surface of immune cells. Similarly, drozitumab also requires FcγR binding to trigger tumor cell apoptosis.[44] Therefore, insufficient antibody cross-linking could contribute to a diminished antitumor response mediated by death receptor agonist antibodies.

TABLE 12.1

Selected Clinical Trials of Death Receptor Agonists

Agent/Target	Setting	Intervention	Results
Conatumumab Fully human DR5 agonist antibody	Colorectal cancer	Combination with bevacizumab/ FOLFOX	Saltz[128]
		Combination with FOLFIRI	Cohn[129]
		Combination with panitumumab	Peeters[130]
	Non-small cell lung cancer	Combination with carboplatin/paclitaxel	Paz-Ares L, 2009[131]
	Pancreatic cancer	Combination with gemcitabine	Kindler H, 2012[132]
	Sarcoma	Combination with doxorubicin	Demetri[133]
	Solid tumors or lymphoma	Monotherapy	Herbst[37]
		Combination with bortezomib or vorinostat	Younes[134]
		Combination with ganitumab	Chawla[135]
Drozitumab Fully human DR5 agonist antibody	Colorectal cancer	Combination with bevacizumab/ FOLFOX	Rocha Lima[136]
		Combination with cetuximab/irinotecan	Completed
	NHL	Combination with rituximab	Wittebol[137]
	Non-small cell lung cancer	Combination with bevacizumab/ carboplatin/paclitaxel	Karapetis[138]
	Sarcoma	Monotherapy	Chawla[139]
	Solid tumors	Monotherapy	Camidge[40]
Dulanermin Recombinant human ligand DR4, DR5 dual agonist,	Colorectal cancer	Combination with bevacizumab/ FOLFOX	Ongoing
		Combination with cetuximab/irinotecan	Yee[140]
	NHL	Combination with rituximab	Completed
	Non-small cell lung cancer	Combination with bevacizumab/ carboplatin/paclitaxel	Soria[141]
	Solid tumors	Monotherapy	Herbst[35]
Lexatumumab Fully human DR5 agonist antibody	Solid tumors or lymphoma	Monotherapy	Plummer[142] Merchant M[143]
		Combination with multiple chemotherapy regimens	Sikic[144]
		Combination with interferon gamma	Ongoing
Mapatumumab Fully human DR4 agonist antibody	Cervical cancer	Combination with cisplatin/radiation	Ongoing
	Colorectal cancer	Monotherapy	Trarbach[145]
	Hepatocellular carcinoma	Combination with sorafenib	Sun[146]
	Multiple myeloma	Combination with bortezomib	Belch[147]
	NHL	Monotherapy	Younes[36]
	Non-small cell lung cancer	Monotherapy	Greco F[148]
		Combination with carboplatin/paclitaxel	Von Pawel[149]
	Solid tumors	Monotherapy	Tolcher[38] Hotte[39]

TABLE 12.1 (continued)
Selected Clinical Trials of Death Receptor Agonists

Agent/Target	Setting	Intervention	Results
TAS266 Tetrameric DR5 nanobody	Solid tumors	Monotherapy	Ongoing
Tigatuzumab	Breast cancer	Combination with nab-paclitaxel	Ongoing
Humanized	Colorectal cancer	Combination with FOLFIRI	Ongoing
DR5 agonist antibody	Hepatocellular carcinoma	Combination with sorafenib	Ongoing
	Non-small cell lung cancer	Combination with carboplatin/paclitaxel	Von Pawel[150]
	Ovarian cancer	Combination with carboplatin/paclitaxel	Completed
	Pancreatic cancer	Combination with gemcitabine	Completed
	Solid tumors or lymphoma	Monotherapy	Forero-Torres[41]

The effects of antibody cross-linking may be multifactorial. Importantly, cross-linking enhances death receptor clustering on the tumor cell surface to generate robust caspase activation. In addition, antibody effector function might also contribute to the mechanism of action of death receptor agonist antibodies. For example, the DR4 antibody mapatumumab was reported to mediate antibody-dependent cellular cytotoxicity (ADCC) against DR4-expressing target cells in vitro.[45] The DR5 antibody conatumumab can also induce ADCC of target cells in vitro, and this is influenced by the allelic polymorphism of FcγR,[46] which leads to high- or low-affinity forms of the receptor. Collectively, this raises the possibility that death receptor agonist antibodies may bring additional immune-mediated mechanisms to bear on the tumor. In this respect, an agonist antibody directed against the mouse TRAIL death receptor can also induce tumor-specific effector and memory T cells.[47] It is worth noting that in randomized phase 2 trials conducted with conatumumab in patients with both advanced non-small cell lung cancer and metastatic colorectal cancer, trends toward a stronger treatment effect on overall survival were observed in patients carrying a high-affinity allele of the FcγR, suggesting that the high-affinity form of the receptor may be associated with enhanced responsiveness to conatumumab.[46]

The limited efficacy observed with soluble recombinant Apo2L/TRAIL ligand (dulanermin) could be attributed to its limited exposure. Dulanermin has a half-life of less than 1 h in humans.[35] In addition, some soluble forms of TNF family ligands have been shown to have different activity profiles than the corresponding membrane form. For example, the soluble form of FasL has limited apoptosis-inducing activity.[48–50] The soluble form of Apo2L/TRAIL has been reported to retain receptor-activating potential for DR4 but is a weak inducer of apoptosis mediated through DR5.[51–54]

These findings have prompted investigators to explore alternative methodologies to improve efficacy of death receptor agonists. Some of these approaches include the use of adenoviral therapies, Apo2L/TRAIL peptide mimetics, receptor-selective Apo2L/TRAIL variants, and Apo2L/TRAIL fusion proteins.[53,55-59] Promoting oligomerization or mimicking the membrane-bound forms of FasL and Apo2L/TRAIL has been achieved by the fusion of a soluble ligand to a single-chain fragment of a variable region (scFv) antibody fragment. In an analogous manner, a single-chain variant of soluble human TNF (scTNF) consisting of three human TNF monomers covalently linked via two glycine serine linkers has been reported.[60] Fusion to a tumor-specific target antigen can also make these agents tumor selective. The scFv-targeted ligand is inactive but becomes activated upon antibody-mediated binding and cross-linking to the tumor cell surface.[58,59,61] Using a gene immunotherapy approach, Apo2L/TRAIL-overexpressing lymphocytes were combined with an EpCAMxCD3 bi-specific antibody to enhance antitumor responsiveness.[62] Although only evaluated preclinically to date, one related DR5 agonist is reported to be entering clinical trials in 2012 (www.clinicaltrials.gov). TAS266 is described as a tetrameric nanobody, consisting of a single, heavy chain domain (V_{HH}) antibody that occurs naturally in the camelid species. TAS266 is humanized and linked to form a tetrameric structure, which should not be dependent on cross-linking by Fcγ receptors in the tumor microenvironment for activity.[63]

Our increased knowledge surrounding the non-apoptotic roles for TNF family death receptor signaling, in combination with advances in methodologies to promote receptor clustering in a tumor-selective and receptor-selective manner, provides the potential for superior clinical activity over first-generation approaches to target death receptors that have been tested to date.

INTRINSIC PATHWAY

The critical event that commits a cell to death by the intrinsic apoptotic pathway is permeabilization of the outer mitochondrial membrane with the subsequent release of cytochrome C. Activation of the intrinsic pathway occurs via multiple cellular stress signals, including DNA damage, growth factor deprivation, oncogene activation, and microtubule disruption. Many of these cytotoxic stress signals feed into the intrinsic pathway via the activation of p53 (Figure 12.3). In some cells, cross talk with the extrinsic pathway may also promote intrinsic pathway activation. The events leading up to cytochrome C release from the mitochondria are tightly regulated by the pro- and anti-apoptotic BCL-2 family members. Mitochondrial membrane permeabilization also releases the mitochondrial factor SMAC/DIABLO, which binds to and neutralizes inhibitor of apoptosis (IAP) proteins to promote caspase 3 activation.[64] Cytochrome C and dATP bind to the adaptor protein APAF1 to form the apoptosome, which recruits and activates caspase 9. Active caspase 9 can then activate the effector caspases 3 and 7[65] (Figure 12.3).

Many of the factors regulating the life–death switch in the intrinsic pathway are overexpressed or dysregulated in disease settings such as cancer, including the pro-survival BCL-2 family members and IAP proteins. Moreover, mutation or inactivation of p53 leads to resistance to many drugs aimed at indirectly activating the

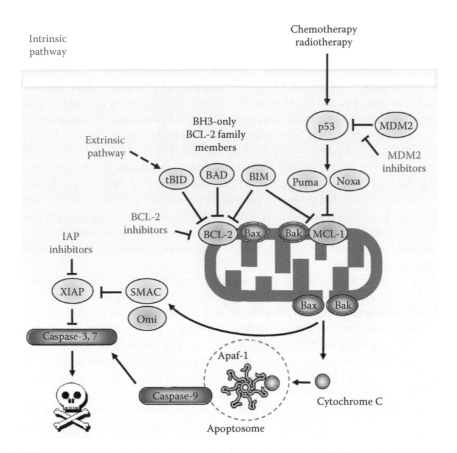

FIGURE 12.3 The intrinsic signaling pathway. The intrinsic or BCL-2-regulated mitochondrial pathway is responsive to a variety of cellular stresses, including chemotherapy and targeted agents that antagonize growth and survival pathways. In response to DNA-damaging agents, the tumor suppressor p53 initiates the intrinsic pathway by upregulating PUMA and NOXA. This results in the inactivation of BCL-2 family members like BCL-2 and MCL-1 and allows BAX and BAK to be activated. Either together or indirectly, BAX, BAK, and matrix metalloproteases (MMPs) promote formation of pores in the mitochondrial membrane. This facilitates the release of pro-apoptotic factors such as cytochrome C and SMAC/ DIABLO from the mitochondria. Once cytochrome C is released, it is incorporated into the apoptosome, a multimeric complex consisting of cytochrome C, dATP, and the adaptor protein APAF1. The apoptosome then recruits and activates caspase 9, leading to the activation of caspases 3 and 7 and the death response. The extrinsic and intrinsic pathways communicate with one another and, in many cells, work together to regulate cell survival. The BCL-2 member BID is cleaved by caspase 8 upon extrinsic pathway activation, and both pathways converge on the effector caspases 3 and 7. Therapeutic targets aimed at promoting intrinsic pathway activation include the MDM2 inhibitors, BCL-2 inhibitors, and IAP inhibitors.

intrinsic pathway, including chemotherapy and radiotherapy. This has provided the biological rationale for the development of agents to restore signaling through the intrinsic pathway.

p53

The tumor suppressor p53 is a DNA-binding protein that responds to diverse cellular stresses to regulate target genes that induce cell cycle arrest, apoptosis, senescence, DNA repair, or changes in metabolism. The induction of irreparable DNA or microtubule damage by chemotherapy and radiotherapy is one mechanism by which the intrinsic pathway is activated via p53 (Figure 12.3).[65] However, p53 is mutated and inactivated in half of all human cancers, underscoring its importance in cancer surveillance. Inactivation of p53 also occurs by binding to MDM2, an E3 ubiquitin ligase that promotes proteasome-mediated p53 degradation. MDM2 is amplified or overexpressed in several human tumor types, supporting a role for its involvement in cancer.[66] Therefore, one attractive therapeutic strategy has been to disrupt the p53–MDM2 interaction, which should stabilize p53 and enable its apoptotic function.

The x-ray structure of the p53–MDM2 complex showed how p53 interacts with MDM2 and aided in the design of p53 mimetics.[67] Early attempts to discover MDM2 inhibitors identified compounds that bound tightly to the p53-interacting cleft in MDM2 but had poor drug-like properties. The first class of compounds reported to function as MDM2 antagonists in vivo was a class of cis-imidazole compounds or nutlins.[68] Nutlins inhibit tumor growth in xenograft models without significant toxicities and display increased activity in tumor cells bearing wild-type p53.[68] Nutlin-3 has been shown to synergize with a wide variety of cytotoxic agents as well as with Apo2L/TRAIL.[69,70] Together, these studies support the development of nutlins for use in cancer therapy either as single agents or in combination with chemotherapy.

MDM2 inhibitors have entered phase 1 clinical trials (Table 12.2). RG7112 is a related pharmacophore of the nutlin family with improved potency, selectivity, and pharmacological properties. It is 15-fold more selective for wild type compared to p53 mutant cells and demonstrated activity in a panel of solid tumor cells

TABLE 12.2
Clinical Trials of MDM2 Antagonists

Agent	Setting	Intervention	Results
MK-8242	AML	Monotherapy and combination with cytarabine	Ongoing
	Solid tumors	Monotherapy	Ongoing
RG7112	Hematologic malignancies	Monotherapy	Andreeff[73]
	Solid tumors	Monotherapy	Kurzrock[72]
RO5503781	Solid tumors	Monotherapy	Ongoing
Serdemetan	Solid tumors	Monotherapy	Tabernero[151]

with the best responses in cells with MDM2 gene amplification.[71] Phase 1 studies were conducted in subjects with wild-type p53 advanced solid tumors[72] and hematologic malignancies.[73] Dose-limiting toxicities included diarrhea, hyponatremia, neutropenia, and thrombocytopenia in the solid tumor study. Evidence of p53 pathway activation was demonstrated in both studies and included a concentration-dependent increase in plasma macrophage inhibitory cytokine-1 (MIC-1) and an increase in p53, p21, and MDM2 levels in posttreatment biopsies. Biologic activity included partial responses in patients with MDM2-amplified liposarcoma and a complete remission in a subject with relapsed acute myelogenous leukemia (AML). A neoadjuvant study in well-differentiated and dedifferentiated liposarcoma with MDM2 amplification and wild-type p53 also demonstrated p53 pathway activation, and there was one partial response out of 20 subjects.[74] Phase 1 studies of additional MDM2 antagonists R05503781 and MK-8242 have been recently initiated. Optimization of the exposure–response relationship and examination of determinants of sensitivity beyond wild-type tumor p53 status will be important for development of these agents.

Preclinical studies have demonstrated that simultaneous targeting of the related homolog MDM4/MDMX may be needed for maximal efficacy.[75] This has led to the development of dual MDM2–MDM4 inhibitors using structure-based peptide design or to the combination of nutlins with MDM4-specific inhibitors.[76,77]

Another p53 activator that blocks MDM2 function is the small-molecule RITA (reactivation of p53 and induction of tumor cell apoptosis).[78] Unlike the nutlins that bind MDM2, RITA binds directly to p53, blocking its ability to interact with MDM2 but not its ability to activate p53-dependent apoptosis. RITA overcomes resistance to nutlin-based MDM2 inhibitors in vitro and shows preclinical activity in tumor xenograft models, but is not yet in clinical trials.[78–81]

Genetic models have demonstrated that restoration of p53 activity in established tumor cells is highly effective in mediating tumor regression, prompting the search for therapeutic agents that can reactivate p53 in human tumors.[69,82–85] One approach is to identify small molecules that bind to the mutant p53 core DNA-binding domain in order to stabilize p53 in its active biological conformation. Some tumor-associated mutations have been shown to thermally destabilize p53.[86,87] In another approach, cell-based screening methods have been used to identify molecules or combinations that selectively kill by activating mutant or wild-type p53. The most advanced compound to come from these types of approaches is APR-246/PRIMA (Aprea, Sweden), a small molecule that activates mutant p53. APR-246 was shown to protect several p53 mutants from unfolding in vitro and restore p53-dependent transcription in cell lines expressing p53 mutants.[88,89] In a first-in-human study in refractory hematologic malignancies and prostate cancer, APR-246 was safe at predicted therapeutic plasma levels, and one p53 mutant AML patient showed a 20% blast reduction in the bone marrow.[90]

The observations that cancer patients make antibodies to p53 and a large number of patients produce p53-reactive T cells have provided the rationale for attempts to vaccinate patients using p53-derived peptides, and a number of clinical trials are in progress.[69,91] To date, however, no significant clinical responses have been observed, although evidence of p53 vaccine-induced immunological responses was noted.[91] The use of dendritic cell-delivered p53 vaccines to boost responses is now being examined.[92] Finally, the concept of cyclotherapy, in which wild-type 53 acts as a chemoprotectant in normal tissues while p53 mutant tumor cells are selectively eradicated with an antimitotic drug, has garnered considerable interest.[69] In one preclinical study, the combination of nutlin with the polo-like kinase (PLK) inhibitor BI-2536 showed that nutlin could protect against neutropenia associated with PLK inhibitor administration without impacting its antitumor activity.[93]

Although numerous clinical trials involving p53 are ongoing, there is only one approved agent to date. A p53 recombinant adenovirus (Gendicine) was approved in China in 2003 to treat head and neck squamous cell carcinoma but remains in extended preregistration trials in the United States.[94,95] Therapy involves local injection into the tumor site and may not be effective in all patients. However, the ongoing progress in demonstrating that mutant inactive p53 can be rescued by a variety of novel approaches to promote intrinsic pathway activation suggests that these methods could make an impact on future p53-based cancer therapy.

BCL-2 FAMILY

The BCL-2 family of proteins serves as the gatekeepers of programmed cell death at the mitochondrion. The BCL-2 gene was initially cloned from the breakpoint of the t(14:18) chromosomal translocation found in the vast majority of follicular lymphomas.[96] Unlike conventional oncogenes, expression of BCL-2 alone does not promote cell proliferation but instead blocks cell death following numerous cellular insults and thus provided early evidence that suppression of apoptosis is a crucial step in tumorigenesis.[96]

In the ten years following the cloning of BCL-2, an entire family of related proteins was identified. Although all have related sequence homology in up to four conserved BCL-2 homology (BH) regions, these proteins have either anti- or pro-apoptotic functions and can be grouped into three classes (Figure 12.4). One class with BH1–BH4 homology inhibits apoptosis (BCL-2, BCL-XL, BCL-w, MCL-1, and A1), whereas a second class with BH1–BH3 homology promotes apoptosis (BAX, BAK, BOK). A third divergent class of BH3-only proteins has a conserved BH3 region that can bind and regulate the anti-apoptotic BCL-2 proteins to promote apoptosis (Figure 12.4). BAX and BAK are critical for inducing mitochondrial membrane permeabilization, and BH3-only proteins function as initial sensors of apoptotic signals that emanate from various cellular processes.[96]

Analysis of the 3D structures of several BCL-2 family proteins reveals a conserved structure consisting of two central predominantly hydrophobic α-helices surrounded by six or seven amphipathic helices. A hydrophobic groove on the surface of the anti-apoptotic BCL-2 proteins forms the binding site for the BH3 region of pro-apoptotic BCL-2 family members.[97] Based on these insights, several small-molecule BCL-2 inhibitors, designed to bind to the same hydrophobic groove that interacts with pro-apoptotic BAK and BAD proteins, have been developed.

Small molecules that target the BH3-binding groove of anti-apoptotic BCL-2 proteins are now in clinical development (Table 12.3). Prominent among these is the drug navitoclax (ABT-263), in multiple clinical trials for small cell lung cancer,

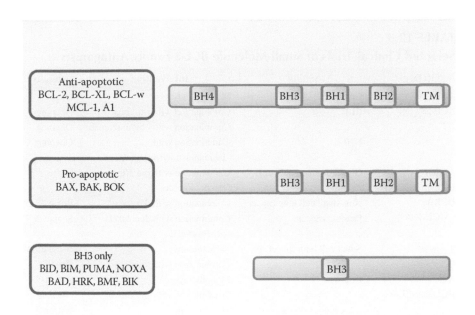

FIGURE 12.4 Structure of the BCL-2 protein family. The anti-apoptotic BCL-2 family members, including BCL-2, BCL-XL, BCL-w, MCL-1, and A1, have sequence homology in four alpha-helical BH (BCL-2 *h*omology) regions (BH1-BH4) and function to block cell death by binding and sequestering the pro-apoptotic BCL-2 family members. The pro-apoptotic BCL-2 proteins can be divided into those that have sequence homology to the BH1, BH2, and BH3 regions or the BH3-only proteins that only have homology with the BH3 region. BAX, BAK, and BOK make up the pro-apoptotic multi-domain BH1–BH3 proteins. Upon activation, BAX and BAK undergo a conformational change that facilitates their oligomerization and promotes the formation of pores in the outer mitochondrial membrane, inducing the release of cytochrome C and other pro-apoptotic proteins. Whereas BAX and BAK are essential for death induced by BH3 proteins, BOK expression is restricted to reproductive tissues. The BH3-only pro-apoptotic proteins, which include BID, BIM, PUMA, NOXA, BAD, HRK, BMF, and BIK, function either by directly inducing the oligomerization of BAK and BAX or by binding to and inhibiting the anti-apoptotic BCL-2 proteins. The BH3-only proteins become active through many mechanisms, including increased transcription, protein stabilization, and posttranslational modification.

lymphoma, chronic lymphocytic leukemia (CLL), and solid tumors. Navitoclax is an orally available modification of a related compound, ABT-737, which selectively antagonizes BCL-2, BCL-XL, and BCL-w and has been evaluated extensively in preclinical models.[98–100] In a phase 1 study in patients with relapsed or refractory CLL, durable partial responses were seen in 35% of patients and prolonged stable disease in 27% receiving continuous treatment at a dose >110 mg per day. The dose-limiting toxicity was thrombocytopenia. This provides strong proof of clinical activity for targeting BCL-2 in CLL as BCL-XL and BCL-w are not significantly expressed. Low MCL-1 expression and high BIM/MCL-1

TABLE 12.3

Selected Clinical Trials of Small-Molecule BCL-2 Family Antagonists

Agent/Target	Setting	Intervention	Results
ABT-199	CLL/NHL	Monotherapy	Ongoing
BCL-2	CLL	Combination with rituximab	Ongoing
		Combination with obinutuzumab	Ongoing
	NHL	Combination with bendamustine/rituximab	Ongoing
AT-101	Glioblastoma multiforme	Combination with radiation/ temozolomide	Fiveash[152]
BCL-2, BCL-XL,			
BCL-w,	Non-small cell lung cancer	Combination with docetaxel	Ready[153]
MCL-1, A1	Prostate cancer	Combination with docetaxel/ prednisone	Sonpavde[154]
	Small cell lung cancer	Monotherapy	Baggstrom[155]
		Combination with topotecan	Heist[156]
Navitoclax	CLL	Monotherapy	Roberts[101]
BCL-2, BCL-XL		Combination with rituximab	Ongoing
	Lymphoid malignancies	Monotherapy	Wilson[102]
	Small cell lung cancer	Monotherapy	Gandhi[157]
Obatoclax	AML	Monotherapy	Ongoing
BCL-2, BCL-XL,	CLL	Monotherapy	O'Brien[158]
BCL-w,	Hematologic malignancies	Monotherapy	Schimmer[159]
MCL-1, A1	Hodgkin lymphoma	Monotherapy	Oki[160]
	NHL	Monotherapy	Hwang[161]
		Combination with bendamustine/rituximab	Ongoing
	Small cell lung cancer	Combination with carboplatin/ etoposide	Langer[162]

or BIM/BCL-2 ratios in leukemic cells correlated with response, while levels of BCL-2 did not.[101]

One common feature of agents that inhibit BCL-XL is their capacity to induce rapid thrombocytopenia in preclinical models and in humans.[102–105] Inhibition of BCL-XL leads to a marked reduction in platelet life span and can induce severe thrombocytopenia at high concentrations. To address this, a new orally available and BCL-2-selective inhibitor, ABT-199, has recently entered clinical trials for CLL and NHL (www.clinicaltrials.gov). This may allow more complete BCL-2 inhibition and lead to improved clinical outcomes.

Another feature of most BCL-2 inhibitors is that they can be extremely potent inhibitors of BCL-2 and BCL-XL but bind with reduced affinity to other anti-apoptotic family members such as MCL-1. This is attributed to the fact that some BH3-only proteins bind promiscuously to all pro-survival BCL-2 proteins, whereas others display marked selectivity, accounting for the differences in the pro-apoptotic activity of BH3-only proteins.[106] For example, BCL-2 and BCL-XL bind to BAD with high affinity, but MCL-1 does not. In contrast, MCL-1 interacts strongly with NOXA, but BCL-2 and BCL-XL do not. This has prompted efforts to develop MCL-1-specific inhibitors and also raises questions about whether development of a pan-BCL-2 inhibitor is feasible and whether it would be tolerated.[107] Some pan-BCL-2 inhibitors that bind all anti-apoptotic family members have been developed but have relatively low affinity.[108] The results from ongoing and future clinical trials with BCL-2 family inhibitors that display various degrees of selectivity will provide insight on the relative clinical benefit from these agents.

There have been other approaches to target BCL-2. Oblimersen is a BCL-2 anti-sense oligonucleotide that targets BCL-2 mRNA. It exerts pro-apoptotic effects through an increase in BAX and PARP and may also promote tumor immunity through the binding of CpG motifs to toll-like receptor 9.[109] Oblimersen has been evaluated in phase 2 and 3 studies in multiple tumor types. In a randomized phase 3 trial in combination with fludarabine/cyclophosphamide, oblimersen significantly improved the complete response rate and nodular partial response rate but not over-all response rate or time to progression in patients with relapsed or refractory CLL.[110] Oblimersen also improved progression-free survival and overall response rate but not overall survival in advanced melanoma.[111]

INHIBITORS OF APOPTOSIS PROTEINS

The IAP proteins are major regulators of apoptosis, and the IAP protein family is characterized by the presence of one or more baculoviral IAP repeat (BIR) protein domains, which are important for binding caspases.[112] Some IAP members, including XIAP, cIAP1, and cIAP2, which are the focus of this chapter, also contain RING domains, which have been shown to possess E3 ubiquitin ligase activity.[113]

XIAP plays an important role in blocking both extrinsic and intrinsic pathway activation by directly binding and blocking caspase 3 and caspase 9 activity.[5] Although cIAP1 and cIAP2 can bind to caspases, their ability to directly inhibit caspases has been controversial.[114] Despite a poor understanding of how cIAP1 and cIAP2 function in blocking cell death, overexpression of IAP proteins has been noted in a variety of solid tumors and hematologic malignancies and is associated with poor prognosis.[115] Moreover, cIAP1 is a target of genetic amplification, and cIAP2 undergoes chromosomal translocation to the MALT1 locus, resulting in constitutive activation of NFkB in MALT lymphomas.[115] These findings have established a role for IAP proteins in contributing to human malignancies.

In cells, the inhibitory activity of XIAP is antagonized by the mitochondrial protein SMAC, which is released into the cytoplasm in response to pro-apoptotic stimuli (Figure 12.3).[64] The pro-apoptotic function of SMAC is dependent on a conserved four-residue IAP protein-interaction motif (A–V–P–I) found at the amino-terminus of the mature, posttranslationally processed protein.[116,117] This motif binds to a surface groove on the BIR domains of IAP proteins and competes for binding with caspases.[116] These findings led to the development of SMAC mimetics, which mimic the SMAC amino-terminus AVPI motif and thus interfere with IAP–caspase interactions.[112]

Characterization of the function of SMAC mimetics has yielded considerable insight into understanding how cIAP1 and cIAP2 block apoptosis.[118,119] Similar to endogenous SMAC, administration of SMAC mimetics to cells leads to the rapid degradation of cIAP1 and in some cases cIAP2, mediated via the E3 ligase activity of the IAPs.[120] This results in constitutive recruitment of the kinase RIP1 and subsequent activation of NFkB via the canonical pathway (Figure 12.2). In sensitive cells, activation of NFkB by an IAP antagonist causes an increase in TNF levels, leading to autocrine signaling and TNF-mediated cell death. In contrast to their positive role in the regulation of canonical NFkB signaling, cIAP proteins negatively regulate noncanonical NFkB signaling by mediating degradative ubiquitination of the NFkB-inducing kinase (NIK) (Figure 12.5). Therefore, the depletion of cIAP1 and cIAP2 by a SMAC mimetic leads to stabilization and accumulation of NIK, leading to activation of IKKα and NFkB.[115,119] Consistent with this, deletions of cIAP1 and cIAP2 in multiple myeloma have been found to cause constitutive aberrant NFkB activation through the noncanonical pathway via stabilization of NIK.[121,122] Thus, loss of IAPs is also associated with the development of certain types of cancer.

Several clinical trials testing SMAC mimetics are in progress (Table 12.4).[115] Agents being investigated include monovalent and bivalent antagonists, which tend to have different relative potencies and, in some cases, differential affinities for cIAP1 vs. cIAP2 and XIAP. The route of administration also differs. The monovalent IAP antagonist LCL-161 has been evaluated in a phase 1 study, in which a maximum tolerated dose was not reached.[123] Evidence of pharmacodynamic activity included reduction of cIAP1 levels in peripheral blood mononuclear cells, skin punch biopsies, and tumor biopsies as well as increases in serum MCP-1 and IL-8. However, no objective responses were observed. Bivalent antagonists are more potent in some preclinical models.[119] Phase 1 results of the bivalent IAP antagonists HGS1029[124] and TL32711[125] have also been reported. Dose-limiting fatigue, amylase/lipase elevation, and facial palsy were observed in the HGS1029 trial. Although pharmacodynamic activity was observed in both trials, there were no objective responses reported. Preclinical studies suggest that IAP antagonists may function optimally in combination settings, when administered with conventional chemotherapeutics or death receptor agonists. Understanding which IAP protein should be targeted in particular combinations as well as investigating other determinants of sensitivity is critical for future development. To this aim, a randomized phase 2 study of neoadjuvant LCL161 in triple-negative breast cancer is selecting patients based on a predefined pattern of gene expression.

FUTURE DIRECTIONS

The last decade has brought forth significant advances in our understanding of the mechanisms of cell death and evasion of apoptosis as a tumor survival mechanism. From this, many novel therapeutics aimed at restoring apoptosis induction in cancer cells have emerged and are currently undergoing clinical evaluation. Although a foundation to support apoptosis induction as a therapeutic strategy is in place, much remains to be learned about the underlying molecular intricacies and regulatory components. Ongoing research continues to provide additional insight into the

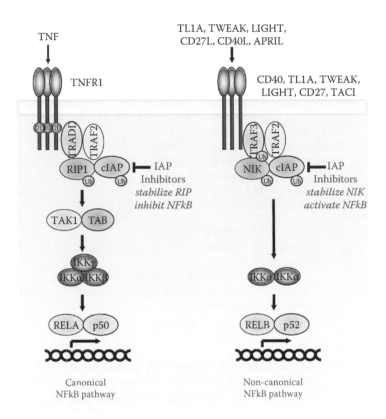

FIGURE 12.5 Opposing roles of IAP antagonists on canonical and noncanonical NFkB signaling pathways. In the canonical pathway, the binding of TNF to TNFR1 triggers the formation of a signaling complex with the adaptor protein TRAF2, RIP1 kinase, and cIAP1 and cIAP2, mediated via the adaptor protein TRADD. cIAP proteins ubiquitinate RIP1 and are themselves ubiquitinated, and this recruits TAK1, TAB, and the IKK complex. This leads to activation of the IKK complex and NFkB (p50-RELA). Administration of an IAP antagonist leads to cIAP1 and cIAP2 inactivation and degradation, resulting in elevated and prolonged association of RIP1 with TNFR1. In the absence of cIAPs, RIP1 forms a cytoplasmic complex with FADD and caspase 8 followed by induction of apoptosis. IAP antagonists therefore block NFkB activation through the canonical pathway. In the noncanonical NFkB pathway, cIAP proteins normally suppress NFkB activity and IAP inhibitors promote NFkB activity. Multiple TNF family ligands can signal through the noncanonical NFkB pathway, including TL1A (TNFSF15), TWEAK (TNFSF12), LIGHT (TNFSF14), CD27L (TNFSF7), CD40L (TNFSF5), and APRIL (TNFSF13).[115] Under resting conditions, cIAP proteins keep NIK levels low by promoting its ubiquitination and degradation. cIAP-mediated degradation of NIK requires the adaptor proteins TRAF2 and TRAF3. Engagement of ligand leads to cIAP-mediated degradation of TRAF3, which no longer recruits the TRAF2–cIAP complex to the receptor, leading to accumulation of NIK. This in turn activates IKKα and subsequently NFkB (p52–RELB) activation and target gene expression. Treatment with IAP antagonists leads to degradation and inactivation of cIAP1 and cIAP2. This prevents cIAP-mediated degradation of NIK, allowing for its stabilization and accumulation, resulting in activation of IKKα and NFkB (p52–RELB). Thus, IAP antagonists enhance NFkB signaling through the noncanonical pathway.

TABLE 12.4
Clinical Trials of IAP Antagonists

Agent	Setting	Intervention	Results
Monovalent inhibitors			
AT-406	AML	Combination with cytarabine/daunorubicin	Ongoing
	Solid tumors	Monotherapy	Ongoing
LCL161	Breast cancer	Combination with paclitaxel	Ongoing
	Solid tumors	Monotherapy	Infante[123]
		Combination with paclitaxel	Ongoing
GDC-0917	Solid tumors	Monotherapy	Ongoing
Bivalent inhibitors			
Birinapant	AML	Monotherapy	Ongoing
	Ovarian cancer	Monotherapy	Ongoing
	Solid tumors	Monotherapy	Amaravadi[125]
		Combination with multiple chemotherapy regimens	Ongoing
		Combination with gemcitabine	Ongoing
HGS1029	Solid tumors	Monotherapy	Sickic[124]

functions of proteins that regulate cell death. For example, emerging evidence for the growth-promoting functions of TNF family ligands such as FasL or the opposing roles of IAP proteins in canonical and noncanonical NFkB signaling are key issues to be considered. Increased understanding of the settings that dictate these contrasting outcomes warrants continued examination of these pathways in the context of tumor therapy.

Parallel to our increased understanding about the mechanisms of apoptosis has been a growing knowledge about other forms of cell death, including autophagy and necroptosis. It is likely that dysregulation of these forms of death also contributes to cancer progression. How these different forms of cell death are coordinated is poorly understood, but reports of the interplay between them are emerging. For example, both BCL-2 and BCL-XL bind to the tumor suppressor Beclin, and this reaction has been shown to inhibit autophagy, and BCL-2 antagonists can stimulate autophagy.[126,127] Future studies on the relationships between various cell death pathways should provide translational advances in the improved design of tumor-selective cell death therapies.

Many challenges remain in our ability to effectively treat cancer and deliver a durable response. Interdiction in one pathway can often lead to upregulation of compensatory mechanisms that drive resistance to targeted therapeutics. Therefore, effective treatment for most tumors may require that agents be given in combination with other compounds. Identifying those agents that result in potent synergistic activity and lower the threshold for tumor cell death induction will be critical for successful management of tumor resistance and relapse. Indeed, preclinical studies of apoptosis-promoting therapies such as death receptor agonists have shown a broad spectrum of cooperativity with other agents, suggesting there may be many therapeutic strategies to explore clinically, provided no additive safety signal is observed in a combination setting. Positive interactions may be achieved in combination with agents that target different points in the same pathway, kill tumor cells via different pathways, or target other cells within the tumor microenvironment. In addition, identifying patients with the greatest likelihood of response by the application of informative, validated biomarkers will be key to the success of these strategies. In conclusion, the results from ongoing trials with various apoptosis-promoting cancer therapies are eagerly awaited, as is an increased understanding of the molecular complexities between cell death networks, particularly in the context of cancer.

REFERENCES

1. Aggarwal BB, Gupta SC, Kim JH. Historical perspectives on tumor necrosis factor and its superfamily: 25 years later, a golden journey. *Blood* 2012;119:651–665.
2. Locksley RM, Killeen N, Lenardo MJ. The TNF and TNF receptor superfamilies: Integrating mammalian biology. *Cell* 2001;104:487–501.
3. Song JH, Tse MC, Bellail A et al. Lipid rafts and nonrafts mediate tumor necrosis factor related apoptosis-inducing ligand induced apoptotic and nonapoptotic signals in non small cell lung carcinoma cells. *Cancer Res* 2007;67:6946–6955.
4. Ashkenazi A. Targeting death and decoy receptors of the tumour-necrosis factor superfamily. *Nat Rev Cancer* 2002;2:420–430.
5. Gyrd-Hansen M, Meier P. IAPs: From caspase inhibitors to modulators of NF-kappaB, inflammation and cancer. *Nat Rev Cancer* 2010;10:561–574.
6. Varfolomeev E, Maecker H, Sharp D et al. Molecular determinants of kinase pathway activation by Apo2 ligand/tumor necrosis factor-related apoptosis-inducing ligand. *J Biol Chem* 2005;280:40599–40608.
7. Peter ME, Legembre P, Barnhart BC. Does CD95 have tumor promoting activities? *Biochim Biophys Acta* 2005;1755:25–36.
8. Balkwill F. Tumour necrosis factor and cancer. *Nat Rev Cancer* 2009;9:361–371
9. Schutze S, Tchikov V, Schneider-Brachert W. Regulation of TNFR1 and CD95 signalling by receptor compartmentalization. *Nat Rev Mol Cell Biol* 2008;9:655–662.
10. O'Malley WE, Achinstein B, Shear MJ. Action of bacterial polysaccharide on tumors. III. Repeated response of Sarcoma 37, in tolerant mice, to Serratia Marcescens Endotoxin. *Cancer Res* 1963;23:890–895.
11. Carswell EA, Old LJ, Kassel RL et al. An endotoxin-induced serum factor that causes necrosis of tumors. *Proc Natl Acad Sci USA* 1975;72:3666–3670.
12. Saks S, Rosenblum M. Recombinant human TNF-alpha: Preclinical studies and results from early clinical trials. *Immunol Ser* 1992;56:567–587.
13. Hersh EM, Metch BS, Muggia FM et al. Phase II studies of recombinant human tumor necrosis factor alpha in patients with malignant disease: A summary of the Southwest Oncology Group experience. *J Immunother* 1991;10:426–431.
14. de Wilt JH, ten Hagen TL, de Boeck G et al. Tumour necrosis factor alpha increases melphalan concentration in tumour tissue after isolated limb perfusion. *Br J Cancer* 2000;82:1000–1003.
15. van Horssen R, Ten Hagen TL, Eggermont AM. TNF-alpha in cancer treatment: Molecular insights, antitumor effects, and clinical utility. *Oncologist* 2006;11:397–408.
16. de Roos WK, de Wilt JH, van Der Kaaden ME et al. Isolated limb perfusion for local gene delivery: Efficient and targeted adenovirus-mediated gene transfer into soft tissue sarcomas. *Ann Surg* 2000;232:814–821.
17. Fraker DL. Management of in-transit melanoma of the extremity with isolated limb perfusion. *Curr Treat Options Oncol* 2004;5:173–184.

18. Olieman AF, Lienard D, Eggermont AM et al. Hyperthermic isolated limb perfusion with tumor necrosis factor alpha, interferon gamma, and melphalan for locally advanced nonmelanoma skin tumors of the extremities: A multicenter study. *Arch Surg* 1999;134:303–307.

19. Sethi G, Sung B, Aggarwal BB. TNF: A master switch for inflammation to cancer. *Front Biosci* 2008;13:5094–5107.

20. Moore RJ, Owens DM, Stamp G et al. Mice deficient in tumor necrosis factor-alpha are resistant to skin carcinogenesis. *Nat Med* 1999;5:828–831.

21. Balkwill F, Mantovani A. Cancer and inflammation: Implications for pharmacology and therapeutics. *Clin Pharmacol Ther* 2010;87:401–406.

22. Nagata S, Suda T. Fas and Fas ligand: lpr and gld mutations. *Immunol Today* 1995;16:39–43.

23. Rieux-Laucat F, Le Deist F, Fischer A. Autoimmune lymphoproliferative syndromes: genetic defects of apoptosis pathways. *Cell Death Differ* 2003;10:124–133.

24. Karray S, Kress C, Cuvellier S et al. Complete loss of Fas ligand gene causes massive lymphoproliferation and early death, indicating a residual activity of gld allele. *J Immunol* 2004;172:2118–2125.

25. Ogasawara J, Watanabe-Fukunaga R, Adachi M et al. Lethal effect of the anti-Fas antibody in mice. *Nature* 1993;364:806–809.

26. Eisele G, Roth P, Hasenbach K et al. APO010, a synthetic hexameric CD95 ligand, induces human glioma cell death in vitro and in vivo. *Neuro Oncol*;13:155–164.

27. Tanaka M, Suda T, Haze K et al. Fas ligand in human serum. *Nat Med* 1996;2:317–322.

28. Chen L, Park SM, Tumanov AV et al. CD95 promotes tumour growth. *Nature* 2010;465:492–496.

29. Kleber S, Sancho-Martinez I, Wiestler B et al. Yes and PI3K bind CD95 to signal invasion of glioblastoma. *Cancer Cell* 2008;13:235–248.

30. Tuettenberg J, Seiz M, Debatin KM et al. Pharmacokinetics, pharmacodynamics, safety and tolerability of APG101, a CD95-Fc fusion protein, in healthy volunteers and two glioma patients. *Int Immunopharmacol*;13:93–100.

31. Ashkenazi A, Pai RC, Fong S et al. Safety and antitumor activity of recombinant soluble Apo2 ligand. *J Clin Invest* 1999;104:155–162.

32. Lum JJ, Pilon AA, Sanchez-Dardon J et al. Induction of cell death in human immunodeficiency virus-infected macrophages and resting memory CD4 T cells by TRAIL/Apo2l. *J Virol* 2001;75:11128–11136.

33. Ashkenazi A, Holland P, Eckhardt SG. Ligand-based targeting of apoptosis in cancer: The potential of recombinant human apoptosis ligand 2/Tumor necrosis factor-related apoptosis-inducing ligand (rhApo2L/TRAIL). *J Clin Oncol* 2008; 26:3621–3630.

34. Wiezorek J, Holland P, Graves J. Death receptor agonists as a targeted therapy for cancer. *Clin Cancer Res* 2010;16:1701–1708.

35. Herbst RS, Eckhardt SG, Kurzrock R et al. Phase I dose-escalation study of recombinant human Apo2L/TRAIL, a dual proapoptotic receptor agonist, in patients with advanced cancer. *J Clin Oncol* 2010;28:2839–2846.

36. Younes A, Vose JM, Zelenetz AD et al. A Phase 1b/2 trial of mapatumumab in patients with relapsed/refractory non-Hodgkin's lymphoma. *Br J Cancer* 2010;103: 1783–1787.

37. Herbst RS, Kurzrock R, Hong DS et al. A first-in-human study of conatumumab in adult patients with advanced solid tumors. *Clin Cancer Res* 2010;16:5883–5891.

38. Tolcher AW, Mita M, Meropol NJ et al. Phase I pharmacokinetic and biologic correlative study of mapatumumab, a fully human monoclonal antibody with agonist activity to tumor necrosis factor-related apoptosis-inducing ligand receptor-1. *J Clin Oncol* 2007;25:1390–1395.

39. Hotte SJ, Hirte HW, Chen EX et al. A phase 1 study of mapatumumab (fully human monoclonal antibody to TRAIL-R1) in patients with advanced solid malignancies. *Clin Cancer Res* 2008;14:3450–3455.

40. Camidge DR, Herbst RS, Gordon MS et al. A phase I safety and pharmacokinetic study of the death receptor 5 agonistic antibody PRO95780 in patients with advanced malignancies. *Clin Cancer Res* 2010;16:1256–1263.

41. Forero-Torres A, Shah J, Wood T et al. Phase I trial of weekly tigatuzumab, an agonistic humanized monoclonal antibody targeting death receptor 5 (DR5). *Cancer Biother Radiopharm* 2010;25:13–19.

42. Pan Y, Xu R, Peach M et al. Evaluation of pharmacodynamic biomarkers in a phase 1a trial of dulanermin (rhApo2L/TRAIL) in patients with advanced tumours. *Br J Cancer* 2011;105:1830–1838.

43. Kaplan-Lefko PJ, Graves JD, Zoog SJ et al. Conatumumab, a fully human agonist antibody to death receptor 5, induces apoptosis via caspase activation in multiple tumor types. *Cancer Biol Ther* 2010;9:618–631.

44. Wilson NS, Yang B, Yang A et al. An Fcgamma receptor-dependent mechanism drives antibody-mediated target-receptor signaling in cancer cells. *Cancer Cell* 2011;19:101–113.

45. Maddipatla S, Hernandez-Ilizaliturri FJ, Knight J et al. Augmented antitumor activity against B-cell lymphoma by a combination of monoclonal antibodies targeting TRAIL-R1 and CD20. *Clin Cancer Res* 2007;13:4556–4564.

46. Pan Y, Haddad V, Sabin T et al. Predictive value of Fc gamma receptor IIIa genotype in response to conatumumab in three phase II studies. *J Clin Oncol* 2011;29(Suppl): Abstract 3103.

47. Takeda K, Yamaguchi N, Akiba H et al. Induction of tumor-specific T cell immunity by anti-DR5 antibody therapy. *J Exp Med* 2004;199:437–448.

48. Suda T, Hashimoto H, Tanaka M et al. Membrane Fas ligand kills human peripheral blood T lymphocytes, and soluble Fas ligand blocks the killing. *J Exp Med* 1997;186:2045–2050.

49. Schneider P, Holler N, Bodmer JL et al. Conversion of membrane-bound Fas(CD95) ligand to its soluble form is associated with downregulation of its proapoptotic activity and loss of liver toxicity. *J Exp Med* 1998;187:1205–1213.

50. O'Reilly L, Tai L, Lee L et al. Membrane-bound Fas ligand only is essential for Fas-induced apoptosis. *Nature* 2009;461:659–663.

51. Muhlenbeck F, Schneider P, Bodmer JL et al. The tumor necrosis factor-related apoptosis-inducing ligand receptors TRAIL-R1 and TRAIL-R2 have distinct cross-linking requirements for initiation of apoptosis and are non-redundant in JNK activation. *J Biol Chem* 2000;275:32208–32213.

52. Wajant H, Moosmayer D, Wuest T et al. Differential activation of TRAIL-R1 and -2 by soluble and membrane TRAIL allows selective surface antigen-directed activation of TRAIL-R2 by a soluble TRAIL derivative. *Oncogene* 2001;20:4101–4106.

53. Kelley RF, Totpal K, Lindstrom SH et al. Receptor-selective mutants of apoptosis-inducing ligand 2/tumor necrosis factor-related apoptosis-inducing ligand reveal a greater contribution of death receptor (DR) 5 than DR4 to apoptosis signaling. *J Biol Chem* 2005;280:2205–2212.

54. Berg D, Lehne M, Muller N et al. Enforced covalent trimerization increases the activity of the TNF ligand family members TRAIL and CD95L. *Cell Death Differ* 2007;14:2021–2034.

55. Newsom-Davis T, Prieske S, Walczak H. Is TRAIL the holy grail of cancer therapy? *Apoptosis* 2009;14:607–623.

56. Pavet V, Beyrath J, Pardin C et al. Multivalent DR5 peptides activate the TRAIL death pathway and exert tumoricidal activity. *Cancer Res* 2010;70:1101–1110.

57. de Bruyn M, Wei Y, Wiersma VR et al. Cell surface delivery of TRAIL strongly augments the tumoricidal activity of T cells. *Clin Cancer Res* 2010;17:5626–5637.

58. Pfizenmaier K, Szymkowski DE. Workshop summary: Introduction to rational design of new means for therapeutic modulation of function of the TNF family. *Adv Exp Med Biol* 2011;691:487–491.

59. de Bruyn M, Bremer E, Helfrich W. Antibody-based fusion proteins to target death receptors in cancer. *Cancer Lett* 2013;332:175–183.

60. Krippner-Heidenreich A, Grunwald I, Zimmermann G et al. Single-chain TNF, a TNF derivative with enhanced stability and antitumoral activity. *J Immunol* 2008;180:8176–8183.

61. Stieglmaier J, Bremer E, Kellner C et al. Selective induction of apoptosis in leukemic B-lymphoid cells by a CD19-specific TRAIL fusion protein. *Cancer Immunol Immunother* 2008;57:233–246.

62. Groth A, Salnikov AV, Ottinger S et al. New gene-immunotherapy combining TRAIL-lymphocytes and EpCAMxCD3 bispecific antibody for tumor targeting. *Clin Cancer Res* 2012;18:1028–1038.

63. Huet H, Schuller A, Li J et al. TAS266, a novel tetrameric nanobody agonist targeting death receptor 5 (DR5), elicits superior antitumor efficacy than conventional DR5-targeted approaches. *Cancer Res* 2012;72:Abstract 3853.

64. Salvesen GS, Duckett CS. IAP proteins: Blocking the road to death's door. *Nat Rev Mol Cell Biol* 2002;3:401–410.

65. Fesik SW. Promoting apoptosis as a strategy for cancer drug discovery. *Nat Rev Cancer* 2005;5:876–885.

66. Momand J, Wu HH, Dasgupta G. MDM2—Master regulator of the p53 tumor suppressor protein. *Gene* 2000;242:15–29.

67. Kussie PH, Gorina S, Marechal V et al. Structure of the MDM2 oncoprotein bound to the p53 tumor suppressor transactivation domain. *Science* 1996;274:948–953.

68. Vassilev LT, Vu BT, Graves B et al. In vivo activation of the p53 pathway by small-molecule antagonists of MDM2. *Science* 2004;303:844–848.

69. Cheok CF, Verma CS, Baselga J et al. Translating p53 into the clinic. *Nat Rev Clin Oncol* 2011;8:25–37.

70. Secchiero P, Vaccarezza M, Gonelli A et al. TNF-related apoptosis-inducing ligand (TRAIL): A potential candidate for combined treatment of hematological malignancies. *Curr Pharm Des* 2004;10:3673–3681.

71. Tovar C, Filipovic Z, Thompson T et al. Antitumor activity of the MDM2 antagonist, RG7112. *Cancer Res* 2012;72:4727.

72. Kurzrock R, Jean-Yves B, Nguyen BB et al. A phase I study of MDM2 antagonist RG7112 in patients (pts) with relapsed/refractory solid tumors. *J Clin Oncol* 2012;30:e13600.

73. Andreeff M, Kojima K, Padmanabhan S et al. A multi-center, open-label, phase I study of single agent RG7112, a first in class p53-MDM2 antagonist, in patients with relapsed/refractory acute myeloid and lymphoid leukemias (AML/ALL) and refractory chronic lymphocytic leukemia/small cell lymphocytic lymphomas (CLL/SCLL). *ASH Annu Meet Abst* 2010;116:657.

74. Ray-Coquard IL, J. B, Italiano A, et al. Neoadjuvant MDM2 antagonist RG7112 for well-differentiated and dedifferentiated liposarcomas (WD/DD LPS): A pharmacodynamic (PD) biomarker study. *J Clin Oncol* 2011;29:100007b.

75. Hu B, Gilkes DM, Farooqi B et al. MDMX overexpression prevents p53 activation by the MDM2 inhibitor Nutlin. *J Biol Chem* 2006;281:33030–33035.

76. Phan J, Li Z, Kasprzak A et al. Structure-based design of high affinity peptides inhibiting the interaction of p53 with MDM2 and MDMX. *J Biol Chem* 2010;285:2174–2183.

77. Reed D, Shen Y, Shelat AA et al. Identification and characterization of the first small molecule inhibitor of MDMX. *J Biol Chem* 2010;285:10786–10796.

78. Issaeva N, Bozko P, Enge M et al. Small molecule RITA binds to p53, blocks p53-HDM-2 interaction and activates p53 function in tumors. *Nat Med* 2004;10:1321–1328.
79. Grinkevich VV, Nikulenkov F, Shi Y et al. Ablation of key oncogenic pathways by RITA-reactivated p53 is required for efficient apoptosis. *Cancer Cell* 2009;15:441–453.
80. Jones RJ, Bjorklund CC, Baladandayuthapani V et al. Drug resistance to inhibitors of the human double minute-2 E3 ligase is mediated by point mutations of p53, but can be overcome with the p53 targeting agent RITA. *Mol Cancer Ther* 2012;11:2243.
81. Saha MN, Yang Y, chang H. Targeting p53 by small molecule p53 activators in multiple myeloma. *J Hematol Oncol* 2012;5(Suppl 1):A7.
82. Martins CP, Brown-Swigart L, Evan GI. Modeling the therapeutic efficacy of p53 restoration in tumors. *Cell* 2006;127:1323–1334.
83. Ventura A, Kirsch DG, McLaughlin ME et al. Restoration of p53 function leads to tumour regression in vivo. *Nature* 2007;445:661–665.
84. Xue W, Zender L, Miething C et al. Senescence and tumour clearance is triggered by p53 restoration in murine liver carcinomas. *Nature* 2007;445:656–660.
85. Brown CJ, Lain S, Verma CS et al. Awakening guardian angels: Drugging the p53 pathway. *Nat Rev Cancer* 2009;9:862–873.
86. Terzian T, Suh YA, Iwakuma T et al. The inherent instability of mutant p53 is alleviated by Mdm2 or p16INK4a loss. *Genes Dev* 2008;22:1337–1344.
87. Joerger AC, Ang HC, Fersht AR. Structural basis for understanding oncogenic p53 mutations and designing rescue drugs. *Proc Natl Acad Sci USA* 2006;103:15056–15061.
88. Bykov VJ, Issaeva N, Shilov A et al. Restoration of the tumor suppressor function to mutant p53 by a low-molecular-weight compound. *Nat Med* 2002;8:282–288.
89. Lambert JM, Gorzov P, Veprintsev DB et al. PRIMA-1 reactivates mutant p53 by covalent binding to the core domain. *Cancer Cell* 2009;15:376–388.
90. Lehmann S, Bykov VJ, Ali D et al. Targeting p53 in Vivo: A first-in-human study with p53-targeting compound APR-246 in refractory hematologic malignancies and prostate cancer. *J Clin Oncol* 2012;30:3633–3639.
91. Vermeij R, Leffers N, van der Burg SH et al. Immunological and clinical effects of vaccines targeting p53-overexpressing malignancies. *J Biomed Biotechnol* 2011;2011:702146.
92. Chiappori AA, Soliman H, Janssen WE et al. INGN-225: A dendritic cell-based p53 vaccine (Ad.p53-DC) in small cell lung cancer: Observed association between immune response and enhanced chemotherapy effect. *Expert Opin Biol Ther* 2010;10:983–991.
93. Sur S, Pagliarini R, Bunz F, et al. A panel of isogenic human cancer cells suggests a therapeutic approach for cancers with inactivated p53. *Proc Natl Acad Sci USA* 2009;106:3964–3969
94. Peng Z. Current status of gendicine in China: Recombinant human Ad-p53 agent for treatment of cancers. *Hum Gene Ther* 2005;16:1016–1027.
95. Pearson S, Jia H, Kandachi K. China approves first gene therapy. *Nat Biotechnol* 2004;22:3–4.
96. Youle RJ, Strasser A. The BCL-2 protein family: Opposing activities that mediate cell death. *Nat Rev Mol Cell Biol* 2008;9:47–59.
97. Petros AM, Olejniczak ET, Fesik SW. Structural biology of the Bcl-2 family of proteins. *Biochim Biophys Acta* 2004;1644:83–94.
98. Konopleva M, Contractor R, Tsao T et al. Mechanisms of apoptosis sensitivity and resistance to the BH3 mimetic ABT-737 in acute myeloid leukemia. *Cancer Cell* 2006;10:375–388.
99. Oltersdorf T, Elmore SW, Shoemaker AR et al. An inhibitor of Bcl-2 family proteins induces regression of solid tumours. *Nature* 2005;435:677–681.
100. Tahir SK, Yang X, Anderson MG et al. Influence of Bcl-2 family members on the cellular response of small-cell lung cancer cell lines to ABT-737. *Cancer Res* 2007;67:1176–1183.

101. Roberts AW, Seymour JF, Brown JR et al. Substantial susceptibility of chronic lympho-cytic leukemia to BCL2 inhibition: Results of a phase I study of navitoclax in patients with relapsed or refractory disease. *J Clin Oncol* 2012;30:488–496.

102. Wilson WH, O'Connor OA, Czuczman MS et al. Navitoclax, a targeted high-affinity inhibitor of BCL-2, in lymphoid malignancies: A phase 1 dose-escalation study of safety, pharmacokinetics, pharmacodynamics, and antitumour activity. *Lancet Oncol*;11:1149–1159.

103. Mason KD, Carpinelli MR, Fletcher JI et al. Programmed a nuclear cell death delimits platelet life span. *Cell* 2007;128:1173–1186.

104. Tse C, Shoemaker AR, Adickes J et al. ABT-263: A potent and orally bioavailable Bcl-2 family inhibitor. *Cancer Res* 2008;68:3421–3428.

105. Zhang H, Nimmer PM, Tahir SK et al. Bcl-2 family proteins are essential for platelet survival. *Cell Death Differ* 2007;14:943–951.

106. Chen L, Willis SN, Wei A et al. Differential targeting of prosurvival Bcl-2 proteins by their BH3-only ligands allows complementary apoptotic function. *Mol Cell* 2005;17:393–403.

107. Quinn BA, Dash R, Azab B et al. Targeting Mcl-1 for the therapy of cancer. *Expert Opin Investig Drugs* 2011;20:1397–1411.

108. Zhai D, Jin C, Satterthwait AC et al. Comparison of chemical inhibitors of antiapoptotic Bcl-2-family proteins. *Cell Death Differ* 2006;13:1419–1421.

109. Kang MH, Reynolds CP. Bcl-2 inhibitors: Targeting mitochondrial apoptotic pathways in cancer therapy. *Clin Cancer Res* 2009;15:1126–1132.

110. O'Brien S, Moore JO, Boyd TE et al. Randomized phase III trial of fludarabine plus cyclophosphamide with or without oblimersen sodium (Bcl-2 antisense) in patients with relapsed or refractory chronic lymphocytic leukemia. *J Clin Oncol* 2007; 25:1114–1120.

111. Bedikian AY, Millward M, Pehamberger H et al. Bcl-2 antisense (oblimersen sodium) plus dacarbazine in patients with advanced melanoma: The Oblimersen Melanoma Study Group. *J Clin Oncol* 2006;24:4738–4745.

112. LaCasse EC, Mahoney DJ, Cheung HH et al. IAP-targeted therapies for cancer. *Oncogene* 2008;27:6252–6275.

113. Vaux DL, Silke J. IAPs—The ubiquitin connection. *Cell Death Differ* 2005;12:1205–1207.

114. Eckelman BP, Salvesen GS. The human anti-apoptotic proteins cIAP1 and cIAP2 bind but do not inhibit caspases. *J Biol Chem* 2006;281:3254–3260.

115. Fulda S, Vucic D. Targeting IAP proteins for therapeutic intervention in cancer. *Nat Rev Drug Discov* 2012;11:109–124.

116. Liu Z, Sun C, Olejniczak ET et al. Structural basis for binding of Smac/DIABLO to the XIAP BIR3 domain. *Nature* 2000;408:1004–1008.

117. Wu G, Chai J, Suber TL et al. Structural basis of IAP recognition by Smac/DIABLO. *Nature* 2000;408:1008–1012.

118. Vince JE, Wong WW, Khan N et al. IAP antagonists target cIAP1 to induce TNFalpha-dependent apoptosis. *Cell* 2007;131:682–693.

119. Varfolomeev E, Blankenship JW, Wayson SM et al. IAP antagonists induce autoubiq-uitination of c-IAPs, NF-kappaB activation, and TNFalpha-dependent apoptosis. *Cell* 2007;131:669–681.

120. Yang QH, Du C. Smac/DIABLO selectively reduces the levels of c-IAP1 and c-IAP2 but not that of XIAP and livin in HeLa cells. *Drug News Perspect* 2004;17:127–134.

121. Keats JJ, Fonseca R, Chesi M et al. Promiscuous mutations activate the noncanonical NF-kappaB pathway in multiple myeloma. *Cancer Cell* 2007;12:131–144.

122. Annunziata CM, Davis RE, Demchenko Y et al. Frequent engagement of the classi-cal and alternative NF-kappaB pathways by diverse genetic abnormalities in multiple myeloma. *Cancer Cell* 2007;12:115–130.

123. Infante JRE, Dees EC, Burris HA et al. A phase I study of LCL161, an oral IAP inhibitor, in patients with advanced cancer. *Proceedings of the 101st Annual Meeting of the American Association for Cancer Research,* Washington, DC 2010;70:Abstract 2775.

124. Sikic BI, Eckhardt SG, Gallant G et al. Safety, pharmacokinetics (PK), and pharmacodynamics (PD) of HGS1029, an inhibitor of apoptosis protein (IAP) inhibitor, in patients (Pts) with advanced solid tumors: Results of a phase I study. *J Clin Oncol* 2011;29:Abstract 3008.

125. Amaravadi RK, Schilder RJ, Dy GK et al. Phase 1 study of the Smac mimetic TL32711 in adult subjects with advanced solid tumors and lymphoma to evaluate safety, pharmacokinetics, pharmacodynamics, and antitumor activity. *Proceedings of the 102nd Annual Meeting of the American Association for Cancer Research,* Orlando, FL 2011:LB-406.

126. Maiuri MC, Le Toumelin G, Criollo A et al. Functional and physical interaction between Bcl-X(L) and a BH3-like domain in Beclin-1. *EMBO J* 2007;26:2527–2539.

127. Levine B, Kroemer G. Autophagy in the pathogenesis of disease. *Cell* 2008;132:27–42.

128. Saltz L, Infante J, Schwartzberg L et al. Safety and efficacy of AMG 655 plus modified FOLFOX6 (mFOLFOX6) and bevacizumab (B) for the first-line treatment of patients (pts) with metastatic colorectal cancer (mCRC). *J Clin Oncol* 2009;27:Abstract 4079.

129. Cohn AL, Tabernero J, Maurel J et al. Conatumumab (CON) plus FOLFIRI (F) or ganitumab (GAN) plus F for second-line treatment of mutant (MT) KRAS metastatic colorectal cancer (mCRC). *J Clin Oncol* 2012;30(Suppl 4): Abstract 534.

130. Peeters M, Infante JR, Rougier P et al. Phase Ib/II trial of conatumumab and panitumumab (pmab) for the treatment (tx) of metastatic colorectal cancer (mCRC): Safety and efficacy. *J Clin Oncol* 2010;2010 *Gastrointestinal Cancers Symp*:Abstract 443.

131. Paz-Ares L, Sánchez Torres JM, Diaz-Padilla I et al. Safety and efficacy of AMG 655 in combination with paclitaxel and carboplatin (PC) in patients with advanced non-small cell lung cancer (NSCLC). *J Clin Oncol* 2009;27: Abstract 19048.

132. Kindler HL, Richards DA, Garbo LE et al. A randomized, placebo-controlled phase 2 study of ganitumab (AMG 479) or conatumumab (AMG 655) in combination with gemcitabine in patients with metastatic pancreatic cancer. *Ann Oncol* 2012;23:2834–2842.

133. Demetri GD, Le Cesne A, Chawla SP et al. First-line treatment of metastatic or locally advanced unresectable soft tissue sarcomas with conatumumab in combination with doxorubicin or doxorubicin alone: A phase I/II open-label and double-blind study. *Eur J Cancer* 2012;48:547–563.

134. Younes A, Kirschbaum M, Sokol L et al. Safety and tolerability of conatumumab in combination with bortezomib or vorinostat in patients with relapsed or refractory lymphoma Presented at the *American Society of Hematology 51st Annual Meeting and Exposition,* December 5–8, New Orleans, LA 2009: Abstract 1708.

135. Chawla SP, Tabernero J, Kindler HL et al. Phase I evaluation of the safety of conatumumab (AMG 655) in combination with AMG 479 in patients (pts) with advanced, refractory solid tumors. *J Clin Oncol* 2010;28(Suppl): Abstract 3102.

136. Rocha Lima CM, Bayraktar S, Flores AM et al. Phase Ib study of drozitumab combined with first-line mFOLFOX6 plus bevacizumab in patients with metastatic colorectal cancer. *Cancer Invest* 2012;30:727–731.

137. Wittebol S, Ferrant A, Wickham NW et al. Phase II study of PRO95780 plus rituximab in patients with relapsed follicular non-Hodgkin's lymphoma (NHL). *J Clin Oncol* 2010;28(Suppl): Abstract e18511.

138. Karapetis CS, Clingan PR, Leighl NB et al. Phase II study of PRO95780 plus paclitaxel, carboplatin, and bevacizumab (PCB) in non-small cell lung cancer (NSCLC). *J Clin Oncol* 2010;28(Suppl): Abstract 7535.

139. Chawla S, Demetri G, Desai J et al. Initial results of a phase II study of the safety and efficacy of the Apomab DR5 agonist antibody in advanced chondrosarcoma and synovial sarcoma patients. *Presented at the Connective Tissue Oncology Society Annual Meeting,* London, U.K., 2008: Abstract # 35010.
140. Yee L, Burris HA, Kozloff M et al. Phase Ib study of recombinant human Apo2L/TRAIL plus irinotecan and cetuximab or FOLFIRI in metastatic colorectal cancer (mCRC) patients (pts): Preliminary results. *J Clin Oncol* 2009;27:Abstract 4129.
141. Soria JC, Mark Z, Zatloukal P et al. Randomized phase II study of dulanermin in combination with paclitaxel, carboplatin, and bevacizumab in advanced non-small-cell lung cancer. *J Clin Oncol* 2011;29:4442–4451.
142. Plummer R, Attard G, Pacey S et al. Phase 1 and pharmacokinetic study of lexatumumab in patients with advanced cancers. *Clin Cancer Res* 2007;13:6187–6194.
143. Merchant MS, Geller JI, Baird K et al. Phase I trial and pharmacokinetic study of lexatumumab in pediatric patients with solid tumors. *J Clin Oncol* 2012;30:4141–4147.
144. Sikic BI, Wakelee HA, von Mehren M et al. A phase Ib study to assess the safety of lexatumumab, a human monoclonal antibody that activates TRAIL-R2, in combination with gemcitabine, pemetrexed, doxorubicin or FOLFIRI. *J Clin Oncol* 2007;25: Abstract 14006.
145. Trarbach T, Moehler M, Heinemann V et al. Phase II trial of mapatumumab, a fully human agonistic monoclonal antibody that targets and activates the tumour necrosis factor apoptosis-inducing ligand receptor-1 (TRAIL-R1), in patients with refractory colorectal cancer. *Br J Cancer* 2010;102:506–512.
146. Sun W, Nelson D, Alberts SR et al. Phase Ib study of mapatumumab in combination with sorafenib in patients with advanced hepatocellular carcinoma (HCC) and chronic viral hepatitis. *J Clin Oncol* 2011;29(Suppl 4); Abstract 261.
147. Belch A, Sharma A, Spencer A et al. A multicenter randomized phase II trial of mapatumumab, a TRAIL-R1 agonist monoclonal antibody, in combination with bortezomib in patients with relapsed/refractory multiple myeloma (MM). *ASH Annu Meet Abstract* 2010;116: Abstract 5031.
148. Greco FA, Bonomi P, Crawford J et al. Phase 2 study of mapatumumab, a fully human agonistic monoclonal antibody which targets and activates the TRAIL receptor-1, in patients with advanced non-small cell lung cancer. *Lung Cancer* 2008;61:82–90.
149. Von Pawel J, Harvey JH, Spigel DR et al. A randomized phase II trial of mapatumumab, a TRAIL-R1 agonist monoclonal antibody, in combination with carboplatin and paclitaxel in patients with advanced NSCLC. *J Clin Oncol* 2010;28(suppl): Abstract LBA7501.
150. Von Pawel J, Hadler D, Fox T et al. A randomized, double-blind, placebo-controlled phase II study of tigatuzumab (CS-1008) in combination with carboplatin/paclitaxel in patients with chemotherapy-naive metastatic/unresectable non-small cell lung cancer (NSCLC). *J Clin Oncol* 2012;30: Abstract 7536.
151. Tabernero J, Dirix L, Schoffski P et al. A phase I first-in-human pharmacokinetic and pharmacodynamic study of serdemetan in patients with advanced solid tumors. *Clin Cancer Res* 2011;17:6313–6321.
152. Fiveash JB, Chowdhary SA, Peereboom D et al. NABTT-0702: A phase II study of R-(-)-gossypol (AT-101) in recurrent glioblastoma multiforme (GBM). *J Clin Oncol* 2009;27:A2010.
153. Ready N, Karaseva NA, Orlov SV et al. Double-blind, placebo-controlled, randomized phase 2 study of the proapoptotic agent AT-101 plus docetaxel, in second-line non-small cell lung cancer. *J Thoracic Oncol Official Publ Intl Assoc Study Lung Cancer* 2011;6:781–785.

154. Sonpavde G, Matveev V, Burke JM et al. Randomized phase II trial of docetaxel plus prednisone in combination with placebo or AT-101, an oral small molecule Bcl-2 family antagonist, as first-line therapy for metastatic castration-resistant prostate cancer. *Ann Oncol* 2012;23:1803–1808.
155. Baggstrom MQ, Qi Y, Koczywas M et al. A phase II study of AT-101 (Gossypol) in chemotherapy-sensitive recurrent extensive-stage small cell lung cancer. *J Thoracic Oncol Official Publ Intl Assoc Study Lung Cancer* 2011;6:1757–1760.
156. Heist RS, Fain J, Chinnasami B et al. Phase I/II study of AT-101 with topotecan in relapsed and refractory small cell lung cancer. *J Thoracic Oncol Official Publ Intl Assoc Study Lung Cancer* 2010;5:1637–1643.
157. Gandhi L, Camidge DR, Ribeiro de Oliveira M et al. Phase I study of navitoclax (ABT-263), a novel Bcl-2 family inhibitor, in patients with small-cell lung cancer and other solid tumors. *J Clin Oncol* 2011;29:909–916.
158. O'Brien SM, Claxton DF, Crump M et al. Phase I study of obatoclax mesylate (GX15–070), a small molecule pan-Bcl-2 family antagonist, in patients with advanced chronic lymphocytic leukemia. *Blood* 2009;113:299–305.
159. Schimmer AD, O'Brien S, Kantarjian H et al. A phase I study of the pan bcl-2 family inhibitor obatoclax mesylate in patients with advanced hematologic malignancies. *Clin Cancer Res* 2008;14:8295–8301.
160. Oki Y, Copeland A, Hagemeister F et al. Experience with obatoclax mesylate (GX15–070), a small molecule pan–Bcl-2 family antagonist in patients with relapsed or refractory classical Hodgkin lymphoma. *Blood* 2012;119:2171–2172.
161. Hwang JJ, Kuruvilla J, Mendelson D et al. Phase I dose finding studies of obatoclax (GX15–070), a small molecule pan-BCL-2 family antagonist, in patients with advanced solid tumors or lymphoma. *Clin Cancer Res* 2010;16:4038–4045.
162. Langer CJ, Albert I, Kovacs P et al. A randomized phase II study of carboplatin (C) and etoposide (E) with or without pan-BCL-2 antagonist obatoclax (Ob) in extensive-stage small cell lung cancer (ES-SCLC). *J Clin Oncol* 2011;29:A7011.

13 Targeting Angiogenesis

Sophie Postel-Vinay
Institut Gustave Roussy

Jean-Pierre Armand
Institut Gustave Roussy

CONTENTS

INTRODUCTION

In 1970, Folkman first hypothesized that angiogenesis was essential for tumor growth, proliferation, and development, and could as such represent a promising target for anticancer therapies. This followed the observation that tumors require oxygen and nutrients to be able to grow beyond 1–2 mm^3, which is achieved through the formation of dedicated neo-vessels, a process known as "angiogenic switch."[1–3]

Subsequent preclinical research confirmed that growth, invasion, and metastasis required a functional vasculature, and that targeting the latter—rather than the cancer cell itself—could represent an effective anticancer therapy.[4,5]

Agents targeting tumor vasculature can be classified into two main categories: (1) antiangiogenic agents, which aim at preventing the angiogenic switch, that is, inhibit the formation of new vessels, and (2) vascular disrupting agents, which occlude or destroy the established tumor vasculature to interrupt blood supply (see corresponding chapter). This chapter will focus on antiangiogenic agents, which have been the subject of intense research and literature over the past 30 years with more than 20,000 publications on the topic.

The cloning of the vascular endothelial growth factor (VEGF) by Ferrera et al. in 1989[6] represented a key step in the development of antiangiogenic agents. This was followed by the clinical development and eventually approval by regulatory authorities of several VEGF-targeting agents, the first of which was the monoclonal antibody bevacizumab in 2004. Besides monoclonal antibodies, multiple tyrosine kinase inhibitors (TKIs), targeting either VEGF receptors (VEGFRs) or other tyrosine kinase receptors involved in angiogenesis, have been developed and are currently in the early or late clinical stage. TKIs, contrary to monoclonal antibodies, do not only target endothelial cells or tumor vasculature but also have intrinsic antiproliferative effects on the tumor cell itself, through collateral inhibition of essential growth factor receptors.

As VEGF is expressed in most, if not all, human cancers and associated with poor prognosis, antiangiogenic therapies have initially been described as "universal therapies."[7] This chapter will discuss mechanism of action of licensed drugs or compounds in development that target angiogenesis, as well as evidence of benefit and mechanisms of resistance that have been described so far. Current challenges, including how to overcome resistance and the development of predictive biomarkers of response, will also be exposed.

TARGETING ANGIOGENESIS

Multiple mechanisms have been involved in tumor angiogenesis, including the VEGF–VEGFR pathway,[4] the delta-like ligand 4 (Dll4)—notch signaling pathway, and the role of circulating bone marrow-derived cells and pericytes.[3] Among them, the VEGF–VEGFR pathway plays a pivotal role in the angiogenic switch (Figure 13.1).

The VEGF ligand family includes four different forms of circulating VEGF (VEGF-A, B, C, and D) and two placenta growth factors (PlGF-1 and 2).[8] They can bind three main transmembrane receptors (VEGFR-1, 2, and 3), which do either homo- or heterodimerize. Overall, VEGF-A preferentially binds to VEGFR-1 and 2, VEGF-B and PlGFs activate VEGFR-1, and VEGFs-C and D preferentially bind VEGFR-3. Importantly, VEGF usually refers to the circulating isoforms of VEGF-A ($VEGF_{121}$ and $VEGF_{185}$), which are the major contributors to tumor neoangiogenesis through the binding to VEGFR-2.[9] Although the binding affinity of VEGF to VEGFR-1 is approximately 10 times higher than its binding affinity to VEGFR-2, the signal-transducing properties of VEGFR-1 receptor are extremely weak. This latter receptor is also able to inhibit VEGFR-2 downstream signaling when they heterodimerize together. As VEGFR-1 exists as well as a soluble inactive form,

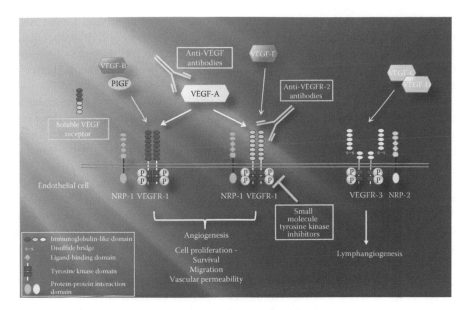

FIGURE 13.1 VEGF pathway and therapeutic strategies. VEGF-A, also called VEGF, preferentially binds VEFR-1 and VEGFR-2, the latter being responsible for the strongest proangiogenic signaling. VEGFR-3 is mainly involved in lymphangiogenesis. Strategies inhibiting the VEGF / VEGFR pathway include anti-VEGF antibodies, anti-VEGFR-2 antibodies, soluble VEGF receptors, and small molecule tyrosine kinase inhibitors. Abbreviations: NRP, neuropilin; PlGF,: placenta growth factor; VEGF, vascular endothelial growth factor.

which binds circulating VEGF, its role has sometimes been described as a negative regulator of VEGF activity.[10] VEGFR-3 mainly plays a role in lymphangiogenesis but has also been involved in neoangiogenesis, notably in breast cancer, melanoma, and some types of leukemia.[11]

Neuropilins (NRP-1 and 2) are two co-receptors of some specific isoforms of circulating VEGF, such as VEGF$_{165}$, which are able to modify their binding affinity to their receptors. Their exact role is still poorly understood, but they could represent interesting therapeutic opportunities to modulate the activity of the antiangiogenic agents or overcome resistance.[12]

The binding of VEGF to VEGFR-2 leads to the dimerization of the receptor, which activates a cascade of signaling pathways, resulting in increased vascular permeability, cell growth, proliferation, and invasion.[13] It has been commonly described that VEGF mainly acts through a paracrine mechanism, where tumor cells produce VEGF but do not have VEGFRs, and endothelial cells express numerous receptors but produce little VEGF. However, evidence is gathering that VEGF can also act through autocrine mechanisms[14] (where tumor cells express VEGFRs on their surface) as well as intracrine mechanisms (where the intracellular expression of the receptor can promote cell survival[15–17]). Overall, the pleiotropic actions of VEGF on its receptor can be summarized as follows: (1) the activation of the phospholipase C gamma—nitric oxide synthase pathway leads to increased vascular permeability; (2) the activation of the mitogen-activated protein kinase (MAPK) and phosphoinositide 3-kinase-AKT-mammalian target of rapamycin (PI3K-AKT-mTOR) pathways result in endothelial activation, increased proliferation, and cellular migration following reorganization of the actin cytoskeleton; and (3) the inhibition of the B-cell lymphoma-2 (Bcl-2)-associated death promoter and caspase signaling promotes cell survival.[4,18-21]

Increased VEGF expression has been described in multiple tumor types and associated with a less favorable prognosis. Both epigenetic and genetic factors can contribute to the induction of VEGF expression, following either environmental factors (such as hypoxia or low pH), increased circulating growth factors, sexual hormones or chemokines, or oncogenes/tumor suppressor genes activation/inactivation.[4,22,23]

Given the pivotal role of VEGF in promoting neoangiogenesis, the vast majority of antiangiogenic agents have originally been developed against the canonical VEGF–VEGFR pathway; they represent the focus of this chapter. However, multiple complementary mechanisms have been described as contributing to tumor neoangiogenesis, such as the Dll4–notch pathway for the growth of capillary sprouts,[3,24] the platelet-derived growth factor (PDGF)–PDGF receptor (PDGFR) pathway of the pericyte—an accessory cell that closely interacts with endothelial cells at the basal membrane,[25] and the role of bone marrow-derived endothelial progenitors.[16,26-28] These mechanisms have, to date, been considered as accessory proangiogenic pathways, but they may also represent important therapeutic targets. Finally, compounds targeting the established tumor vasculature—namely "vascular disrupting agents"—to interrupt blood supply have also been developed (see corresponding chapter).

AGENTS TARGETING THE VEGF–VEGFR PATHWAY

Although the crucial role of angiogenesis in tumor growth and metastasis had been described since the late 1960s, the first report of the clinical efficacy of antiangiogenic drugs was presented at the ASCO 2003 Annual Meeting, with the observation of a survival benefit following the adjunction of bevacizumab to conventional chemotherapy in patients with metastatic colorectal cancer (mCRC).[29] This triggered the exponential development of antiangiogenic agents, both monoclonal antibodies and small molecule TKIs (Figure 13.1 and Table 13.1).

MONOCLONAL ANTIBODIES

Initial preclinical experiments demonstrated that antibodies directed against VEGF or VEGFR could cause tumor regression in mice xenografts. This launched the development of several antibodies inhibiting VEGFR-2 or its ligand.

Bevacizumab

Bevacizumab (Avastin, Roche) is a humanized monoclonal IgG_1 directed against VEGF-A. Although IgG_1 usually display shorter half-lives $(T_{1/2})$ than IgG_2, bevacizumab displays a particularly long $T_{1/2}$, which allows administering the drug every 2–3 weeks only. Interestingly, the original phase I study did not manage to reach the maximum tolerated dose (MTD) and provide an optimal schedule recommendation.[30] This explains why the dose and schedule of administration of

TABLE 13.1
Antiangiogenic Drugs in Development

Drug (Company)	Target	Administration	Clinical Status	Disease (Metastatic Setting)
Antibodies				
Bevacizumab (Avastin, Roche)	VEGF-A	5 or 10 mg/kg q2w	FDA approved	CRC (+ 5-FU-based chemotherapy)
		7.5 or 15 mg/kg q3w		NSCLC (+ platinum-based chemotherapy)
		7.5 or 15 mg/kg q3w		RCC (+INF-α)
		10 mg/kg q2w		Glioblastoma
		10 mg/kg q2w	I/II/III	Solid tumors
VEGF-Trap (Zaltrap, Ziv-aflibercept, Sanofi)	VEGF-A	4 mg/kg q2w	FDA approved	CRC (+ 5-FU-irinotecan chemotherapy)
			I/II/III	Solid tumors
Ramucirumab (IMC-1121B, Eli Lilly)	VEGFR-2	8 mg/kg q2w	I/II/III	Solid tumors (OGJ)
Small molecule tyrosine kinase inhibitors				
VEGFR (and PDGFR) inhibitors				
Axitinib (AG-013736, Pfizer)	VEGFR-1, 2, 3/c-kit/PGDFR-β	5 mg bd	FDA approved	RCC
			I/II/III	Solid tumors
Brivanib alaninate (BMS-582664; Bristol Meyer Squibb)	VEGFR-1, 2/FGFR-1	800 mg od	I/II/III	Solid tumors
Cediranib (AZD2171; AstraZeneca)	VEGFR-1, 2, 3/PDGFR-α/c-kit	30–45 mg od	I/II/III	Solid tumors
Linifanib (ABT869, Abbott)	VEGFR-2/PDGFR-β	17.5 mg od	II	CRC
Motesanib (AMG 706, Amgen)	VEGFR-1, 2, 3/PDGFR-α/c-kit/ rearranged during transfection (RET)		I/II	Breast cancer, pancreatic cancer
Pazopanib (GlaxoSmithKline)	VEGFR1, 2, 3	800 mg od	FDA approved	RCC
				STS
			I/II/III	Solid tumors

(continued)

TABLE 13.1 (continued)

Antiangiogenic Drugs in Development

Drug (Company)	Target	Administration	Clinical Status	Disease (Metastatic Setting)
Regorafenib	**RET, VEGFR-1, 2, 3, KIT, PDGFR-α and PDGFR-β, FGFR-1 and 2**	**160 mg od 21d/28**	**FDA approved**	**CRC**
			II/III	Solid tumors (GIST, CRC, HCC)
Sorafenib (Bayer)	**VEGFR-2, 3/PDGFR-α/FLT-3/c-kit**	**400 mg bd**	**FDA approved**	**RCC**
				HCC
SU014813	VEGFR-1, 2, 3/PDGFR/FLT-3/c-kit	100 mg od	I/II/III	Solid tumors
			II	Breast cancer
Sunitinib (Pfizer)	**VEGFR-1, 2/c-kit/FLT-3/PDGFR-α**	**50 mg od 4w/6**	**FDA approved**	**PNET**
				RCC
				GIST
Vargatef (BIBF 1120, Boehringer-Ingelheim)	VEGFR-1, 2, 3/FGFR-3/PDGFR-α	200 mg bd	I/II/III	Solid tumors
			I/II/III	Solid tumors (ovarian cancer, NSCLC)
EGFR (and VEGFR inhibitors)				
Vandetanib	**EGFR/VEGFR-2/RET**	**300 mg od**	**FDA approved**	**Medullary thyroid carcinoma**
			I/II/III	Solid tumors
VEGFR (and c-met) inhibitors				
MGCD265 (MethylGene)	VEGFR/C-MET	To be determined	I/II	Solid tumors/NSCLC
Compounds of which development is currently halted				
BAY 57–9352 (Bayer)	VEGFR-2, 3/PDGFR/c-kit			
BMS-690514 (Bristol Meyer Squibb)	Pan-HER/VEGFR			
Vatalanib (PTK787/ZK222584)	VEGFRs/PDGFR-α/c-kit/c-fos			

Abbreviations: CRC, colorectal cancer; NSCLC, non-small cell lung cancer; RCC, renal cell carcinoma; STS, soft tissue sarcoma; HCC, hepatocellular carcinoma; PNET, pancreatic neuroendocrine tumor; GIST, gastrointestinal stromal tumor; in bold: drug approved by the FDA in at least one tumor type; in brackets: tumor types for which a pivotal/registration trial is currently ongoing.

bevacizumab are currently mainly based on the tumor type and associated chemotherapy regimen (Table 13.1). In 2004, bevacizumab was the first antiangiogenic drug approved by the Food and Drug Administration (FDA) followed by European Medicine Agencies (EMEA) in 2005.

Colorectal Cancer

Two major phase III studies have evaluated the use of bevacizumab in first-line mCRC. The first pivotal study, AVF2107g, included 923 patients who were randomized between (1) bevacizumab (5 mg/kg q2w) + 5-fluorouracil (5-FU) + irinotecan (IFL); (2) bevacizumab + 5-FU; and (3) placebo + IFL. The study met its primary objective, with a significant benefit in overall survival (OS) in the bevacizumab + IFL arm compared to the placebo + IFL arm (20.3 vs 15.6 months, $p < .001$, respectively). The progression-free survival (PFS) was also significantly higher in the bevacizumab + IFL arm (10.6 vs 6.2 months, respectively).[29] Interestingly, the OS benefit was observed in all molecular subtypes of colorectal cancer (i.e., whatever the P53, BRAF, and KRAS tumoral status).[31] This study led to the approval of bevacizumab by the FDA for first-line mCRC in association with a 5-FU-based chemotherapy. The second major study evaluating the use of bevacizumab in first-line mCRC, NO16966, included 1401 patients who were randomized between (1) bevacizumab (7.5 mg/kg q3w) + xeloda-oxaliplatine (XELOX); (2) bevacizumab + FOLFOX4; (3) placebo + XELOX; and (4) placebo + FOLFOX4. Although the study met its primary endpoint, with a significant difference in PFS in favor of the bevacizumab arms (9.4 vs 8 months, $p = .0023$), no difference in OS was observed (21.3 vs 19.9 months, $p = .077$).[32]

Bevacizumab has also been evaluated in second-line mCRC, in patients who were initially treated with IFL. The E3200 study included 820 patients who were randomly allocated to receive bevacizumab (10 mg/kg q2w) + FOLFOX4, bevacizumab as monotherapy, or FOLFOX4. A significant difference in OS was reported between the bevacizumab + FOLFOX4 arm and the FOLFOX4 arm (12.9 vs 10.8 months, respectively; $p = .0001$).[33] PFS and overall response rate (ORR) were also significantly improved by the adjunction of bevacizumab.

Breast Cancer

The use of bevacizumab in metastatic breast cancer (mBC) has generated many controversies. After an initial full approval by EMEA in 2007 and accelerated approval by FDA in 2008 for first-line mBC in combination with paclitaxel, the FDA revoked its license at the end of 2011, following the results of a meta-analysis reporting the absence of survival benefit by the adjunction of bevacizumab.[37]

Three main studies evaluated the adjunction of bevacizumab to conventional cytotoxic chemotherapy regimens in mBC. The E2100 trial included 722 patients and evaluated bevacizumab (10 mg/kg q2w) in combination with paclitaxel[34,35]; the AVADO study assessed the adjunction of bevacizumab (15 mg/kg q3w or 7.5 mg/kg/q3w) to docetaxel in human epidermal growth factor receptor 2 (HER2)-negative mBC[36]; finally, 1237 patients were included in the RIBBON-1 study, which evaluated bevacizumab (15 mg/kg q3w) in combination with a taxane-, anthracycline-, or capecitabine-based chemotherapy.[37]

The meta-analysis of the aforementioned three trials, presented by O'Shaughnessy et al. at the ASCO 2010 Annual Meeting, reported a significant benefit in PFS for patients receiving bevacizumab (9.2 vs 6.7 months; $p < .0001$),[38] which was significant in all analyzed subgroups (age > or < 65 years; triple-negative status; number of metastatic sites < or ≥ 3; disease-free interval ≤ or > 24 months; and concomitant neoadjuvant chemotherapy). The response rate was also significantly higher in patients receiving bevacizumab (49% vs 32%). However, this meta-analysis failed to demonstrate a significant difference in OS, leading to the withdrawal of the approval for this indication by the FDA.

The RIBBON-2 trial also evaluated bevacizumab in second-line mBC in combination with gemcitabine-, taxane-, capecitabine-, or vinorelbine-based chemotherapy regimens. Similarly to the results of the studies evaluating bevacizumab in first-line mBC, a significant benefit in PFS was observed in favor of the bevacizumab arm (7.2 vs 5.1 months; $p = .0072$) but no difference in OS was noted.[39]

Non-Small Cell Lung Cancer

The original phase II study evaluating bevacizumab in combination with a carboplatin–paclitaxel chemotherapy in non-small cell lung cancer (NSCLC) reported an increased rate of hemoptysis following tumor necrosis in patients with squamous tumors.[40] These patients have consequently been excluded from subsequent trials, although bevacizumab may be efficient in this histological subtype.

Two main phase III trials have evaluated the adjunction of bevacizumab to conventional chemotherapies in metastatic NSCLC: the E5499 and AVAiL (BO17704) studies. The E5499 study enrolled 878 patients who received a carboplatin–paclitaxel chemotherapy with or without bevacizumab (15 mg/kg q3w). This study reported a significant increase in response rate, PFS, and OS in patients receiving bevacizumab (12.3 vs 10.3 months; $p = .003$). The difference was even more significant for patients with adenocarcinoma.[41] On the other hand, the AVAiL study, which evaluated the adjunction of bevacizumab (15 or 7.5 mg/kg q3w) to a gemcitabine–cisplatin regimen, did not report any significant increase in OS.[42] An increase of 0.6 and 0.4 months in PFS was, however, noted in the 15 mg/kg and 7.5 mg/kg arms, respectively. Several hypotheses have been formulated to explain this discrepancy, including the role of the associated chemotherapy regimen as well as differences in inclusion–exclusion criteria and designs. On the basis of these results, bevacizumab was approved by the FDA in 2006, followed by EMEA in 2007, for first-line treatment of metastatic NSCLC in combination with a platinum-based regimen.

Renal Cell Carcinoma

The use of bevacizumab in combination with interferon (INF)-alpha for the treatment of patients with metastatic renal cell carcinoma (mRCC) was approved by the FDA in July 2009 and by EMEA in 2007. The approval was based on results from the AVOREN (BO17705) trial, which demonstrated a 5-month improvement in median PFS in patients treated with bevacizumab.[43] This randomized study enrolled 649 patients with mRCC who had undergone nephrectomy and compared the combination of bevacizumab plus INF-alpha-2a to INF-2a plus placebo. The median PFS was 10.2 months for the bevacizumab arm compared to 5.4 months for the placebo arm ($p < 0.0001$). No statistically significant advantage in OS was reported.

A similar prolongation in PFS—without improvement in OS—was reported by the CALBG 90206 study, with a median PFS of 8.4 months for patients treated with the bevacizumab in combination with INF-2b versus 4.9 months for patients who received the INF-2b single agent.[44]

Ovarian Cancer

Two large phase III studies (ICON-7 and GOG-0218) have evaluated the use of bevacizumab in combination with carboplatin–paclitaxel chemotherapy in advanced ovarian cancer, followed by bevacizumab maintenance. Both studies have reported a significant increase in PFS (2.4 and 3.9 months for the ICON-7 and GOG-0218 studies, respectively; $p < .005$).[45,46] No statistically significant difference in OS has been reported so far, but full survival data are not mature yet. The European Union approved bevacizumab for front-line treatment of advanced ovarian cancer following surgery in combination with a carboplatin–paclitaxel chemotherapy, but no approval has been granted by the FDA yet. Bevacizumab has also been evaluated in platinum-sensitive recurrent ovarian cancer in combination with carboplatin–gemcitabine followed by bevacizumab maintenance, in the OCEANS study.[47] A significant increase in PFS in favor of the bevacizumab arm was reported (12.4 vs 8.4 months; $p < 0.0001$), without significant difference in OS.

Glioblastoma

The durable response rate observed in two phase II studies was the basis for the FDA approval in 2009 of bevacizumab as a single agent for patients with recurrent glioblastoma (GBM). The first study, AVF3708g, evaluated bevacizumab (10 mg/kg IV) alone in combination with irinotecan in patients who previously received temozolomide plus radiotherapy.[48] The objective response rate of the bevacizumab arm alone (28.2%, 85 patients) was considered as significantly higher than historical control data and led to drug approval. In the NCI 06-C-0064E single-arm study, the ORR was 19.6% and median response duration was 3.9 months.[49] In the AVF3708g study, central nervous system (CNS) hemorrhage occurred in two patients (2.4%; two grade 1 events) in the bevacizumab arm and in three patients (3.8%; one grade 1, one grade 2, and one grade 4 events) in the bevacizumab/ CPT11 arm. In the NCI 06-C-0064E study, certain adverse events (e.g., CNS hemorrhage, wound healing complications, and thromboembolic events) could not be attributed to either bevacizumab, underlying disease status, or both due to the single-arm study design.

Other Tumor Types

Bevacizumab has also been evaluated in several other tumor types, including gastric cancer (AVAGAST study[49]), prostate cancer (CALBG90401 trial), and pancreatic cancer (CALBG80303 and NCT01214720 studies). A significant benefit in PFS was demonstrated in all the aforementioned trials but the CALBG80303 study, without leading to any OS improvement, and bevacizumab is currently not approved for these tumor types.

Toxicities

In phase I studies evaluating bevacizumab in monotherapy, the MTD was not reached and no dose-limiting toxicity (DLT) specific to the drug was described.[30] However, some delayed toxicities related to chronic administration have been described in later phase trials, notably the phase III first bevacizumab antibody trial and Bevacizumab Regimen: Investigation of Treatment Effects and Safety (BRiTE) studies.[50,51] Although most of these toxicities can be labeled as "class effects"—that is, toxicities directly related to the inhibition of the VEGF–VEGFR pathway that are not specific to bevacizumab—some peculiar side effects deserve attention.

The most frequent class effects described with bevacizumab are hypertension (22%–32% of all grades) and asymptomatic proteinuria (27%–38% of all grades).[52–58] Other common toxicities include would healing delay (7%–10%), minor bleeding (3%–5%), and arterial thrombosis (4.5%).[55,59,60] Rare but severe adverse events include posterior leukoencephalopathy (1%–5%),[61,62] fistula formation, and nasal septum perforation (all <1%). Thromboembolic events have been particularly well studied with bevacizumab because of their potential severity. A pooled analysis of five randomized phase III trials (representing a total of 1745 patients) has reported a twofold increase in the risk of arterial thrombosis,[63] highlighting the importance of carefully evaluating cardiovascular risk factors prior to bevacizumab prescription. The enhanced risk of venous thromboembolic events (VTEs) has generated many controversies as contradictory results have been provided. Although the results of the pooled analysis did initially not demonstrate any increased risk of VTE, a meta-analysis including 15 randomized trials (7956 patients) recently reported a 30% increase in the incidence of VTEs. Similarly, recent data from 1401 patients with mCRC who were treated with bevacizumab reported a significantly higher incidence of deep venous thrombosis (13.5% vs 9%) in patients receiving bevacizumab.[64] Importantly, this higher frequency of DVTs persisted despite the use of anticoagulants, suggesting that patients at risk of VTEs should be carefully monitored during bevacizumab administration.

Two main specific side effects of bevacizumab have been reported to date: ovarian failure (which was reported in 32% of patients with mCRC included in a randomized trial evaluating bevacizumab in combination with FOLFOX6, compared to 2% in the placebo arm) and jaw osteonecrosis.[65] This latter side effect was higher in patients who were concomitantly treated with or previously received bisphosphonates, and justifies recommending dental examination and preventive dentistry prior to bevacizumab administration.

Other Monoclonal Antibodies

Alternative strategies targeting the VEGF–VEGFR pathway with antibodies have been developed, such as VEGF-trap and ramucirumab.

VEGF-Trap

VEGF-Trap (Zaltrap, ziv-aflibercept, previously aflibercept, Sanofi) is a chimeric antibody fusing the second binding domain of the VEGFR-1 receptor and the third domain of the VEGFR-2 receptor to the Fc segment of a human IgG backbone, which binds VEGF-A with a very high affinity. The drug was very recently approved by the FDA in August 2012 for use in combination with 5-FU, leucovorin, and irinotecan (FOLFIRI) for the treatment of patients with mCRC following an oxaliplatin-based regimen. This approval is based on the results of the VELOUR trial, which randomized 1226 patients who were allocated (1:1) to receive FOLFIRI with either ziv-aflibercept (4 mg/kg q2w) or placebo. A statistically significant improvement in OS was observed in patients receiving FOLFIRI plus ziv-aflibercept compared to those receiving FOLFIRI plus placebo (HR 0.82 [95% CI: 0.71–0.94], $p = .0032$), with a median OS of 13.5 and 12.06 months for patients on the ziv-aflibercept and placebo arms, respectively (results presented at the ESMO 2012 Annual Meeting). Median PFS in the ziv-aflibercept arm was also significantly better than in the placebo arm (6.9 vs 4.7 months; $p = .00007$). Interestingly, the PFS benefit was similar in patients who did or not previously receive bevacizumab.[66] Other large randomized studies that currently evaluate aflibercept include the VENICE trial (phase III trial assessing aflibercept in first-line metastatic hormone-resistant prostate cancer in combination with docetaxel and prednisone), the AFFIRM study (phase II trial evaluating aflibercept in combination with a 5-FU-oxaliplatine [FOLFOX] regimen in first-line mCRC) and the VITAL trial (phase III study assessing aflibercept in combination with docetaxel as second-line treatment in patients with advanced NSCLC).

The most severe adverse events included grade 3–4 hemorrhage (2.9% vs 1.7% in the ziv-aflibercept arm and placebo arms, respectively). Therefore, the ziv-aflibercept label contains a special warning for the serious adverse reactions gastrointestinal perforation and compromised wound healing—in addition to hemorrhage. Ziv-aflibercept also displays the common class adverse events observed with antiangiogenic agents, including arterial and VTEs, fistula formation, and posterior leukoencephalopathy. In the VELOUR trial, the incidence of ziv-aflibercept-related toxicities was similar whether or not the patient had previously received bevacizumab.

Ramucirumab

Ramucirumab (IMC-1121B, Eli Lilly) is a fully human IgG$_1$ monoclonal antibody targeting VEGF-receptor 2, which is being evaluated in two major phase III studies. The REGARD trial evaluated the safety and efficacy of ramucirumab (8 mg/kg q2w) versus placebo in 335 patients with metastatic gastric or gastroesophageal junction adenocarcinoma progressing on first-line platinum- and/or fluoropyrimidine-containing combination therapy. A significant improvement in OS was reported in October 2012, with a median OS of 5.2 and 3.8 months for the ramucirumab and placebo arms, respectively (95% CI, 0.603–0.998; $p = .0473$) (Lilly, press release Oct 2012). The median PFS was also significantly improved in the ramucirumab arm (2.1 vs 1.3 months; $p < .05$), as well as the disease control rate (49% vs 23%; $p < .0001$). The toxicity profile of ramucirumab was comparable to other VEGF-targeting antibodies, with an increased rate of class effects including hypertension (7.2% vs 2.6% in the ramucirumab and placebo arms, respectively), but also more specific toxicities such as hyponatremia (3.4% vs 0.9% in the ramucirumab vs placebo arms, respectively). RAINBOW, the second major phase III study that currently evaluates ramucirumab in combination with paclitaxel, in the same patient population, has completed enrollment in September 2012 and results are expected shortly. Several phase II and III trials are also evaluating ramucirumab in hepatocellular carcinoma (HCC), breast, gastric, prostate, and colorectal cancer.

SMALL MOLECULE TKIs

Besides antibodies, multiple oral antiangiogenic small molecule TKIs have been developed. If most of them are primarily directed against the intracellular kinase domain of the VEGFR-2, the low specificity of these TKIs allows them to inhibit multiple other kinase receptors, such as the epidermal growth factor receptor family, the PDGFR, c-kit, or fetal liver kinase receptor 3 (FLT-3).[67] This ability to inhibit multiple receptors often involved in cell proliferation may account for the tumor regressions observed in the preclinical models—as opposed to VEGF-targeting antibodies, which only induced tumor stabilizations. Furthermore, the parallel inhibition of the PDGFR also enhances the antiangiogenic effect of these small molecules, by compromising the stabilizing role of the pericyte. These "off-target" effects also account for the unique toxicity profile of each individual antiangiogenic TKI, besides the common backbone of antiangiogenic class effects.

Sunitinib

Sunitinib (SU-11248; Sutent®, Pfizer Inc., USA) is a multikinase inhibitor targeting VEGFR-1, VEGFR-2, PDGFR, c-kit, and FLT-3. Although its main mechanism of action is an antiangiogenic effect, this compound also displays some antiproliferative and proapoptotic properties.[68] Sunitinib is administered at a 50 mg dose once daily on a 4 weeks on/2 weeks off schedule, following the recommendations of the original phase I study.[69] As a meta-analysis of three studies evaluating sunitinib in mRCC reported that continuous drug exposure might enhance the therapeutic effect, more recent trials have evaluated continuous dosing schedules at 37.5 mg once daily.[70,71] Following two initial phase II studies in mRCC,[72,73] a randomized trial comparing both schedules reported a trend toward inferior time to progression with continuous dosing, although response rate, OS, and safety profiles were similar. Ongoing trials are still evaluating the continuous dosing regimen, notably in gastrointestinal stromal tumors (GISTs)—where sunitinib activity is not related to its antiangiogenic properties but to the inhibition of c-kit,[74] cf corresponding chapter—where results between both schedules appeared to be comparable.[75]

Sunitinib was approved by the FDA for the first-line treatment of mRCC based on the highly statistically significant improvement in PFS reported in the pivotal phase III study comparing sunitinib to INF-alpha in 750 patients with advanced renal clear cell carcinoma (11 vs 5 months in the sunitinib and INF-α arms, respectively).[76] This PFS benefit was observed across all subgroups according to the Memorial Sloan-Kettering Cancer Centre (MSKCC) classification. Although the difference in OS failed to reach significance (26.4 vs 21.8 months in favor of the sunitinib arm: $p = .05$) when considering the overall study population, it became significant when performing subgroup analysis on patients that did not crossover nor receive further systemic treatment, with an OS of 28 and 14 months for the sunitinib and INF-α arm, respectively. However, toxicities were more frequent in the sunitinib arm, including fatigue (12% vs 7%; $p < .005$) and grade 3–4 toxicities such as hypertension, diarrhea, hand–foot syndrome, mucositis, and bleeding. Sunitinib was also evaluated in second-line therapy for patients with mRCC who progressed after sorafenib treatment. Interestingly, partial responses or disease stabilizations were observed in 18% and 55% of the patients, respectively, highlighting the potential for using sequentially different therapies targeting the same pathway.[77]

Although sunitinib has also been evaluated in multiple other tumor types, including NSCLC, breast cancer, and prostate cancer, no benefit has been observed in monotherapy, and its use has mainly been associated with increased toxicities in heavily pretreated patients.[78] Several ongoing studies are now evaluating the use of sunitinib in combination with various cytotoxic chemotherapies.

Interestingly, responses observed with sunitinib included not only tumor shrinkage but also central necrosis without any change in tumor volume, suggesting that alternatives to response evaluation criteria in solid tumors (RECIST), such as Choi criteria, could be used to evaluate the therapeutic response to this agent.

In the original phase I study evaluating sunitinib, the reported dose-limiting toxicities were fatigue and hypertension. Interestingly, hypertension has been correlated to clinical efficacy in patients with mRCC treated by sunitinib, suggesting the potential for using this clinical toxicity as a surrogate biomarker of efficacy.[79] Specific sunitinib toxicities include thyroid function abnormalities—that need to systematically be monitored but do not always result in clinical symptoms—, yellow skin pigmentation and hair decoloration (respectively related to some drug metabolites and c-kit inhibition in melanocytes), stomatitis, and hand–foot syndrome.[80]

Sorafenib

Sorafenib (BAY43-9006, Nexavar, Bayer Pharmaceuticals, USA) is a potent inhibitor of VEGFR-2, PDGFR, c-kit, FLT-3, as well as the serine threonine kinases, CRAF and BRAF.[81] Like sunitinib, sorafenib inhibits both serine/threonine and tyrosine kinases and, as such, inhibits both targets on the tumor cell, inducing antiproliferative effects, and targets on the endothelial cell, accounting for its antiangiogenic properties. Sorafenib is an oral multikinase inhibitor administered orally at a 400 mg bd dose.

Sorafenib was originally developed as a BRAF inhibitor and thought to have activity in melanoma. A phase II trial performed in metastatic melanoma failed to demonstrate any efficacy of the drug in this indication, even when only considering the BRAF-mutated subset of patients.[82] However, after initial responses observed in the phase I trial in RCC, the drug's potential for inhibiting VEGFR-2 was exploited, and sorafenib was further developed as an antiangiogenic therapy in RCC and other tumor types such as HCC.[83,84]

The first pivotal phase III study evaluated sorafenib in patients with advanced clear cell carcinoma who received prior immunotherapy. Most of the patients included in this trial presented a low or intermediate prognostic risk tumor according to the MSKCC classification. Results of the trial demonstrated a significant increase in PFS in patients receiving sorafenib (24 vs 12 weeks; $p < .001$), which led to the approval of the drug by the FDA in 2005. The final OS analysis also demonstrated a significant difference between the sorafenib and placebo arms, with median OS of 15.9 and 19.3 months ($p = .015$), respectively.[85] Sorafenib has also been evaluated in combination with INF-α, without showing any increased benefit when combining both drugs.[86]

Several trials are currently ongoing, which evaluate the use of sorafenib in the neo-adjuvant and adjuvant settings (Adjuvant Sorafenib and Sunitinib in Unfavorable Renal Cell Carcinoma trial).

Sorafenib has also demonstrated activity in HCC. The drug was registered by the FDA in November 2007 based on the results of the randomized phase III SHARP trial, which compared sorafenib to placebo in chemonaïve patients with HCC (only prior hor-monotherapy was allowed).[87] The trial was stopped prematurely, following a pre-speci-fied second interim analysis for survival, disclosing a statistically significant advantage for sorafenib (10.7 vs. 7.9 months; $p = .00058$). The final analysis of time-to-tumor pro-gression (TTP) by independent radiologic review also demonstrated a statistically sig-nificant improvement in TTP in the sorafenib arm (5.5 vs. 2.8 months; $p = .000007$).

Specific sorafenib toxicities include hair and nail modifications (100% of patients), hand–foot syndrome (30%), diarrhea (43%), and appearance of naevi (7%). Hypertension and fatigue are also reported in 17% and 37% of the patients, respectively.[80,88]

Likewise, what has previously been described with sunitinib, RECIST criteria do not appropriately evaluate the antitumor efficacy of the drug, and alternative criteria assessing tumor viability or vasculature should probably be used. For example, despite the statistically significant increase in PFS of the TARGET trial, only 10% of the patients displayed objective responses as measured by RECIST criteria. However, doppler ultrasonography was performed in a subset of 30 patients and changes in tumor vasculature positively correlated with PFS and OS from 3 weeks after treatment initiation.[89,90]

Pazopanib

Pazopanib (GW786034, Votrient, GlaxoSmithKline) is a highly potent second-generation inhibitor of all VEGFRs, as well as PDGF-a and c-kit, which is more selec-tive toward VEGFRs than sorafenib or sunitinib.[91] Based on the data of the phase I trial, where the MTD was not reached but the pharmacokinetic profile was similar between 800 and 2000 mg od, the recommended dose of pazopanib is currently 800 mg od.[92]

Pazopanib is currently registered for advanced RCC and soft tissue sarcoma (STS). The registration study evaluating pazopanib in RCC included 435 patients who were chemonaïve or had received prior cytokine therapy. The trial reported a significant increase in PFS (9.2 vs 4.2 months; $p = .001$) in the pazopanib arm, with-out any associated increase in OS.[93]

The approval of the drug for patients with advanced STS is more recent. In April 2012, the FDA approved pazopanib for this tumor type, following the results of a randomized multicenter trial in 369 patients with STS (excluding adipocytic STS and GISTs) who received prior chemotherapy. A statistically significant improvement in PFS was reported in the pazopanib arm (4.6 vs 1.6 months in the pazopanib and pla-cebo arms, respectively; $p < .001$), which was also observed in all subgroups (synovial sarcoma, leiomyosarcoma, and other STS). No statistically significant OS improve-ment (12.6 vs 10.7 months in the pazopanib and placebo arm, respectively; $p > .05$) was noted.[94] Several phase II trials are also currently evaluating pazopanib in combination with chemotherapy in multiple tumor types, including NSCLC and ovarian cancer.

Besides common antiangiogenic side effects, pazopanib displays a specific liver toxicity, which can be life-threatening and needs to be monitored during treatment.

Moderate transaminitis (TA) elevation is usually observed in 60% of the patients within 4 weeks of starting the treatment, but treatment must be interrupted if severe TA elevation occurs. Other pazopanib side effects include fatigue, diarrhea, hair color changes, musculoskeletal pain, and skin hypopigmentation.[95]

Vandetanib

Vandetanib (ZD6474, Zactima, Caprelsa, AstraZeneca), which inhibits VEGFR-2, EGFR, and RET,[96] is the first TKI approved by the FDA for the treatment of medullary thyroid cancer. This approval was based on the results of the ZETA phase III trial that randomized 331 patients with unresectable locally advanced or metastatic medullary thyroid cancer to vandetanib 300 mg od ($n=231$) or placebo ($n=100$). Patients randomized to vandetanib showed a statistically significant improvement in PFS when compared to patients receiving placebo (22.6 vs 16.4 months, respectively; $p<.0001$).[97] No significant OS difference was observed. It should be noted that the efficacy of vandetanib in medullary thyroid cancer is not related to antiangiogenic effects but to the inhibition of RET, a driver tyrosine kinase in this disease.

Vandetanib has also been evaluated as an antiangiogenic agent in several tumor types, notably NSCLC, both in monotherapy or in combination with taxane-, carboplatin-, or pemetrexed-based regimens (ZODIAC,[98] ZEIST, and ZEPHYR[99] trials). As none of these large studies managed to demonstrate a statistically significant benefit in OS, AstraZeneca withdrew in October 2009 the drug application and marketing authorization that had been submitted to the FDA and EMEA. The development of the drug in this indication was subsequently halted. Ongoing clinical trials currently evaluate vandetanib in combination with cytotoxic chemotherapy in glioma and pancreatic adenocarcinoma, and a recent phase I trial (VanSel-1) started evaluating the drug in combination with the MEK inhibitor AZD6244 in solid tumors including NSCLC.

Vandetanib administration has been associated with cardiac toxicities, notably QT prolongation and torsades de pointes, supporting the inclusion of sudden death in the boxed warning for vandetanib.[100] The most common adverse drug reactions reported in the ZETA trial were diarrhea (57%), rash (53%), acne (35%), nausea (33%), hypertension (33%), and headache.[97]

Axitinib

Axitinib (AG-03736, Inlyta, Pfizer) is a potent inhibitor of all VEGFRs, PDGFR, and c-kit, which is administered orally at a 5 mg dose twice daily.

Axitinib was approved by the FDA in January 2012 for patients with advanced RCC after failure of one prior systemic therapy on the basis of the results of the phase III AXIS 1032 study.[101] The PFS analysis demonstrated a statistically significant improvement in median PFS of patients receiving axitinib compared to patients receiving sorafenib (6.7 vs 4.7 months; $p<.0001$). Interestingly, this improvement in PFS was greater in the cytokine-pretreated subgroup compared to the sunitinib-pretreated subgroup. The toxicity profile of axitinib was slightly different from that of sorafenib in the same patient population, with higher incidence of hypertension (40% vs 29%), fatigue (39% vs 32%), dysphonia (31% vs 14%), and hypothyroidism (19% vs 8% for the axitinib- and sorafenib-treated patients, respectively). However, hand–foot syndrome, rash, alopecia, and anemia were more frequently observed with sorafenib (with a respective incidence of 51%/27%, 32%/13%, 32%/4%, and 12%/4% in sorafenib-/axitinib-treated patients). Multiple trials are currently evaluating axitinib in combination with chemotherapy, notably in NSCLC, mesothelioma, hepatocarcinoma, prostate cancer, carcinoid tumors, and nasopharyngeal cancer.

Regorafenib

Regorafenib (and its active metabolites) inhibit(s) multiple membrane-bound and intracellular kinases including RET, VEGFR1–3, KIT, PDGFR-α and PDGFR-β, FGFR-1 and 2, tyrosine kinase with Ig and EGF homology domains-2 (TIE2), discoidin domain receptor family, member 2 (DDR2), Trk2A, Eph2A, RAF-1, BRAF, BRAF[V600E], and Abelson (Abl). It is administered at a dose of 160 mg od continuously for 21 days, followed by an 8 day rest period off-drug (in a 28-day cycle).[102]

Following promising activity in mCRC in the initial Phase IB study,[103] the drug was recently evaluated in a large randomized (2:1) phase III trial. The CORRECT study enrolled 760 patients with mCRC who had received prior treatment with fluoropyrimidine-, oxaliplatin-, and irinotecan-based chemotherapy as well as anti-VEGF therapy. All but one of the patients with *KRAS* wild-type tumors also previously received anti-EGFR therapy (cetuximab or panitumumab). The primary endpoint of OS was met at a preplanned interim analysis, with a median OS of 6.4 months in the regorafenib group versus 5 months in the placebo group ($p = .0052$).[104] Importantly, this benefit was observed in all analyzed subgroups. A statistically significant improvement in PFS in patients who received regorafenib was also noted (2 vs 1.7 months for the regorafenib and placebo arms, respectively; $p < 0.0001$). Regorafenib was subsequently granted approval by the FDA in September 2012, for the treatment of patients with mCRC who have been previously treated with 5-FU-, oxaliplatin-, or irinotecan-based therapy, or with an anti-VEGF therapy, or with an anti-EGFR therapy (if *KRAS* wild-type disease). Interestingly, the mechanism of clinical efficacy of regorafenib in mCRC remains to be elucidated, considering the drug's potential to inhibit multiple kinases that are drivers in this disease. Regorafenib has also shown activity in GIST, where the drug demonstrated significant improvement in PFS and disease control rate in patients who previously failed imatinib or sunitinib therapy (results of the GRID trial[105]). The drug is currently evaluated in multiple phase II or III trials, notably in combination with FOLFIRI as a second-line treatment in patients with mCRC, as well as in monotherapy following sorafenib in patients with HCC.

The most frequently observed adverse drug reactions reported in the CORRECT trial included fatigue (47% all grades/10% grade 3), hand–foot skin reaction (47%/17%), diarrhea (34%/7%), dysphonia (29%/1%), hypertension (28%/7%), mucositis (27%/3%), and rash or desquamation (29%/6%). The most serious adverse drug reaction in patients receiving regorafenib was liver toxicity, leading to an approval with a boxed warning describing the risk of hepatotoxicity.

Other Antiangiogenic TKIs in Development

Several other antiangiogenic TKIs are currently being developed, either as monotherapy or in combination with cytotoxic conventional chemotherapy in multiple solid tumor types. The main compounds evaluated in ongoing phase II or III trials include cediranib[106] (AZD2171, AstraZeneca), motesanib[107] (AMG706, Amgen), vargatef[108] (BIBF1120), brivanib alaninate[109] (BMS-583364), linifanib,[110] (ABT-869) and SU014813. They all differ by their selectivity and potency with regard to VEGFR-1, 2, 3, PDGFR, and fibroblast growth factor (FGFR) inhibition, which account, at least in part, for the variability observed in their clinical efficacy across multiple tumor types.

Cediranib

Cediranib (AZD2171, AstraZeneca) is a potent VEGFR-2 inhibitor, which also inhibits VEGFR-3, PDGFR-α and PDGFR-β, FGFR-1, and c-kit at higher concentrations. Initial phase I and II trials reported interesting activity in GBM multiforme.[101] This was unfortunately not confirmed in a large phase III trial, the REGAL study, which compared (A) cediranib as monotherapy to either (B) lomustine or (C) lomustine + cediranib: the PFS was comparable between all arms (92, 82, and 125 days for arm A, B, and C, respectively) as well as OS (8, 9.8, and 9.4 months for arm A, B, and C, respectively) (2010 Society for Neuro-Oncology Annual Meeting). However, as the dose administered in the phase III trial (30 mg) was lower than in previous studies (45 mg) and as a proportion of patients reported improvements in disease-related symptoms, several studies are currently ongoing.

Vargatef

Vargatef (Nintedanib, BIBF 1120, Boerhinger Ingelheim) is an indolinone derivative, which potently inhibits VEGFR-1, 2, 3, PDGFR, FGFR, and src.[111] Interestingly, this molecule recently demonstrated activity for treating idiopathic pulmonary fibrosis.

A phase II trial evaluating BIBF1120 as monotherapy after failure of first- or second-line chemotherapy in 73 patients with NSCLC reported a median PFS and OS of 6.9 weeks and 21.9 weeks, respectively.[112] When considering only patients with an Eastern Cooperative Oncology Group performance status (ECOG PS) of 0–1, the observed PFS and OS were 2.9 months and 9.5 months, respectively, supporting further development of vargatef in this setting. The phase III development program in NSCLC is currently ongoing with two pivotal studies: the LUME-Lung 1 trial and LUME-Lung 2 trials, which evaluate vargatef in combination with standard docetaxel or pemetrexed therapy, respectively. Following promising results in a phase II trial evaluating BIBF 1120 (nintedanib) in ovarian cancer, a development program is also currently ongoing in this indication. It includes notably a large phase III trial (LUME-Ovar 1, which evaluates nintedanib in combination with carboplatin–paclitaxel standard chemotherapy) and two phase II trials (CHIVA, which evaluates BIBF 1120 in combination to first-line chemotherapy with interval debulking surgery, and a study that assesses vargatef in patients with bevacizumab-resistant ovarian cancer). Several combination phase I trials are also ongoing.

Of note, the toxicity profile of vargatef is closer to that of an EGFR-inhibitor than the one of a VEGFR-inhibitor, with the most frequent adverse events being nausea (11%), diarrhea (11%), and vomiting (6%). Asymptomatic TA elevation has also been frequently described in 20% of patients approximately.

The development of other antiangiogenic TKIs, such as telatinib (BAY57-9352), vatalanib (PTK787/ZK222584), or BMS-690514, has recently been halted.

ANTIANGIOGENIC AGENTS IN COMBINATION

Antiangiogenic Agents in Combination with Conventional Chemotherapy

It was first thought that antiangiogenic drugs, which aim at interrupting or disabling the tumor blood supply, would decrease the efficacy of cytotoxic chemotherapy secondary to a diminished intratumoral drug delivery. However, this hypothesis has been rejected early, following several observations. First, it was demonstrated that antiangiogenic agents were able to induce a "vascular normalization" phenomenon and as such had the capacity to potentiate the effects of chemotherapy.[113,114] Second, antiangiogenic agents could have a preferential efficacy on perivascular niches containing tumor stem cells and render the latter more sensitive to chemotherapy.[28] Finally, antiangiogenic drugs could prevent the "proangiogenic rebound," that is, the mobilization of bone marrow–derived endothelial progenitors, that has been described following the administration of high dose cytotoxic chemotherapy.[115,116] Several other mechanisms have also been evoked,[27,117–119] and the contribution of each of them is still debatable, calling for further research in this area.

Interestingly, it should be noted that, overall, antibodies have demonstrated significant activity—leading to improvements in OS—in combination with chemotherapy, whereas small molecules only demonstrated marginal benefit when combined with cytotoxic agents and are consequently currently prescribed in monotherapy. This could result from the intrinsic antiproliferative effect of TKIs, which could negatively impact the efficacy of cytotoxic agents that are only effective on cycling cells. Several ongoing phase III studies currently evaluating combinations of TKIs with conventional chemotherapy should bring further insight into this question.

Combination of Antiangiogenic Agents

The combination of two antiangiogenic agents has been proposed in order to achieve a maximal inhibition of the proangiogenic pathways, either through a "horizontal" or "vertical" blockade (i.e., either inhibiting two parallel pathways or blocking a single pathway at two levels). The observation that patients who previously received bevacizumab could still benefit from VEGF-targeting TKIs, such as sunitinib,[120] also supported this hypothesis. In the phase I study evaluating the combination of bevacizumab with sorafenib, a significant and dose-limiting increase in class toxicities was observed, including hypertension and proteinuria. The MTD was reached at subtherapeutic doses of sorafenib and bevacizumab (200 mg od and 5 mg/kg q2w, respectively).[121] However, clinical benefit was noted in 34 of 37 patients enrolled in this study, with partial responses observed in patients with ovarian carcinoma, leading to an ongoing phase II study performed in this tumor type (NCT00436215). Several clinical trials evaluating combinations of antiangiogenic agents have been performed or are currently ongoing, notably in HCC (sorafenib + bevacizumab, NCT00881751) or GBM (sorafenib + temsirolimus, NCT00329719). Other combination trials have been prematurely terminated following the occurrence of intolerable dose-limiting toxicities in multiple tumor types, such as RCC[122], colorectal cancer (NCT00779311), or breast cancer (NCT00662641). Therefore, a careful evaluation of the optimal administration sequence and schedule of antiangiogenic agents to optimize their efficacy is currently warranted.

In conclusion, multiple TKIs and antibodies targeting angiogenesis are currently approved for clinical use or being developed. Almost all of them have shown efficacy as monotherapy in advanced RCC, and in combination with cytotoxic chemotherapy in various solid tumor types. The main challenges are currently to determine the optimal administration schedule of these antiangiogenic agents (in terms of therapeutic sequence and choice of the optimal molecule according to its toxicity and efficacy profile) and potentially manage to combine antiangiogenic drugs to achieve a more complete inhibition of the VEGF pathway. The results of the PISCES study, which compared the quality of life of patients with advanced RCC receiving either sunitinib or pazopanib, were recently presented at the ASCO 2012 Annual Meeting.[120] In this study, pazopanib was preferred by 70% of patients, whereas 22% of them preferred sunitinib. Furthermore, adverse-events-related dose reductions and treatment interruptions were less frequent in patients receiving pazopanib (13% and 6%, respectively) compared to sunitinib-treated patients (20% and 12%, respectively). The results of the COMPARZ trial, which included 1110 patients with advanced RCC and compared the efficacy of pazopanib and sunitinib in advanced RCC, were presented at the ESMO 2012 Meeting. Pazopanib demonstrated non-inferiority to sunitinib in terms of PFS and OS, but displayed a different safety profile, including a lower incidence of fatigue, hand–foot syndrome, mucositis, hematological toxicities, but a higher incidence of liver function test abnormalities. Furthermore, the majority of quality of life indicators (11/14) statistically favored pazopanib over sunitinib, though none met the minimally important difference threshold (where applicable). Such efficacy and quality of life comparative studies will certainly bring essential information regarding the management of antiangiogenic TKIs in the future.

Finally, no antiangiogenic therapy has demonstrated efficacy in the adjuvant or neo-adjuvant setting so far. Although the rationale for using antiangiogenic agents at the micrometastatic stage of the disease—that is, where tumor does not need any extra blood supply—has been controversial, it has been advocated that the use of antivascular therapies could delay the angiogenic switch. More information could be available soon, as several trials are currently evaluating the use of bevacizumab in the adjuvant and neo-adjuvant setting (including the ECOG1505 and BEACON studies for NSCLC, the ECOG5205 trial in colorectal cancer, and the NSABP-NCI and BEATRICE studies for breast cancer).

RESISTANCE TO ANTIANGIOGENIC AGENTS

As any tumor requires vascular supply—regardless the primary cell of origin or tumor localization—antiangiogenic therapies have sometimes been described as "universal therapies" that would be effective in all types of cancer. Unfortunately, not all tumors are sensitive to antiangiogenic agents, and several mechanisms of primary or acquired resistance have been described.[123]

PRIMARY RESISTANCE MECHANISMS

The mechanisms of primary resistance to antiangiogenic agents that have been described are mainly related to tumor type, localization, and stage.

Slow growing or quiescent tumor cells do not require important nutrient supply and tend therefore to be insensitive to hypoxia. Other tumors, such as pancreatic ductal adenocarcinoma, often present with an abundant desmoplastic stroma and hypovascularization.[124] Interestingly, molecular characteristics could also play a role in sensitivity to hypoxia: for example, some mutations in *TP53* have been associated in vitro with a relative resistance to hypoxia.[125] Furthermore, preclinical models have demonstrated that when injecting to mice a mix of two populations of tumor cells—one sensitive and one insensitive to antiangiogenic agents—the resulting tumor is intrinsically resistant to antiangiogenic drugs, suggesting that insensitivity to hypoxia confers a selective advantage to tumor cells.

Some tumors also tend to use the normal vasculature that is already in place in the organ where they develop, making them intrinsically resistant to therapies targeting angiogenesis. For example, xenografts of kidney cancer cells are more sensitive to antiangiogenic therapies when they develop in the kidney than in the bone (where they tend to use the normal vasculature).

Finally, it has been suggested that late-stage or heavily pretreated diseases could secondary to the activation of various proangiogenic pathways and increased expression of several ligands (such as PDGF or FGF2) after multiple lines of chemotherapy.[126]

Acquired Resistance Mechanisms

Acquired resistance to antiangiogenic agents mainly results from redundancies and cross-talks between several proliferative and proangiogenic pathways. For example, increased levels of circulating VEGF, PlGF, or FGF2, as well as enhanced intratumoral c-Met expression, have been reported after administration of antiangiogenic agents in humans.[127,128] This could support the sequential administration of different antiangiogenic drugs displaying distinct potencies and selectivity profiles toward the main proangiogenic pathways. In line with this hypothesis, the VELOUR trial reported comparable response rates in patients who received or not prior bevacizumab, and the use of sunitinib as second-line therapy for patients with mRCC who progressed after sorafenib treatment demonstrated partial responses or disease stabilizations in 18% and 55% of the patients, respectively.

Increased mobilization of endothelial precursors, notably trough the induction of G-CSF, SFD-1, or HIF-1a expression, has also been reported.[129] Although still controversial, it has been suggested that such mechanism might account for the proangiogenic rebound sometimes described at treatment cessation.

Increased pericyte coverage and vascular remodeling (i.e., switch from abnormal immature vessels to more mature forms of vasculature that are less sensitive to angiogenesis inhibition) could also explain some forms of acquired resistance.[130] As such, concomitant targeting of the endothelial cell and of the pericyte could be key in overcoming some forms of acquired resistance.

Finally, the role of tumor-stroma interactions, recruitment of vascular progenitor cells and proangiogenic monocytes from the bone marrow,[131] or enhanced invasive capacity of the tumor cell itself[132] have also been reported.

Altogether, several mechanisms may collaborate in the development of secondary resistances. Optimal drug scheduling (sequential administration, combinations of antiangiogenic agents, or combination of antiangiogenic and vascular disrupting agents [VDAs]) might eventually allow overcoming acquired resistances.

PREDICTIVE BIOMARKERS

One of the main current challenges in the development of antiangiogenic agents is the identification of predictive biomarkers that would allow selecting patients who are the most likely to benefit from such therapies.[7,133]

Clinical toxicities secondary to on-target effects of antiangiogenic agents have initially been proposed as biomarker of efficacy, following the report that elevated blood pressure on treatment correlated with increased treatment efficacy in patients with colorectal cancer treated with bevacizumab[134] and patients with RCC treated with axitinib.[135] Other constitutional biomarkers, such as single nucleotide polymorphisms in genes encoding for key proteins of proangiogenic pathways, have been extensively studied, but some discrepancies have been reported between the different studies and different antiangiogenic molecules.[136–139] Furthermore, most data arise from retrospective studies and a prospective validation is required prior to any clinical implementation. However, as genomic DNA is invariant (contrary to tumor DNA), easily accessible through blood test or buccal swab and as single-nucleotide polymorphisms (SNPs) can be analyzed at very low costs, it represents a powerful tool that would be a biomarker of highest interest for clinical use.

Besides these host-related biomarkers, considerable efforts have been put into analyzing several tumor biomarkers[133] (including microvessel density,[140] VEGF or VEGFR expression,[23,141] oncogenes, and tumor suppressor genes mutations[142,143]), either on preclinical models or on tumor samples from patients included in clinical studies. Multiple peripheral blood biomarkers, such as circulating VEGF pre- and on-treatment levels, soluble VEGFR-2 levels, PlGF levels, or cytokines (IL-6, SDF1) levels have also been studied.[7,120,144–146] The variation in treatment of the levels of circulating tumor cells, circulating endothelial cells, and endothelial progenitors has also been evaluated.[147,148] Similarly to what had been observed with host-related biomarkers, most studies reported discordant results, and no reliable biomarker of efficacy has been identified so far.

Another promising approach is the use of functional imaging, which directly evaluates tumor perfusion, oxygen supply, and metabolism.[149] Although the cost and availability of some powerful techniques—including dynamic contrast-enhanced magnetic resonance imaging (DCE-MRI), perfusion computed tomography (CT), or TEP imaging—may represent an important limiting factor for a widespread use of functional, promising results have been obtained with contrast ultrasound, which might as such represent a powerful tool to study early tumor responses to antiangiogenic treatment.[89] Dedicated ongoing clinical trials (such as the NCT 0110564 study) should bring relevant insight to this question.

The main biomarkers that have been studied, their advantages and drawbacks, as well as examples of results that have been obtained so far are summarized in Table 13.2.

TABLE 13.2
Predictive Biomarkers for Antiangiogenic Therapies

Type of Biomarker	Example	Analysis Technique	Advantages	Disadvantages	Existing Data
Patient-related biomarkers					
Clinical biomarkers	Blood pressure	Clinical assessment	Cost Dynamic	Confounding factors Low specificity and sensitivity	Correlation of high blood pressure with efficacy for axitinib[135] and bevacizumab[134]
Constitutional DNA—SNPs	VEGF-A VEGFR-1 VEGFR-2 VEGFR-3 NRP-1 NRP-2 IL-8	Sequencing on buccal swab of blood sample	Cost	Low specificity	SNPs predicting bevacizumab efficacy: VEGF-A in NSCLC,[136] breast cancer,[137] and meta-analysis of three randomized trials[138] VEGFR-1 in pancreatic cancer IL-8, VEGFR-2, VEGFR-3, NRP-1–2 in RCC[139]
Tumor biomarkers					
Tumor biopsy	Microvascular density NRP-1 or VEGF expression	Immunohistochemistry Immunofluorescence	Direct analysis of the tumor	Invasive procedure Sequential assessment not feasible (repeated tumor biopsies)	No statistically significant studies[133] VEGF-A very unspecific as highly expressed by stromal cells,[141] endothelium[23] Microvascular density: prognostic but not predictive[140]

Driver or tumor suppressor genes mutations	VHL, p53, Kras, BRAF	Sequencing		No correlation with VHL mutation in RCC patients[150] No correlation with p53, KRAS, BRAF status in CRC[142] Decreased PFS in RCC patients with HIF-1a deletion[143]
Circulating biomarkers				
Proangiogenic factors and cytokines	VEGF, VEGFR, FGF	ELISA, western blot Proteomics	Reproducible per center/ method Cost (Elisa) Development of platforms: AVANTRAT biochips (decision biomarkers), search light protein array (Aushon), ELISA Quantikine (R1D systems) Few standardized analysis procedures so far No assessment of VEGF bound to plasma proteins VEGF release by leucocytes during sample transport Detection of certain isoforms only	Baseline levels of VEGF-A and VEGFR-2: contradictory results but potential correlation with PFS7'138'144'145 Decrease of VEGF-A, VEGFR-2, and VEGFR-3 levels on treatment correlated with better PFS in mRCC120'146

(continued)

TABLE 13.2 (continued)
Predictive Biomarkers for Antiangiogenic Therapies

Type of Biomarker	Example	Analysis Technique	Advantages	Disadvantages	Existing Data
Circulating endothelial cells		Flow cytometry Veridex		No standardized analysis procedure	Contradictory results147'148
Circulating endothelial progenitors		Immunomagnetic/ microfluid (EpiSep) ISET		Time-consuming	
Functional evaluation					
Functional imaging	Microtubules Iodin Gadolinium H₂ ¹⁵O	Contrast ultrasound Diffusion TDM DCE-MRI positron emission tomography (PET)-scan	Direct functional assessment No radiation (MRI, US) Concomittant tumor assessment (PET, TDM, MRI) Cost (US)	Theoretically reproducible but lack of standardized procedures Cost (TDM, PET, IRM) Irradiation (TDM, PET)	Decrease in perfusion correlated to tumor response: US[89], perfusion CT[145,146], DCE-MRI[147,148], PET-scan
Molecular imaging	αVβ3	Antibody-conjugated label directed against a vascular target, detected by PET or US	High sensitivity and specificity	Cost	

CONCLUSION

Great hopes have been generated by the discovery of tumor neoangiogenesis and subsequent evidence of clinical efficacy of antiangiogenic agents. Numerous clinical successes have been achieved, and both monoclonal antibodies and small molecules targeting angiogenesis are currently licensed in several tumor types. However, modest survival benefits observed in some tumor types, onset of resistance, and drug-related toxicities have limited the development of these therapies, calling for a better understanding of tumor biology. Several questions also remain unanswered, such as the role for antiangiogenic agents in the adjuvant and neo-adjuvant settings and the potential for combining antiangiogenic drugs or antiangiogenic with vascular disrupting agents. Current challenges include the development of an appropriate evaluation method for assessing drug efficacy as well as predictive biomarkers for customizing treatment and optimizing patient outcome.

REFERENCES

1. Folkman J: Tumor angiogenesis: Therapeutic implications. *N Engl J Med* 285: 1182–1186, 1971.
2. Bergers G, Benjamin LE: Tumorigenesis and the angiogenic switch. *Nat Rev Cancer* 3:401–410, 2003.
3. Kerbel RS: Tumor angiogenesis. *N Engl J Med* 358:2039–2049, 2008.
4. Hicklin DJ, Ellis LM: Role of the vascular endothelial growth factor pathway in tumor growth and angiogenesis. *J Clin Oncol* 23:1011–1027, 2005.
5. Dvorak HF: Vascular permeability factor/vascular endothelial growth factor: A critical cytokine in tumor angiogenesis and a potential target for diagnosis and therapy. *J Clin Oncol* 20:4368–4380, 2002.
6. Leung DW, Cachianes G, Kuang WJ et al.: Vascular endothelial growth factor is a secreted angiogenic mitogen. *Science* 246:1306–1369, 1989.
7. Poon RT, Fan ST, Wong J: Clinical implications of circulating angiogenic factors in cancer patients. *J Clin Oncol* 19:1207–1225, 2001.
8. Ellis LM, Hicklin DJ: VEGF-targeted therapy: Mechanisms of anti-tumour activity. *Nat Rev Cancer* 8:579–591, 2008.
9. Ferrara N, Gerber HP, LeCouter J: The biology of VEGF and its receptors. *Nat Med* 9:669–676, 2003.
10. Shibuya M, Claesson-Welsh L: Signal transduction by VEGF receptors in regulation of angiogenesis and lymphangiogenesis. *Exp Cell Res* 312:549–560, 2006.
11. Lohela M, Bry M, Tammela T et al.: VEGFs and receptors involved in angiogenesis versus lymphangiogenesis. *Curr Opin Cell Biol* 21:154–165, 2009.
12. Ellis LM: The role of neuropilins in cancer. *Mol Cancer Ther* 5:1099–1107, 2006.
13. Price DJ, Miralem T, Jiang S et al.: Role of vascular endothelial growth factor in the stimulation of cellular invasion and signaling of breast cancer cells. *Cell Growth Differ* 12:129–135, 2001.
14. Kessler T, Fehrmann F, Bieker R et al.: Vascular endothelial growth factor and its receptor as drug targets in hematological malignancies. *Curr Drug Targets* 8: 257–268, 2007.
15. Lee TH, Seng S, Sekine M et al.: Vascular endothelial growth factor mediates intracrine survival in human breast carcinoma cells through internally expressed VEGFR1/FLT1. *PLoS Med* 4:e186, 2007.

16. Kaplan RN, Riba RD, Zacharoulis S et al.: VEGFR1-positive haematopoietic bone marrow progenitors initiate the pre-metastatic niche. *Nature* 438:820–827, 2005.
17. Gerber HP, Malik AK, Solar GP et al.: VEGF regulates haematopoietic stem cell survival by an internal autocrine loop mechanism. *Nature* 417:954–958, 2002.
18. Koch S, Tugues S, Li X et al.: Signal transduction by vascular endothelial growth factor receptors. *Biochem J* 437:169–183, 2011.
19. Dvorak HF, Brown LF, Detmar M et al.: Vascular permeability factor/vascular endothelial growth factor, microvascular hyperpermeability, and angiogenesis. *Am J Pathol* 146:1029–1039, 1995.
20. Zachary I, Gliki G: Signaling transduction mechanisms mediating biological actions of the vascular endothelial growth factor family. *Cardiovasc Res* 49:568–581, 2001.
21. Gerber HP, McMurtrey A, Kowalski J et al.: Vascular endothelial growth factor regulates endothelial cell survival through the phosphatidylinositol 3'-kinase/Akt signal transduction pathway. Requirement for Flk-1/KDR activation. *J Biol Chem* 273:30336–30343, 1998.
22. Maxwell PH, Wiesener MS, Chang GW et al.: The tumour suppressor protein VHL targets hypoxia-inducible factors for oxygen-dependent proteolysis. *Nature* 399:271–275, 1999.
23. Hlatky L, Tsionou C, Hahnfeldt P et al.: Mammary fibroblasts may influence breast tumor angiogenesis via hypoxia-induced vascular endothelial growth factor upregulation and protein expression. *Cancer Res* 54:6083–6086, 1994.
24. Ridgway J, Zhang G, Wu Y et al.: Inhibition of Dll4 signalling inhibits tumour growth by deregulating angiogenesis. *Nature* 444:1083–1087, 2006.
25. Dong J, Grunstein J, Tejada M et al.: VEGF-null cells require PDGFR alpha signaling-mediated stromal fibroblast recruitment for tumorigenesis. *Embo J* 23:2800–2810, 2004.
26. Asahara T, Murohara T, Sullivan A et al.: Isolation of putative progenitor endothelial cells for angiogenesis. *Science* 275:964–967, 1997.
27. Bertolini F, Shaked Y, Mancuso P et al.: The multifaceted circulating endothelial cell in cancer: Towards marker and target identification. *Nat Rev Cancer* 6:835–845, 2006.
28. Calabrese C, Poppleton H, Kocak M et al.: A perivascular niche for brain tumor stem cells. *Cancer Cell* 11:69–82, 2007.
29. Hurwitz H, Fehrenbacher L, Novotny W et al.: Bevacizumab plus irinotecan, fluorouracil, and leucovorin for metastatic colorectal cancer. *N Engl J Med* 350:2335–2342, 2004.
30. Gordon MS, Margolin K, Talpaz M et al.: Phase I safety and pharmacokinetic study of recombinant human anti-vascular endothelial growth factor in patients with advanced cancer. *J Clin Oncol* 19:843–850, 2001.
31. Hurwitz HI, Yi J, Ince W et al.: The clinical benefit of bevacizumab in metastatic colorectal cancer is independent of K-ras mutation status: Analysis of a phase III study of bevacizumab with chemotherapy in previously untreated metastatic colorectal cancer. *Oncologist* 14:22–28, 2009.
32. Saltz LB, Clarke S, Diaz-Rubio E et al.: Bevacizumab in combination with oxaliplatin-based chemotherapy as first-line therapy in metastatic colorectal cancer: A randomized phase III study. *J Clin Oncol* 26:2013–2019, 2008.
33. Giantonio BJ, Catalano PJ, Meropol NJ et al.: Bevacizumab in combination with oxaliplatin, fluorouracil, and leucovorin (FOLFOX4) for previously treated metastatic colorectal cancer: Results from the Eastern Cooperative Oncology Group Study E3200. *J Clin Oncol* 25:1539–1544, 2007.
34. Miller K, Wang M, Gralow J et al.: Paclitaxel plus bevacizumab versus paclitaxel alone for metastatic breast cancer. *N Engl J Med* 357:2666–2676, 2007.

35. Gray R, Bhattacharya S, Bowden C et al.: Independent review of E2100: A phase III trial of bevacizumab plus paclitaxel versus paclitaxel in women with metastatic breast cancer. *J Clin Oncol* 27:4966–4972, 2009.

36. Pivot X, Schneeweiss A, Verma S et al.: Efficacy and safety of bevacizumab in combination with docetaxel for the first-line treatment of elderly patients with locally recurrent or metastatic breast cancer: Results from AVADO. *Eur J Cancer* 47:2387–2395, 2011.

37. Robert NJ, Dieras V, Glaspy J et al.: RIBBON-1: Randomized, double-blind, placebo-controlled, phase III trial of chemotherapy with or without bevacizumab for first-line treatment of human epidermal growth factor receptor 2-negative, locally recurrent or metastatic breast cancer. *J Clin Oncol* 29:1252–1260, 2011.

38. O'Shaughnessy J, Miles D, Gray RJ et al.: A meta-analysis of overall survival data from three randomized trials of bevacizumab (BV) and first-line chemotherapy as treatment for patients with metastatic breast cancer (MBC). *J Clin Oncol* 18:1005, 2010.

39. Brufsky A, Hoelzer K, Beck T et al.: A randomized phase II study of paclitaxel and bevacizumab with and without gemcitabine as first-line treatment for metastatic breast cancer. *Clin Breast Cancer* 11:211–220, 2011.

40. Johnson DH, Fehrenbacher L, Novotny WF et al.: Randomized phase II trial comparing bevacizumab plus carboplatin and paclitaxel with carboplatin and paclitaxel alone in previously untreated locally advanced or metastatic non-small-cell lung cancer. *J Clin Oncol* 22:2184–2191, 2004.

41. Sandler A, Gray R, Perry MC et al.: Paclitaxel-carboplatin alone or with bevacizumab for non-small-cell lung cancer. *N Engl J Med* 355:2542–2550, 2006.

42. Reck M, von Pawel J, Zatloukal P et al.: Overall survival with cisplatin-gemcitabine and bevacizumab or placebo as first-line therapy for nonsquamous non-small-cell lung cancer: Results from a randomised phase III trial (AVAiL). *Ann Oncol* 21: 1804–1809, 2010.

43. Escudier B, Pluzanska A, Koralewski P et al.: Bevacizumab plus interferon alfa-2a for treatment of metastatic renal cell carcinoma: A randomised, double-blind phase III trial. *Lancet* 370:2103–2111, 2007.

44. Rini BI, Halabi S, Rosenberg JE et al.: Phase III trial of bevacizumab plus interferon alfa versus interferon alfa monotherapy in patients with metastatic renal cell carcinoma: Final results of CALGB 90206. *J Clin Oncol* 28:2137–2143, 2010.

45. Perren TJ, Swart AM, Pfisterer J et al.: A phase 3 trial of bevacizumab in ovarian cancer. *N Engl J Med* 365:2484–2496, 2011.

46. Heitz F, Harter P, Barinoff J et al.: Bevacizumab in the treatment of ovarian cancer. *Adv Ther* 29:723–735, 2012.

47. Aghajanian C, Finkler NJ, Rutherford T et al.: OCEANS: A randomized, double-blinded, placebo-controlled phase III trial of chemotherapy with or without bevacizumab (BEV) in patients with platinum-sensitive recurrent epithelial ovarian (EOC), primary peritoneal (PPC), or fallopian tube cancer (FTC). *J Clin Oncol* 29, 2011.

48. Friedman HS, Prados MD, Wen PY et al.: Bevacizumab alone and in combination with irinotecan in recurrent glioblastoma. *J Clin Oncol* 27:4733–4740, 2009.

49. Kreisl TN, Kim L, Moore K et al.: Phase II trial of single-agent bevacizumab followed by bevacizumab plus irinotecan at tumor progression in recurrent glioblastoma. *J Clin Oncol* 27:740–745, 2009.

50. Grothey A, Sugrue MM, Purdie DM et al.: Bevacizumab beyond first progression is associated with prolonged overall survival in metastatic colorectal cancer: Results from a large observational cohort study (BRiTE). *J Clin Oncol* 26:5326–5334, 2008.

51. Berry SR, Van Cutsem E, Kretzschmar A et al.: Preliminary efficacy of bevacizumab with first-line FOLFOX, XELOX, FOLFIRI, and fluoropyrimidines for mCRC: First BEAT. ASCO GI 2008, Orlando, FL, Abstract 350, 2008.

52. Keefe D, Bowen J, Gibson R et al.: Noncardiac vascular toxicities of vascular endothelial growth factor inhibitors in advanced cancer: A review. *Oncologist* 16:432–444, 2011.
53. Vaklavas C, Lenihan D, Kurzrock R et al.: Anti-vascular endothelial growth factor therapies and cardiovascular toxicity: What are the important clinical markers to target? *Oncologist* 15:130–141, 2010.
54. Yang JC, Haworth L, Sherry RM et al.: A randomized trial of bevacizumab, an anti-vascular endothelial growth factor antibody, for metastatic renal cancer. *N Engl J Med* 349:427–434, 2003.
55. Chen HX, Cleck JN: Adverse effects of anticancer agents that target the VEGF pathway. *Nat Rev Clin Oncol* 6:465–477, 2009.
56. Izzedine H, Massard C, Spano JP et al.: VEGF signalling inhibition-induced proteinuria: Mechanisms, significance and management. *Eur J Cancer* 46:439–448, 2010.
57. Izzedine H, Rixe O, Billemont B et al.: Angiogenesis inhibitor therapies: Focus on kidney toxicity and hypertension. *Am J Kidney Dis* 50:203–218, 2007.
58. Izzedine H, Brocheriou I, Deray G et al.: Thrombotic microangiopathy and anti-VEGF agents. *Nephrol Dial Transplant* 22:1481–1482, 2007.
59. Zangari M, Fink LM, Elice F et al.: Thrombotic events in patients with cancer receiving antiangiogenesis agents. *J Clin Oncol* 27:4865–4873, 2009.
60. Scappaticci FA, Skillings JR, Holden SN et al.: Arterial thromboembolic events in patients with metastatic carcinoma treated with chemotherapy and bevacizumab. *J Natl Cancer Inst* 99:1232–1239, 2007.
61. Glusker P, Recht L, Lane B: Reversible posterior leukoencephalopathy syndrome and bevacizumab. *N Engl J Med* 354:980–982; discussion 980–982, 2006.
62. Martin G, Bellido L, Cruz JJ: Reversible posterior leukoencephalopathy syndrome induced by sunitinib. *J Clin Oncol* 25:115–124, 2007.
63. Schutz FA, Je Y, Azzi GR et al.: Bevacizumab increases the risk of arterial ischemia: A large study in cancer patients with a focus on different subgroup outcomes. *Ann Oncol* 22:1404–1412, 2011.
64. Nalluri SR, Chu D, Keresztes R et al.: Risk of venous thromboembolism with the angiogenesis inhibitor bevacizumab in cancer patients: A meta-analysis. *JAMA* 300:2277–2285, 2008.
65. Guarneri V, Miles D, Robert N et al.: Bevacizumab and osteonecrosis of the jaw: Incidence and association with bisphosphonate therapy in three large prospective trials in advanced breast cancer. *Breast Cancer Res Treat* 122:181–188, 2010.
66. Wang TF, Lockhart AC: Aflibercept in the treatment of metastatic colorectal cancer. *Clin Med Insights Oncol* 6:19–30, 2012.
67. Gotink KJ, Verheul HMW: Anti-angiogenic tyrosine kinase inhibitors: What is their mechanism of action? *Angiogenesis* 13:1–14, 2010.
68. Schueneman AJ, Himmelfarb E, Geng L et al.: SU11248 maintenance therapy prevents tumor regrowth after fractionated irradiation of murine tumor models. *Cancer Res* 63:4009–4016, 2003.
69. Faivre S, Delbaldo C, Vera K et al.: Safety, pharmacokinetic, and antitumor activity of SU11248, a novel oral multitarget tyrosine kinase inhibitor, in patients with cancer. *J Clin Oncol* 24:25–35, 2006.
70. Houk BE, Bello CL, Poland B et al.: Relationship between exposure to sunitinib and efficacy and tolerability endpoints in patients with cancer: Results of a pharmacokinetic/pharmacodynamic meta-analysis. *Cancer Chemother Pharmacol* 66:357–371, 2010.
71. Houk BE, Bello CL, Kang D et al.: A population pharmacokinetic meta-analysis of sunitinib malate (SU11248) and its primary metabolite (SU12662) in healthy volunteers and oncology patients. *Clin Cancer Res* 15:2497–2506, 2009.

72. Escudier B, Roigas J, Gillessen S et al.: Phase II study of sunitinib administered in a continuous once-daily dosing regimen in patients with cytokine-refractory metastatic renal cell carcinoma. *J Clin Oncol* 27:4068–4075, 2009.
73. Barrios CH, Hernandez-Barajas D, Brown MP et al.: Phase II trial of continuous once-daily dosing of sunitinib as first-line treatment in patients with metastatic renal cell carcinoma. *Cancer* 118:1252–1259, 2012.
74. Demetri GD, van Oosterom AT, Garrett CR et al.: Efficacy and safety of sunitinib in patients with advanced gastrointestinal stromal tumour after failure of imatinib: A randomised controlled trial. *Lancet* 368:1329–1338, 2006.
75. George S, Blay JY, Casali PG et al.: Clinical evaluation of continuous daily dosing of sunitinib malate in patients with advanced gastrointestinal stromal tumour after imatinib failure. *Eur J Cancer* 45:1959–1968, 2009.
76. Motzer RJ, Hutson TE, Tomczak P et al.: Sunitinib versus interferon alfa in metastatic renal-cell carcinoma. *N Engl J Med* 356:115–124, 2007.
77. Motzer RJ, Rini BI, Bukowski RM et al.: Sunitinib in patients with metastatic renal cell carcinoma. *JAMA* 295:2516–2524, 2006.
78. Gan HK, Seruga B, Knox JJ: Sunitinib in solid tumors. *Expert Opin Investig Drugs* 18:821–834, 2009.
79. Rixe O, Billemont B, Izzedine H: Hypertension as a predictive factor of Sunitinib activity. *Ann Oncol* 18:1117–1125, 2007.
80. Sulkes A: Novel multitargeted anticancer oral therapies: Sinitinib and sorafenib as a paradigm. *IMAJ* 12:628–632, 2010.
81. Wilhelm SM, Adnane L, Newell P et al.: Preclinical overview of sorafenib, a multikinase inhibitor that targets both Raf and VEGF and PDGF receptor tyrosine kinase signaling. *Mol Cancer Ther* 7:3129–3140, 2008.
82. Eisen T, Ahmad T, Flaherty KT et al.: Sorafenib in advanced melanoma: A phase II randomised discontinuation trial analysis. *Br J Cancer* 95:581–586, 2006.
83. Strumberg D, Richly H, Hilger RA et al.: Phase I clinical and pharmacokinetic study of the Novel Raf kinase and vascular endothelial growth factor receptor inhibitor BAY 43–9006 in patients with advanced refractory solid tumors. *J Clin Oncol* 23:965–972, 2005.
84. Awada A, Hendlisz A, Gil T et al.: Phase I safety and pharmacokinetics of BAY 43–9006 administered for 21 days on/7 days off in patients with advanced, refractory solid tumours. *Br J Cancer* 92:1855–1861, 2005.
85. Escudier B, Eisen T, Stadler WM et al.: Sorafenib in advanced clear-cell renal-cell carcinoma. *N Engl J Med* 356:125–134, 2007.
86. Ryan CW, Goldman BH, Lara PN, Jr. et al.: Sorafenib with interferon alfa-2b as first-line treatment of advanced renal carcinoma: A phase II study of the Southwest Oncology Group. *J Clin Oncol* 25:3296–3301, 2007.
87. Llovet JM, Ricci S, Mazzaferro V et al.: Sorafenib in advanced hepatocellular carcinoma. *N Engl J Med* 359:378–390, 2008.
88. Lacouture ME, Wu S, Robert C et al.: Evolving strategies for the management of hand-foot skin reaction associated with the multitargeted kinase inhibitors sorafenib and sunitinib. *Oncologist* 13:1001–1011, 2008.
89. Lassau N, Lamuraglia M, Koscielny S et al.: Prognostic value of angiogenesis evaluated with high-frequency and colour Doppler sonography for preoperative assessment of primary cutaneous melanomas: Correlation with recurrence after a 5 year follow-up period. *Cancer Imaging* 6:24–29, 2006.
90. Lamuraglia M, Escudier B, Chami L et al.: To predict progression-free survival and overall survival in metastatic renal cancer treated with sorafenib: Pilot study using dynamic contrast-enhanced Doppler ultrasound. *Eur J Cancer* 42:2472–2479, 2006.

91. Schutz FA, Choueiri TK, Sternberg CN: Pazopanib: Clinical development of a potent anti-angiogenic drug. *Crit Rev Oncol Hematol* 77:163–171, 2011.

92. Hurwitz HI, Dowlati A, Saini S et al.: Phase I trial of pazopanib in patients with advanced cancer. *Clin Cancer Res* 15:4220–4227, 2009.

93. Sternberg CN, Davis ID, Mardiak J et al.: Pazopanib in locally advanced or metastatic renal cell carcinoma: Results of a randomized phase III trial. *J Clin Oncol* 28: 1061–1068, 2010.

94. Endo M, Nielsen TO: Pazopanib for metastatic soft-tissue sarcoma. *Lancet* 380:801; author reply 801, 2012.

95. Pick AM, Nystrom KK: Pazopanib for the treatment of metastatic renal cell carcinoma. *Clin Ther* 34:511–520, 2012.

96. Holden SN, Eckhardt SG, Basser R et al.: Clinical evaluation of ZD6474, an orally active inhibitor of VEGF and EGF receptor signaling, in patients with solid, malignant tumors. *Ann Oncol* 16:1391–1397, 2005.

97. Wells SA, Jr., Gosnell JE, Gagel RF et al.: Vandetanib for the treatment of patients with locally advanced or metastatic hereditary medullary thyroid cancer. *J Clin Oncol* 28:767–772, 2010.

98. Herbst RS, Sun Y, Eberhardt WE et al.: Vandetanib plus docetaxel versus docetaxel as second-line treatment for patients with advanced non-small-cell lung cancer (ZODIAC): A double-blind, randomised, phase 3 trial. *Lancet Oncol* 11:619–626, 2010.

99. Lee JS, Hirsh V, Park K et al.: Vandetanib versus placebo in patients with advanced non-small-cell lung cancer after prior therapy with an epidermal growth factor receptor tyrosine kinase inhibitor: A randomized, double-blind phase III trial (ZEPHYR). *J Clin Oncol* 30:1114–1121, 2012.

100. Heymach JV, Paz-Ares L, De Braud F et al.: Randomized phase II study of vandetanib alone or with paclitaxel and carboplatin as first-line treatment for advanced non-small-cell lung cancer. *J Clin Oncol* 26:5407–5415, 2008.

101. Rini BI, Escudier B, Tomczak P et al.: Comparative effectiveness of axitinib versus sorafenib in advanced renal cell carcinoma (AXIS): A randomised phase 3 trial. *Lancet* 378:1931–1939, 2011.

102. Strumberg D, Schultheis B: Regorafenib for cancer. *Expert Opin Investig Drugs* 21: 879–889, 2012.

103. Strumberg D, Scheulen ME, Schultheis B et al.: Regorafenib (BAY 73–4506) in advanced colorectal cancer: A phase I study. *Br J Cancer* 106:1722–1727, 2012.

104. Grothey A, Van Cutsem E, Sobrero A et al.: Regorafenib monotherapy for previously treated metastatic colorectal cancer (CORRECT): An international, multicentre, randomised, placebo-controlled, phase 3 trial. *Lancet* 381:303–312, 2013.

105. Demetri GD, Reichardt P, Kang YK et al. Efficacy and safety of regofafenib for advanced gastrointestinal stromal tumours after failure of imatinib and sunitinib (GRID): An international, multicentre, randomised, placebo-controlled phase 3 trial. *Lancet* 381(9863):295–302, 2013.

106. Goss GD, Arnold A, Shepherd FA et al.: Randomized, double-blind trial of carboplatin and paclitaxel with either daily oral cediranib or placebo in advanced non-small-cell lung cancer: NCIC clinical trials group BR24 study. *J Clin Oncol* 28:49–55, 2010.

107. Raghav KP, Blumenschein GR: Motesanib and advanced NSCLC: Experiences and expectations. *Expert Opin Investig Drugs* 20:859–869, 2011.

108. Reck M: BIBF 1120 for the treatment of non-small cell lung cancer. *Expert Opin Investig Drugs* 19:789–794, 2010.

109. Diaz-Padilla I, Siu LL: Brivanib alaninate for cancer. *Expert Opin Investig Drugs* 20:577–586, 2011.

110. Zhou J, Goh BC, Albert DH et al.: ABT-869, a promising multi-targeted tyrosine kinase inhibitor: From bench to bedside. *J Hematol Oncol* 2:33, 2009.

111. Gori B, Ricciardi S, Fulvi A et al.: New antiangiogenics in non-small cell lung cancer treatment: Vargatef (BIBF 1120) and beyond. *Ther Clin Risk Manag* 7:429–440, 2011.

112. Reck M, Kaiser R, Eschbach C et al.: A phase II double-blind study to investigate efficacy and safety of two doses of the triple angiokinase inhibitor BIBF 1120 in patients with relapsed advanced non-small-cell lung cancer. *Ann Oncol* 22:1374–1381, 2011.

113. Yang AD, Bauer TW, Camp ER et al.: Improving delivery of antineoplastic agents with anti-vascular endothelial growth factor therapy. *Cancer* 103:1561–1570, 2005.

114. Teicher BA, Sotomayor EA, Huang ZD: Antiangiogenic agents potentiate cytotoxic cancer therapies against primary and metastatic disease. *Cancer Res* 52:6702–6704, 1992.

115. Shaked Y, Ciarrocchi A, Franco M et al.: Therapy-induced acute recruitment of circulating endothelial progenitor cells to tumors. *Science* 313:1785–1787, 2006.

116. Shaked Y, Bertolini F, Emmenegger U et al.: On the origin and nature of elevated levels of circulating endothelial cells after treatment with a vascular disrupting agent. *J Clin Oncol* 24:4040; author reply 4040–4041, 2006.

117. Miller KD, Sweeney CJ, Sledge GW, Jr.: Redefining the target: Chemotherapeutics as antiangiogenics. *J Clin Oncol* 19:1195–1206, 2001.

118. Kerbel RS, Kamen BA: The anti-angiogenic basis of metronomic chemotherapy. *Nat Rev Cancer* 4:423–436, 2004.

119. Pasquier E, Kavallaris M, Andre N: Metronomic chemotherapy: New rationale for new directions. *Nat Rev Clin Oncol* 7:455–465, 2010.

120. Rini BI, Michaelson MD, Rosenberg JE et al.: Antitumor activity and biomarker analysis of sunitinib in patients with bevacizumab-refractory metastatic renal cell carcinoma. *J Clin Oncol* 26:3743–3748, 2008.

121. Azad NS, Posadas EM, Kwitkowski VE et al.: Combination targeted therapy with sorafenib and bevacizumab results in enhanced toxicity and antitumor activity. *J Clin Oncol* 26:3709–3714, 2008.

122. Feldman DR, Baum MS, Ginsberg MS et al.: Phase I trial of bevacizumab plus escalated doses of sunitinib in patients with metastatic renal cell carcinoma. *J Clin Oncol* 27:1432–1439, 2009.

123. Bergers G, Hanahan D: Modes of resistance to anti-angiogenic therapy. *Nat Rev Cancer* 8:592–603, 2008.

124. Sofuni A, Iijima H, Moriyasu F et al.: Differential diagnosis of pancreatic tumors using ultrasound contrast imaging. *J Gastroenterol* 40:518–525, 2005.

125. Yu JL, Rak JW, Coomber BL et al.: Effect of p53 status on tumor response to antiangiogenic therapy. *Science* 295:1526–1528, 2002.

126. Marty M, Pivot X: The potential of anti-vascular endothelial growth factor therapy in metastatic breast cancer: Clinical experience with anti-angiogenic agents, focusing on bevacizumab. *Eur J Cancer* 44:912–920, 2008.

127. Fernando NT, Koch M, Rothrock C et al.: Tumor escape from endogenous, extracellular matrix-associated angiogenesis inhibitors by up-regulation of multiple proangiogenic factors. *Clin Cancer Res* 14:1529–1539, 2008.

128. Batchelor TT, Sorensen AG, di Tomaso E et al.: AZD2171, a pan-VEGF receptor tyrosine kinase inhibitor, normalizes tumor vasculature and alleviates edema in glioblastoma patients. *Cancer Cell* 11:83–95, 2007.

129. Petit I, Jin D, Rafii S: The SDF-1-CXCR4 signaling pathway: A molecular hub modulating neo-angiogenesis. *Trends Immunol* 28:299–307, 2007.

130. Jain RK, Booth MF: What brings pericytes to tumor vessels? *J Clin Invest* 112:1134–1136, 2003.

131. Du R, Lu KV, Petritsch C et al.: HIF1alpha induces the recruitment of bone marrow-derived vascular modulatory cells to regulate tumor angiogenesis and invasion. *Cancer Cell* 13:206–220, 2008.

132. Xian X, Hakansson J, Stahlberg A et al.: Pericytes limit tumor cell metastasis. *J Clin Invest* 116:642–651, 2006.
133. Jubb AM, Oates AJ, Holden S et al.: Predicting benefit from anti-angiogenic agents in malignancy. *Nat Rev Cancer* 6:626–635, 2006.
134. Scartozzi M, Galizia E, Chiorrini S et al.: Arterial hypertension correlates with clinical outcome in colorectal cancer patients treated with first-line bevacizumab. *Ann Oncol* 20:227–230, 2009.
135. Rini BI, Schiller JH, Fruehauf JP et al.: Diastolic blood pressure as a biomarker of axitinib efficacy in solid tumors. *Clin Cancer Res* 17:3841–3849, 2011.
136. Heist RS, Zhai R, Liu G et al.: VEGF polymorphisms and survival in early-stage non-small-cell lung cancer. *J Clin Oncol* 26:856–862, 2008.
137. Schneider BP, Wang M, Radovich M et al.: Association of vascular endothelial growth factor and vascular endothelial growth factor receptor-2 genetic polymorphisms with outcome in a trial of paclitaxel compared with paclitaxel plus bevacizumab in advanced breast cancer: ECOG 2100. *J Clin Oncol* 26:4672–4678, 2008.
138. Lambrechts D, Claes B, Delmar P et al.: VEGF pathway genetic variants as biomarkers of treatment outcome with bevacizumab: An analysis of data from the AViTA and AVOREN randomised trials. *Lancet Oncol* 13:724–733, 2012.
139. Kim JJ, Vaziri SA, Rini BI et al.: Association of VEGF and VEGFR2 single nucleotide polymorphisms with hypertension and clinical outcome in metastatic clear cell renal cell carcinoma patients treated with sunitinib. *Cancer* 118:1946–1954, 2012.
140. Hlatky L, Hahnfeldt P, Folkman J: Clinical application of antiangiogenic therapy: Microvessel density, what it does and doesn't tell us. *J Natl Cancer Inst* 94:883–893, 2002.
141. Fukumura D, Xavier R, Sugiura T et al.: Tumor induction of VEGF promoter activity in stromal cells. *Cell* 94:715–725, 1998.
142. Ince WL, Jubb AM, Holden SN et al.: Association of k-ras, b-raf, and p53 status with the treatment effect of bevacizumab. *J Natl Cancer Inst* 97:981–989, 2005.
143. Klatte T, Seligson DB, Riggs SB et al.: Hypoxia-inducible factor 1 alpha in clear cell renal cell carcinoma. *Clin Cancer Res* 13:7388–7393, 2007.
144. Jubb AM, Hurwitz HI, Bai W et al.: Impact of vascular endothelial growth factor-A expression, thrombospondin-2 expression, and microvessel density on the treatment effect of bevacizumab in metastatic colorectal cancer. *J Clin Oncol* 24:217–227, 2006.
145. Dowlati A, Gray R, Sandler AB et al.: Cell adhesion molecules, vascular endothelial growth factor, and basic fibroblast growth factor in patients with non-small cell lung cancer treated with chemotherapy with or without bevacizumab—An Eastern Cooperative Oncology Group Study. *Clin Cancer Res* 14:1407–1412, 2008.
146. Siegel AB, Cohen EI, Ocean A et al.: Phase II trial evaluating the clinical and biologic effects of bevacizumab in unresectable hepatocellular carcinoma. *J Clin Oncol* 26:2992–2998, 2008.
147. Willett CG, Boucher Y, Duda DG et al.: Surrogate markers for antiangiogenic therapy and dose-limiting toxicities for bevacizumab with radiation and chemotherapy: Continued experience of a phase I trial in rectal cancer patients. *J Clin Oncol* 23:8136–8139, 2005.
148. Norden-Zfoni A, Desai J, Manola J et al.: Blood-based biomarkers of SU11248 activity and clinical outcome in patients with metastatic imatinib-resistant gastrointestinal stromal tumor. *Clin Cancer Res* 13:2643–2650, 2007.
149. Ocak I, Baluk P, Barrett T et al.: The biologic basis of in vivo angiogenesis imaging. *Front Biosci* 12:3601–3616, 2007.
150. Cowey CL, Rathmell WK: VHL gene mutations in renal cell carcinoma: Role as a biomarker of disease outcome and drug efficacy. *Curr Oncol Rep* 11:94–101, 2009.

14 Antivascular Agents

Gianluca Del Conte
Ospedale San Raffaele

Cristiana Sessa
Istituto Oncologico della Svizzera Italiana
Ospedale San Raffaele

CONTENTS

INTRODUCTION

All tumors need to generate their own blood supply in order to obtain sufficient oxygen and nutrients to grow beyond a volume of approximately 1 mm^3.[1] They achieve this through the complex processes of angiogenesis whereby endothelial cells proliferate in response to growth factors and invade the basal lamina, resulting in the budding of new vessels from the existing vasculature.[2,3] The endothelial cells of tumor blood vessels are attractive targets for drug development because of their pivotal role in cancer cell survival, growth and metastasis and because they are more genetically stable, and potentially less likely to develop resistance to therapeutic agents than the tumor cells themselves.[3] Furthermore, because endothelial cell targets are different from those targeted by chemotherapy agents, the potential for combination treatment can be evaluated.

Tumor vasculature differs from normal vasculature because tumor vessels are immature with incomplete pericyte coverage and increased tortuosity, permeability, and fragility. A number of compounds that target components of the angiogenesis pathways are now routinary used and others are in development (currently the most important of these is the vascular endothelial growth factor (VEGF) signaling pathway). This chapter will focus on the development of compounds that target and occlude the established tumor vasculature to interrupt blood supply. Those compounds have been previously defined "anti-vascular" or "vascular targeting agents," but it has

TABLE 14.1

VDAs in Clinical Development

Compound	Trade Name	Company	Clinical Development	$t_{1/2}$	References
CA4P	Fosbretabulin	OxiGene	Ongoing	33 min	Stevenson et al.[13]
Oxi4503		OxiGene	Ongoing	20 h	Patterson et al.[21]
AVE8062	Ombrabulin	Sanofi-Aventis	Ongoing	15 min	Tolcher et al.[23]
EPC2407	Crinobulin	Epicept	Ongoing	~2 h	Read et al.[29]
MPC6827	Verubulin	Myrexis	Ongoing	3.8–7.5 h	Tsimberidou et al.[30]
CYT997	Lexibulin	YM BioScience	Ongoing	3.17 h	Burge[39]
BNC105P		Bionomics	Ongoing	0.13 h	Rischin et al.[34]
NPI2358	Plinabulin	Nereus			
ASA404	Vadimezan	Novartis	Discontinued		
ABT-751		Abbott	Discontinued		
Dolastatin 10		Marine Biotech	Discontinued		
TZT1027	Soblidotin	Daiichi Sankyo	Discontinued		
ZD6126		AstraZeneca	Discontinued		
MN029	Denibulin	MediciNova	Discontinued		

been proposed that the most useful term to distinguish their mechanism of action from anti-angiogenic compounds is vascular disrupting agents (VDAs)[4] (Table 14.1).

MECHANISM OF ACTION

Microtubules are key components of the cytoskeleton and are vital for a number of essential cellular functions; they form the cytoskeleton of endothelial cells and are required for the maintenance of cellular shape, the formation of the mitotic spindle and movement of organelles, receptors, and transporters through the cytoplasm.[5] Microtubules are composed of α-tubulin and β-tubulin heterodimers and are dynamic structures, growing by polymerization. Inhibition of microtubular function results in poor alignment of chromosomes during mitosis, mitotic arrest, and apoptosis[6]; this is the basis of the mechanism of action of a number of chemotherapy drugs, specifically vinca alkaloids and taxanes. At high doses, vinca alkaloids, taxanes, and colchicine have all demonstrated anti-vascular effects in preclinical models because binding to tubulin alters the cytoskeleton and shape of endothelial cells. This shape change increases vascular permeability and ultimately leads to their detachment from the basal lamina, vascular wall collapse, and occlusion of tumor blood flow.[7,8] Those compounds have a narrow therapeutic window, and the anti-vascular effect is achieved at doses that are associated to severe toxicities in animals, in particular gastro-intestinal and peripheral neuropathy.

Successful attempts have been made to increase the therapeutic window either by enveloping taxanes within lipid complexes that target endothelial cells to improve selectivity or by generating novel tubulin binding agents with a more favorable safety profile than taxanes and vinca alkaloids.

VDAs act rapidly after administration by disrupting vascular wall with increase of interstitial pressure, followed by inhibition of blood flow, ischemia, and then collapse of the existing tumor blood vessels, starving areas of tumors of their blood supply. The result is marked ischemia, necrosis, and hemorrhage in tumors.[9,10] These effects are more marked in the central areas of tumors. By contrast, a thin, viable rim of tumor cells remains at the periphery, where the cells are nourished either by diffusion of nutrients from normal adjacent tissue or from host blood vessels in close proximity that are less susceptible to the agents than the tumor.

The clinical development programs for VDAs have focused on the development of combinations of VDA with a variety of anti-cancer therapies, including chemotherapy and radiotherapy.[10] Whereas anti-angiogenesis agents may be expected to be most effective when started in the early stages of cancer, VDAs may be still used when tumors are at more advanced stages. Also, while chronic dosing of anti-angiogenics may be required for sustaining the angiogenic effect, VDAs have an acute effect, and intermittent dosing schedules appear effective. The two approaches may therefore be complementary, and combinations of anti-angiogenics with VDAs are under investigation.

Fosbretabulin (Combretastatin A4 Diphosphate)

The initial phase I development of fosbretabulin consisted of three monotherapy studies to investigate the safety, tolerability, and pharmacokinetic profile of the compound and identify an optimum treatment schedule. The first study[11,12] investigated single doses given at three weekly intervals in 25 patients with advanced cancers. The study monitored effects on tumor blood flow using dynamic contrast-enhanced magnetic resonance imaging (DCE-MRI) and changes in plasma levels of cell adhesion molecules in patients treated at the higher-dose levels. Four dose levels were examined from 18 to 90 mg/m^2. The maximum tolerated dose (MTD) was defined at 60 mg/m^2. Dose limiting toxicities (DLTs) above this dose were pain at the tumor site and two episodes of reversible acute coronary syndrome. Pharmacokinetic analysis showed a short plasma half-life of approximately 30 min. Significant reductions in tumor blood flow by DCE-MRI were observed in six of seven patients treated at 60 mg/m^2. Three patients had prolonged disease stabilization, and one patient with anaplastic thyroid cancer had a durable complete response.

In another study, 37 patients with solid malignancies received fosbretabulin daily for 5 days repeated every 3 weeks.[13] Again, the only dose limiting toxicity was tumor pain at 75 mg/m^2. Cardiovascular DLTs (syncope and dyspnea or hypoxia) were observed at this dose, and the MTD was defined as 52 mg/m^2, a dose with which a decrease in the tumor perfusion was observed by DCE-MRI. A partial response was reported in a patient with metastatic soft tissue sarcoma.

In the third phase I study, fosbretabulin was given weekly for 3 weeks followed by a 1 week interval.[14] The only drug-related toxicity up to 40 mg/m^2 was tumor pain. Overall, fosbretabulin was considered to be tolerable at doses of 52 or 68 mg/m^2.

Further phase I studies of fosbretabulin focused on combination therapy with a number of agents including radiotherapy, chemotherapy, and radio-immunotherapy. In a phase Ib trial, fosbretabulin at a dose of 50 mg/m^2 was given in combination with different radiotherapy schedules.[15] The most common drug-related toxicities were grade 1 hypertension, mild bradycardia and QTc prolongation (13 ms), lymphopenia, and severe tumor pain that often required opioids. There was no increase in the number or severity of reactions to radiotherapy and no accumulation of toxicity with repeated doses. Tumor blood flow was assessed using perfusion computed tomography (CT) and demonstrated a sustained reduction in tumor blood volume.

Following a phase I study of fosbretabulin in combination with carboplatin,[16] a three-center phase Ib/II trial of fosbretabulin in combination with carboplatin and paclitaxel, both alone and together, was carried out in patients with advanced ovarian cancer and other solid tumors.[17,18] The adverse effects in the phase Ib portion of the study were mild and self-limiting with no cardiac toxicity, indicating that fosbretabulin added no additional toxicity to the chemotherapy alone. DLTs of hypertension and ataxia occurred at a fosbretabulin dose of 72 mg/m². Objective tumor responses were observed in a number of patients. In advanced ovarian cancer, response evaluation criteria in solid tumors (RECIST) or CA-125 responses were observed in 10 of 15 patients and 4 others had prolonged disease stabilization. In a phase II study in patients with platinum resistant ovarian cancer, fosbretabulin was combined with paclitaxel and carboplatin. Treatment was well tolerated and produced a higher response rate than the standard chemotherapy. Grade ≥ 2 toxic effects were neutropenia (75%) and thrombocytopenia (9%); tumor pain, fatigue, hypertension, and neuropathy were also observed. The response rate by RECIST was 13.5% and by Gynecologic Cancer InterGroup CA125 criteria 34%.

In non-small cell lung cancer, a randomized phase 2 trial was conducted to determine the safety, tolerability, and efficacy of fosbretabulin in combination with bevacizumab, carboplatin, and paclitaxel in chemotherapy naïve patients.

In a phase 1 trial combining fosbretabulin with bevacizumab, patients with advanced solid malignancies received combretastatin A4 diphosphate (CA4P) at 45, 54, or 63 mg/m² on day 1, day 8, and then every 2 weeks and bevacizumab (10 mg/kg) on day 8 and then every 2 weeks at subsequent cycles, 4 h after fosbretabulin. The recommended phase II dose of CA4P was 63 mg/m². DLTs were grade 3 asymptomatic atrial fibrillation and grade 4 liver hemorrhage in one patient each. Other common toxicities were hypertension (73%), headache, lymphopenia, pruritus, and pyrexia. DCE-MRI showed significant reductions in tumor perfusion, which reversed after fosbretabulin alone but were sustained following bevacizumab.[19]

Objective responses were seen in advanced anaplastic thyroid cancer and a clinical program in this disease was initiated.

OXI4503 (COMBRETASTATIN A1 PHOSPHATE, CA1P; OXIGENE)

Oxi4503 is the more potent phosphorylated prodrug of combretastatin A4, causing a greater reduction in tumor blood flow and greater tumor shrinkage than the parent compound.[20]

Oxi4503 has a peculiar mechanism of action, being a VDA but also a cytotoxic agent due to the metabolic production of reactive cytotoxics ortho-quinones, which bind to nucleophiles and form free radicals.

In phase I in patients with advanced solid tumors, DLTs were atrial fibrillation, increased troponin, blurred vision, diplopia, and tumor lysis with GI fistula formation. Common adverse events (AEs) were hypertension (59%), tumor pain (59%), anemia (45%), fatigue (47%), and QTc prolongation (31%). The MTD was 8.5 mg/m^2, but the escalation of the dose to 14 mg/m^2 was feasible excluding patients with pre-existing hypertension. Dynamic contrast enhanced magnetic resonance imaging (DCEMRI) and positron emission tomography (PET) showed a significant reduction in tumor perfusion at doses of 11 mg/m^2 or higher, and the recommended dose (RD) was defined in the range of 11–14 mg/m^2. Anti-tumor activity was seen at 14 mg/m^2 (one partial response (PR) in a heavily pre-treated patient with ovarian cancer).[21]

Overall, Oxi4503 showed a less favorable toxicity profile than the parent compound, while the potential overlapping vascular toxicities might preclude the development of combinations with anti-angiogenics.

Another single agent phase 1 was performed in patients with primary or secondary hepatic tumor. The rationale of the study is that Oxi4503 is bioactivated to its reactive orthoquinone metabolite by oxidative enzymes, in particular by myeloperoxidase, tyrosinase, and hepatic peroxidases, so that the drug should be more active in tissues with high levels of these enzymes like the liver.

An ongoing phase 1 is testing Oxi4503 in patients with relapsed or refractory acute myeloid leukemia (AML) and myelodysplastic syndrome (MDS). In preclinical studies, OXi4503 was shown to be cytotoxic to leukemic cells, with regression of leukemic cell engraftment in bone marrow and induction of phenotypic and molecular remissions.[22]

OMBRABULIN (AVE-8062)

Ombrabulin, a water-soluble analogue of combretastatin A4, underwent a similar phase I development program. The first phase I study investigated a weekly schedule for 3 out of 4 weeks.[23] Patients received doses ranging from 4.5 to 30 mg/m^2, and the 30 mg/m^2 cohort was expanded due to a DLT consisting of asymptomatic systolic hypotension without evidence of creatine phosphokinase (CPK), troponin I, or electrocardiogram (ECG) changes. Reductions in tumor vascular flow by DCE-MRI were observed at and above 15.5 mg/m^2. Ombrabulin was rapidly eliminated with a $t_{1/2}$ of 15 min although an active metabolite was identified with a $t_{1/2}$ of 7 h.

In a second phase I study, ombrabulin was given for five consecutive days every 3 weeks, while a third investigated a single intermittent schedule every 3 weeks.[24] Because of the occurrence of four potentially drug-related vascular events (myocardial ischemia, transient asymptomatic hypotension, transient cerebral ischemia, and asymptomatic ventricular tachycardia) without residual clinical deficits, in the 5 day and weekly schedule studies, all trials were temporarily interrupted. No vascular events were observed in the every 3 week schedule up to a dose of 22 mg/m^2, and this trial was later resumed at the same dose, with restricted eligibility criteria and increased cardiovascular monitoring (continuous 24 h ECG, continual ambulatory blood pressure [BP] monitoring, serial CPK, troponin, ECG, ventriculographies and echocardiograms).

Phase 1 combination studies with platinum and taxanes have been performed, but results have not been published yet. Ombrabulin was administered on day 1 followed by docetaxel on day 2 every 3 weeks in two cohorts with docetaxel at 75 or 100 mg/m^2, respectively. In the first cohort, the MTD was 35/75 mg/m^2 with two DLTs (grade 3 headache and asthenia) reported at 42/75 mg/m^2. Second cohort MTD was 30/100 mg/m^2 with grade 3 asthenia and deep vein thrombosis. The pharmacokinetics (PK) profiles of the drugs were similar to those found in monotherapy studies. Preliminary anti-tumor activity was observed with three partial responses (breast cancer) and 20 stable diseases (including two prostate cancer with biological response and five patients who received more than 10 cycles).[25]

A phase II randomized trial is ongoing to evaluate whether the addition of ombrabulin to carboplatin and paclitaxel improves outcomes in patients with platinum-sensitive recurrent ovarian cancer. Patients are randomized (1:1) to receive either ombrabulin 35 mg/m^2 or placebo plus carboplatin and paclitaxel every 3 weeks. The primary endpoint is progression-free survival stratified by the time of first disease recurrence (6–12 or >12 months). One hundred and fifty patients from 45 sites will be randomized. Sixty-five patients have been randomized as of January 2012.[26]

Recent data have shown that the combination of ombrabulin with bevacizumab is feasible and with promising anti-tumor activity in ovarian cancer.[27]

OTHERS

There are many "VDAs" still at an early stage of clinical development.

EPC2407 (crinobulin) is a novel 4-aryl chromene, single isomer microtubulin inhibitor of high potency, causing tumor apoptosis and vessel disruption. Two phase 1 trials were conducted with the single agent in patients with advanced solid tumors. In one trial, EPC2407 was administered as 1 h infusions daily for 3 days on a 21 day cycle; at 21 mg/m^2 dose, DLTs were tumor pain and increases of BP and QTc. MTD was 13 mg/m^2.[28] In the second trial, the infusion duration was prolonged to 4 h, and the doses were escalated from 13 to 30 mg/m^2 with determination of MTD at 24 mg/m^2. Stabilization and clinical benefit were seen in two patients with hepatocellular carcinoma.[29] A phase I/II of EPC2407 plus cisplatin in adults with solid tumors with a focus on anaplastic thyroid cancer is ongoing.

MPC-6827 (verubulin) is a 4-arylaminoquinazoline causing both microtubule destabilization and vascular disruption at nanomolar concentrations. In the phase 1 in patients with solid tumors, verubulin was administered once-weekly, as a 1–2 h intravenous infusion for three consecutive weeks every 4 weeks (one cycle). There were two cases of myocardial infarction, and the MTD was determined at 3.3 mg/m^2. Common AEs were nausea, fatigue, flushing, and hyperglycemia.[30] Because of the high concentrations achieved in the brain, a phase 1 of verubulin and carboplatin was performed in patients with relapsed glioblastoma multiforme (GBM). Three doses (2.1, 2.7, and 3.3 mg/m^2) and two regimens were evaluated: 2.1 mg/m^2 every other week of a 6 week cycle, 2.7 and 3.3 mg/m^2 for 3 weeks in a 4 week cycle. Nineteen patients were enrolled and four experienced a drug-related AE (hyperesthesia cerebral ischemia, anemia, and thrombocytopenia). Mean plasma hal-life was 3.2 h. Two partial responses were seen according to Macdonald criteria. The combination looked safe with no cases of cerebral hemorrhage.[31]

A combination of verubulin with bevacizumab was tested in a phase II study in patients with recurrent treatment-naïve glioblastoma with acceptable toxicity but modest activity. The 6 months progression-free survival (PFS) was 14% (90% CI: 3%–25%) with a median PFS time of 1.8 months (90% CI: 1.8–1.9), and a median overall survival of 9.9 months (90% CI: 8.3–11.6).[32]

The potent tubulin polymerization inhibitor CYT997 has also a double mechanism of action causing tubulin accumulation in the cells and vascular disruption. In a phase 1 trial in patients with advanced solid tumors, CYT997 was administered as a continuous intravenous infusion over 24 h every 3 weeks at 12 dose levels (7–358 mg/m^2). DLTs were a prolonged QT interval in two patients and dyspnea in one patient at 269 and 358 mg/m^2, respectively. The PK was linear, and DCE-MRI showed significant changes in tumor perfusions.[33]

BNC105P is an inhibitor of tubulin polymerization with a vascular disruption action and direct anti-proliferative effects. The phosphorylated parent agent is rapidly converted to the active compound BNC105. Preclinically BNC105 shows a good therapeutic index with a large window between effective dose and toxic dose, in fact in mice the therapeutic index for BNC105 is 26 times greater than that for Combretastatin A4. The recommended dose is 16 mg/m^2, and the administration is associated to pharmacodynamic effects such as blood flow changes by DCE-MRI and dose-dependent reduction in the PBMCs levels of polymerized tubulin.[34] In a phase 2 trial as second-line chemotherapy for advanced malignant pleural mesothelioma, 30 subjects were enrolled with 1 PR and 13 stable disease (SD) as best response; the authors concluded that the treatment with BNC105P failed to meet the primary endpoint of interest despite a good toxicity profile. BNC105P is currently in phase II also in kidney cancer, in combination with everolimus or following everolimus in patients treated with prior tyrosine kinase inhibitors.

DISCUSSION

The development of VDAs has provided an exciting new approach for the treatment of cancer. The preclinical and clinical studies outlined in this chapter illustrate the effectiveness of these agents in multiple tumor types. Since no single approach is likely to be effective in the treatment of cancer, the potential of VDAs to be synergistic with a number of other anti-cancer modalities of treatment including chemotherapy, radiotherapy, and anti-angiogenic agents is of primary importance.

The study of the pharmacodynamic effects in early clinical studies is essential for a rational clinical development of molecularly targeted agents. With VDAs, the first challenge is the assessment of the changes in tumor perfusion. Alternative imaging methods such as DCE-MRI, dynamic contrast CT or ultrasounds to assess the reduction of the tumor blood flow had to be implemented.

The limits in the applicability of these techniques are the high intra- and inter-patient variability and the lack of a direct relationship between the reduction of blood flow and the efficacy. Other technical challenges are the identification of the optimum contrast agents suitable for clinical use and the limited inter-institutional reproducibility of the results. These techniques should be evaluated in larger efficacy studies in single tumor types, even if DCE-MRI cannot yet be definitely accepted as valid biomarker for anti-vascular effect.[35]

Another important pharmacodynamic tool may be the measurement of circulating endothelial cells (CECs) and bone marrow-derived precursor cells (CECPs). CECPs are recruited to cancer sites to promote tumor progression, while increased numbers of CECs and CECPs are observed in the blood of cancer patients.[36] Different populations of CECPs are recognized in tumor sites: endothelial cell progenitors, monocyte-like cells infiltrating the stroma and able to produce vascular growth factors, and pericyte precursors attracted to tumor sites able to stabilize tumor vessels. An increased count of CECPs is associated with angiogenesis in mice,[37] while anti-angiogenic therapies cause a decrease of CECPs.[38] Despite the outstanding scientific results, the true clinical value of CEC and CECP as biomarkers of angiogenesis is still to be defined.

Another major challenge is the selection of the dose and schedule for VDAs. In most of the clinical studies of individual VDAs, the toxicity is neither clearly dose-related nor consistent among phase I studies. VDAs cause a unique adverse event of tumor pain, presumably due to ischemia and necrosis, but this has not been sufficient to guide dose escalation. VDAs have a spectrum of adverse events which differ from the ones observed with conventional cytotoxic agents, the major class effect being cardiovascular toxicity, possibly because of drug-induced microvessel vasoconstriction and/or endothelial cell activation leading to the formation of micro-thrombi in the coronary circulation and decrease of the blood supply to the cardiac muscle. Many clinical studies with VDAs have reported asymptomatic elevations of troponin or creatine kinase MB (CK-MB), indicative of myocardial damage, acute coronary syndrome, QTc prolongation, and reduction in left ventricular ejection fraction. In most cases, agents have a short half-life and effects are quickly reversible; however, pulmonary embolism and myocardial infarction have also been reported.

A further challenge is the choice of dose and schedule when combining a VDA to conventional chemotherapy. In this particular case, the choice of schedule may be limited, for practical as well as scientific reasons, by the need to align with the chemotherapy cycles.

In summary, VDAs represent an exciting new class of anti-angiogenic agents, some of which are nowadays well defined in terms of cardiovascular, neurological, and hematological toxicities with relevant signs of clinical activity in solid tumors. Their efficacy can be increased by adding standard chemotherapy or other biologic compounds with an acceptable safety profile. The most important challenge is to define validated predictive biomarkers for selecting the patients most likely to benefit from this class of drugs.

REFERENCES

1. Folkman J. How is blood vessel growth regulated in normal and neoplastic tissue? *Cancer Res* 1986; 46: 467–473.
2. Ellis LM, Liu W, Ahmad SA et al. Overview of angiogenesis: Biologic implications for anti-angiogenic therapy. *Semin Oncol* 2001; 28: 94–104.

3. Kerbel R, Folkman J. Clinical translation of angiogenesis inhibitors. *Nat Rev Cancer* 2002; 2: 727–739.
4. Siemann DW, Bibby MC, Dark GB et al. Differentiation and definition of vascular-targeted therapies. *Clin Cancer Res* 2005; 11: 416–420.
5. Jordan MA, Wilson L. Microtubules as a target for anticancer drugs. *Nat Rev Cancer* 2004; 4: 253–265.
6. Jordan MA, Wendell K, Gardiner S et al. Mitotic bock induced in HeLa cells by low concentrations of paclitaxel (Taxol) results in abnormal mitotic exit and apoptotic cell death. *Cancer Res* 1996; 56: 816–825.
7. Seed L, Slaughter DP, Limarzi LR. Effect of colchicine on human carcinoma. *Surgery* 1940; 7: 696–709.
8. Hill SA, Sampson LE, Chaplin DJ. Anti-vascular approaches to solid tumor therapy: Evaluation of vinblastine and flavone acetic acid. *Int J Cancer*. 1995; 63: 119–123.
9. Arap W, Pasqualini R, Ruoslahti E. Cancer treatment by targeted drug delivery to tumor vasculature in a mouse model. *Science* 1998; 279: 377–380.
10. Landuyt W, Ahmed B, Nuyts S et al. In vivo antitumor effect of vascular targeting agents combined with either ionizing radiation or anti-angiogenesis treatment. *Int J Radiat Oncol Biol Phys* 2001; 49: 443–450.
11. Dowlati A, Robertson K, Cooney M et al. A phase I pharmacokinetic and translational study of the novel vascular targeting agent combretastatin A-4 phosphate on a single-dose intravenous schedule in patients with advanced cancer. *Cancer Res* 2002; 62: 3408–3416.
12. Cooney M, Radivoyevitch T, Dowlati A et al. Cardiovascular safety profile of combretastatin A4 phosphate in a single-dose phase I study in patients with advanced cancer. *Clin Cancer Res* 2004; 10: 96–100.
13. Stevenson JP, Rosen M, Sun W et al. Phase I trial of the antivascular agent combretastatin A4 phosphate on a 5-day schedule to patients with cancer: Magnetic resonance imaging evidence for altered tumor blood flow. *J Clin Oncol* 2003; 21: 4428–4438.
14. Rustin GJ, Galbraith SM, Anderson H et al. Phase I clinical trial of weekly combretastatin A4 phosphate: Clinical and pharmacokinetic results. *J Clin Oncol* 2003; 21: 2815–2822.
15. Ng QS, Carnell D, Milner J et al. Phase Ib trial of combretastatin A4 phosphate (CA4P) in combination with radiotherapy (RT): Initial clinical results. *Proc Am Soc Clin Oncol* 2005; 23: Abstract 3117.
16. Bilenker JH, Flaherty KT, Rosen M et al. Phase I trial of combretastatin A-4 phosphate with carboplatin. *Clin Cancer Res* 2005; 11: 1527–1533.
17. Zweifel M, Jayson GC, Reed NS et al. Phase II trial of combretastatin A4 phosphate, carboplatin, and paclitaxel in patients with platinum-resistant ovarian cancer. *Ann Oncol* 2011; 22(9): 2036–2041. Epub January 27, 2011.
18. Rustin GJ, Shreeves G, Nathan PD. A phase Ib trial of CA4P (combretastatin A-4 phosphate), carboplatin, and paclitaxel in patients with advanced cancer. *Br J Cancer* 2010; 102(9): 1355–1360. Epub April 13, 2010.
19. Nathan P, Zweifel M, Padhani AR et al. Phase I trial of combretastatin A4 phosphate (CA4P) in combination with bevacizumab in patients with advanced cancer. *Clin Cancer Res* 2012 15; 18(12): 3428–3439. Epub May 29, 2012.
20. Kirwan IG, Loadman PM, Swaine DJ et al. Comparative preclinical pharmacokinetic and metabolic studies of the combretastatin prodrugs combretastatin A4 phosphate and A1 phosphate. *Clin Cancer Res* 2004; 10(4): 1446–1453.
21. Patterson DM, Zweifel M, Middleton MR et al. Phase I clinical and pharmacokinetic evaluation of the vascular-disrupting agent OXi4503 in patients with advanced solid tumors. *Clin Cancer Res* 2012; 18(5): 1415–1425. Epub January 10, 2012.
22. Madlambayan GJ, Meacham AM, Hosaka K et al. Leukemia regression by vascular disruption and antiangiogenic therapy. *Blood* 2010; 116(9): 1539–1547. Epub May 14, 2010.

23. Tolcher AW, Forero L, Celio P. Phase I, pharmacokinetic, and DCE-MRI correlative study of AVE8062A, an antivascular combretastatin analogue, administered weekly for 3 weeks every 28-days. *Proc Am Soc Clin Oncol* 2003; 22: Abstract 834.

24. Sessa C, LoRusso P, Tolcher AW. A pharmacokinetic and DCE-MRI-dynamic phase I study of the antivascular combretastatin analogue AVE8062A administered every 3 weeks. *Proc Am Soc Clin Oncol* 2005: Abstract 5827.

25. Tresca P, Tosi D, van Doorn L et al. Phase I and pharmacologic study of the vascular disrupting agent ombrabulin (Ob) combined with docetaxel (D) in patients (pts) with advanced solid tumors. *J Clin Oncol* 2010; 28: 15s, (suppl; Abstract 3023).

26. Pujade-Lauraine E, Vergote I, Allard A et al. OPSALIN: A phase II placebo-controlled randomized study of ombrabulin in patients with platinum-sensitive recurrent ovarian cancer treated with carboplatin (Cb) and paclitaxel (P). *J Clin Oncol* 2012; 30 (suppl): Abstract TPS5112.

27. Del Conte G, Bahleda R, Moreno V et al. A phase I study of ombrabulin (O) combined with bevacizumab (B) in patients with advanced solid tumors. *J Clin Oncol* 2012; 30 (suppl): Abstract 3080.

28. Anthony SP, Read W, Rosen PJ et al. Initial results of a first-in-man phase I study of EPC2407, a novel small molecule microtubule inhibitor anticancer agent with tumor vascular endothelial disrupting activity. *J Clin Oncol* 2008; 26 (May 20 suppl): Abstract 2531.

29. Read WL, Rosen P, Lee P et al. Pharmacokinetic and pharmacodynamic results of a 4-hr IV administered phase I study with EPC2407, a novel vascular disrupting agent. *J Clin Oncol* 2009; 27: 15s (suppl) Abstract 3569.

30. Tsimberidou AM, Akerley W, Schabel MC et al. Phase I clinical trial of MPC-6827 (Azixa), a microtubule destabilizing agent, in patients with advanced cancer. *Mol Cancer Ther* 2010 Dec; 9(12): 3410–3419.

31. Grossmann KF, Colman H, Akerley WA et al. Phase I trial of verubulin (MPC-6827) plus carboplatin in patients with relapsed glioblastoma multiforme. *J Neurooncol* 2012; 110(2): 257–264. doi: 10.1007/s11060–012–0964–7. Epub August 30, 2012.

32. Kim LJ, Chamberlain MC, Zhu J et al. Phase II study of verubulin (MPC-6827) for the treatment of subjects with recurrent glioblastoma naïve to treatment with bevacizumab. *J Clin Oncol* 2011; 29 (suppl): Abstract 2088.

33. Lickliter JD, Francesconi AB, Smith G et al. Phase I trial of CYT997, a novel cytotoxic and vascular-disrupting agent. *Br J Cancer* 2010; 103(5): 597–606.

34. Rischin D, Bibby DC, Chong G et al. Clinical, pharmacodynamic, and pharmacokinetic evaluation of BNC105P: A phase I trial of a novel vascular disrupting agent and inhibitor of cancer cell proliferation. *Clin Cancer Res* 2011; 17(15): 5152–5160. Epub June 20, 2011.

35. O'Connor JP, Jackson A, Parker GJ et al. Dynamic contrast-enhanced MRI in clinical trials of antivascular therapies. *Nat Rev Clin Oncol* 2012; 9(3): 167–177.

36. Bertolini F, Shaked Y, Mancuso P. The multifaceted circulating endothelial cell in cancer: Towards marker and target identification. *Nat Rev Cancer* 2006; 6(11): 835–845. Epub October 5, 2006.

37. Lyden D, Hattori K, Dias S et al. Impaired recruitment of bone-marrow-derived endothelial and hematopoietic precursor cells blocks tumor angiogenesis and growth. *Nat Med* 2001; 7(11): 1194–1201.

38. Sessa C, Guibal A, Del Conte G et al. Biomarkers of angiogenesis for the development of antiangiogenic therapies in oncology: Tools or decorations? *Nat Clin Pract Oncol* 2008; 5(7): 378–391. Epub June 17, 2008.

39. Burge M, Francesconi AB, Kotasek D. Phase I, pharmacokinetic and pharmacodynamic evaluation of CYT997, an orally-bioavailable cytotoxic and vascular-distrupting agent. *Invest New Drugs* 2013 Feb; 31(1):126–135. doi: 10.1007/s10637-012-9813-y. Epub March 27, 2012.

15 Immunotherapy
CTLA4, PD-1, PD-L1, IL-18, and IL-21

Patrick M. Forde
Sidney Kimmel Comprehensive Cancer
Center at Johns Hopkins

Julie R. Brahmer
Sidney Kimmel Comprehensive Cancer
Center at Johns Hopkins

CONTENTS

INTRODUCTION

Host immunity is fundamental to the suppression of human cancer. Conversely, host immune evasion by tumor cells is an essential pathway in the development of human cancer. The concept of cancer immune editing is well described in animal models whereby tumors are capable of subverting host immunity despite developing frequent genetic aberrations with the potential to generate immunogenic neo-antigens.[1] The three phases of immune editing are as follows: elimination (host immune system responds to tumor neo-antigens and destroys tumor cells), equilibrium (immune evasive tumor cells persist; however, growth and metastasis are restrained by residual host immunity), and escape (tumor cells overcome immune control and can develop into clinically evident cancers). The development of clinically apparent tumors indicates failure of the host immune system to recognize and destroy incipient cancers.

Consequently, strategies aimed at augmenting host anti-tumor immunity are attractive with potential for long-term tumor control or even cure if persistent immune responsiveness can be engendered, particularly in earlier stages of disease.

Attempts have been made over many years to potentiate the host immune response to human cancer with limited success until recently, and in some cases significant toxicity.[2-4] While occasional dramatic tumor responses have been seen with interleukin (IL)-2 treatment in melanoma and renal cell cancer (RCC), in particular, these responses are difficult to predict based on clinical criteria, and a dependable biological marker of response in the patient or tumor has yet to be described.[5-7]

Recent breakthroughs have led to the approval of two new immune activating agents for the treatment of advanced solid tumors, the autologous dendritic cell vaccine, sipuleucel-T, for castration-resistant prostate cancer (CRPC), and the anti-cytotoxic T lymphocyte antigen-4 (anti-CTLA-4) immune checkpoint inhibitory antibody, ipilimumab, for the treatment of advanced melanoma.[8,9]

This chapter will focus on anti-CTLA-4 and other novel immunotherapeutic agents that are currently undergoing clinical trial investigation for the treatment of cancer reviewing preclinical and clinical data and exploring future directions in this exciting field of cancer drug development.

CANCER IMMUNOTHERAPY: IMMUNE CHECKPOINT INHIBITION AND NOVEL CYTOKINES

Strategies to augment the T cell immune response to tumor have long been a focus of cancer immunotherapy building on the knowledge that increased T cell infiltration of tumor may be predictive of improved clinical outcome.[10] Non-specific T cell immune-stimulating cytokines, such as interferon (IFN) and recombinant interleukin (IL)-2, demonstrated early promise, however, have also been associated with significant acute toxicity and tumor responses in 10%–20% of highly selected advanced renal cell carcinoma and melanoma patients.[11,12] IL-2 treatment is reserved for good performance status patients with preserved cardiac and renal function and is delivered as an inpatient with therapy frequently requiring intensive care monitoring and inotrope support due to cytokine-induced capillary leak syndrome. High dose IL-2 has remained part of the treatment paradigm for advanced melanoma and renal cell carcinoma patients because of the tantalizing finding that approximately 2%–5% of patients achieve long-term cure of their disease with IL-2 treatment.[13,14]

Regulation of the T cell immune response to tumor cell antigen is mediated through a balance between co-stimulatory and co-inhibitory signaling molecules known as immune checkpoints (Figure 15.1).[15] Expression of co-inhibitory immune checkpoint molecules is induced by T cell activation, leading to down-regulation of T cell responses and allowing maintenance of self-tolerance in the absence of disease.[16] Tumors have the ability to induce expression of co-inhibitory immune checkpoints both on tumor cells and infiltrating immune cells essentially blocking the innate immune response to tumor and potentiating neoplastic growth and spread.[17,18] Mechanisms of tumor induced immune evasion include increased levels

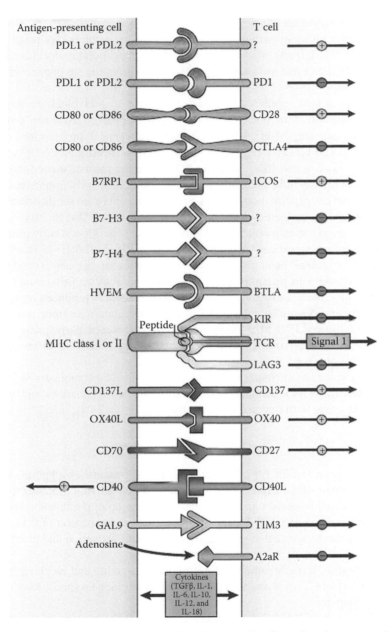

FIGURE 15.1 Ligand–receptor interactions between T cells and antigen-presenting cells (APCs) that regulate the T cell response to antigen. (Reprinted with permission from Macmillan Publishers Ltd. *Nat. Rev. Cancer*, Pardoll, D.M. The blockade of immune checkpoints in cancer immunotherapy, 22, 12(4), 252–264, copyright 2012.)

of T-regulatory lymphocytes that suppress tumor specific effector T lymphocytes and natural killer (NK) cells. Additionally, tumor induction of myeloid suppressor cells leads to T-lymphocyte apoptosis and accumulation of tumor-associated macrophages that can enhance tumor growth and invasion. Finally, up-regulation of programmed death ligand-1 (PD-L1) and other inhibitory immune checkpoint molecules and their ligands on both tumor and inflammatory cells has a profoundly suppressive effect on antitumor immunity.[16]

Several monoclonal antibodies (mAbs) that bind to and block co-inhibitory immune checkpoints, thus potentiating the T cell response, have been produced; and molecules targeting B7-H3, lymphocyte-activation gene 3, programmed death-1 (PD-1), PD-L1, and CTLA-4 have entered clinical trial investigation.[9,19-23] Of these agents, anti-CTLA-4, anti-PD-1, and anti-PD-L1 are the most advanced in clinical development with the fully human anti-CTLA-4 antibody, ipilimumab, becoming the first immune checkpoint modulating antibody to be approved for the treatment of advanced melanoma by the Food and Drug Administration (FDA) in 2011.[24]

Next generation recombinant human cytokines have also shown early promise in the treatment of advanced cancer including IL-18 and IL-21.[25,26] IL-18 is an immunostimulatory cytokine belonging to the IL-1 family that can act synergistically with other cytokines to promote IFN-γ secretion and activate inflammatory cells including T cells, B cells, monocytes, and NK cells.[27] IL-21 is produced by activated CD4+T cells and NK cells and acts to potently stimulate antitumor immunity.[28] Recombinant human IL (rhIL)-18 and rIL-21 have entered early phase clinical investigation, and data from these clinical studies are discussed in the relevant sections of this chapter.

Promising strategies currently under investigation include combinatorial immune checkpoint studies, cytokine/immune checkpoint inhibitor combinations, and sequencing of chemotherapy with immune targeting therapy.

CTLA-4 ANTIBODIES

CTLA-4, first described in 1987,[29] is the prototypical immune checkpoint, a transmembrane receptor whose expression is induced by T cell activation leading to down-regulation of T cell responses and consequent suppression of the innate response to foreign tumor neo-antigen.[16,30] T cell activation induces expression of CTLA-4 on the T cell membrane where it negatively regulates T cell activation and proliferation (Figure 15.2).[31]

Two antibodies, tremelimumab and ipilimumab, targeting and blocking the constitutive activity of CTLA-4 and thus potentiating the immune response have entered clinical development.

Tremelimumab (CP-675,206, Medimmune) is a fully human IgG$_2$ mAb that binds CTLA-4 with high affinity, preventing inhibition of T cell activation.[30,32] In preclinical studies, tremelimumab was shown to enhance production of cytokines including IL-2 and led to substantial tumor regression in a range of murine solid tumor models.[33,34] Preclinical toxicology studies demonstrated good tolerance overall, however, suggested possible gastrointestinal and endocrine effects, which would be borne out in clinical studies. Phase I investigation of tremelimumab was

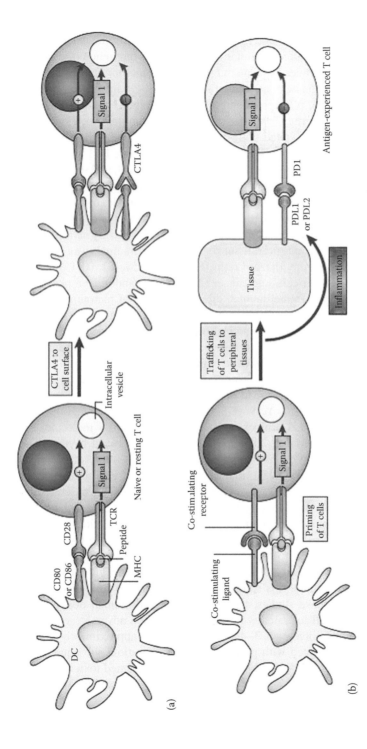

FIGURE 15.2 (a) Regulation of CTLA-4 and (b) regulation of PD1/PD-L1. (Reprinted with permission from Macmillan Publishers Ltd. *Nat. Rev. Cancer*, Pardoll, D.M. The blockade of immune checkpoints in cancer immunotherapy, 22, 12(4), 252–264, copyright 2012.)

conducted in 39 patients with advanced solid tumors; dose-limiting toxicities noted included grade 3 diarrhea in 13% of patients and other less common toxicities felt to be related to immune activation including dermatitis, vitiligo, and endocrine abnormalities affecting thyroid and pituitary tissues.[35] Anti-tumor activity was noted with four responses in advanced melanoma patients. Tremelimumab continued through phase I/II investigation demonstrating further activity in melanoma.[36] Despite these early positive results, phase III comparison of single-agent tremelimumab versus single-agent chemotherapy (dacarbazine or temozolomide) failed to demonstrate a survival advantage associated with tremelimumab.[37] This first-line study enrolled 655 stage IIIB/IV melanoma patients who were randomized 1:1 to tremelimumab or chemotherapy with a primary endpoint of overall survival, and secondary endpoints included response rate and progression-free survival (PFS). Toxicities associated with tremelimumab treatment included diarrhea (14% grade 3–4), pruritus and rash, and endocrine side effects (hypopituitarism, hypoadrenalism, or hypothyroidism) were noted in 4% of patients. The study was stopped for futility at the second interim analysis when the median overall survival for tremelimumab was 11.8 versus 10.7 months for chemotherapy (hazard ratio [HR]: 1.04; 95% CI: 0.84–1.28). Similarly, in advanced non-small-cell lung cancer (NSCLC), a randomized phase II first-line study of maintenance tremelimumab after four cycles of platinum doublet chemotherapy failed to demonstrate a PFS advantage for the maintenance arm compared to placebo.[38] These negative studies, which were conducted prior to our current understanding of the unique kinetics of response to immune checkpoint inhibition,[39] led to the discontinuation of clinical development of tremelimumab as a single agent in melanoma; however, its single agent activity for mesothelioma[40] and combination studies for melanoma[41] continue to be investigated.

Ipilimumab (MDX-010, Yervoy; Bristol-Myers Squibb) is a fully human IgG$_1$ mAb that binds to CTLA-4 blocking its interaction with B7 molecules on antigen presenting cells.[42] In March 2011, ipilimumab was approved by the FDA for the treatment of metastatic melanoma based on a phase III study of ipilimumab with or without a peptide vaccine.[9] Initial phase I studies of ipilimumab demonstrated sustained responses in refractory solid tumor patients in some cases lasting several years without requirement for ongoing treatment and associated with toxicities similar to those seen with tremelimumab.[43] A dose response relationship was noted up to 10 mg/kg with best response rates seen at the higher dose levels. In the phase III study,[9] which enrolled 676 pretreated advanced melanoma patients, ipilimumab was given at 3 mg/kg every 21 days for four cycles either with or without a gp100 peptide vaccine; of note, this study commenced prior to final dose recommendations from early phase studies, hence the lower ipilimumab dose used. Overall, ipilimumab was well tolerated with the most common adverse events (AEs) being immune related; of note, grade 3–4 colitis occurred in approximately 4% of patients, in some cases associated with gastrointestinal perforation, subsequently treatment algorithms have been developed to mitigate immune-related toxicity including colitis.[39] Median survival was significantly increased for the patients who received ipilimumab plus gp100 vaccine at 10 months compared with 6.4 months for gp100 alone ($P < .001$). Of note, there appeared to be a substantial tail on the survival curve consistent with immune-mediated response, this has also been noted with longer follow-up of patients who have received ipilimumab suggesting that up to 10% may achieve 5 year survival.[44] Subsequently, ipilimumab, when combined with dacarbazine chemotherapy, has shown improved survival for previously untreated advanced melanoma patients compared with dacarbazine alone.[45] This study randomized 502 patients with advanced cutaneous melanoma to ipilimumab 10 mg/kg every 3 weeks for four cycles with or without dacarbazine every 3 weeks for eight cycles. Patients with stable or responsive disease at 24 weeks were eligible for maintenance ipilimumab or placebo given once every 12 weeks until disease progression. Overall survival was significantly prolonged for patients who received ipilimumab/dacarbazine at 11.2 months compared with 9.1 months for dacarbazine alone, $P < .001$. Patients who received ipilimumab were almost twice as likely to be alive at 3 years (20.8% vs. 12.2%), and all analyzed subgroups appeared to receive benefit. Toxicities seen more commonly in the ipilimumab/dacarbazine arm included transaminitis, diarrhea, rash, and pruritus with grade 3–4 toxicities occurring twice as frequently in the combination arm (56.3% vs. 27.5%); however, no gastrointestinal perforations or treatment-related deaths were observed probably due to enhanced awareness and prompt management of immune-related toxicities and possible mitigation of some toxicities by the immunosuppressive effect of concurrent chemotherapy. Overall, however, while this study demonstrated that ipilimumab is an improvement over dacarbazine for newly diagnosed advanced melanoma patients, the role of combination treatment with chemotherapy and the need for the higher 10 mg/kg dosing is controversial with many experts continuing to utilize ipilimumab 3 mg/kg every 3 weeks for four doses in both the first- and second-line settings.[46] Important future questions in melanoma immunotherapy include sequencing and combinatorial studies with B-rapidly accelerated fibrosarcoma (B-Raf) targeting agents such as vemurafenib and dabrafenib, and combinations with cytokines and other immune checkpoint antibodies.

Other recent studies incorporating ipilimumab have been reported in advanced NSCLC and extensive disease-small cell lung cancer (ED-SCLC). Of note, these studies utilized immune-related response criteria, which are tailored to the unique nature of solid tumor response to immunotherapy where tumors may initially increase in size or new tumors develop before regressing, or tumor regression may be very slow and continue for many months after cessation of treatment.[47] In a recent multicenter international phase II study, 130 patients with untreated ED-SCLC were randomized in a 1:1:1 design to one of three regimens, control— up to six cycles of carboplatin/paclitaxel chemotherapy with placebo, concurrent ipilimumab—four doses of ipilimumab/paclitaxel/carboplatin followed by two doses of placebo/paclitaxel/carboplatin or phased ipilimumab—two doses of placebo/paclitaxel/carboplatin followed by four doses of ipilimumab/paclitaxel/ carboplatin.[48] The endpoints for the ED-SCLC cohort in this study were exploratory and included PFS by immune response (irPFS), PFS, and overall survival. Phased ipilimumab but not concurrent ipilimumab improved irPFS compared with control (HR: 0.64; $P = 0.03$). No improvement in traditional RECIST-defined progression-free or overall survival was noted. Overall rates of grade 3–4 immune-related AEs were 17%, 21%, and 19% for phased ipilimumab, concurrent ipilimumab, and control, respectively. The combination of cisplatin/etoposide with concurrent ipilimumab is currently under investigation in a phase III first-line study in ED-SCLC that plans to enroll 1100 patients utilizing a phased schedule similar to the phase II study.[49] In NSCLC, a phase II study of 204 chemotherapy-naïve patients assigned patients to carboplatin/paclitaxel chemotherapy with placebo or combined with concurrent or phased ipilimumab.[50] The primary endpoint was irPFS. The phased ipilimumab regimen of two cycles of chemotherapy following by four cycles of chemotherapy with ipilimumab demonstrated improved irPFS compared with the control arm of chemotherapy plus placebo (5.7 vs. 4.6 months, $P=0.05$) and a trend was noted toward improved OS, which did not meet statistical significance (12.2 vs. 8.3 months, $P=0.23$). Interestingly, in subgroup analysis, the effect of phased ipilimumab appeared to be confined to patients with squamous histology, leading to a phase III trial currently being conducted in this group.[51]

PD-1 ANTIBODIES

PD-1 is a co-inhibitory molecule expressed on the surface of activated T-cells, antigen specific T-cells after chronic antigen exposure, B-cells, and myeloid cells (Figure 15.2).[52] PD-L1, one of two ligands of PD-1, can be expressed in human tumors and has been associated with a poor prognosis.[53,54] PD-1 has been shown to inhibit CD-28-mediated upregulation of the immune activating cytokines IL-2, IL-10, IL-13, IFN-γ, and Bcl-xL. PD-1 expression has also been noted to inhibit T cell activation and expansion of previously activated cells (Figure 15.3).[55] Blockade of the PD-1/PD-L1 pathway by mAbs has led to augmented antitumor immunity and tumor regression in murine models, providing the rationale for further exploration of these agents in the clinic.[56]

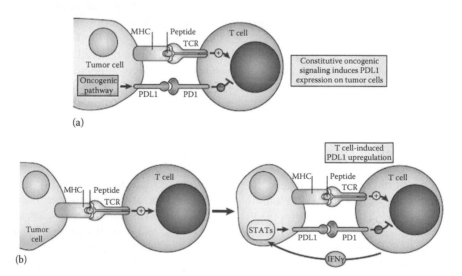

FIGURE 15.3 Mechanisms of expression of immune checkpoints: (a) innate immune resistance and (b) adaptive immune resistance. (Reprinted with permission from Macmillan Publishers Ltd. *Nat. Rev. Cancer*, Pardoll, D.M. The blockade of immune checkpoints in cancer immunotherapy, 22, 12(4), 252–264, copyright 2012.)

Currently, three molecules targeting PD-1, nivolumab (BMS-936558/ONO-5438/ MDX-1106, Bristol Myers-Squibb), lambrolizumab (MK-3475, Merck), and AMP-224 (Amplimmune, GlaxoSmithKline) are under investigation in clinical trials, with the most extensive clinical experience involving nivolumab. Nivolumab (ONO-5438, MDX-1106) is a fully human, IgG4 (kappa) mAb that binds PD-1 with high affinity, blocking its interactions with its ligands PD-L1 (B7-H1) and PD-L2 (B7-DC) and increasing tumor antigen specific T cell proliferation and cytokine secretion.[57]

A phase 1 single dose, dose-escalation study of nivolumab in 39 heavily pretreated solid tumor patients demonstrated good tolerance and signals of efficacy.[58] Toxicity was mild with most frequent AEs being hematologic (notably a grade 3 reduction in CD4 count in 17.9% of patients), fatigue, and mild musculoskeletal symptoms. Maximum tolerated dose (MTD) was not reached. Immune-related colitis, well described with CTLA-4 inhibition, was described in one patient and resolved after treatment with steroids and infliximab. Grade 2 hypothyroidism and grade 2 polyarthritis were noted in one and two patients, respectively. Efficacy was promising with a durable complete response (CR) in a colorectal cancer (CRC) patient, two partial responses (PRs) in renal cell cancer (RCC) and melanoma patients and a sustained response not meeting PR criteria in an NSCLC patient. Pharmacodynamic analyses suggested that high level occupancy of the PD-1 receptor persisted for up to 85 days after a single dose.

Updated safety, efficacy, and immune correlative data from the multicenter phase 1b multi-dose study of nivolumab confirmed efficacy and tolerability in melanoma, RCC, and NSCLC.[22] Nivolumab was administered as an intravenous infusion every 2 weeks of an 8 week treatment cycle. Patients with PR or stable disease (SD) received treatment for up to 2 years (12 cycles); after 2 years of treatment, patients were followed for up to 1 year and offered retreatment for an additional year in the event of disease progression. MTD was not reached in this study, five expansion cohorts of 16 patients each were enrolled at the 10 mg/kg dose for melanoma, NSCLC, RCC, metastatic CRPC (mCRPC), and CRC. After initial assessment of activity, additional expansion cohorts of 16 patients each were enrolled for melanoma (0.1, 0.3, 1.0, and 3.0 mg/kg) NSCLC (squamous and non-squamous, 1.0, 3.0, and 10.0 mg/kg), and RCC (1.0 mg/kg). This study enrolled 296 patients between October 2008 and February 2012. The cohort was heavily pretreated, with the majority of melanoma (64%) and RCC (59%) patients having received prior immunotherapy. Tolerance in general was good with grade 3 or grade 4 treatment-related AEs (most commonly fatigue, diarrhea, and rash) noted in 14% of patients. Of note, drug-related pneumonitis occurred in 3% of patients with three (1%) drug-related deaths due to pneumonitis. Tumor response and prolonged stabilization of disease were seen in 28% of melanoma patients, 27% of kidney cancer patients and 18% of lung cancer patients. No responses to nivolumab were noted in patients with CRC or mCRPC. In a subgroup of 42 patients for whom PD-L1 expression in pretreatment tumor biopsy was evaluated, 9 of 25 patients tumors responded in the PD-L1 positive group, whereas none of 17 patients with PD-L1 negative tumors had a response suggesting tumor PD-L1 expression as a candidate predictive marker for future investigation. Further studies of nivolumab currently in progress or being planned include phase III trials compared with chemotherapy in NSCLC, with anti-angiogenic therapy in RCC, and as a single-agent compared with dacarbazine chemotherapy for advanced melanoma.[59-61]

Lambrolizumab is a humanized monoclonal IgG4 antibody against PD-1. Early toxicity, pharmacological, and efficacy data from a multicenter phase I study of lambrolizumab in advanced solid tumors including NSCLC, CRC, melanoma, sarcoma, and carcinoid was presented at ASCO 2012.[62] At the time of report, 17 patients had received lambrolizumab (4 patients at the 1 mg/kg dose level, 3 patients at 3 mg/kg, and 10 patients at 10 mg/kg). Pharmacologic assessment indicated a half-life of 14–21 days and a C_{max} that increased linearly with dose. Lambrolizumab was, overall, well tolerated. Grade 2 pneumonitis responsive to steroid therapy occurred in one patient. Grade 1–2 pruritus was noted in 4 of 17 patients, and grade 1–2 pneumonitis was noted in one patient. No grade 3–4 toxicities were reported to date. Two confirmed PRs were reported in patients with melanoma along with one unconfirmed PR in NSCLC. SD exceeding 5 months was noted in three patients (tumor types—NSCLC, soft tissue sarcoma, and carcinoid). An expansion cohort of melanoma patients is currently being enrolled at the 10 mg/kg dose level every 2 weeks with four responses from 10 patients evaluated by RECIST thus far, while a NSCLC expansion cohort is also planned.[63]

PD-L1 ANTIBODIES

Currently, several clinical studies are ongoing utilizing mAbs targeting PD-L1; these include BMS-936559 (MDX-1105, Bristol Myers-Squibb) and MPDL3280A (RG7446, Genentech). BMS-936559 (MDX-1105), the first PD-L1 targeted antibody to enter clinical trials, is a fully human IgG4 mAb to PD-L1 and inhibits the binding of PD-L1 to both PD-1 and CD80 (a ligand of CTLA-4).[64] Safety, pharmacological, and clinical activity data from a multicenter phase I study of BMS-936559 in patients with advanced solid tumors were recently reported.[23] In this study, patients with advanced solid tumors (NSCLC, melanoma, RCC, ovarian cancer, CRC, pancreatic cancer, gastric cancer, and breast cancer) refractory to at least one standard systemic therapy received BMS-936559 as an intravenous infusion on day 1, 15, and 29 of a 42 day cycle for a total of up to 16 cycles. Patients with melanoma, NSCLC, RCC, CRC, and ovarian cancer were enrolled in a dose escalation portion of the study, which assessed safety of BMS-936559 at 0.3, 1, 3, and 10 mg/kg dose levels. Expansion cohorts of patients with these tumor types were also enrolled at selected dose levels. At the time of report, 207 patients were evaluable for safety analysis, while 160 were included in the efficacy analysis. In this study, 56% of melanoma and 41% of RCC patients had previously received immunotherapy. MTD was not reached and treatment-related grade 3 or grade 4 AEs occurred in 9% of patients. The most common drug-related AEs included fatigue (16%), infusion reactions (10%), and diarrhea (9%). AEs of special interest (potential immune etiology) occurred in 39% of patients; however, these were generally mild, requiring systemic glucocorticoid therapy in only nine patients. BMS-936559 demonstrated promising activity in melanoma and NSCLC and responses were also observed in RCC and ovarian cancer. No responses were seen in CRC or pancreatic cancer.

INTERLEUKIN-18

IL-18 belongs to the IL-1 cytokine family and is a potent stimulator of cellular anti-tumor immunity through a variety of mechanisms including NK cell activation, activation of Th1 cells, induction of IFN-γ production and up-regulation of Fas ligand on NK and T cells.[65,66]

rhIL-18, SB-485232, demonstrated safety in a single dose study of 28 subjects with advanced RCC, melanoma, or Hodgkin lymphoma.[67] MTD was not reached and two unconfirmed PRs in melanoma and RCC patients were noted. In a phase II first-line study of 64 patients with advanced melanoma, rhIL-18 was well tolerated, but had limited efficacy, with one patient achieving a confirmed PR, two patients unconfirmed PR's, and four subjects with SD for >6 months.[68] Common toxicities included chills, pyrexia, and fatigue, which were acute and resolved on discontinuation of treatment. The study was terminated without proceeding to the second stage for lack of efficacy.

SB-485232 has been combined with pegylated liposomal doxorubicin in a phase I dose escalation study of 16 patients with platinum-resistant advanced epithelial ovarian cancer.[69] Maximal SB-485232 biological activity, assessed by peripheral blood NK and T cell markers, was observed at 10–100 mg/kg. Tumor response was observed in 6% of patients, and 38% of patients presented SD.

Given the relatively limited clinical anti-tumor activity seen to date, it is likely that further investigation of rhIL-18 will involve combination with other immune modulating agents such as anti-CTLA-4 and anti-PD-1.

INTERLEUKIN-21

IL-21 is produced by activated CD4+ T cells and leads to stimulation of T cells, B cells, and NK cells.[70] In preclinical studies, IL-21 induced regression of several solid tumor types in murine models.[71]

rIL-21 was studied in an open-label dose escalation study of 29 advanced melanoma patients.[72] IL-21 was well tolerated with the principal toxicities encountered being transaminitis and flu-like symptoms; at higher dose levels myelosuppression was noted. MTD was reached at 30 mcg/kg; and one partial tumor response, which later became complete, was noted. Another phase I study included 43 patients (24 melanoma and 19 RCC) and confirmed the most common AEs to be grade 1–2 flu-like symptoms, pruritus, and rash.[73] Dose-limiting toxicities were transient laboratory abnormalities including grade 3 transaminitis, and MTD was confirmed at 30 mcg/kg. Tumor responses were observed in both melanoma (1 CR and 11 patients with SD) and in RCC (4 PRs and 13 SD). In a third phase I study, subcutaneous rIL-21 was administered to 26 patients with advanced melanoma or RCC.[74] MTD for the subcutaneous form was found to be 200 mcg/kg, and three patients (one melanoma and one RCC) had PRs.

In an Australian first-line phase IIa study of 24 patients with advanced melanoma at a 30 mcg/kg dose, one CR, and one PR, both in patients with lung metastases, were observed and treatment was well tolerated.[75] Most recently, a Canadian multicenter first-line phase II study enrolled 40 patients with advanced melanoma to one of three different dose schedules.[76] The overall response rate was 22.5%, and nine confirmed PRs were seen with 16 patients having SD. Two patients had responses lasting 22 months. The median duration of both response and SD was 5.3 months. No relationship was seen between IL-21 expression levels or B-Raf mutation status and response. Median PFS was 4.3 months, and overall survival was 12.4 months.

In hematologic malignancies, rIL-21 has been combined with rituximab in a phase I study of 21 patients with relapsed and refractory low grade B-cell leukemia or lymphoma.[77] The MTD for rIL-21 was 100 mcg/kg and toxicities included nausea, hypotension, and electrolyte abnormalities. Clinical responses were seen in eight patients with half of these responses lasting longer than the patient's previous response to rituximab-based treatment.

rIL-21 has been combined with the epidermal growth factor receptor antibody, cetuximab, in a phase I study of 15 patients with chemotherapy-naïve metastatic CRC.[78] This study was terminated early following sponser's decision; however, the combination appeared to be well tolerated with no increased skin toxicity. The only dose-limiting reported was a grade 3 diarrhea at the 100mcg/kg dose-level. Nine subjects had SD as their best response with no objective responses noted.

Phase II randomized studies evaluating rIL-21 combined with dacarbazine in melanoma[79], or combined with antiangiogenic TKIs[80,81] in RCC have completed enrollment; however, results have not been reported as yet.

Studies are ongoing combining rIL-21 with anti-PD-1 in patients with advanced solid tumors[82] and with ipilimumab in melanoma.[83] Future challenges include developing optimal sequencing as well as combinatorial strategies and developing predictive markers of response and toxicity.

CONCLUSION

Immunotherapy for cancer has undergone a renaissance in recent years with important breakthroughs in immune checkpoint inhibition using anti-CTLA-4 and anti-PD-1/PD-L1 leading to durable remissions and in some cases effective cure for patients with advanced melanoma or other solid tumors. Despite these advances, many challenges remain, including determining the optimal sequencing of immune targeting agents and combinatorial strategies with other immune-based treatments, cytotoxic chemotherapy, and non-immune targeted agents. While experience in managing the unique toxicities of these agents is growing, these also represent additional challenges and highlight the need for collaboration between oncologists and organ specialists. Finally, the development of predictive biomarkers of response and toxicity will be crucial for a successful development of these agents.

REFERENCES

1. Dunn GP, Bruce AT, Ikeda H et al. Cancer immunoediting: From surveillance to tumor escape. *Nat Immunol* 2002;3(11):991–998.
2. Retsas S, Priestman TJ, Newton KA et al. Evaluation of human lymphoblastoid interferon in advanced malignant melanoma. *Cancer* 1983;51(2):273–276.
3. West WH, Tauer KW, Yannelli JR et al. Constant-infusion recombinant interleukin-2 in adoptive immunotherapy of advanced cancer. *N Engl J Med* 1987;316(15):898–905.

4. Tao MH, Levy R. Idiotype/granulocyte-macrophage colony-stimulating factor fusion protein as a vaccine for B-cell lymphoma. *Nature* 1993;362(6422):755–758.

5. Phan GQ, Attia P, Steinberg SM et al. Factors associated with response to high-dose interleukin-2 in patients with metastatic melanoma. *J Clin Oncol* 2001; 19(15):3477–3482.

6. Sabatino M, Kim-Schulze S, Panelli MC et al. Serum vascular endothelial growth factor and fibronectin predict clinical response to high-dose interleukin-2 therapy. *J Clin Oncol* 2009;27(16):2645–2652.

7. Joseph RW, Sullivan RJ, Harrell R et al. Correlation of NRAS mutations with clinical response to high-dose IL-2 in patients with advanced melanoma. *J Immunother* 2012;35(1):66–72.

8. Kantoff PW, Higano CS, Shore ND et al. Sipuleucel-T immunotherapy for castration-resistant prostate cancer. *N Engl J Med* 2010;363(5):411–422.

9. Hodi FS, O'Day SJ, McDermott DF et al. Improved survival with ipilimumab in patients with metastatic melanoma. *N Engl J Med* 2010;363(8):711–723.

10. Bhan AK, DesMarais CL. Immunohistologic characterization of major histocompatibility antigens and inflammatory cellular infiltrate in human breast cancer. *J Natl Cancer Inst* 1983;71(3):507–516.

11. Retsas S, Priestman TJ, Newton KA et al. Evaluation of human lymphoblastoid interferon in advanced malignant melanoma. *Cancer* 1983;51(2):273–276.

12. West WH, Tauer KW, Yannelli JR et al. Constant-infusion recombinant interleukin-2 in adoptive immunotherapy of advanced cancer. *N Engl J Med* 1987;316(15):898–905.

13. Hess V, Herrmann R, Veelken H. Interleukin-2-based biochemotherapy for patients with stage IV melanoma: Long-term survivors outside a clinical trial setting. *Oncology* 2007;73(1–2):33–40.

14. Atkins MB, Lotze MT, Dutcher JP et al. High-dose recombinant interleukin 2 therapy for patients with metastatic melanoma. Analysis of 270 patients treated between 1985 and 1993. *J Clin Oncol* 1999;17(7):2105–2116.

15. Pardoll DM. The blockade of immune checkpoints in cancer immunotherapy. *Nat Rev Cancer* 2012;12(4):252–264.

16. Krummel MF, Allison JP. CD28 and CTLA-4 have opposing effects on the response of T cells to stimulation. *J Exp Med* 1995;182(2):459–465.

17. Konishi J, Yamazaki K, Azuma M et al. B7-H1 expression on non-small cell lung cancer cells and its relationship with tumor-infiltrating lymphocytes and their PD-1 expression. *Clin Cancer Res* 2004;10(15):5094–5100.

18. Dong H, Chen L. B7-H1 pathway and its role in the evasion of tumor immunity. *J Mol Med* (Berl). 2003;81(5):281–287.

19. http://www.clinicaltrials.gov/ct2/show/NCT01391143?term=MGA271&rank=1

20. Wang-Gillam A, Plambeck-Suess S, Goedegebuure P et al. A phase I study of IMP321 and gemcitabine as the front-line therapy in patients with advanced pancreatic adenocarcinoma. *Invest New Drugs* June 2013;31(3):707–713.

21. Brignone C, Gutierrez M, Mefti F et al. First-line chemoimmunotherapy in metastatic breast carcinoma: Combination of paclitaxel and IMP321 (LAG-3Ig) enhances immune responses and antitumor activity. *J Transl Med* 2010 Jul 23;8:71.

22. Topalian SL, Hodi FS, Brahmer JR et al. Safety, activity, and immune correlates of anti-PD-1 antibody in cancer. *N Engl J Med* 2012;366(26):2443–2454.

23. Brahmer JR, Tykodi SS, Chow LQ et al. Safety and activity of anti-PD-L1 antibody in patients with advanced cancer. *N Engl J Med* 2012;366(26):2455–2465.

24. http://www.accessdata.fda.gov/drugsatfda_docs/label/2011/125377s0000lbl.pdf

25. Tarhini AA, Millward M, Mainwaring P et al. A phase 2, randomized study of SB-485232, rhIL-18, in patients with previously untreated metastatic melanoma. *Cancer* 2009;115(4):859–868.

26. Petrella TM, Tozer R, Belanger K et al. Interleukin-21 has activity in patients with meta-static melanoma: A phase II study. *J Clin Oncol* 2012;30(27):3396–3401.
27. Srivastava S, Salim N, Robertson MJ et al. Interleukin-18: Biology and role in the immunotherapy of cancer. *Curr Med Chem* 2010;17(29):3353–3357.
28. Spolski R, Leonard WJ. Interleukin-21: Basic biology and implications for cancer and autoimmunity. *Annu Rev Immunol* 2008;26:57–79.
29. Brunet JF, Denizot F, Luciani MF et al. A new member of the immunoglobulin super-family—CTLA-4. *Nature* 1987;328(6127):267–270.
30. Leach DR, Krummel MF, Allison JP. Enhancement of anti-tumor immunity by CTLA-4 blockade. *Science* 1996;271(5256):1734–1736.
31. Chambers CA, Krummel MF, Boitel B et al. The role of CTLA-4 in the regulation and initiation of T-cell responses. *Immunol Rev* 1996;153:27–46.
32. Ribas A, Hanson DC, Noe DA et al. Tremelimumab (CP-675,206), a cytotoxic T lym-phocyte associated antigen 4 blocking monoclonal antibody in clinical development for patients with cancer. *Oncologist* 2007;12(7):873–883.
33. van Elsas A, Hurwitz AA, Allison JP. Combination immunotherapy of B16 melanoma using anti-cytotoxic T lymphocyte-associated antigen 4 (CTLA-4) and granulocyte/macrophage colony-stimulating factor (GM-CSF)-producing vaccines induces rejection of subcutaneous and metastatic tumors accompanied by autoimmune depigmentation. *J Exp Med* 1999;190(3):355–366.
34. Hurwitz AA, Foster BA, Kwon ED et al. Combination immunotherapy of primary prostate cancer in a transgenic mouse model using CTLA-4 blockade. *Cancer Res* 2000;60(9):2444–2448.
35. Ribas A, Camacho LH, Lopez-Berestein G et al. Antitumor activity in melanoma and anti-self responses in a phase I trial with the anti-cytotoxic T lymphocyte-associated antigen 4 monoclonal antibody CP-675,206. *J Clin Oncol* 2005;23(35):8968–8977.
36. Camacho LH, Antonia S, Sosman J et al. Phase I/II trial of tremelimumab in patients with metastatic melanoma. *J Clin Oncol* 2009;27(7):1075–1081.
37. Ribas A, Hauschild R, Kefford J et al. Phase III, open-label, randomized, compara-tive study of tremelimumab (CP-675,206) and chemotherapy (temozolomide [TMZ] or dacarbazine [DTIC]) in patients with advanced melanoma. *J Clin Oncol* 26(suppl):485s, abstr LBA9011.
38. Zatloukal P, Heo DS, Park K et al. Randomized phase II clinical trial comparing treme-limumab (CP-675,206) with best supportive care following first-line platinum-based therapy in patients with advanced non-small cell lung cancer. *ASCO Meeting Abstracts*, 2009:8071.
39. Weber JS, Kähler KC, Hauschild A. Management of immune-related adverse events and kinetics of response with ipilimumab. *J Clin Oncol* 2012;30(21):2691–2697.
40. ClinicalTrials.gov Identifier: NCT01655888.
41. ClinicalTrials.gov Identifier: NCT01103635.
42. Keler T, Halk E, Vitale L et al. Activity and safety of CTLA-4 blockade combined with vaccines in cynomolgus macaques. *J Immunol* 2003;171(11):6251–6259.
43. Weber JS, O'Day S, Urba W et al. Phase I/II study of ipilimumab for patients with meta-static melanoma. *J Clin Oncol* 2008;26(36):5950–5956.
44. Prieto PA, Yang JC, Sherry RM et al. CTLA-4 blockade with ipilimumab: Long-term follow-up of 177 patients with metastatic melanoma. *Clin Cancer Res* 2012;18(7):2039–2047.
45. Robert C, Thomas L, Bondarenko I et al. Ipilimumab plus dacarbazine for previously untreated metastatic melanoma. *N Engl J Med* 2011;364(26):2517–2526.
46. Wolchok J. How recent advances in immunotherapy are changing the standard of care for patients with metastatic melanoma. *Ann Oncol* 2012;23 Suppl 8:viii15– viii21.

47. Wolchok JD, Hoos A, O'Day S et al. Guidelines for the evaluation of immune therapy activity in solid tumors: Immune-related response criteria. *Clin Cancer Res* 2009;15(23):7412–7420.
48. Reck M, Bondarenko I, Luft A et al. Ipilimumab in combination with paclitaxel and carboplatin as first-line therapy in extensive-disease-small-cell lung cancer: Results from a randomized, double-blind, multicenter phase 2 trial. *Ann Oncol* 2013;24:75–83.
49. Spigel DR, Zielinski C, Maier S et al. CA184–156: A randomized, multicenter, double-blind, phase III trial comparing the efficacy of ipilimumab plus etoposide/platinum (EP) versus EP in subjects with newly diagnosed extensive-stage disease small cell lung cancer. *ASCO Meeting Abstracts*, 2012:TPS7113.
50. Lynch TJ, Bondarenko I, Luft A et al. Ipilimumab in combination with paclitaxel and carboplatin as first-line treatment in stage IIIB/IV non-small-cell lung cancer: Results from a randomized, double-blind, multicenter phase II study. *J Clin Oncol* 2012;30(17):2046–2054.
51. ClinicalTrials.gov Identifier: NCT01285609.
52. Zhang X, Schwartz JC, Guo X et al. Structural and functional analysis of the costimulatory receptor programmed death-1. *Immunity* 2004;20(3):337–347.
53. Dong H, Strome SE, Salomao DR et al. Tumor-associated B7-H1 promotes T-cell apoptosis: A potential mechanism of immune evasion. *Nat Med* 2002;8(8):793–800.
54. Thompson RH, Kuntz SM, Leibovich BC et al. Tumor B7-H1 is associated with poor prognosis in renal cell carcinoma patients with long-term follow-up. *Cancer Res* 2006;66(7):3381–3385.
55. Chemnitz JM, Parry RV, Nichols KE et al. SHP-1 and SHP-2 associate with immunoreceptor tyrosine-based switch motif of programmed death-1 upon primary human T cell stimulation, but only receptor ligation prevents T cell activation. *J Immunol* 2004;173(2):945–954.
56. Hirano F, Kaneko K, Tamura H et al. Blockade of B7-H1 by monoclonal antibodies potentiates cancer therapeutic immunity. *Cancer Res* 2005;65(3):1089–1096.
57. Wong RM, Scotland RR, Lau RL et al. Programmed death-1 blockade enhances expansion and functional capacity of human melanoma antigen-specific CTLs. *Int Immunol* 2007;19(10):1223–1234.
58. Brahmer JR, Drake CG, Wollner I et al. Phase I study of single-agent anti-programmed death-1 (MDX-1106) in refractory solid tumors: Safety, clinical activity, pharmacodynamics, and immunologic correlates. *J Clin Oncol* 2010;28(19):3167–3175.
59. Gettinger SN, Rizvi NA, Shepherd FA et al. A phase I study of BMS-936558 in combination with gemcitabine/cisplatin, pemetrexed/cisplatin or carboplatin/paclitaxel in patients with treatment naïve, stage IIIB/IV non-small-cell lung cancer. *J Clin Oncol (Meeting Abstracts)* 2012;30(15)suppl 2615.
60. Hammers HJ, Rini BI, Hudes GR et al. A phase I study of BMS-936558 plus pazopanib or sunitinib in patients with metastatic renal cell carcinoma. *J Clin Oncol (Meeting Abstracts)* 2012;30(15)suppl 2614.
61. ClinicalTrials.gov Identifier: NCT01721772.
62. Patnaik A, Kang SP, Tolcher AW et al. Phase I study MK-3475 (anti-PD-1 monoclonal antibody) in patients with advanced solid tumors. *J Clin Oncol (Meeting Abstracts)* 2012;30(15)suppl 2512.
63. ClinicalTrials.gov Identifier: NCT01295827.
64. Lucas JA, Menke J, Rabacal WA. Programmed death ligand 1 regulates a critical checkpoint for autoimmune myocarditis and pneumonitis in MRL mice. *J Immunol* 2008;181(4):2513–2521.
65. Osaki T, Péron JM, Cai Q et al. IFN-gamma-inducing factor/IL-18 administration mediates IFN-gamma- and IL-12-independent antitumor effects. *J Immunol* 1998;160(4):1742–1749.

66. Nagai H, Hara I, Horikawa T et al. Antitumor effects on mouse melanoma elicited by local secretion of interleukin-12 and their enhancement by treatment with interleukin-18. *Cancer Invest* 2000;18(3):206–213.
67. Robertson MJ, Mier JW, Logan T et al. Clinical and biological effects of recombinant human interleukin-18 administered by intravenous infusion to patients with advanced cancer. *Clin Cancer Res* 2006;12(14 Pt 1):4265–4273.
68. Tarhini AA, Millward M, Mainwaring P et al. A phase 2, randomized study of SB-485232, rhIL-18, in patients with previously untreated metastatic melanoma. *Cancer* 2009;115(4):859–868.
69. Simpkins F, Flores AM, Chu C et al. A phase I, dose escalation trial to assess the safety and biological activity of recombinant human interleukin-18 (SB-485232) in combination with pegylated liposomal doxorubicin in platinum-resistant recurrent ovarian cancer. *J Clin Oncol. 2012 ASCO Annual Meeting Proceedings (Post-Meeting Edition).* 2012;30(15; May 20 Supplement): 5065.
70. Parrish-Novak J, Dillon SR, Nelson A et al. Interleukin 21 and its receptor are involved in NK cell expansion and regulation of lymphocyte function. *Nature* 2000;408(6808):57–63.
71. Moroz A, Eppolito C, Li Q et al. IL-21 enhances and sustains CD8+T cell responses to achieve durable tumor immunity: Comparative evaluation of IL-2, IL-15, and IL-21. *J Immunol* 2004;173(2):900–909.
72. Davis ID, Skrumsager BK, Cebon J et al. An open-label, two-arm, phase I trial of recombinant human interleukin-21 in patients with metastatic melanoma. *Clin Cancer Res* 2007;13(12):3630–3636.
73. Thompson JA, Curti BD, Redman BG et al. Phase I study of recombinant interleukin-21 in patients with metastatic melanoma and renal cell carcinoma. *J Clin Oncol* 2008;26(12):2034–2039.
74. Schmidt H, Brown J, Mouritzen U et al. Safety and clinical effect of subcutaneous human interleukin-21 in patients with metastatic melanoma or renal cell carcinoma: A phase I trial. *Clin Cancer Res* 2010;16(21):5312–5319.
75. Davis ID, Brady B, Kefford RF et al. Clinical and biological efficacy of recombinant human interleukin-21 in patients with stage IV malignant melanoma without prior treatment: A phase IIa trial. *Clin Cancer Res* 2009;15(6):2123–2129.
76. Petrella TM, Tozer R, Belanger K et al. Interleukin-21 has activity in patients with metastatic melanoma: A phase II study. *J Clin Oncol* 2012;30(27):3396–3401.
77. Timmerman JM, Byrd JC, Andorsky DJ et al. A phase I dose-finding trial of recombinant interleukin-21 and rituximab in relapsed and refractory low grade B-cell lymphoproliferative disorders. *Clin Cancer Res* 2012;18(20):5752–5760.
78. Steele N, Anthony A, Saunders M et al. A phase 1 trial of recombinant human IL-21 in combination with cetuximab in patients with metastatic colorectal cancer. *Br J Cancer* 2012;106(5):793–798.
79. ClinicalTrials.gov Identifier: NCT01152788.
80. ClinicalTrials.gov Identifier: NCT00617253.
81. ClinicalTrials.gov Identifier: NCT00389285.
82. ClinicalTrials.gov Identifier: NCT01629758.
83. ClinicalTrials.gov Identifier: NCT01489059.

16 Vaccine Therapy and Integration with Other Modalities

Benedetto Farsaci
National Institutes of Health

Peter S. Kim
National Institutes of Health

James W. Hodge
National Institutes of Health

Claudia Palena
National Institutes of Health

James L. Gulley
National Institutes of Health

Jeffrey Schlom
National Institutes of Health

CONTENTS

INTRODUCTION

The aim of tumor vaccines is to trigger or enhance an immune response against antigens expressed by tumor cells (designated as tumor-associated antigens (TAAs)) [1,2]. TAAs are presented to the immune system by a network of specialized cells known as professional antigen-presenting cells (APCs), such as dendritic cells (DCs). Upon exposure to TAAs by APCs, naïve T lymphocytes differentiate into effector and memory T cells. Effector T cells can, in turn, lyse tumor cells that express the antigens. Memory T cells might provide immune protection against tumor recurrence [2]. This mechanism of action differentiates immunotherapies from conventional chemotherapy and radiotherapy, which affect highly proliferative tumor cells, and from targeted therapies, which target the molecular pathways on which cancer cells depend for survival and expansion.

Clinical trials have evaluated numerous vaccine platforms that differ in terms of targeted disease, targeted TAAs, clinical end points, and method of administration (Table 16.1). A detailed review of these vaccine platforms was recently published by Schlom [3]. This chapter delineates the factors and concepts currently being evaluated in the effort to develop therapeutic vaccines, either as monotherapies or in combination with other therapies, for a wide range of human cancers and cancer stages.

VACCINE TARGETS

Common TAAs include oncoproteins, oncofetal antigens, differentiation-associated proteins, and viral proteins (Table 16.2).

ONCOPROTEINS

Oncoproteins are proteins derived from overexpressed or mutated genes (oncogenes) that have the potential to promote cancer. Among the targets being investigated in

TABLE 16.1
Vaccine Platforms in Phase II/III Clinical Trials

Vaccine Platform	Examples	Cancer	References
Peptides/proteins			
Peptide	gp100, MUC-1, and HER2/neu	Melanoma, lung, and breast	[4–6,112]
Protein	MAGE-A3 and NY-ESO	Melanoma	[13]
Antibody	Anti-idiotype	Lymphoma	[33,36,37]
Glycoproteins	STn-KLH	Melanoma	[121,122]
Recombinant vectors			
Poxvirus	rV and rF PSA-TRICOM (PROSTVAC)	Prostate	[1,38–40,60,82,104]
Saccharomyces cerevisiae (yeast)	Yeast-Ras, yeast-CEA	Pancreatic and carcinoma	[43,44,123]
Listeria	Listeria-mesothelin	Pancreatic	[45]
Alpha- and adenoviruses	Adeno-CEA and Alpha-CEA	Carcinoma	[41]
Tumor cells			
Autologous	Adeno-CD40L and colon (BCG)	CLL, colon, and melanoma	[42]
DC/autologous tumor cell infusion		Multiple myeloma	[49]
Allogeneic	GVAX (+ GM-CSF)	Pancreatic and prostate	[50–52]
DC/APCs			
APC-protein	Sipuleucel-T (PAP GM-CSF)	Prostate	[32,66]
DC/peptide	Glioma peptides	Glioma and melanoma	[114]
DC/infected vector	rV and rF CEA-MUC1-TRICOM (PANVAC DC)	Colorectal	[115]

Source: Adapted from Schlom, J., *J. Natl. Cancer Inst.*, 104, 599, 2012.

APC, antigen-presenting cell; BCG, bacillus Calmette–Guerin; CD40L, CD40 ligand; CEA, carcinoembryonic antigen; CLL, chronic lymphocytic leukemia; DC, dendritic cell; gp100, glycoprotein 100; GM-CSF, granulocyte-macrophage colony-stimulating factor; GVAX, GM-CSF gene vaccine; MAGE-A3, melanoma-associated antigen 3; MUC-1, mucin 1; NY-ESO, New York esophageal carcinoma antigen; PAP, prostatic acid phosphatase; PSA, prostate-specific antigen; rF, recombinant fowlpox; rV, recombinant vaccinia; STn-KLH, sialyl-TN-keyhole limpet hemocyanin.

TABLE 16.2
Tumor-Associated Antigens

Types	Examples	References
Oncoprotein	Point mutated: ras, BRAF, frame shift mutations, undefined unique tumor mutations; HER2/neu, MUC-1 C-terminus, and p53	[4–6]
Oncofetal antigen	CEA and MUC-1	[29,30,82,124,125]
Cancer–testis	MAGE-A3, BAGE, SEREX-defined, and NY-ESO	[8,13,126]
Tissue lineage	PAP, PSA, gp100, tyrosinase, and glioma antigen	[1,32,60,112,114,127]
Stem cell/EMT	Brachyury, SOX-2, OCT-4, TERT, CD44^{high}/CD24^{low}, and CD133$^+$	[19,22,24]
Viral	HPV and HCV	[128]
Glycopeptides	STn-KLH	[121,122]
Antiangiogenic	VEGF-R	[27]
B-cell lymphoma	Anti-idiotype	[33,36,37]

Source: Adapted from Schlom, J., *J. Natl. Cancer Inst.*, 104, 599, 2012.

BAGE, B melanoma antigen; CEA, carcinoembryonic antigen; EMT, epithelial to mesenchymal transition; gp100, glycoprotein 100; HCV, hepatitis C virus; HPV, human papillomavirus; MAGE-A3, melanoma-associated antigen-A3; MUC-1, mucin 1; NY-ESO, New York esophageal carcinoma antigen 1; OCT-4, octamer-binding transcription factor 4; PAP, prostatic acid phosphatase; PSA, prostate-specific antigen; SOX-2, (sex-determining region Y)-box-2; STn-KLH: sialyl-Tn–keyhole limpet hemocyanin; TERT, telomerase reverse transcriptase; VEGF-R, vascular endothelial growth factor receptor.

vaccine clinical trials are amplified or overexpressed HER2/neu (ErbB2) [4], protein 53 (p53), the c-terminus of mucin-1 (MUC-1c) [5,6], the product of mutated *ras* genes in colorectal and pancreatic cancer, and mutated *BRAF* genes in melanoma. A BRAF inhibitor has been shown to enhance expression of TAAs on melanoma cells containing a *BRAF* gene mutation, resulting in enhanced T-cell lysis of tumor cells in vitro [7].

Unfortunately, multiple genetic mutations of a given gene that generate a large number of different protein constructs, such as the mutated exons of the *P53* gene that produce innumerable mutant p53 proteins, would require numerous vaccine constructs and are therefore not practical candidates for immunotherapies. This is also true of frameshift mutations and the unique mutations that occur in individual tumors.

Oncofetal Antigens

Oncofetal antigens are normally produced in the early stages of embryonic development and disappear by the time the immune system is fully developed; thus, self-tolerance may not develop against these antigens [8]. Examples are carcinoembryonic antigen (CEA), which is elevated in a variety of cancers such as colorectal, pancreatic, gastric, lung, breast, and medullary thyroid, and alpha-fetoprotein, which is produced by hepatocellular carcinoma and some germ cell tumors.

Another oncofetal antigen is the trophoblast glycoprotein, also known as TPBG or 5T4, expressed in colorectal, gastric, and ovarian cancer. It is the target of the cancer vaccine TroVax®, which is in clinical trials for the treatment of a range of different solid tumor types [9].

TISSUE-SPECIFIC ANTIGENS AND OTHER OVEREXPRESSED PROTEINS

Some tumors express tissue-lineage antigens that are not expressed or are poorly expressed on vital organs, which can be targeted by specific vaccine platforms. Examples of these antigens include prostatic acid phosphatase (PAP), prostate-specific antigen (PSA), prostate-specific membrane antigen (PSMA), and the melanoma-associated antigens glycoprotein 100 (gp100) and tyrosinase [10,11]. Other examples of oncoproteins are cancer/testis antigens such as the ovarian cancer-associated New York esophageal carcinoma antigen-1 [12,13], L antigen family member-1, preferentially expressed antigen of melanoma, and the melanoma-associated antigen 3 and B melanoma antigen [14].

ANTIGENS EXPRESSED BY CANCER STEM CELLS AND EPITHELIAL TO MESENCHYMAL TRANSITION

Cancer stem cells (CSCs), also known as tumor-initiating cells, are believed to be responsible for the repopulation of tumors after cytoreductive therapy. Telomerase, the enzyme responsible for maintaining the extremities of chromosomes (telomeres), is critical for the integrity of stem cells [15]. CSCs can be potentially targeted by vaccines that induce the expansion and cytotoxicity of telomerase-specific T lymphocytes [16,17]. One limitation to targeting CSCs is that their markers are also expressed in some normal tissues, such as bone marrow stem cells (CD133 and telomerase), fibroblasts (CD44), and B-lymphocytes (CD24).

The metastatic process can also potentially be targeted by vaccines that stimulate an immune response against cells in the process of epithelial to mesenchymal transition (EMT) [18]. EMT and cancer stemness are associated with the transcription factor sex-determining region Y-box 2. Each of these gene products is being evaluated for its ability to generate human T-cell responses in vitro [19–21]. The T-box transcription factor brachyury, a major driver of EMT, is selectively expressed in both primary and metastatic carcinomas [19,22–24]. Unlike some of the other transcription factors shown to be involved in EMT, brachyury is selectively expressed on tumors but not on normal adult human tissues. T-cell epitopes have been shown to elicit the generation of brachyury-specific human cytotoxic T lymphocytes (CTLs) that can lyse a range of carcinoma cells [20]. An antibrachyury vaccine is currently being evaluated in a clinical trial [25].

ANTIGENS EXPRESSED BY TUMOR VASCULATURE

Vaccines targeting receptors for vascular endothelial growth factor (VEGF-Rs) have shown promising results in preclinical studies [26,27]. As a result, a phase I clinical trial evaluating the effect of the VEGFR2 DNA vaccine VXM01 in stage IV pancreatic cancer is currently in the accrual stage [28].

VACCINE PLATFORMS

Multiple vaccine platforms have been evaluated in clinical trials as described in the following and outlined in Table 16.1.

PEPTIDE AND PROTEIN VACCINES

Some polypeptide vaccines contain potential epitopes in their amino acid sequence that can stimulate both CD4 and CD8 T lymphocytes. For example, the therapeutic cancer vaccine Stimuvax® contains both kinds of epitopes for MUC-1, a cell-surface proteoglycan associated with several tumor types [29,30]. Many peptide and protein vaccines are used as part of a DC vaccine platform.

DENDRITIC CELL VACCINES

DCs are immune cells whose role is the recognition, processing, and presentation of foreign antigens to T lymphocytes. DC vaccines involve using DCs from the cancer patient to stimulate immune responses. DC therapy requires harvesting peripheral blood mononuclear cells (PBMCs) from a patient and processing them in a laboratory in large amounts while exposing them to antigens from the patient's own cancer. DCs are then reinfused back into the patient in order to allow massive activation of the immune system [31]. The most successful example of a DC vaccine is sipuleucel-T, which has been approved by the US Food and Drug Administration (US FDA) for the treatment of metastatic castration-resistant prostate cancer (mCRPC) [32].

ANTI-IDIOTYPE VACCINES

Anti-idiotype (anti-id) vaccines, which are made of antibodies directed against other antibodies, have shown clinical benefit in clinical trials [33]. Anti-id vaccines can stimulate the immune system to produce antibodies against tumor cells. The immune network model proposed by Lindenmann [34] and Jerne [35] describes the immune system as a network of interacting antibodies and lymphocytes and can help to understand the mechanism involved in the activity of this vaccine platform. Antibodies directed against TAAs (Ab1) are targeted by anti-id antibodies (Ab2), which bind to the antigen-combining site of Ab1; as a consequence, Ab2 can induce anti-anti-id antibodies (Ab3) that specifically bind to the tumor antigen recognized by Ab1. Ab2, mimicking tumor antigens, have been shown to induce anti-anti-id proliferative T helper and suppressor lymphocytes, as well as CTLs [36,37]. While anti-id vaccines have the disadvantage of being patient-specific, some can be produced in less than a month [37].

RECOMBINANT VECTOR VACCINES

Recombinant vectors used in therapeutic vaccines are derived mainly from the Poxviridae family, including vaccinia, modified vaccinia Ankara (MVA), and the avipoxviruses fowlpox and canarypox. An advantage of poxviral vectors is that they can accept large inserts of foreign DNA and thus can accommodate multiple genes.

As a vaccine vector, vaccinia virus, used in vaccines for smallpox, can express genes within the cytoplasm of mammalian cells. Intracellular expression of a transgene allows for processing of the tumor antigen by both the class I and II major histocompatibility complex (MHC) pathways [38]. Because poxviral replication and transcription are restricted to the cytoplasm, there is minimal risk to the host of insertional mutagenesis. The local inflammatory response mediated by Toll-like receptors (TLRs) of poxviruses increases the immunogenicity of the inserted transgenes for the TAAs. However, when transgenes for TAAs are inserted in nonavian poxviruses (i.e., vaccinia and MVA), the host's immune response neutralizes the virus, limiting the use of some poxviral-based vaccines to no more than two administrations. In contrast, recombinant avipoxviruses (i.e., fowlpox) can be used multiple times because their late viral coat proteins are not produced in mammalian cells [39,40]. Thus, vaccinia and MVA are often used as priming vaccines, while avipoxviruses, such as fowlpox, are used as boosts for repeated vaccinations.

Alphaviruses, such as Venezuelan equine encephalitis virus, can also be used as vectors for TAAs. Once the virus replicates its RNA within the cytoplasm of infected host cells, it can express high levels of a transgene [41]. Recombinant adenovirus vectors, which are easy to engineer, have also shown utility as vaccines and gene therapy agents [42], but clinical evaluation has been hindered by high levels of preexisting antiviral immunity. New variants of adenoviruses are being developed and evaluated that may potentially be less immunogenic.

Heat-killed recombinant *Saccharomyces cerevisiae*, the yeast commonly used in winemaking, baking, and brewing, is inherently nonpathogenic, easily propagated and purified, and very stable. However, yeast vectors are not able to accept large inserts of foreign DNA and thus can only accommodate a single gene. Recombinant yeasts have been shown to activate maturation of human DCs and to present both class I and II epitopes of transgenes [43]. Yeast vectors can be administered multiple times without eliciting host-neutralizing activity [44]. Several recombinant yeast vaccines are currently being evaluated in phase I and II trials. Attenuated recombinant *Listeria monocytogenes* bacteria have also been shown to target DCs and, like viral and yeast vectors, can stimulate both innate and adaptive immune responses [45].

DNA Vaccines

DNA vaccines have entered into a variety of human clinical trials for various diseases, including cancer. They are well tolerated and have an excellent safety profile. Nonetheless, results from these clinical trials have been disappointing [27], indicating that DNA vaccines require much improvement in antigen expression and delivery methods to make them sufficiently effective in the clinic [46]. DNA vaccine immunogenicity can be attributed to its immunostimulatory CpG motifs acting as an inside adjuvant recognized by TLR9. Recent research, however, has indicated that the adjuvant effect of plasmid DNA can be mediated by its double-stranded structure, which activates TANK-binding kinase-1 (TBK1)-dependent innate immune signaling pathways in the absence of TLRs [47]. TBK1-signaling may mediate antigen presentation through distinct types of cells *in vivo*, which in turn elicit antigen-specific CD4$^+$ and CD8$^+$ T cells.

WHOLE TUMOR-CELL VACCINES

Whole tumor-cell vaccines have the advantage of presenting the immune system with a range of both known and undefined TAAs as immunogens. However, this same property also potentially diminishes the relative level of expression of a particular TAA (or group of TAAs) and its presentation and processing by APCs. A killed whole tumor-cell vaccine is usually accompanied by an immune stimulant such as granulocyte-macrophage colony-stimulating factor (GM-CSF), bacillus Calmette–Guerin adjuvant, or CD40 ligand.

Autologous tumor-cell vaccines present a unique set of TAAs, such as particular point mutations or fusion gene products, from a patient's own tumor [48]. Unfortunately, because this technology depends on the availability of tumor biopsies, it is feasible for only some tumor types and stages. In one variation of this technique, DCs and autologous tumor cells are fused before the patient is immunized [49]. DC/tumor-cell fusions combine the unique properties of whole tumor-cell vaccines with the enhanced antigen-presenting power of DCs.

Alternatively, allogeneic whole tumor-cell vaccines, which typically contain two or three established and characterized human tumor-cell lines of a given tumor type, may be used to overcome many logistical limitations of autologous tumor-cell vaccines. The GVAX vaccine platforms [50–52], which contain allogeneic pancreatic, prostate, or breast tumor cells, are a testament to the ability to provide such a vaccine for multicenter evaluation.

EFFECTS OF THERAPEUTIC CANCER VACCINES AND CONSEQUENCES FOR ANALYSIS OF DATA

While interest in harnessing the immune system to defeat cancer has grown, many clinical trials of cancer vaccines have shown only marginal antitumor activity [53,54]. International organizations such as the Cancer Immunotherapy Consortium of the Cancer Research Institute have collaborated with clinical centers to systematically investigate the reasons for these outcomes. Their conclusions identify the need for better understanding of human tumor immunology and improved clinical trial design, including more refined criteria for trial end points [55]. Understanding the dynamics of therapeutic cancer vaccines is fundamental not only for determining the optimal dose and timing of administration but also for interpreting outcomes.

RESPONSE TO CANCER VACCINES

It has been hypothesized that the immune system responds to a cancer vaccine in three stages. Soon after initial vaccine administration, there is a cellular response involving immune activation and proliferation of T lymphocytes (cellular response). Over the following weeks or months, activated immune cells can mediate cytotoxic tumor-cell killing, causing clinically measurable or nonmeasurable antitumor effects such as tumor shrinkage. Several months after the initial vaccination, there is a delayed effect, whereby antitumoral immune memory maintains immune surveillance and tumor-cell killing, potentially resulting in increased overall survival (OS) (Figure 16.1). This dynamic is specific to immunotherapy. Cytotoxic agents affect the tumor only

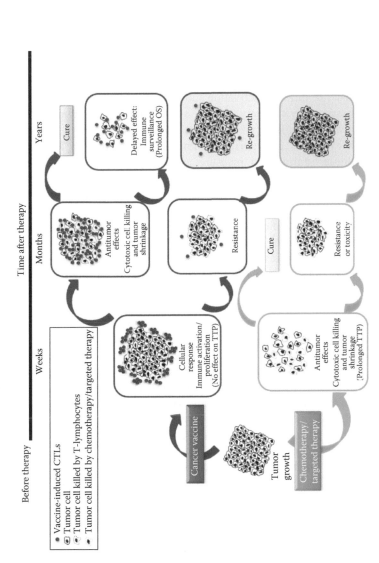

FIGURE 16.1 Cancer vaccines can potentially result in delayed detection of clinical response and improved OS. Within a few weeks of initial administration of cancer vaccines, there is immune activation and proliferation of antigen-specific T lymphocytes (cellular response). Over months, activated immune cells can mediate clinically measurable antitumor effects (cytotoxic cell killing and tumor shrinkage). Several months after vaccine administration, antitumoral immune memory can maintain immune surveillance and tumor-cell killing, causing prolonged OS (delayed effect). Cytotoxic agents affect the tumor only during the period of administration. If the tumor is not eliminated, prolonged therapy may be necessary. Soon after the drug is discontinued, because of recurrence or toxicity, antitumor activity ceases and tumor growth rate will increase. CTL, cytotoxic T lymphocytes; TPP, time to progression.

during the period of administration; soon after the agent is discontinued, antitumor activity ceases and the tumor growth rate can return to pretreatment levels. In contrast, the different mechanism of action and kinetics of therapeutic vaccines [56] mean that immune responses can take time to develop and can be potentially enhanced by continued booster vaccinations. As a consequence, the RECIST criteria for evaluating clinical response, which were designed to assess the effects of cytotoxic agents, often cannot adequately assess the effects of immunotherapy.

TOOLS FOR ASSESSING IMMUNE RESPONSE

The quality and intensity of immune activation soon after vaccination (initial cellular response) can be assessed by a variety of bioassays, including the enzyme-linked immunosorbent spot assay, cytometry-based tests such as intracellular cytokine staining to measure cytokines as interferon-gamma (IFN-γ), human leukocyte antigen–peptide multimer staining to measure antigen-specific CTLs, and carboxyfluorescein succinimidyl ester to assess the proliferation of T lymphocytes. The Cancer Vaccine Clinical Trial Working Group, representing academia and the pharmaceutical and biotechnology industries, with participation from the US FDA [57], has designed a series of proficiency tests for executing these immunoassays and interpreting data derived from them to ensure that they are reproducible and technically validated in laboratories around the world [55]. They have also developed guidelines for laboratory protocols that limit interlaboratory variability, so that results from these laboratory tests can be compared with clinical outcomes.

Recent studies have conducted more comprehensive analyses of immune-cell subsets from PBMCs, including, in addition to T-cell responses, analyses of T regulatory cells (Tregs), myeloid-derived suppressor cells, natural killer cells, DCs, and antibodies to TAAs [58,59]. Ratios of effector to regulatory cells have also been analyzed [60]. Numerous studies have also analyzed multiple serum cytokines and chemokines. These bioassay studies have occasionally found an association between clinical outcome and a specific immune assay; however, these results sometimes fall far short of identifying any one assay as a surrogate for clinical response. Potential reasons for this outcome may be that (a) PBMC analyses may not reflect which immune cells are actually at the tumor site; (b) few studies have actually analyzed the antigen cascade phenomenon, where the true biomarker may be a T-cell population directed against a TAA not in the vaccine but generated via cross-priming [4,61]; (c) the diversity of the immune response may not allow for any one marker or set of markers to be a true surrogate for clinical response; and (d) OS benefit has only recently emerged as a prominent end point in vaccine studies, and thus adequate samples may not yet be available for comprehensive correlative analyses.

DELAYED DETECTION OF CLINICAL RESPONSE MAY EXPLAIN IMPROVED OVERALL SURVIVAL WITHOUT INCREASED TIME TO PROGRESSION

Because it is a consequence of a cellular response, it may take time for a clinical response to vaccine to be measurable. Thus, clinical response in terms of OS can be considered a late or delayed effect of therapy (Figure 16.1).

Immune responses can potentially be enhanced by continued booster vaccinations. Any resulting tumor-cell lysis can lead to cross-priming of additional TAAs, thus broadening the immune repertoire (a phenomenon known as antigen cascade or epitope spreading) [4,61]. This broader immune response may take some time to develop. Another peculiar effect of cancer vaccines is that, although they may not induce any substantial reduction in tumor burden, they have the potential to promote antitumor activity over a long period of time, resulting in a slower tumor growth rate. This deceleration in growth rate may continue for months or years and, more importantly, through subsequent therapies. This process can lead to clinically significant improved OS, often with little or no difference in time to progression (TTP) and a low rate of, or lack of, objective response [1,32]. This aspect is well reviewed by Madan et al. [62]. Thus, treating patients with a vaccine when they have a lower tumor burden may result in better outcomes. It is hypothesized that the combined use of vaccine and cytotoxic therapy may result in both tumor regression via the cytotoxic therapy and reduced tumor growth rate via the vaccine therapy (Figure 16.2) [56,62,63].

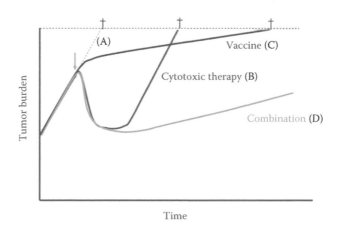

FIGURE 16.2 Tumor growth rates in patients with metastatic prostate cancer, from four trials with chemotherapy and one with PROSTVAC (PSA-TRICOM). (Adapted from data in Stein, W.D. et al., *Clin. Cancer Res.*, 17, 907, 2011. With permission; Madan, R.A. et al., *Oncologist*, 15, 969, 2010. With permission; Gulley, J.L. et al., *Curr. Oncol.*, 18, e150, 2011. With permission; and *Seminars in Oncology*, 39, Madan, R.A. et al., Clinical evaluation of TRICOM vector therapeutic cancer vaccines, 296–304, Copyright (2012), with permission from Elsevier.) (A) Tumor growth rate with no therapy. (B) Chemotherapy induced initial tumor reduction, but tumor growth rate at relapse was similar to pretreatment tumor growth rate. (C) PROSTVAC vaccine reduced tumor growth rate, following therapy. Thus, patients who received vaccine showed little if any tumor reduction (and virtually no increase in TTP) but showed an increase in OS. Dagger denotes time of death. (D) Predictions of enhanced OS for patients treated with both vaccine and chemotherapy. This phenomenon could potentially be enhanced if vaccine were initiated earlier in the disease process or in patients with low tumor burden.

PROSTATE CANCER AS A MODEL FOR
UNDERSTANDING VACCINE THERAPY

Prostate cancer can serve as a prototype disease for the evaluation of therapeutic cancer vaccines for several reasons [64]. First, prostate cancer is generally an indolent disease that may not lead to metastasis or death for over a decade, thus allowing the time necessary to generate a sufficient immune response. Second, because prostate cancer cells express numerous TAAs, including PSA, PAP, PSMA, and prostate stem cell antigen, they can be targeted by multiple TAA-specific lymphocytes. Third, serum concentrations of PSA can be used to identify patients with minimal tumor burden as well as patients who are responding to therapy. Finally, the validated Halabi nomogram [65] can be used at presentation of metastatic disease to predict a patient's probable response to standard chemotherapy and/or hormonal therapy.

In April 2010, the US FDA approved the therapeutic cancer vaccine sipuleucel-T for the treatment of nonsymptomatic or minimally symptomatic mCRPC. Although a few small phase III trials failed to meet their primary end point of improved TTP, they did show evidence of prolonged OS in mCRPC [66]. A larger (n = 512) phase III trial of sipuleucel-T [32] was subsequently conducted with OS as the primary end point. Sipuleucel-T consists of APCs from PBMCs that have been incubated with PAP that has been fused with GM-CSF. PBMCs obtained from patients by leukapheresis are processed in a central facility where the PAP fusion protein is added to the APCs. These cells are then reinfused into the patient to confer immunity. This process is repeated three times at biweekly intervals (Figure 16.3A). In this trial, as in the smaller trials, no change in TTP was seen; however, OS was improved in the vaccine arm (25.8 vs. 21.7 months; $P = 0.032$) (Figure 16.3B). One obvious drawback of DC vaccines is the requirement for leukapheresis and cell culture processing of PBMCs, limiting the number of vaccinations that can be given.

A second prostate cancer vaccine, PROSTVAC®, has been evaluated in mCRPC. This off-the-shelf platform consists of a recombinant vaccinia priming vaccination and multiple fowlpox booster vaccinations. Each vector contains transgenes for PSA and three costimulatory molecules: CD80, intercellular adhesion molecule 1, and lymphocyte function-associated antigen 3, collectively designated TRICOM (Figure 16.3C) [67,68]. A 43-center randomized placebo-controlled phase II trial enrolled 125 minimally symptomatic patients with mCRPC [1]. As seen with sipuleucel-T, treatment with PROSTVAC did not alter TTP; however, it did improve median OS relative to placebo (25.1 vs. 16.6 months; $P = 0.006$) (Figure 16.3D). Over the course of follow-up, patients who received PROSTVAC had a 44% lower rate of death compared with patients in the control cohort (hazard ratio [HR] = 0.56) [1]. The median OS in a second PROSTVAC single-arm phase II study [60] was 26.6 months, which was similar to that observed in the PROSTVAC arm of the larger randomized trial. Outcomes with sipuleucel-T and PROSTVAC compared favorably with chemotherapeutic agents and hormonal therapies US FDA approved for mCRPC, with fewer serious adverse events.

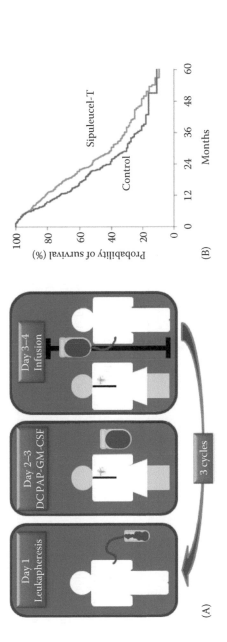

FIGURE 16.3 Prostate cancer vaccines sipuleucel-T (US FDA approved) and PROSTVAC (in phase II clinical trial) for patients with mCRPC. (A) The procedure for harvesting and processing PBMCs and reinfusing the cancer vaccine sipuleucel-T. (1) Leukapheresis is performed at an apheresis center. (2) At a company (Dendreon) facility, the patient's DCs are cocultured with PAP and GM-CSF. (3) The vaccine is reinfused into the patient at the doctor's office. This procedure is repeated three times at biweekly intervals. (B) Primary efficacy analysis of treatment with sipuleucel-T vs. placebo, showing that sipuleucel-T improved OS (HR for death=0.78; 95%; confidence interval=0.61–0.98; *P*=.03). (Adapted from Kantoff, P.W. et al., *N. Engl. J. Med.*, 363, 411, 2010. With permission.) The placebo control consisted of cultured APCs from leukapheresis, without PAP GM-CSF antigen. Per the trial protocol, the control group could receive cryopreserved APCs with antigen upon disease progression.

(*continued*)

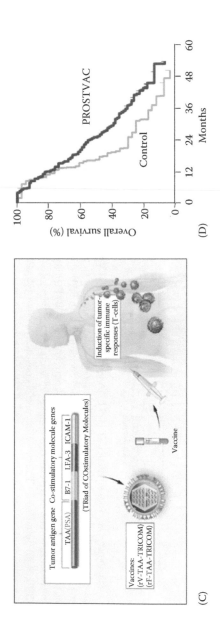

FIGURE 16.3 (continued) Prostate cancer vaccines sipuleucel-T (US FDA approved) and PROSTVAC (in phase II clinical trial) for patients with mCRPC. (C) A second prostate cancer vaccine evaluated in the same population of patients with mCRPC. PROSTVAC, an off-the-shelf vaccine platform, consists of a recombinant vaccinia virus priming vaccination and multiple fowlpox booster vaccinations. Each vector contains transgenes for PSA and three costimulatory molecules (CD80, ICAM-1, and LFA-3; designated TRICOM). (Adapted from *Seminars in Oncology*, 39, Madan, R.A. et al., Clinical evaluation of TRICOM vector therapeutic cancer vaccines, 296, Copyright (2012), with permission from Elsevier.) (D) A randomized, placebo-controlled 43-center trial of PROSTVAC vs. empty vector showed an OS advantage of 8.5 months (25.1 vs. 16.6 months; $P=.006$) and a 44% reduction in death in the vaccine arm. (Adapted from Kantoff, P.W. et al., *J. Clin. Oncol.*, 28, 1099, 2010. With permission.)

ENHANCED AGONIST EPITOPES

It is possible to enhance the immunogenicity of a TAA by altering its amino acid sequence. This alteration allows for the development of agonist epitopes designed to enhance binding to either MHC or T-cell receptors, resulting in higher levels of T-cell responses and/or higher-avidity T lymphocytes [69–73]. Agonist epitopes are employed in the gp100 melanoma vaccine [74], the PROSTVAC vaccine (PSA agonist) [72], and the PANVAC vaccine (agonists for CEA and MUC-1) [75].

IMMUNE STIMULANTS FOR POTENTIATING IMMUNOTHERAPIES

Multiple preclinical studies have shown that vaccines combined with immune stimulants or inhibitors of immune suppression can enhance antitumor responses. However, the availability of many of these agents is limited. In 2007, a National Cancer Institute (NCI) workshop identified 12 such agents [76], most of which are still unavailable for use in vaccine combination therapies. Preclinical studies have demonstrated that some of these agents, when given with vaccine at doses far below the maximum tolerated dose, or at lower doses locally with vaccine, can greatly enhance vaccine efficacy [77]. A preclinical study that used two diverse recombinant CEA vaccine platforms (poxviral and yeast) demonstrated that each vector processed TAA epitopes differentially and activated a different T-cell repertoire and cytokine profile, resulting in enhanced antitumor activity [78]. The potential of combination vaccine therapies is also evidenced in results from preclinical and clinical studies using diversified prime–boost strategies with vaccinia and fowlpox vectors [39].

CYTOKINES

Cytokines such as interleukin (IL)-2, IL-15, IL-7, GM-CSF, and IFNs act as immune stimulants [79]. IL-2 has the disadvantage of enhancing Tregs along with effector cells [80], while IL-15 enhances effector T-cell response but not Tregs [81]. GM-CSF has been used in the GVAX and other vaccine platforms [51,82,83] but may be immunosuppressive at higher dose levels [60]. IFNs have been shown to enhance immune responses and expression of TAAs and MHC on tumor cells [84–86]. Antibody–cytokine fusions, such as hu14.18–IL2, have shown promise in patients with refractory neuroblastoma [87], and similar immunocytokines are currently under development. A range of TLRs has been shown to enhance vaccine efficacy in preclinical studies [7], but most are being evaluated clinically as monotherapies. Classic adjuvants such as incomplete Freund's, immune stimulating complexes, Detox, and chitosan provide both a depot effect for the protein/peptide vaccine (or cytokine) and immune stimulation in regional lymph nodes [88]. Clinical trials will need to carefully evaluate the dose and scheduling of all of these immune stimulants with vaccine.

INHIBITORS OF IMMUNOSUPPRESSANTS

Preclinical and clinical studies of vaccines in combination with immune checkpoint inhibitors and inhibitors of immunosuppressive entities are generating promising data.

Ipilimumab, an inhibitor of CTL-associated antigen 4, has been shown in several pre-clinical models to enhance the avidity of T cells and to enhance antitumor effects in combination with vaccines [89,90]. A recent clinical trial of PROSTVAC in combination with ipilimumab showed prolonged survival in patients with mCRPC compared with what had been seen in previous trials with PSA-TRICOM as monotherapy [21,91]. The recent US FDA approval of ipilimumab for metastatic melanoma [89] may make combination therapies employing this agent with a range of vaccine platforms more feasible. However, the severe side effects seen in some patients receiving ipilimumab may not be conducive to its use in many patient populations. Ongoing clinical studies with anti-PD-1 and anti-PD-1 ligand 1 monoclonal antibodies as monotherapies are also showing promising results [92,93] and may eventually be used with vaccine.

Other agents that can reduce or eliminate immune suppressive factors are also being evaluated. Monoclonal anti-CD25-diptherial toxin (Ontak®) has been shown to reduce Tregs and to enhance vaccine efficacy [94]. Both monoclonal and small-molecule inhibitors of transforming growth factor-beta are also currently in clinical evaluation as monotherapies, but their full potential may be realized in vaccine combination therapy [95].

COMBINING VACCINES WITH OTHER THERAPEUTIC MODALITIES

Preclinical studies and clinical trials have demonstrated that many cytotoxic and small-molecule targeted therapies can be administered concurrently with or subsequent to vaccine therapy, with additive or synergistic effects (Figure 16.4).

IMMUNOGENIC MODULATION OF TUMOR CELLS

Cytotoxic doses of ionizing radiation, the chemotherapy agent oxaliplatin, and anthracyclines such as doxorubicin can induce immunogenic cell death in tumors, which results in enhanced cross-priming of TAAs by DCs and subsequent activation of T cells [96]. Immunogenic cell death is the result of three events. First, dying tumor cells expose calreticulin from the endoplasmic reticulum to the cell membrane. Calreticulin can be bound by a receptor expressed by DCs, thereby stimulating the uptake of apoptotic tumor cells. Second, nonhistone chromatin-binding protein (HMGB-1, high-mobility group protein B-1) is released into the extracellular compartment. HMGB1 binds to the TLR4, inhibiting the lysosomal antigen degradation pathway in DCs and thus favoring tumor antigen processing and presentation, and stimulates the synthesis of the precursor of IL-1β. Third, adenosine triphosphate released by the tumor cell binds to the purinergic receptor P2RX7 at the surface of DCs, causing the assembly and activation of the cryopyrin inflammasome and secretion of IL-1β. As a consequence, APCs such as DCs engulf tumor cells, process them, and cross-prime CTLs, eliciting a tumor-specific immune response [97]. In this case, tumor-cell death is an indispensable factor in immunostimulation.

Another mechanism that can enhance an antitumor response is the immunogenic modulation of tumor phenotype. In this process, the phenotype of cancer cells that remain alive during treatment is altered. These cells upregulate TAAs as well as MHC and costimulatory molecules, making them more immunostimulatory [98,99].

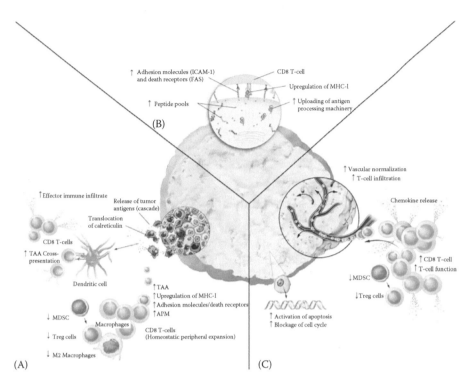

FIGURE 16.4 Mechanisms of synergy between radiation therapy, chemotherapy, or small-molecule inhibitors and vaccine. (Adapted from data in references *Seminars in Oncology*, 39, Hodge, J.W. et al., The tipping point for combination therapy: Cancer vaccines with radiation, chemotherapy, or targeted small molecule inhibitors, 323–339, Copyright 2012, with permission from Elsevier; Hodge, J.W. et al., *Oncology (Williston Park)*, 22, 1064–1070; discussion 75, 80–81, 84, 2008. With permission.) Various immunomodulatory effects of conventional therapies can be exploited to enhance the antitumor activity induced by vaccines. (A) Immunomodulatory effects of chemotherapy: induction of immunogenic tumor-cell death, leading to activation of DCs and facilitating cross-priming and tumor-specific T-cell generation; upregulation of tumor antigens (TAA), adhesion molecules, antigen-processing machinery (APM), and MHC, which increases T-cell recognition and triggers T-cell killing; and induction of leukopenia followed by differential homeostatic peripheral expansion that favors tumor-specific T cells. (B) Radiation therapy's immunomodulatory effects: upregulation of tumor antigens, costimulatory molecules, Fas, and MHC moieties, which makes tumors more susceptible to immune-mediated attack; upregulation of cytokines, chemokines, and adhesion molecules, which enhances T-cell trafficking to the tumor site and prolongs T-cell/tumor contact; and downregulation of Tregs, which facilitates the generation of antigen-specific T cells. (C) Targeted small-molecule inhibitors can increase the number and function of tumor antigen-specific T cells, decrease the number and function of myeloid-derived suppressor cells and Tregs, block the tumor-cell cycle, induce apoptosis, inhibit angiogenesis, modulate hypoxia, and normalize tumor vasculature.

For example, chemotherapy agents such as the taxane docetaxel have been shown to increase the expression of TAAs, peptide–MHC complexes, adhesion molecules, and death receptors such as Fas on the surface of tumor cells, rendering them more susceptible to vaccine-induced T-cell killing [100]. This same phenomenon has been observed in tumor cells exposed to noncytotoxic doses of external beam radiation, radiolabeled monoclonal antibodies, and bone-seeking radionuclides [101–103]. Clinical trials of a vaccine plus docetaxel in patients with prostate cancer [104] have been completed. A trial of the recombinant vaccinia/fowlpox CEA-MUC-1/TRICOM vaccine (PANVAC) in combination with docetaxel in patients with metastatic breast cancer has recently been completed. A trial of PROSTVAC in combination with a bone-seeking chelated radionuclide in patients with prostate cancer metastatic to bone is in progress [105,106].

ACTIVATION OF EFFECTOR CELLS AND INHIBITION OF IMMUNOSUPPRESSIVE ELEMENTS

Certain chemotherapeutic regimens, such as cisplatin with vinorelbine, have shown, in preclinical models, a differential recovery of diverse immune subsets as a consequence of immune homeostatic proliferation, resulting in an enhanced effector/Treg ratio [107]. In clinical studies, low-dose cyclophosphamide has been shown to decrease Treg levels [52]. Lenalidomide has been shown to stimulate T-cell proliferation and to enhance production of IL-2 and IFN-γ [108]. Small-molecule targeted therapeutics can enhance vaccine-mediated T-cell lysis of tumors. In preclinical studies, both a B cell lymphoma-2 inhibitor [109] and the tyrosine kinase inhibitor sunitinib [110,111] enhanced the ratio of TAA-specific T cells to Tregs, resulting in enhanced vaccine efficacy. The mTOR inhibitor rapamycin has been shown to enhance IL-12 production and the generation of memory $CD8^+$ T cells [99]. The HER2/neu inhibitor trastuzumab, in combination with vaccine, enhanced HER2/neu-specific immune responses in patients with breast cancer [98].

Hormonal therapies used in the treatment of several different stages of prostate cancer have been shown to induce thymic regeneration as well as naïve T cells [4]. Vaccine therapy may be most effective at this stage of treatment [82,112]. A clinical study has demonstrated increased levels of infiltrating T cells in prostate cancer biopsies post- vs. prehormonal therapy [113]. Randomized clinical trials of vaccine in combination with either nilutamide or flutamide hormonal therapy in patients with nonmetastatic prostate cancer have been completed and others are ongoing [114,115].

CONCLUSIONS AND FUTURE PERSPECTIVES

Since the approval of sipuleucel-T by the US FDA in 2010 for the treatment of patients with mCRPC, immunotherapy for cancer treatment has become a valid clinical alternative [32]. The two most relevant peculiarities of cancer vaccines are their ability to (1) improve OS and (2) cause significantly less toxicity than other agents. Nonetheless, a major concern about the benefits of immunotherapy is the lack of effect on TTP. Mathematical tumor growth models have demonstrated that immunologic therapies act by slowing tumor growth and thus prolonging survival [116] (Figure 16.2). This differs from most standard-of-care therapies, which cause initial tumor shrinkage due to the sensitivity of cancer cells to the therapy. This period of shrinkage, however, is sometimes followed by a rebound of tumor growth velocity when tumors become resistant to the treatment or extreme toxicity is observed. The finding that tumor growth rates measured during clinical trials may correlate with OS provides a novel strategy for evaluating clinical trial data [116,117]. More importantly, tumor regression and growth rates determined in five intramural NCI prostate cancer trials employing chemotherapy vs. vaccine confirmed that the growth rate constant could be a valid indicator of therapeutic efficacy, suggesting that the effectiveness of immunotherapy can be more accurately determined by improved OS than by TTP [56].

In addition to aiding the generation of an immune response, combination therapy may also allow clinical benefits to be achieved with lower drug concentrations, if these concentrations also induce immunogenic cell death or immunogenic tumor-cell modulation. An example of how a low-dose targeted therapy can reprogram the tumor microenvironment away from immunosuppression toward potentiation of cancer vaccine therapies comes from a recent preclinical investigation from Huang et al. [118]. The authors showed that combining a whole cancer cell vaccine with low-dose anti-VEGF-R2 therapy enhanced anticancer efficacy in two murine breast cancer models. This was the result of a homogeneous redistribution of functional tumor vessels, along with a polarization of tumor-associated macrophages from an immune inhibitory M2-like phenotype toward an immune stimulatory M1-like phenotype, which in turn facilitated T-cell tumor infiltration. The use of low-dose chemotherapy can have significant clinical consequences, since toxicities from chemotherapy or radiotherapy are the major cause of dose reduction or treatment interruption in patients with cancer [119]. Validating the safety and efficacy of combination therapy will support the practice of administering vaccines earlier in the disease process, as does the fact that better results are seen in patients with more indolent disease [1].

A number of preclinical and clinical reports have shown that conventional chemotherapies, radiotherapies, or small-molecule inhibitors can synergistically potentiate vaccine-mediated immune attack against tumor cells. The direct antitumor effect mediated by cytotoxic therapies can decrease tumor volume, diminishing tumor-produced immune suppression and leaving a smaller tumor mass for the immune system to attack (Figure 16.1). The destruction of tumor cells by these therapies can also lead to exposure of additional TAAs [120], resulting in a larger antigen pool that, in turn, induces a more robust immune response.

As a therapeutic modality, cancer vaccines are unique in their ability to initiate a dynamic process of immune system activation, along with low toxicity and the potential for combination with lower-dose chemotherapy or radiotherapy. Ongoing phase II and III trials could establish the flexibility and efficacy of cancer vaccines, alone and in combination with other therapies, and support their use as standard-of-care therapy for numerous types of cancer.

ACKNOWLEDGMENT

The authors thank Bonnie L. Casey for editorial assistance in the preparation of this chapter.

REFERENCES

1. Kantoff PW, Schuetz TJ, Blumenstein BA et al. Overall survival analysis of a phase II randomized controlled trial of a poxviral-based PSA-targeted immunotherapy in metastatic castration-resistant prostate cancer. *J Clin Oncol* 2010;28:1099–1105.
2. Henry F, Boisteau O, Bretaudeau L et al. Antigen-presenting cells that phagocytose apoptotic tumor-derived cells are potent tumor vaccines. *Cancer Res* 1999;59:3329–3332.
3. Schlom J. Therapeutic cancer vaccines: Current status and moving forward. *J Natl Cancer Inst* 2012;104:599–613.
4. Disis ML, Wallace DR, Gooley TA et al. Concurrent trastuzumab and HER2/neu-specific vaccination in patients with metastatic breast cancer. *J Clin Oncol* 2009; 27:4685–4692.
5. Kufe DW. Mucins in cancer: Function, prognosis and therapy. *Nat Rev Cancer* 2009;9:874–885.
6. Raina D, Kosugi M, Ahmad R et al. Dependence on the MUC1-C oncoprotein in non-small cell lung cancer cells. *Mol Cancer Ther* 2011;10:806–816.
7. Adams S. Toll-like receptor agonists in cancer therapy. *Immunotherapy* 2009;1:949–964.
8. Gnjatic S, Ritter E, Buchler MW et al. Seromic profiling of ovarian and pancreatic cancer. *Proc Natl Acad Sci USA* 2010;107:5088–5093.
9. Kim DW, Krishnamurthy V, Bines SD et al. TroVax, a recombinant modified vaccinia Ankara virus encoding 5T4: Lessons learned and future development. *Hum Vaccin* 2010;6:784–791.
10. Madan RA, Aragon-Ching JB, Gulley JL et al. From clinical trials to clinical practice: Therapeutic cancer vaccines for the treatment of prostate cancer. *Expert Rev Vac* 2011;10:743–753.
11. Boni A, Muranski P, Cassard L et al. Adoptive transfer of allogeneic tumor-specific T cells mediates effective regression of large tumors across major histocompatibility barriers. *Blood* 2008;112:4746–4754.
12. Gnjatic S, Nishikawa H, Jungbluth AA et al. NY-ESO-1: Review of an immunogenic tumor antigen. *Adv Cancer Res* 2006;95:1–30.
13. Karbach J, Neumann A, Atmaca A et al. Efficient in vivo priming by vaccination with recombinant NY-ESO-1 protein and CpG in antigen naive prostate cancer patients. *Clin Cancer Res* 2011;17:861–870.
14. Dyrskjot L, Zieger K, Kissow Lildal T et al. Expression of MAGE-A3, NY-ESO-1, LAGE-1 and PRAME in urothelial carcinoma. *Br J Cancer* 2012;107:116–122.
15. Shay JW, Keith WN. Targeting telomerase for cancer therapeutics. *Br J Cancer* 2008; 98:677–683.
16. Ning N, Pan Q, Zheng F et al. Cancer stem cell vaccination confers significant antitumor immunity. *Cancer Res* 2012;72:1853–1864.
17. Azvolinsky A. Cancer stem cells: Getting to the root of cancer. *J Natl Cancer Inst* 2012;104:893–895.
18. Palena C, Fernando RI, Litzinger MT et al. Strategies to target molecules that control the acquisition of a mesenchymal-like phenotype by carcinoma cells. *Exp Biol Med (Maywood)* 2011;236:537–545.
19. Palena C, Polev DE, Tsang KY et al. The human T-box mesodermal transcription factor Brachyury is a candidate target for T-cell-mediated cancer immunotherapy. *Clin Cancer Res* 2007;13:2471–2478.
20. Roselli M, Fernando RI, Guadagni F et al. Brachyury, a driver of the epithelial-mesenchymal transition, is overexpressed in human lung tumors: An opportunity for novel interventions against lung cancer. *Clin Cancer Res* 2012;18:3868–3879.
21. Madan RA, Mohebtash M, Arlen PM et al. Ipilimumab and a poxviral vaccine targeting prostate-specific antigen in metastatic castration-resistant prostate cancer: A phase 1 dose-escalation trial. *Lancet Oncol* 2012;13:501–508.

22. Fernando RI, Litzinger M, Trono P et al. The T-box transcription factor Brachyury promotes epithelial-mesenchymal transition in human tumor cells. *J Clin Invest* 2010; 120:533–544.

23. Hamilton DH, Litzinger MT, Fernando RI et al. Cancer vaccines targeting the epithelial-mesenchymal transition: Tissue distribution of brachyury and other drivers of the mesenchymal-like phenotype of carcinomas. *Semin Oncol* 2012;39:358–366.

24. Fernando RI, Castillo MD, Litzinger M et al. IL-8 signaling plays a critical role in the epithelial-mesenchymal transition of human carcinoma cells. *Cancer Res* 2011;71:5296–5306.

25. Open Label Study to Evaluate the Safety and Tolerability of GI-6301 a Vaccine Consisting of Whole Heat-Killed Recombinant Yeast Genetically Modified to Express Brachyury Protein in Adults With Solid Tumors. [October 03, 2012]; Available from: http://clinicaltrials.gov/ct2/show/NCT01519817?term=brachyury&rank=1.

26. Xiang R, Luo Y, Niethammer AG et al. Oral DNA vaccines target the tumor vasculature and microenvironment and suppress tumor growth and metastasis. *Immunol Rev* 2008;222:117–128.

27. Kaplan CD, Kruger JA, Zhou H et al. A novel DNA vaccine encoding PDGFRbeta suppresses growth and dissemination of murine colon, lung and breast carcinoma. *Vaccine* 2006;24:6994–7002.

28. VXM01 Phase I Dose Escalation Study in Patients with Locally Advanced, Inoperable and Stage IV Pancreatic Cancer. [August 27, 2012]; Available from: http://clinicaltrials.gov/ct2/show/NCT01486329?term=VXM01&rank=1.

29. Pejawar-Gaddy S, Rajawat Y, Hilioti Z et al. Generation of a tumor vaccine candidate based on conjugation of a MUC1 peptide to polyionic papillomavirus virus-like particles. *Cancer Immunol Immunother* 2010;59:1685–1696.

30. Finn OJ, Gantt KR, Lepisto AJ et al. Importance of MUC1 and spontaneous mouse tumor models for understanding the immunobiology of human adenocarcinomas. *Immunol Res* 2011;50:261–268.

31. Palucka K, Ueno H, Fay J et al. Dendritic cells and immunity against cancer. *J Intern Med* 2011;269:64–73.

32. Kantoff PW, Higano CS, Shore ND et al. Sipuleucel-T immunotherapy for castration-resistant prostate cancer. *N Engl J Med* 2010;363:411–422.

33. Inoges S, Rodriguez-Calvillo M, Zabalegui N et al. Clinical benefit associated with idiotypic vaccination in patients with follicular lymphoma. *J Natl Cancer Inst* 2006; 98:1292–1301.

34. Lindenmann J. Speculations on idiotypes and homobodies. *Ann Immunol (Paris)* 1973; 124:171–184.

35. Jerne NK. Towards a network theory of the immune system. *Ann Immunol (Paris)* 1974;125C:373–389.

36. Schuster SJ, Neelapu SS, Gause BL et al. Vaccination with patient-specific tumor-derived antigen in first remission improves disease-free survival in follicular lymphoma. *J Clin Oncol* 2011;29:2787–2794.

37. Bendandi M. Idiotype vaccines for lymphoma: Proof-of-principles and clinical trial failures. *Nat Rev Cancer* 2009;9:675–681.

38. Moss B. Genetically engineered poxviruses for recombinant gene expression, vaccination, and safety. *Proc Natl Acad Sci USA* 1996;93:11341–11348.

39. Hodge JW, Higgins J, Schlom J. Harnessing the unique local immunostimulatory properties of modified vaccinia Ankara (MVA) virus to generate superior tumor-specific immune responses and antitumor activity in a diversified prime and boost vaccine regimen. *Vaccine* 2009;27:4475–4482.

40. Hodge JW, Grosenbach DW, Aarts WM et al. Vaccine therapy of established tumors in the absence of autoimmunity. *Clin Cancer Res* 2003;9:1837–1849.

41. MacDonald GH, Johnston RE. Role of dendritic cell targeting in Venezuelan equine encephalitis virus pathogenesis. *J Virol* 2000;74:914–922.
42. Okur FV, Yvon E, Biagi E et al. Comparison of two CD40-ligand/interleukin-2 vaccines in patients with chronic lymphocytic leukemia. *Cytotherapy* 2011;13:1128–1139.
43. Remondo C, Cereda V, Mostbock S et al. Human dendritic cell maturation and activation by a heat-killed recombinant yeast (*Saccharomyces cerevisiae*) vector encoding carcinoembryonic antigen. *Vaccine* 2009;27:987–994.
44. Wansley EK, Chakraborty M, Hance KW et al. Vaccination with a recombinant *Saccharomyces cerevisiae* expressing a tumor antigen breaks immune tolerance and elicits therapeutic antitumor responses. *Clin Cancer Res* 2008;14:4316–4325.
45. Singh R, Paterson Y. Listeria monocytogenes as a vector for tumor-associated antigens for cancer immunotherapy. *Expert Rev Vac* 2006;5:541–552.
46. Fioretti D, Iurescia S, Fazio VM et al. DNA vaccines: Developing new strategies against cancer. *J Biomed Biotechnol* 2010;2010:174378.
47. Coban C, Koyama S, Takeshita F et al. Molecular and cellular mechanisms of DNA vaccines. *Hum Vaccin* 2008;4:453–456.
48. Hoover HC, Jr., Brandhorst JS, Peters LC et al. Adjuvant active specific immunotherapy for human colorectal cancer: 6.5-year median follow-up of a phase III prospectively randomized trial. *J Clin Oncol* 1993;11:390–399.
49. Avigan D, Vasir B, Gong J et al. Fusion cell vaccination of patients with metastatic breast and renal cancer induces immunological and clinical responses. *Clin Cancer Res* 2004;10:4699–4708.
50. Laheru D, Lutz E, Burke J et al. Allogeneic granulocyte macrophage colony-stimulating factor-secreting tumor immunotherapy alone or in sequence with cyclophosphamide for metastatic pancreatic cancer: A pilot study of safety, feasibility, and immune activation. *Clin Cancer Res* 2008;14:1455–1463.
51. Lutz E, Yeo CJ, Lillemoe KD et al. A lethally irradiated allogeneic granulocyte-macrophage colony stimulating factor-secreting tumor vaccine for pancreatic adenocarcinoma. A Phase II trial of safety, efficacy, and immune activation. *Ann Surg* 2011; 253:328–335.
52. Emens LA, Asquith JM, Leatherman JM et al. Timed sequential treatment with cyclophosphamide, doxorubicin, and an allogeneic granulocyte-macrophage colony-stimulating factor-secreting breast tumor vaccine: A chemotherapy dose-ranging factorial study of safety and immune activation. *J Clin Oncol* 2009;27:5911–5918.
53. Dalgleish AG. Therapeutic cancer vaccines: Why so few randomised phase III studies reflect the initial optimism of phase II studies. *Vaccine* 2011;29:8501–8505.
54. Copier J, Dalgleish A. Whole-cell vaccines: A failure or a success waiting to happen? *Curr Opin Mol Ther* 2010;12:14–20.
55. Hoos A, Eggermont AM, Janetzki S et al. Improved endpoints for cancer immunotherapy trials. *J Natl Cancer Inst* 2010;102:1388–1397.
56. Stein WD, Gulley JL, Schlom J et al. Tumor regression and growth rates determined in five intramural NCI prostate cancer trials: The growth rate constant as an indicator of therapeutic efficacy. *Clin Cancer Res* 2011;17:907–17.
57. Hoos A, Parmiani G, Hege K et al. A clinical development paradigm for cancer vaccines and related biologics. *J Immunother* 2007;30:1–15.
58. Disis ML. Immunologic biomarkers as correlates of clinical response to cancer immunotherapy. *Cancer Immunol Immunother* 2011;60:433–442.
59. Butterfield LH, Palucka AK, Britten CM et al. Recommendations from the iSBTc-SITC/FDA/NCI Workshop on Immunotherapy Biomarkers. *Clin Cancer Res* 2011; 17:3064–3076.
60. Gulley JL, Arlen PM, Madan RA et al. Immunologic and prognostic factors associated with overall survival employing a poxviral-based PSA vaccine in metastatic castrate-resistant prostate cancer. *Cancer Immunol Immunother* 2010;59:663–674.

61. Kudo-Saito C, Schlom J, Hodge JW. Induction of an antigen cascade by diversified sub-cutaneous/intratumoral vaccination is associated with antitumor responses. *Clin Cancer Res* 2005;11:2416–2426.
62. Madan RA, Gulley JL, Fojo T et al. Therapeutic cancer vaccines in prostate cancer: The paradox of improved survival without changes in time to progression. *Oncologist* 2010;15:969–975.
63. Gulley JL, Madan RA, Schlom J. Impact of tumour volume on the potential efficacy of therapeutic vaccines. *Curr Oncol* 2011;18:e150–e157.
64. Madan RA, Mohebtash M, Schlom J et al. Therapeutic vaccines in metastatic castration-resistant prostate cancer: Principles in clinical trial design. *Expert Opin Biol Ther* 2010;10:19–28.
65. Halabi S, Small EJ, Kantoff PW et al. Prognostic model for predicting survival in men with hormone-refractory metastatic prostate cancer. *J Clin Oncol* 2003;21:1232–1237.
66. Higano CS, Schellhammer PF, Small EJ et al. Integrated data from 2 randomized, double-blind, placebo-controlled, phase 3 trials of active cellular immunotherapy with sipuleucel-T in advanced prostate cancer. *Cancer* 2009;115:3670–3679.
67. Hodge JW, Chakraborty M, Kudo-Saito C et al. Multiple costimulatory modalities enhance CTL avidity. *J Immunol* 2005;174:5994–6004.
68. Hodge JW, Sabzevari H, Yafal AG et al. A triad of costimulatory molecules synergize to amplify T-cell activation. *Cancer Res* 1999;59:5800–5807.
69. Dzutsev AH, Belyakov IM, Isakov DV et al. Avidity of CD8 T cells sharpens immuno-dominance. *Int Immunol* 2007;19:497–507.
70. Tsang KY, Palena C, Gulley J et al. A human cytotoxic T-lymphocyte epitope and its agonist epitope from the nonvariable number of tandem repeat sequence of MUC-1. *Clin Cancer Res* 2004;10:2139–2149.
71. Palena C, Schlom J, Tsang KY. Differential gene expression profiles in a human T-cell line stimulated with a tumor-associated self-peptide versus an enhancer agonist peptide. *Clin Cancer Res* 2003;9:1616–1627.
72. Terasawa H, Tsang KY, Gulley J et al. Identification and characterization of a human agonist cytotoxic T-lymphocyte epitope of human prostate-specific antigen. *Clin Cancer Res* 2002;8:41–53.
73. Salazar E, Zaremba S, Arlen PM et al. Agonist peptide from a cytotoxic t-lymphocyte epitope of human carcinoembryonic antigen stimulates production of tc1-type cyto-kines and increases tyrosine phosphorylation more efficiently than cognate peptide. *Int J Cancer* 2000;85:829–838.
74. Clay TM, Custer MC, McKee MD et al. Changes in the fine specificity of gp100(209–217)-reactive T cells in patients following vaccination with a peptide modified at an HLA-A2.1 anchor residue. *J Immunol* 1999;162:1749–1755.
75. Gulley J, Arlen PM, Dahut WL et al. A pilot study of a PANVAC-V and PANVAC-F in patients (pts) with metastatic carcinoma. *J Clin Oncol* 2006;24(18S):abstr 2512.
76. Cheever MA. Twelve immunotherapy drugs that could cure cancers. *Immunol Rev* 2008;222:357–368.
77. Grosenbach DW, Barrientos JC, Schlom J et al. Synergy of vaccine strategies to amplify antigen-specific immune responses and antitumor effects. *Cancer Res* 2001;61:4497–4505.
78. Boehm AL, Higgins J, Franzusoff A et al. Concurrent vaccination with two distinct vaccine platforms targeting the same antigen generates phenotypically and functionally distinct T-cell populations. *Cancer Immunol Immunother* 2010;59:397–408.
79. Gulley JL, Arlen PM, Hodge JW et al. Vaccines and immunostimulants. In: Hong W, editor. *Cancer Medicine*, vol. 8. Shelton, CT: AACR; 2010. pp. 725–736.
80. Burchill MA, Yang J, Vang KB et al. Interleukin-2 receptor signaling in regulatory T cell development and homeostasis. *Immunol Lett* 2007;114:1–8.

81. Becker TC, Wherry EJ, Boone D et al. Interleukin 15 is required for proliferative renewal of virus-specific memory CD8 T cells. *J Exp Med* 2002;195:1541–1548.
82. Marshall JL, Hoyer RJ, Toomey MA et al. Phase I study in advanced cancer patients of a diversified prime-and-boost vaccination protocol using recombinant vaccinia virus and recombinant nonreplicating avipox virus to elicit anti-carcinoembryonic antigen immune responses. *J Clin Oncol* 2000;18:3964–3973.
83. Borrello IM, Levitsky HI, Stock W et al. Granulocyte-macrophage colony-stimulating factor (GM-CSF)-secreting cellular immunotherapy in combination with autologous stem cell transplantation (ASCT) as postremission therapy for acute myeloid leukemia (AML). *Blood* 2009;114:1736–1745.
84. Greiner JW, Guadagni F, Goldstein D et al. Intraperitoneal administration of interferon-gamma to carcinoma patients enhances expression of tumor-associated glycoprotein-72 and carcinoembryonic antigen on malignant ascites cells. *J Clin Oncol* 1992;10:735–746.
85. Greiner JW, Guadagni F, Noguchi P et al. Recombinant interferon enhances monoclonal antibody-targeting of carcinoma lesions in vivo. *Science* 1987;235:895–898.
86. Greiner JW, Hand PH, Noguchi P et al. Enhanced expression of surface tumor-associated antigens on human breast and colon tumor cells after recombinant human leukocyte alpha-interferon treatment. *Cancer Res* 1984;44:3208–3214.
87. Shusterman S, London WB, Gillies SD et al. Antitumor activity of hu14.18-IL2 in patients with relapsed/refractory neuroblastoma: A Children's Oncology Group (COG) phase II study. *J Clin Oncol* 2010;28:4969–4975.
88. Zaharoff DA, Rogers CJ, Hance KW et al. Chitosan solution enhances the immunoadjuvant properties of GM-CSF. *Vaccine* 2007;25:8673–8686.
89. Hodi FS, O'Day SJ, McDermott DF et al. Improved survival with ipilimumab in patients with metastatic melanoma. *N Engl J Med* 2010;363:711–723.
90. Chakraborty M, Schlom J, Hodge JW. The combined activation of positive costimulatory signals with modulation of a negative costimulatory signal for the enhancement of vaccine-mediated T-cell responses. *Cancer Immunol Immunother* 2007;56:1471–1484.
91. Madan RA, Mohebtash M, Arlen PM et al. Overall survival (OS) analysis of a phase 1 trial of a vector-based vaccine (PSA-TRICOM) and ipilimumab (Ipi) in the treatment of metastatic castration-resistant prostate cancer (mCRPC). *J Clin Oncol* 2010;28(15S):abstr 2550.
92. Brahmer JR, Drake CG, Wollner I et al. Phase I study of single-agent anti-programmed death-1 (MDX-1106) in refractory solid tumors: Safety, clinical activity, pharmacodynamics, and immunologic correlates. *J Clin Oncol* 2010;28:3167–3175.
93. Kline J, Gajewski TF. Clinical development of mAbs to block the PD1 pathway as an immunotherapy for cancer. *Curr Opin Investig Drugs* 2010;11:1354–1359.
94. Litzinger MT, Fernando R, Curiel TJ et al. IL-2 immunotoxin denileukin diftitox reduces regulatory T cells and enhances vaccine-mediated T-cell immunity. *Blood* 2007; 110:3192–3201.
95. Morris JC, Shapiro GI, Tan AR et al. Phase I/II study of GC1008: A human anti-transforming growth factor-beta (TGFβ) monoclonal antibody (MAb) in patients with advanced malignant melanoma (MM) or renal cell carcinoma (RCC). *J Clin Oncol* 2008; 26(May 20 Suppl):abstr 9028.
96. Zitvogel L, Kroemer G. Anticancer immunochemotherapy using adjuvants with direct cytotoxic effects. *J Clin Invest* 2009;119:2127–2130.
97. Kepp O, Galluzzi L, Martins I et al. Molecular determinants of immunogenic cell death elicited by anticancer chemotherapy. *Cancer Metastasis Rev* 2011;30:61–69.
98. Kwilas A, Donahue R, Bernstein M et al. In the field: Exploiting the untapped potential of immunogenic modulation by radiation in combination with immunotherapy for the treatment of cancer. *Front Oncol* 2012;2:104.

99. Hodge JW, Ardiani A, Farsaci B et al. The tipping point for combination therapy: Cancer vaccines with radiation, chemotherapy, or targeted small molecule inhibitors. *Semin Oncol* 2012;39:323–339.

100. Garnett CT, Schlom J, Hodge JW. Combination of docetaxel and recombinant vaccine enhances T-cell responses and antitumor activity: Effects of docetaxel on immune enhancement. *Clin Cancer Res* 2008;14:3536–3544.

101. Chakraborty M, Gelbard A, Carrasquillo JA et al. Use of radiolabeled monoclonal antibody to enhance vaccine-mediated antitumor effects. *Cancer Immunol Immunother* 2008;57:1173–1183.

102. Gelbard A, Garnett CT, Abrams SI et al. Combination chemotherapy and radiation of human squamous cell carcinoma of the head and neck augments CTL-mediated lysis. *Clin Cancer Res* 2006;12:1897–1905.

103. Chakraborty M, Wansley EK, Carrasquillo JA et al. The use of chelated radionuclide (samarium-153-ethylenediaminetetramethylenephosphonate) to modulate phenotype of tumor cells and enhance T cell-mediated killing. *Clin Cancer Res* 2008;14:4241–4249.

104. Arlen PM, Gulley JL, Parker C et al. A randomized phase II study of concurrent docetaxel plus vaccine versus vaccine alone in metastatic androgen-independent prostate cancer. *Clin Cancer Res* 2006;12:1260–1269.

105. Docetaxel Alone or in Combination with Vaccine to Treat Breast Cancer. [August 27, 2012]; Available from: http://clinicaltrials.gov/ct2/show/NCT00179309?term=docetaxel+vaccine+breast&rank=1.

106. 153Sm-EDTMP with or without a PSA/TRICOM Vaccine to Treat Men with Androgen-Insensitive Prostate Cancer. [August 27, 2012]; Available from: http://clinicaltrials.gov/ct2/show/NCT00450619

107. Fridman WH, Galon J, Pages F et al. Prognostic and predictive impact of intra- and peritumoral immune infiltrates. *Cancer Res* 2011;71:5601–5605.

108. Corral LG, Haslett PA, Muller GW et al. Differential cytokine modulation and T cell activation by two distinct classes of thalidomide analogues that are potent inhibitors of TNF-alpha. *J Immunol* 1999;163:380–386.

109. Farsaci B, Sabzevari H, Higgins JP et al. Effect of a small molecule BCL-2 inhibitor on immune function and use with a recombinant vaccine. *Int J Cancer* 2010; 127:1603–1613.

110. Bose A, Taylor JL, Alber S et al. Sunitinib facilitates the activation and recruitment of therapeutic anti-tumor immunity in concert with specific vaccination. *Int J Cancer* 2011;129:2158–2170.

111. Farsaci B, Higgins JP, Hodge JW. Consequence of dose scheduling of sunitinib on host immune response elements and vaccine combination therapy. *Int J Cancer* 2012; 130:1948–1959.

112. Schwartzentruber DJ, Lawson DH, Richards JM et al. gp100 peptide vaccine and interleukin-2 in patients with advanced melanoma. *N Engl J Med* 2011;364:2119–2127.

113. Mercader M, Bodner BK, Moser MT et al. T cell infiltration of the prostate induced by androgen withdrawal in patients with prostate cancer. *Proc Natl Acad Sci USA* 2001; 98:14565–14570.

114. Okada H, Kalinski P, Ueda R et al. Induction of CD8 + T-cell responses against novel glioma-associated antigen peptides and clinical activity by vaccinations with {alpha}-type 1 polarized dendritic cells and polyinosinic-polycytidylic acid stabilized by lysine and carboxymethylcellulose in patients with recurrent malignant glioma. *J Clin Oncol* 2011;29:330–336.

115. Morse M, Niedzwiecki D, Marshall J et al. Survival rates among patients vaccinated following resection of colorectal cancer metastases in a phase II randomized study compared with contemporary controls. *J Clin Oncol* 2011;29:abstr 3557.

116. Stein WD, Figg WD, Dahut W et al. Tumor growth rates derived from data for patients in a clinical trial correlate strongly with patient survival: A novel strategy for evaluation of clinical trial data. *Oncologist* 2008;13:1046–1054.
117. Stein WD, Yang J, Bates SE et al. Bevacizumab reduces the growth rate constants of renal carcinomas: A novel algorithm suggests early discontinuation of bevacizumab resulted in a lack of survival advantage. *Oncologist* 2008;13:1055–1062.
118. Huang Y, Yuan J, Righi E et al. Vascular normalizing doses of antiangiogenic treatment reprogram the immunosuppressive tumor microenvironment and enhance immunotherapy. *Proc Natl Acad Sci USA* 2012;109:17561–17566.
119. Eng C. Toxic effects and their management: Daily clinical challenges in the treatment of colorectal cancer. *Nat Rev Clin Oncol* 2009;6:207–218.
120. Garnett CT, Greiner JW, Tsang KY et al. TRICOM vector based cancer vaccines. *Curr Pharm Des* 2006;12:351–361.
121. Gilewski TA, Ragupathi G, Dickler M et al. Immunization of high-risk breast cancer patients with clustered sTn-KLH conjugate plus the immunologic adjuvant QS-21. *Clin Cancer Res* 2007;13:2977–2985.
122. Ragupathi G, Damani P, Srivastava G et al. Synthesis of sialyl Lewis(a) (sLe (a), CA19-9) and construction of an immunogenic sLe(a) vaccine. *Cancer Immunol Immunother* 2009;58:1397–1405.
123. Open Label Phase I Study to Evaluate the Safety and Tolerability of Vaccine (GI-6207) Consisting of Whole, Heat-Killed Recombinant Saccharomyces Cerevisiae Genetically Modified to Express CEA Protein in Adults with Metastatic CEA-Expressing Carcinoma. [October 03, 2012]; Available from: http://clinicaltrials.gov/ct2/show/record/NCT00924092?term=yeast-cea&rank=1.
124. Butts C, Murray N, Maksymiuk A et al. Randomized phase IIB trial of BLP25 liposome vaccine in stage IIIB and IV non-small-cell lung cancer. *J Clin Oncol* 2005;23:6674–6681.
125. Marshall JL, Gulley JL, Arlen PM et al. Phase I study of sequential vaccinations with fowlpox-CEA(6D)-TRICOM alone and sequentially with vaccinia-CEA(6D)-TRICOM, with and without granulocyte-macrophage colony-stimulating factor, in patients with carcinoembryonic antigen-expressing carcinomas. *J Clin Oncol* 2005;23:720–731.
126. Gnjatic S, Wheeler C, Ebner M et al. Seromic analysis of antibody responses in non-small cell lung cancer patients and healthy donors using conformational protein arrays. *J Immunol Methods* 2009;341:50–58.
127. Kaufman HL, Wang W, Manola J et al. Phase II randomized study of vaccine treatment of advanced prostate cancer (E7897): A trial of the Eastern Cooperative Oncology Group. *J Clin Oncol* 2004;22:2122–2132.
128. Kemp TJ, Hildesheim A, Safaeian M et al. HPV16/18 L1 VLP vaccine induces cross-neutralizing antibodies that may mediate cross-protection. *Vaccine* 2011;29:2011–2014.
129. Madan RA, Bilusic M, Heery C et al. Clinical evaluation of TRICOM vector therapeutic cancer vaccines. *Semin Oncol* 2012;39:296–304.
130. Hodge JW, Guha C, Neefjes J et al. Synergizing radiation therapy and immunotherapy for curing incurable cancers. Opportunities and challenges. *Oncology (Williston Park)* 2008;22:1064–1070; discussion 75, 80–81, 84.

17 Histone Deacetylase Inhibitors as Targeted Therapies

Alexandra Zimmer
National Cancer Institute

Arup R. Chakraborty
National Cancer Institute

Robert W. Robey
National Cancer Institute

Susan E. Bates
National Cancer Institute

CONTENTS

INTRODUCTION

Histone deacetylase inhibitors (HDIs) belong to the broader category of epigenetic agents, which also include the DNA methyltransferase inhibitors (5-azacytidine and decitabine), and several other agents in clinical development. Vorinostat and romidepsin were the first HDIs to be approved for the treatment of cancer and were approved based on their activity in T-cell lymphomas. Although these agents cause rapid and durable disease response in T-cell lymphoma, the mechanism underlying this is not entirely clear, as the agents induce an array of biological effects. Some of these have been studied for potential roles in combination therapies.

An octomer of histone proteins surrounded by 140 bp DNA form the nucleosome observed in chromatin as "beads on a string" [1]. The 5′ regions of the various histone proteins, inaccurately referred to as "histone tails," are lysine rich and classically thought to determine the accessibility of DNA to transcription factor complexes through modification of the recurring lysines and other amino acids by acetylation, methylation, and phosphorylation, among others. The precise sequence of these histone modifications is termed the "histone code." Increasingly, mutation, overexpression, or rearrangement of genes encoding proteins that control these modifications has been recognized as important in tumorigenesis. These findings have led to drug development efforts targeting the enzymes responsible [2]. This chapter will focus on agents that increase acetylation of histone proteins, through inhibition of histone deacetylase (HDAC) activity. Of unknown relative importance is the acetylation of nonhistone proteins that also follows HDAC inhibition.

HISTONE ACETYLTRANSFERASES

Histone acetylation on various target lysines is a posttranslational modification generally associated with gene expression. Histone acetyltransferases (HATs) are the enzymes that catalyze the addition of an acetyl group from acetyl CoA to conserved lysines to form ε-N-acetyl lysine. On the basis of sequence similarities, these enzymes are grouped into several families; the most extensively studied HAT families are GCN5-related N-acetyltransferase (GNAT), EIA binding protein p300/CREB-binding protein (p300/CBP), Moz, ybf2/Sas3, Sas2, Tip60 (MYST), and the Rtt109 family [3]. In complexes with other HATs, transcription co-activators, and co-repressors, HATs function to preferentially acetylate specific histone lysine substrates and induce gene-specific transcriptional activation [4–7]. Because these enzymes play a key role in the regulation of cell proliferation and differentiation, genetic alterations are implicated in carcinogenesis [8].

HISTONE DEACETYLASES

HDACs cause transcriptional repression of genes, in part, by deacetylation of the repeating lysine residues in the amino terminus of histones. In addition, the structure or stability of numerous cytoplasmic proteins is altered by acetylation. To date, 18 different human HDACs have been described and are divided into four classes based on homology with yeast proteins [9]. Class I, II, and IV HDACs require an active site zinc (Zn^{2+}) to carry out deacetylation, while class III HDACs require nicotinamide adenine dinucleotide (NAD^+) [2]. HDACs 1–3 and 8 are 40–55 kDa proteins, belong to class I, and are ubiquitously expressed [10]. HDACs 1–3 are localized in the nucleus, while HDAC 8 is located in both cytoplasm and nucleus [9]. The class I HDACs are involved in many cellular processes including development, proliferation, cell cycle progress, DNA damage response, and smooth muscle differentiation [11–14]. Class II HDACs are 70–130 kDa proteins and are further subdivided into classes IIa and IIb. HDAC4, 5, 7, and 9 belong to class IIa, whereas HDAC6 and 10 are of class IIb. These HDACs are expressed in a tissue-specific manner, localizing to both nucleus and cytoplasm. HDAC6 is primarily localized in the cytoplasm. Class III HDACs, also known as sirtuins, are structurally similar to yeast SirT2 and require NAD^+ as a cofactor for enzymatic activity [15]. This class of HDAC is associated with deacetylation of histone and nonhistone proteins or transcription factors including p53 and c-myc [16,17]. The only known HDAC of class IV is the nuclear HDAC11 [9].

HATs AND HDACs IN CANCER

With the increasing genomic data available for cancers, it has become clear that genes encoding proteins regulating chromatin, including histone-modifying enzymes, are often mutated or aberrantly expressed. While it is tempting to view these changes as oncogenic, it is likely that many of the aberrations are permissive, with mutation required to avoid normal regulatory controls. Table 17.1 lists some of the genetic alterations identified in HDAC and HAT enzymes. Interestingly, mutation of HATs is common, while mutation of HDACs appears to be rare. Overexpression of HDACs is pro-oncogenic, resulting in transcriptional quiescence of genes involved in differentiation, apoptosis, and cell cycle arrest [2,18]. HAT enzymes function in opposition to the HDACs. The classical explanation that lysine acetylation allows relaxation of DNA thereby increasing accessibility is being replaced by a more nuanced understanding in which specific modifications of specific residues constitute an epigenetic code that can be read by bridging or chromatin-modifying proteins. Acetylation sites are read by proteins with bromodomains. Many cancers display molecular alterations that diminish or dampen HAT activity or shift the balance toward HDAC activity. Chromosomal translocations involving HAT proteins are frequent in leukemias and lymphomas, and inactivating mutations have been identified in colorectal, breast, and ovarian cancer [19–22].

Increasing information regarding the histone code makes it clear that the mechanisms regulating gene transcription are quite complex. Histone acetylation appears to give a general "go" signal, while histone methylation provides greater specificity. For example, among lysines found on the histone H3 tail, K4 methylation is associated with gene activation and transcription, K9 methylation with gene repression and inactivation, K27 methylation with repression—but also found to be associated with K4 acetylation such that genes bearing this mark may be "poised" for transcription—and K79 methylation associated with transcriptional elongation [23]. These lysines are candidates for mono-, di-, or trimethylation, as well as for

TABLE 17.1

Evidence of Altered Histone Acetyl Transferase (HAT) or Histone Deacetylase (HDAC) Activity in Cancer

HAT/HDAC	Molecular Abnormality	Chromosomal Abnormality (Gene Product)	Cancer	Reference
CBP (CREB-binding proteins)	Point mutations, translocations and micro-deletions	16p13.3	Neural Crest and developmental Ca[a]	[174]
	Fusion	t(11;16) MLL/CBP	MDS	[175]
	Fusion	t(11;16) MLL/CBP	AML	[20]
	Fusion	t(8;16) MOZ-CBP	M4/5 AML	[176]
	Inactivating mutation		Relapsed acute lymphoblastic leukemia	[177]
	Inactivating mutation		Diffuse large B cell lymphoma	[178]
	Inactivating mutation		Follicular lymphoma	[178]
	Truncation mutation		Ovarian Ca	[22]
p300	Fusion	t(11;22) MLL/p300	t(11;22) AML	[19]
	Mutations and LOH	22q13	Gastric (intestinal type)	[179]
	Mutations, Deletions		B-cell non-Hodgkin lymphoma	[178]
	Insertion		Breast Ca colorectal Ca	[21]
	Missense mutation			
TIP 60	Underexpression		Colorectal Ca	[180]
HDAC1	Recruitment	t(15;17) RARa-PML t(11;17) RARz-PLZF	APL APL	[181]
	Recruitment	t(8;21) AML1-ETO	AML	[182]
HDAC2	Mutation		Polyps and colorectal Ca	[183]
HDAC4	Somatic Mutation		Breast Ca	[184]

[a] Rubinstein–Taybi syndrome with increased risk of oligodendroglioma, medulloblastoma, neuroblastoma, benign meningioma, pheochromocytoma, nasal rhabdomyosarcoma, leiomyosarcoma, seminoma, and embryonal carcinoma.

acetylation, and are thus points at which there may be constraints on gene modulation induced by acetylation.

HDAC INHIBITORS

HDIs were first described as differentiating agents, and studied together with agents such as retinoic acid that were able to block cell growth and increase the expression of markers of differentiation. A number of the HDIs in clinical development (as defined by trials listed in http://www.clinicaltrials.gov) are provided in Table 17.2, and structures of many of these agents are provided in Figure 17.1. Many HDIs are structurally unrelated, but generally contain a zinc-binding domain, a capping group, and a linker [24].

The first class of agents recognized as HDAC inhibitors and tested clinically were the short-chain and aromatic fatty acids, sodium butyrate [25], phenylbutyrate [26], and valproic acid [27]. Sodium phenylbutyrate has been approved for the treatment of urea cycle disorders and valproic acid for seizure disorders, bipolar disorders, and in migraine prophylaxis. The short-chain fatty acids are far less potent than the HDIs in development or approved for use in oncology.

TABLE 17.2
HDIs Currently in Clinical Trials

Class	Compound	HDAC Specificity	Clinical Trial Stage
Aliphatic acids	Valproic acid	Classes I and IIa	Phase II, as a single agent or in combination
Hydroxamic acids	Vorinostat (SAHA)	Pan-inhibitor	Approved for CTCL, phase III alone or phase I/II in combination
	Panobinostat (LBH589)	Classes I and II	Phase III, as a single agent or in combination
	Belinostat (PDX-101)	Pan-inhibitor	Phase II, as a single agent or in combination
	Resminostat (4SC-201)	Pan-inhibitor	Phase II, as a single agent or in combination
	Abexinostat (PCI24781)	Classes I and II	Phase II alone, phase I in combination
	JNJ-26481585	Class I	Phase I in combination
	ACY-1215	Class II, HDAC 6	Phase II as a single agent or in phase I in combination
Benzamides	AR-42	Pan-inhibitor	Phase I as a single agent
	Entinostat (MS-275)	Class I	Phase I as a single agent or in combination
	4SC-202	Class I	As a single agent in phase I
Cyclic peptide	Romidepsin	Class I	Approved for CTCL and PTCL, phase III as a single agent or in combination

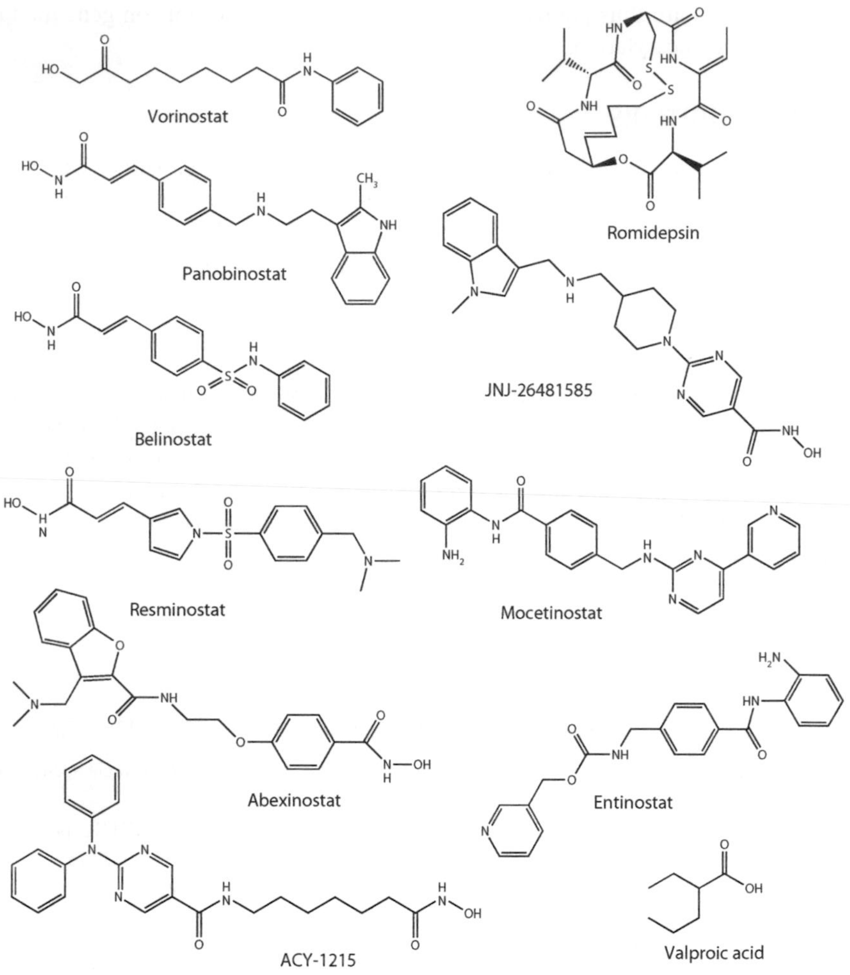

FIGURE 17.1 Chemical structures of selected HDIs.

The discovery of vorinostat began with the observation that dimethyl sulfoxide induced the synthesis of hemoglobin and differentiation of murine erythroleukemia cells [28]. Screening of related polar compounds led to the selection of vorinostat as the lead compound [29]. Vorinostat (suberoylanilide hydroxamic acid [SAHA]) is structurally similar to trichostatin A and belongs to the hydroxamic acid class of HDIs that includes abexinostat (PCI-24781), givinostat (ITF2357), panobinostat (LBH589), and belinostat (PXD101). The hydroxamic acids are generally active against both class I and II HDACs. As discussed subsequently, the class II HDACs are involved in deacetylation of a number of cytoplasmic proteins. Indeed, ACY-1215 is a hydroxamic acid derivative being developed specifically to target HDAC6 [30]. It seems probable that differences in clinical activity will exist among compounds with different inhibitory profiles.

Romidepsin (also FK228 and depsipeptide) is a bicyclic peptide isolated from the fermentation broth of *Chromobacterium violaceum* [31,32]. Clinical development at the National Cancer Institute was initiated following studies by the NCI drug screen that revealed a unique cytotoxicity profile among the 60-cell line panel. The disulfide bond of romidepsin must be reduced to yield the drug's active form [33]. Romidepsin is able to inhibit both class I and class II HDACs, but the high potency against the class I HDACs makes it predominantly a class I inhibitor. The benzamide class of HDIs, including entinostat (MS-275), tacedinaline (CI-994), and mocetinostat (MGCD0103), inhibit only class I HDACs.

MECHANISM OF ACTION

While inhibition of the HDAC enzymes constitutes the therapeutic target, a myriad of downstream biological effects have been observed, and which one(s) constitute the dominant mechanism by which cell death is mediated is not known. These downstream effects target both proliferating and nonproliferating cells, preferentially affecting tumor cells over normal cells [34].

Indeed, the array of putative mechanisms highlights the fact that we do not know how HDIs induce cell death. One possibility is that a unifying mechanism of action exists—generalized effects on acetylation lead to aberrant gene transcription and cell death, depending on the readiness of the cell to undergo apoptosis. In this model, the cell senses aberrant gene expression as DNA damage. The limited activity of the HDIs in solid tumors, as opposed to hematological malignancies, would support this model. Another possibility is that cell death is due to one or more among the following mechanisms (or an as yet undescribed mechanism) creating an intolerable milieu for cell survival.

Effects on Gene Expression

The most commonly observed molecular effect of the HDIs is increased acetylation [35,36]. HDIs bind the HDAC enzymes, inhibit ongoing deacetylation, and allow acetylation by HATs. The classical mechanism of action posits that this increase in acetylation neutralizes the positively charged histone tails, decreasing the electrostatic forces with the negative DNA phosphate backbone, opening the chromatin, and providing increased transcription factor access to DNA [36]. This leads to increased transcription of, for example, *CDKN1A*, which encodes p21 and in turn causes cell cycle arrest [36]. Other genes, such as *CCND1*, show reduced expression. Indeed, studies of cancer cell lines using cDNA array have shown that the expression of only 2%–5% of genes is altered upon exposure to an HDI and that as many genes are repressed as induced [37–40]. Whether gene downregulation is a primary or secondary effect of the HDIs is a point of active investigation. Interestingly, a cell type-specific set of differentiation markers is often included among those upregulated. For example, the sodium–iodide symporter is increased in thyroid cancer cells [41], and fetal hemoglobin is induced in erythroleukemia cells [42].

Because gene transcription is physiologically much more complex, involving multiple transcription factors binding in a dynamic and highly regulated fashion, the extent to which the global acetylation following HDAC inhibition is responsible for gene induction and cell cycle arrest is not clear, nor is the contribution of acetylation to the stability or activity of transcription factors and nuclear hormone receptors [43,44].

Effects on Cell Cycle

HDIs typically arrest cells in the G2/M or G1/S phase of the cell cycle, or both [45,46], depending, in part, on whether or not cell cycle checkpoints are intact or activated. As noted earlier, G1/S phase arrest has been ascribed to p21 induction and cyclins D and A repression. Multiple other genes involved in cell cycle progression are also modulated [40,47,48]. Cell cycle arrest in G2 may also result from activation of mitotic checkpoints following HDI-mediated acetylation of pericentromeric chromatin and impairment of kinetochore assembly [49].

Release of Reactive Oxygen Species

Several studies have reported enhanced production of reactive oxygen species (ROS) as a mechanism of HDI cytotoxicity. Treatment of cancer cells with HDIs results in release of ROS followed by ceramide generation, mitochondrial injury, and activation of the apoptotic caspase cascade [50,51]. Free radical scavengers can prevent cellular apoptosis [50,51], supporting a ROS-mediated mechanism of cell death caused by HDIs.

Nonhistone Protein Acetylation

Acetylation of nonhistone proteins also occurs following inhibition of the cytoplasmic HDACs; some of these protein targets are listed in Table 17.3. In some cell types, this may be the principal mechanism of action. For example, following HDI exposure, acetylation of p53 is increased, reducing its proteasomal degradation, thereby increasing its activity [52]. Acetylation can alter the stability and function of multiple other proteins, including c-myc, pRb, and STAT-3 [24,53–57]. Tubulin is deacetylated by HDAC6, and HDAC6 inhibition promotes tubulin acetylation.

TABLE 17.3
Effects of HDIs on Nonhistone Proteins

Proteins	HDI Effects
STAT1 and STAT3	Phosphorylation is inhibited by acetylation [185,186]
p53	Acetylation activates DNA binding [187]
NF-kappaB	Enhance RelA/p65 acetylation leading to activation of NF-kappaB [56]
E2F	Acetylation facilitates transcription of proapoptotic proteins [188]
Rb	Causes dephosphorylation of Rb [45]
Ku70	Acetylation in DNA-binding domains diminishes DNA-repair ability [189]
Hsp90	ATP-binding ability as well as chaperone activity become impaired by acetylation [190]
RUNX3	Stability and transcriptional activity of RUNX3 is enhanced by acetylation [191]
Androgen receptor	Acetylation enhances binding with p300 [192]
Estrogen receptor alpha	Transcriptional activity is increased by acetylation [193]

We have shown that romidepsin acetylates histone proteins but not tubulin, at equipotent doses with vorinostat where tubulin is readily acetylated [58]. HDAC6 is also involved in the transport of ubiquitinated proteins to the aggresome, a pro-survival mechanism utilized in cells with an excess production of protein or in cells producing a mutated protein that fails to be properly processed [59].

Another nonhistone protein of interest undergoing acetylation is protein chaperone Hsp90 [60]. Acetylation of Hsp90 disrupts the interaction of the chaperone with its client proteins, which are then susceptible to degradation [61]. The long list of Hsp90 client proteins (http://www.picard.ch/downloads/Hsp90 interactors) includes many proteins implicated in cancer. Prominent client proteins include HER-2, the BCR-ABL fusion protein, mutant FLT-3, and mutant EGFR; cells dependent on the activity of these proteins are sensitive to both Hsp90 inhibitors and to HDIs [62–65]. Thus, HDIs may have particular efficacy where proliferation is controlled by an Hsp90 client protein, and where the HDI is able to disrupt that Hsp90-client protein interaction.

Inhibition of DNA Repair

HDIs disrupt DNA repair processes through acetylation or downregulation of repair proteins such as Ku70, Ku86, BRCA1, and RAD51. This is likely the mechanism of synergy between DNA damaging agents and HDIs when the two are used in combination [66,67]. Enhanced gamma-H2AX foci, associated with double-strand DNA repair, have been reported [68,69].

Apoptosis Induction

Apoptosis can proceed via the intrinsic, mitochondria-mediated pathway, or the extrinsic pathway, in which death receptors trigger apoptosis via a death-inducing signaling complex. HDIs upregulate one or more factors in this complex, including TRAIL, DR-5, DR-4, Fas, and Fas-L [70–72]. They may also downregulate c-FLIP [70,73], a protein associated with TRAIL resistance [74]. In the intrinsic pathway, cytochrome c release from mitochondria leads to activation of caspase 9, which activates caspase 3 and elicits apoptosis [75]. HDIs downregulate mitochondrial antiapoptotic proteins including BCL-2, Mcl-1, and BCL-XL and upregulate proapoptotic proteins such as Bax, Puma, and Noxa [64,76,77]. Upregulation of Bim may be a key event in mediating HDI-induced apoptosis [78].

FINAL COMMENTS ON MECHANISM OF ACTION

HDI mechanism of action likely depends upon specific cellular context. A T-cell lymphoma may find induction of death receptors intolerable and undergo rapid apoptosis. A cell with HER-2 amplification or epidermal growth factor pathway activation may undergo cell death following the loss of Hsp90 chaperone function and client protein degradation [61,64]. A myeloma cell filled with paraproteins may be more sensitive to the loss of HDAC6-mediated transport to the aggresome [79]. Thus, the various unique mechanisms offer a spectrum of possibilities for the use of HDIs in the clinic, and differing HDAC affinities may portend some selectivity for the different clinical settings.

HDIs IN CLINICAL TRIALS

Impressive responses to romidepsin in T-cell lymphoma, first reported by Piekarz et al. [80], were confirmed in subsequent phase II testing and extended to other HDIs, as shown in Table 17.4. To date, all HDIs tested have shown efficacy in cutaneous T-cell lymphoma (CTCL) [81–84], and both vorinostat and romidepsin received FDA approval for treatment of this disease. Romidepsin and belinostat have significant activity in peripheral T-cell lymphoma (PTCL), a heterogeneous class of mature T-cell lymphomas with a historically poor overall prognosis [84,85]; romidepsin received accelerated approval for this indication. Despite preclinical evidence for activity in both solid malignancies and hematological disorders, HDIs have had little success in trials of patients with solid malignancies, and the way forward appears to be in combination studies, as discussed in the subsequent sections.

SINGLE AGENT STUDIES

Vorinostat is approved for patients with advanced CTCL at an oral dose of 400 mg once daily [86]. The pivotal trial in CTCL enrolled 74 patients, 61 stage IIB or higher, and noted objective response and pruritus relief in 30% of patients, with a >6 month response duration [87]. Phase I trials also suggested some antitumor activity in B-cell non-Hodgkin and Hodgkin lymphomas [88–90]. However, activity in DLBCL was not sufficient to support continued development [91]. Phase I studies of vorinostat in other hematological malignancies such as acute myelogenous leukemia (AML), myelodysplastic syndrome (MDS), chronic lymphocytic leukemia (CLL), and multiple myeloma (MM) revealed activity that has been subsequently pursued in combination studies [92,93].

Romidepsin is approved for patients with CTCL who have received at least one prior systemic therapy at 14 mg/m^2 on days 1, 8, and 15 of a 28 day cycle. The first sign of activity in T-cell lymphoma was observed in the phase I study of romidepsin administered on days 1 and 5 of a 21 day cycle, at which the maximum tolerated dose (MTD) was 17.8 mg/m^2 [94,95]. Results in 4 of 10 patients subsequently enrolled were reported in 2001 [80], prior to the start of a phase II trial enrolling patients with either CTCL or PTCL. Ultimately, the schedule was changed to that first studied at Georgetown University [94,95]. Among 71 patients with CTCL, 4 patients achieved a complete response (CR) and 20 a partial response (PR), for an overall response rate of

TABLE 17.4
Activity against T-Cell Lymphomas Is a Class Effect for the HDIs

	Vorinostat (SAHA)	Romidepsin (Depsipeptide)	Panobinostat (LBH589)	Belinostat (PDX 101)
CTCL	24% (8/33) [82]	34% (24/71) [81]	17.3% (24/139) [195]	14% (4/29) [84]
	30% (22/74)(88)	35% (33/96) [194]	60% (6/10) [83]	
PTCL	—	38% (17/45) [85]	—	25% (5/20) [84]
		25% (33/130) [97]		

34% and a 13.7 month median response duration [81]. In an international trial, 6 of 96 patients enrolled experienced a CR and 27 patients a PR for an overall response rate of 34% [96]. Among 47 patients enrolled with PTCL in the NCI study, 7 had a CR and 11 patients a PR for an overall response rate of 38% and a 10.3 month median response duration [85]. Responses were noted in multiple T-cell lymphoma subtypes, in patients with multiple prior regimens, and in patients who were post stem-cell transplant. These results were confirmed in a pivotal trial that enrolled 130 patients with PTCL [97].

Responses in CTCL or PTCL have also been observed with panobinostat and belinostat [83,84]. In phase I/II studies with hematological malignancies, such as AML, and in refractory Hodgkin's disease, panobinostat demonstrated some antitumor activity [98,99]. Belinostat produced responses in PTCL [84], leading to a pivotal phase II study of belinostat in PTCL in which 129 patients have been enrolled (NCT00865969 at www.clinicaltrials.gov). Efficacy results are awaited. Mocetinostat has clinical activity in non-Hodgkin lymphoma (one CR and four PRs) [100] and in relapsed or refractory Hodgkin lymphoma (two CR and six PR in 23 evaluable patients). A phase II study of abexinostat in patients with follicular or mantle cell lymphoma gave promising results in follicular lymphoma with a 64% response rate and several durable responses [101], confirming results in an earlier phase I study [102].

Results in solid tumors have been much less promising. Vorinostat was tested in phase II trials in various solid tumors, including breast, colorectal, ovarian, head and neck, and thyroid cancer, as well as mesothelioma and glioblastoma multiforme, yielding few responses [103–108]. While romidepsin gave evidence of antileukemic effects in two AML trials [109,110], few responses were observed in patients with CLL, renal cell, prostate, colorectal, or lung cancer [111–115]. A phase I study of entinostat demonstrated an unexpected long half-life requiring change in schedule [116,117]. A prolonged PR was noted in one patient with melanoma [118], but no objective responses in melanoma were seen in a follow-up study [119]. As monotherapy, belinostat did not show significant activity in solid tumors, such as malignant pleural mesothelioma [120].

Given the low activity of HDIs in solid tumors, the way forward for exploiting the unique activities of this therapeutic class will be to combine HDIs with other agents. The question is which combinations are most likely to be effective and truly synergistic; numerous clinical trials testing "rational" combination approaches are already underway. It will be very important that these trials determine whether the molecular effect hypothesized to create synergy between two agents has actually occurred. To this end, laboratory correlates will be an essential component of future HDI clinical trials.

PHARMACODYNAMICS

Although there are no predictive markers for HDI efficacy to enable selection of patients for treatment, pharmacodynamic markers confirm inhibition of the HDACs. Increased histone acetylation is readily demonstrated in peripheral blood mononuclear cells (PMBCs) and post-treatment biopsies. Despite no standardized assay, remarkably similar levels of induced acetylation have been observed in PBMCs from patients treated with vorinostat [89], belinostat [121], panobinostat [83], romidepsin [122], and entinostat [118]. With romidepsin the one exception, acetylation levels have not correlated with response.

Our group demonstrated increased histone acetylation, increased gene expression, and an increase in hemoglobin F in samples obtained from patients with T-cell lymphoma treated with romidepsin [122]. *MDR1*, known to be directly upregulated by HDIs, was selected as a surrogate for gene induction. Induction of both acetylation and MDR1 gene expression was seen in most PBMC samples within 4 h of treatment, and in ≈40% of patients persisted to 24 h [122]. Most patients also had a greater than fourfold increase in hemoglobin F detected in red blood cells. Associating pharmacokinetic parameters and disease response with these biomarkers, we observed that induced histone acetylation correlated with C_{max} and AUC. Furthermore, the increase in histone acetylation in PBMCs at the 24 h time point correlated with response [122]. These data suggest that for romidepsin, a threshold may exist for drug activity; this could relate to the need to activate the pro-drug form. One implication of this observation is that lower drug levels could confer a pharmacologic mechanism of resistance.

Gene expression profiling using patient derived samples has been incorporated in some studies. Genes involved in apoptosis, cell proliferation, immune regulation, and angiogenesis are altered as early as 4 h after drug administration [83,92,115]. Notably, gene expression profiling studies have consistently shown that as many (or more) genes are downregulated as upregulated; microarray studies in the NCI samples revealed similar findings. The importance of these downregulated genes is not known.

TOXICITY

The toxicities of the HDIs appear to be class effects, implying that they are on-target effects of inhibiting the HDACs, since similar toxicity is observed with structurally different HDIs. The major side effects are fatigue, nausea and vomiting, and thrombocytopenia. Confirmation that these side effects are due to class I inhibition may come from the development of class II specific agents.

Anorexia, dysgeusia, nausea, and vomiting are common in patients receiving HDIs [89,95,121,123,124]. Antiemetic prophylaxis is standard supportive care for these agents, although it may be discontinued if symptoms are absent. The orally administered agents have additional gastrointestinal side effects including constipation or diarrhea [88,89,123]. Fatigue and occasional fever have been observed [89,95,121,124]; an increase in serum IL-6 levels may play a role in producing fatigue [121]. Leukopenia, granulocytopenia, and especially thrombocytopenia occur, but are rapidly reversible. No cumulative thrombocytopenia has been reported, and prolonged bone marrow suppression, such as that following cytotoxic therapy, has not been observed. Thrombocytopenia following panobinostat was recently attributed to impairment of megakaryocytic maturation mediated by tubulin acetylation [125].

The early development of HDIs, including romidepsin, was characterized by a concern about cardiac toxicity and QT prolongation [87,121,124,126–129]. Careful studies of this question have concluded that there are no major concerns regarding QT prolongation [130,131]. However, avoidance of concomitant use of agents that significantly prolong the QT (e.g., antiarrhythmics) is recommended. ECG changes, primarily ST and T wave changes, have been reported in clinical trials with the HDIs vorinostat, romidepsin, dacinostat, panobinostat, belinostat, and entinostat, and may be considered a class effect [129,132–136]. Cardiac assessments following romidepsin showed no impact on myocardial wall motion or on left ventricular ejection fraction, or serum troponin, despite the ECG changes [127,137].

While careful studies have shown no clinically significant cardiac abnormalities, atrial fibrillation was reported as a dose limiting toxicity in several phase I studies [95,112,120,121,124]. Potassium and magnesium monitoring and replacement prior to HDI therapy, as recommended in the package inserts for both vorinostat and romidepsin, have ensured a margin of safety. The authors observed that roughly half of patients with T-cell lymphoma require potassium or magnesium supplementation prior to romidepsin infusion [138]. Notably, *pre-study* ambulatory monitoring demonstrated significant ectopy in patients with T-cell lymphoma [127]. Clinical trials exclude patients with pre-existing cardiac disorders, long QT syndrome, or other risk factors for arrhythmia or sudden death, and package inserts for the approved agents recommend caution in these patient populations.

HDIs in Combination Therapy Trials

To exploit the promising preclinical activity of HDIs, the field has turned to the development of rational combination of HDIs with other agents based on one or more putative mechanisms of action to develop new approaches to solid tumors, overcome resistance mechanisms, or capitalize on preclinical evidence of synergy. A selection of these studies is shown in Tables 17.5 and 17.6.

Combination with other agents that affect gene expression has been attempted. Combination with DNMT inhibitors 5-azacytidine and decitabine, retinoids, and PPAR agonists showed encouraging but mixed results involving AML/MDS and combinations of valproate or mocetinostat with 5-azacytidine and/or ATRA [139–142]. Phase I and II trials evaluating advanced solid tumors, however, had more disappointing results combining HDIs with other epigenetic agents [143–145].

Cytotoxic agents combined with HDIs have been evaluated in phase I and II trials without great success except perhaps for hematologic malignancies. A phase II trial combining vorinostat with idarubicin and Ara-C for treatment of high-risk MDS or recently diagnosed AML reached an overall response rate of 85%, of which 76% were complete responses [146]. In advanced solid tumors, trials combining vorinostat with doxorubicin or 5-FU–leucovorin had poor responses [147,148]. Combination of belinostat with carboplatin, for ovarian and fallopian tube cancers showed an overall response rate of only 7.4% [149]. Another phase I and II study added paclitaxel to the combination of carboplatin with belinostat generating an overall response rate of 31% in patients previously treated with platinum-based regimens [150]. Considering that an active agent was combined with the HDIs, these numbers suggest that the preclinical evidence of synergy was not borne out in the clinic. However, the unknown factor in these studies is how refractory were the tumors in patients enrolled. No major responses were observed when HDIs (panobinostat and romidepsin) were added to gemcitabine [151,152]. These studies reported stable disease but without a randomized trial, the meaning of stable disease cannot be assessed. There was, however, important toxicity involving

TABLE 17.5

Selected Phase I Studies: HDIs in Combination with Other Therapies

HDI	Combined with	Diseases	Study	Results	Reference
Valproate sodium	Epirubicin	Advanced solid tumors	Phase I	PR 22%, SD 39%	[196]
	ATRA-liposomal	Advanced solid tumors	Phase I	SD 11%	[142]
Sodium phenylbutyrate	5-azacytidine	AML-MDS	Phase I	OR 28%	[197]
Vorinostat	Erlotinib	Erlotinib-refractory NSCLC with EGFR mutations	Phase I	6 of 9 SD	[154]
	Gemcitabine and cisplatin	Advanced NSCLC	Phase I	PR 47%, SD 42%	[198]
	FOLFOX	Advanced colorectal cancer	Phase I	SD 5 of 21	[199]
	13-cis-retinoic acid	Refractory neuroblastomas, medulloblastomas, primitive neuroectodermal tumors and atypical teratoid rhabdoid tumor	Phase I	No DLT's	[200]
	Doxorubicin	Advanced solid tumors	Phase I	PR 2, SD 2	[147]
	Bexarotene	Advanced CTCL	Phase I	OR 18%	[201]
	Bortezomib	Relapsed/refractory multiple myeloma	Phase I	Clinical benefit 32%, OR 42%	[202]
	5FU	Colorectal tumor	Phase I	MTD not obtained	[203]
	Radiation	Colorectal/stomach tumors	Phase I	PR 26%	[204]
	Bevacizumab and CPT-11	Glioblastoma	Phase I	PFS 3.6m, OS 7.3m	[205]

	Combination	Tumor type	Phase	Response	Ref.
	Idarubicin	Leukemias	Phase I	OR 17%	[206]
	5FU-LV	Advanced solid tumors	Phase I	SD 55% PR 2.6% (1 patient)	[207]
	Docetaxel	Advanced solid tumors	Phase I	No response Excessive toxicities	[208]
	Flavopiridol	Advanced solid tumors	Phase I	SD 19%	[209]
	Decitabine	Advanced solid tumors (n=39) and NHL (n=4)	Phase I	SD 29%	[145]
Romidepsin	Gemcitabine	Advanced solid tumors	Phase I	PR 7% SD 52%	[152]
Belinostat	Carboplatin and/or paclitaxel	Advanced solid tumors	Phase I	OR 13% CR 1/23, PR 2/23 SD 6/23	[210]
Mocetinostat	Gemcitabine	Advanced solid tumors	Phase I	PR 2/5 pancreatic cancer	[211]
Entinostat	13-cis-retinoic acid	Advanced solid tumors	Phase I	SD 37%	[143]
Panobinostat	Bevacizumab	Glioma	Phase I	PR 25% SD 58%	[212]
	Docetaxel (armB)	Prostate tumor	Phase I (parallel 2 arm)	PR 2/7 SD 4/7	[213]
	Gemcitabine	Advanced solid tumors	Phase I	SD 47%	[151]

Abbreviations: HDI, histone deacetylase inhibitors; OR, objective or overall response rate; CR, complete response/remission; SD, stable disease; PR, partial response/remission; CTCL, cutaneous T-cell lymphoma; NSCLC, non-small cell lung cancer; AML, acute myelogenous leukemia; MDS, myelodysplasia; ATRA, all-trans retinoic acid; FOLFOX, 5-fluorouracil, leucovorin and oxaliplatin; 5 FU, fluorouracil; 5FU-LV fluorouracil and leucovorin.

TABLE 17.6

Selected Phase II Studies: HDIs in Combination with Other Therapies

HDI	Combined with	Diseases	Study	Results	N	Reference
Valproate	5-aza-2'-ç-deoxycytidine	Advanced leukemia	Phase I/II	OR 22% CR 19%	54	[139]
	5-azacytidine and ATRA	AML-MDS	Phase I/II	OR 42%–52%	53	[141]
	Doxorubicin	Mesothelioma	Phase II	PR 16% SD 22%	45	[214]
Vorinostat	Carboplatin and paclitaxel	Advanced NSCLC	Phase II randomized placebo control trial	Confirmed response rates vorinostat 34%, placebo 12.5%	94	[152]
	Idarubicin and Ara-C	Advanced MDS or AML	Phase II	OR 85% CR 76%	75	[146]
	Paclitaxel and Bevacizumab	Breast tumor	Phase I/II	OR 49% SD 30%	54	[215]
	Tamoxifen	Breast tumor	Phase II	OR 19% SD 21%	43	[216]
	5FU-LV	Colorectal tumor	Phase II	2mo PFS 53%, 1 PR	58	[148]
	Bortezomib	Glioblastoma	Phase II	6mo PFS 0/37	38	[217]

Romidepsin	Bortezomib and dexamethasone	Relapsed or refractory multiple myeloma	Phase I/II	OR 72% CR 8% PR 52%	25	[156]
	Low-dose electron beam radiation	CTCL	Phase II	PR 4 of 5 patients	5	[218]
Belinostat	Carboplatin and paclitaxel	Relapsed epithelial ovarian cancer	Phase II	OR 31%	35	[150]
	Carboplatin	Ovary, fallopian, and primary peritoneal carcinoma	Phase II	OR 7.4% SD 44%	27	[149]
Mocetinostat	5-Azacytidine	Advanced MDS or AML	Phase I/II	OR 30% 11% CR	24	[140]
Entinostat	Erlotinib	Advanced NSCLC	Phase I Phase II	PR 1 SD 1 OR 3%	132	[155]
	5-Azacytidine	Relapsed NSCLC	Phase I/II	OR 6% SD 22%	45	[144]

Abbreviations: HDI, histone deacetylase inhibitors; OR, objective or overall response rate; CR, complete response/remission; SD, stable disease; PR, partial response/remission; VGPR, very good partial response/remission; CTCL, cutaneous T cell lymphoma; NSCLC, non-small cell lung cancer; AML, acute myelogenous leukemia; MDS, myelodysplasia; ATRA, all-trans retinoic acid; 5FU-LV fluorouracil and leucovorin.

TABLE 17.7
HDI Combinations Requiring Dose Reductions

HDI	Combined with	Diseases	Study	Results	Reference
Vorinostat	5FU	Colorectal tumor	Phase I	Terminated, excessive toxicity: myelosuppression/ gastrointestinal	[203]
	Docetaxel	Advanced solid tumors	Phase I	Terminated, excessive toxicity: myelosuppression/ gastrointestinal	[208]
Romidepsin	Gemcitabine	Advanced solid tumors	Phase I	Amendment for dose adjustment, excessive thrombocytopenia	[152]
Panobinostat	Gemcitabine	Advanced solid tumors	Phase I	Amendment for dose adjustment, excessive myelosuppression	[151]

myelosuppression and gastrointestinal symptoms. Because of major toxicity, treatment protocols in several studies had to be amended and initial planned doses downgraded (Table 17.7). This may indicate synergy in bone marrow cells—or a drug–drug interaction. Pharmacokinetic studies are needed to evaluate such combinations. The most promising result obtained so far was that in a phase I/II clinical trial with vorinostat combined with carboplatin and paclitaxel in the treatment of advanced NSCLC. A randomized phase II study against placebo found response rates of 34% vs. 12.5% in favor of vorinostat [153]. Unfortunately, a phase III trial with this combination was terminated after interim analysis found no difference between the arms (NCT00473889 at www.clinicaltrial.gov).

Trials have also been organized to exploit the loss of client proteins due to degradation following Hsp90 acetylation and impairment of chaperone function. Loss of EGFR or HER-2, or other mutant or overexpressed proteins should allow synergy in combination with gefitinib or trastuzumab [64]. However, phase I/II trials combining vorinostat or entinostat with erlotinib in EGFR-mutated NSCLC [154,155] were unsuccessful. A phase I-II study with vorinostat and trastuzumab was terminated early, after no responses in 10 patients (NCT00258349 at www. clinicaltrials.gov).

HDAC6 inhibition, in addition to effects on Hsp90, prevents trafficking of ubiquitinated proteins to the aggresome. Combination of proteasome inhibitors with HDIs may exploit this latter activity in cells dependent on the aggresome pathway for survival after proteasome inhibition. Vorinostat and romidepsin have been used in combination with bortezomib in multiple myeloma and have shown more promising results. The combination of romidepsin, bortezomib, and dexamethasone in 25 previously treated patients showed 2 CR and 13 PR with median TTP of 7.2 months and median OS of more than 36 months [156]. The phase III Vantage trial (NCT00773747) showed a 23% reduction in the risk of disease progression combining bortezomib with vorinostat vs. bortezomib with placebo: median progression-free survival 7.63 months vs. 6.83 months and 56% response rate vs. 41%, respectively [157]. Development of vorinostat in myeloma is continuing in combination with lenalidomide in newly diagnosed patients in a maintenance arm (NCT01554852).

RESISTANCE TO HDIs

Despite the fact that HDIs have been in clinical development for some time, relatively little is known about mechanisms of resistance [58,158]. Most data have been derived from in vitro models, and relatively little clinical data have been gathered. One of the first recognized mechanisms of resistance to romidepsin was overexpression of the ATP-binding cassette transporter, P-glycoprotein (Pgp; encoded by the *MDR-1/ABCB1* gene). During preclinical development, romidepsin was identified as a Pgp substrate in profiles generated with the National Cancer Institute Anticancer Drug Screen cell lines [159]. Induction of Pgp seems to be a class effect of the HDIs [160,161]; however, romidepsin is unique in that it is also a substrate for Pgp-mediated transport. While in vitro selection with romidepsin has been shown to result in development of Pgp as the resistance mechanism [162–164], we found no correlation between *ABCB1* expression and clinical resistance in tumor biopsies obtained from a series of patients with CTCL treated with romidepsin [123], thus suggesting other mechanisms predominate.

Cell line models have identified multiple other potential mechanisms of resistance. A link between increased levels of the reactive oxygen scavenger, thioredoxin, and resistance to HDI treatment was reported [165]. Enforced expression of the proapoptotic proteins BCL-2 or BCL-XL has been shown to confer resistance to HDIs, and increased apoptosis has been observed when HDIs are combined with BCL-2 inhibitors such as ABT-737 [166–168]. We found that increased insulin receptor expression and MAPK signaling correlated with resistance to romidepsin and other HDIs in a T-cell lymphoma cell line selected for non-Pgp-mediated resistance to romidepsin [169]. Other groups have also suggested that activation of the MAP kinase as well as the PI3 kinase pathway is a factor in resistance to HDIs [170–172]. High nuclear staining of phosphorylated STAT3 was found to correlate with resistance to vorinostat treatment in a series of skin biopsy samples [173]. Despite these promising leads, further studies are necessary to determine their ability to predict clinical resistance to HDI treatment and to identify approaches to overcome that resistance.

CONCLUSION

HDIs qualify as targeted therapies in their inhibition of the HDAC enzyme family. In patients, the agents have a unique set of likely on-target side effects and a common efficacy in T-cell lymphomas. Targeted therapies such as imatinib, erlotinib, and vemurafenib for BCR-ABL, mutant EGF receptor or mutant B-Raf are active in tumor types in which the target is expressed, and activity should not be expected where the target is not found. The marked activity in T-cell lymphoma remains unexplained, and studies are desperately needed to unravel that question. Following the targeted therapy paradigm, there ought to be a unique epigenetic lesion that sensitizes T-cell lymphomas to the HDIs. However, the effects of these agents in cells in the laboratory are as diverse as the effects of more classical cytotoxic agents, and this diversity has generated a clinical trial effort far broader than would be needed for a single target. This has the potential of identifying disease entities in which the drugs can be active but also the potential of creating disillusionment when the majority of the clinical trials fail. Indeed, no other signals of great activity have been identified beyond the hematologic malignancies.

Perhaps the HDIs should not be viewed as true targeted therapies. They are after all epigenetic agents, and they induce global changes in acetylation and gene expression that some cells are likely to not find very tolerable. Viewing the agents as more like DNA damaging agents could create a better therapeutic paradigm. Regardless of which paradigm is finally proven correct, investigators participating in studies of these agents should avoid home-run designs and instead opt for trials that include diligent correlative investigations. In the case of combination studies, the putative mechanism of synergy has to be examined in clinical samples. HDIs hold the promise that they can be more than targeted therapies. It remains to the scientific community to sort out exactly what that means.

REFERENCES

1. Annunziato AT. Assembling chromatin: The long and winding road. *Biochim Biophys Acta*. 2012;1819:196–210.
2. Lane AA, Chabner BA. Histone deacetylase inhibitors in cancer therapy. *J Clin Oncol*. 2009;27:5459–5468.
3. Dekker FJ, Haisma HJ. Histone acetyl transferases as emerging drug targets. *Drug Discov Today*. 2009;14:942–948.
4. Marks P, Rifkind RA, Richon VM, Breslow R, Miller T, Kelly WK. Histone deacetylases and cancer: Causes and therapies. *Nat Rev Cancer*. 2001;1:194–202.
5. Nagy Z, Tora L. Distinct GCN5/PCAF-containing complexes function as co-activators and are involved in transcription factor and global histone acetylation. *Oncogene*. 2007;26:5341–5357.
6. Vogelauer M, Wu J, Suka N, Grunstein M. Global histone acetylation and deacetylation in yeast. *Nature*. 2000;408:495–498.
7. Anamika K, Krebs AR, Thompson J, Poch O, Devys D, Tora L. Lessons from genome-wide studies: An integrated definition of the coactivator function of histone acetyl transferases. *Epigenetics Chromatin*. 2010;3:18.
8. Kouzarides T. Histone acetylases and deacetylases in cell proliferation. *Curr Opin Genet Dev*. 1999;9:40–48.
9. Schrump DS. Cytotoxicity mediated by histone deacetylase inhibitors in cancer cells: Mechanisms and potential clinical implications. *Clin Cancer Res*. 2009;15:3947–3957.
10. Witt O, Deubzer HE, Milde T, Oehme I. HDAC family: What are the cancer relevant targets? *Cancer Lett*. 2009;277:8–21.
11. Haberland M, Montgomery RL, Olson EN. The many roles of histone deacetylases in development and physiology: Implications for disease and therapy. *Nat Rev Genet*. 2009;10:32–42.

12. Zupkovitz G, Grausenburger R, Brunmeir R, Senese S, Tischler J, Jurkin J et al. The cyclin-dependent kinase inhibitor p21 is a crucial target for histone deacetylase 1 as a regulator of cellular proliferation. *Mol Cell Biol.* 2010;30:1171–1181.

13. Bhaskara S, Chyla BJ, Amann JM, Knutson SK, Cortez D, Sun ZW et al. Deletion of histone deacetylase 3 reveals critical roles in S phase progression and DNA damage control. *Mol Cell.* 2008;30:61–72.

14. Waltregny D, Glénisson W, Tran SL, North BJ, Verdin E, Colige A et al. Histone deacetylase HDAC8 associates with smooth muscle alpha-actin and is essential for smooth muscle cell contractility. *FASEB J.* 2005;19:966–968.

15. Vaquero A, Sternglanz R, Reinberg D. NAD+-dependent deacetylation of H4 lysine 16 by class III HDACs. *Oncogene.* 2007;26:5505–5520.

16. Luo J, Nikolaev AY, Imai S, Chen D, Su F, Shiloh A et al. Negative control of p53 by Sir2alpha promotes cell survival under stress. *Cell.* 2001;107:137–148.

17. Vaziri H, Dessain SK, Ng Eaton E, Imai SI, Frye RA, Pandita TK et al. hSIR2(SIRT1) functions as an NAD-dependent p53 deacetylase. *Cell.* 2001;107:149–159.

18. Glozak M, Seto E. Histone deacetylases and cancer. *Oncogene.* 2007;26:5420–5432.

19. Ida K, Kitabayashi I, Taki T, Taniwaki M, Noro K, Yamamoto M et al. Adenoviral E1A-associated protein p300 is involved in acute myeloid leukemia with t(11;22)(q23;q13). *Blood.* 1997;90:4699–4704.

20. Sobulo O, Borrow J, Tomek R, Reshmi S, Harden A, Schlegelberger B et al. MLL is fused to CBP, a histone acetyltransferase, in therapy-related acute myeloid leukemia with a t(11;16)(q23;p13.3). *Proc Natl Acad Sci USA.* 1997;94:8732–8737.

21. Gayther S, Batley S, Linger L, Bannister A, Thorpe K, Chin S et al. Mutations truncating the EP300 acetylase in human cancers. *Nat Genet.* 2000;24:300–303.

22. Ward R, Johnson M, Shridhar V, van Deursen J, Couch F. CBP truncating mutations in ovarian cancer. *J Med Genet.* 2005;42:514–518.

23. Lachner M, O'Sullivan RJ, Jenuwein T. An epigenetic road map for histone lysine methylation. *J Cell Sci.* 2003;116:2117–2124.

24. Marks P, Xu W. Histone deacetylase inhibitors: Potential in cancer therapy. *J Cell Biochem.* 2009;107:600–608.

25. Demary K, Wong L, Spanjaard R. Effects of retinoic acid and sodium butyrate on gene expression, histone acetylation and inhibition of proliferation of melanoma cells. *Cancer Lett.* 2001;163:103–107.

26. Davis T, Kennedy C, Chiew Y, Clarke C, deFazio A. Histone deacetylase inhibitors decrease proliferation and modulate cell cycle gene expression in normal mammary epithelial cells. *Clin Cancer Res.* 2000;6:4334–4342.

27. Phiel C, Zhang F, Huang E, Guenther M, Lazar M, Klein P. Histone deacetylase is a direct target of valproic acid, a potent anticonvulsant, mood stabilizer, and teratogen. *J Biol Chem.* 2001;276:36734–36741.

28. Friend C, Scher W, Holland J, Sato T. Hemoglobin synthesis in murine virus-induced leukemic cells in vitro: Stimulation of erythroid differentiation by dimethyl sulfoxide. *Proc Natl Acad Sci USA.* 1971;68:378–382.

29. Marks PA, Breslow R. Dimethyl sulfoxide to vorinostat: Development of this histone deacetylase inhibitor as an anticancer drug. *Nat Biotechnol.* 2007;25:84–90.

30. Santo L, Hideshima T, Kung AL, Tseng JC, Tamang D, Yang M et al. Preclinical activity, pharmacodynamic, and pharmacokinetic properties of a selective HDAC6 inhibitor, ACY-1215, in combination with bortezomib in multiple myeloma. *Blood.* 2012;119:2579–2589.

31. Nakajima H, Kim YB, Terano H, Yoshida M, Horinouchi S. FR901228, a potent antitumor antibiotic, is a novel histone deacetylase inhibitor. *Exp Cell Res.* 1998;241:126–133.

32. Ueda H, Nakajima H, Hori Y, Goto T, Okuhara M. Action of FR901228, a novel antitumor bicyclic depsipeptide produced by Chromobacterium violaceum no. 968, on Ha-ras transformed NIH3T3 cells. *Biosci Biotech Biochem.* 1994;58:1579–1583.

33. Furumai R, Matsuyama A, Kobashi N, Lee KH, Nishiyama M, Nakajima H et al. FK228 (depsipeptide) as a natural prodrug that inhibits class I histone deacetylases. *Cancer Res.* 2002;62:4916–4921.

34. Burgess A, Ruefli A, Beamish H, Warrener R, Saunders N, Johnstone R et al. Histone deacetylase inhibitors specifically kill nonproliferating tumour cells. *Oncogene.* 2004;23:6693–6701.

35. Bolden J, Peart M, Johnstone R. Anticancer activities of histone deacetylase inhibitors. *Nat Rev Drug Discov.* 2006;5:769–784.

36. Schrump D. Cytotoxicity mediated by histone deacetylase inhibitors in cancer cells: Mechanisms and potential clinical implications. *Clin Cancer Res.* 2009;15:3947–3957.

37. Van Lint C, Emiliani S, Verdin E. The expression of a small fraction of cellular genes is changed in response to histone hyperacetylation. *Gene Expr.* 1996;5:245–253.

38. Della Ragione F, Criniti V, Della Pietra V, Borriello A, Oliva A, Indaco S et al. Genes modulated by histone acetylation as new effectors of butyrate activity. *FEBS Lett.* 2001;499:199–204.

39. Hoshino I, Matsubara H, Akutsu Y, Nishimori T, Yoneyama Y, Murakami K et al. Gene expression profiling induced by histone deacetylase inhibitor, FK228, in human esophageal squamous cancer cells. *Oncol Rep.* 2007;18:585–592.

40. Peart M, Smyth G, van Laar R, Bowtell D, Richon V, Marks P et al. Identification and functional significance of genes regulated by structurally different histone deacetylase inhibitors. *Proc Natl Acad Sci USA.* 2005;102:3697–3702.

41. Kitazono M, Robey R, Zhan Z, Sarlis NJ, Skarulis MC, Aikou T et al. Low concentrations of the histone deacetylase inhibitor, depsipeptide (FR901228), increase expression of the Na(+)/I(−) symporter and iodine accumulation in poorly differentiated thyroid carcinoma cells. *J Clin Endocrinol Metab.* 2001;86:3430–3435.

42. Cao H, Stamatoyannopoulos G. Histone deacetylase inhibitor FK228 is a potent inducer of human fetal hemoglobin. *Am J Hematol.* 2006;81:981–983.

43. Sánchez-Pacheco A, Martínez-Iglesias O, Méndez-Pertuz M, Aranda A. Residues K128, 132, and 134 in the thyroid hormone receptor-alpha are essential for receptor acetylation and activity. *Endocrinology.* 2009;150:5143–5152.

44. Kawamura T, Ono K, Morimoto T, Wada H, Hirai M, Hidaka K et al. Acetylation of GATA-4 is involved in the differentiation of embryonic stem cells into cardiac myocytes. *J Biol Chem.* 2005;280:19682–19688.

45. Sandor V, Senderowicz A, Mertins S, Sackett D, Sausville E, Blagosklonny MV et al. P21-dependent g(1)arrest with downregulation of cyclin D1 and upregulation of cyclin E by the histone deacetylase inhibitor FR901228. *Br J Cancer.* 2000;83:817–825.

46. Atadja P, Gao L, Kwon P, Trogani N, Walker H, Hsu M et al. Selective growth inhibition of tumor cells by a novel histone deacetylase inhibitor, NVP-LAQ824. *Cancer Res.* 2004;64:689–695.

47. Glaser K, Staver M, Waring J, Stender J, Ulrich R, Davidsen S. Gene expression profiling of multiple histone deacetylase (HDAC) inhibitors: Defining a common gene set produced by HDAC inhibition in T24 and MDA carcinoma cell lines. *Mol Cancer Ther.* 2003;2:151–163.

48. Prystowsky M, Adomako A, Smith R, Kawachi N, McKimpson W, Atadja P et al. The histone deacetylase inhibitor LBH589 inhibits expression of mitotic genes causing G2/M arrest and cell death in head and neck squamous cell carcinoma cell lines. *J Pathol.* 2009;218:467–477.

49. Robbins AR, Jablonski SA, Yen TJ, Yoda K, Robey R, Bates SE et al. Inhibitors of histone deacetylases alter kinetochore assembly by disrupting pericentromeric heterochromatin. *Cell Cycle.* 2005;4:717–726.

50. Rosato RR, Maggio SC, Almenara JA, Payne SG, Atadja P, Spiegel S et al. The histone deacetylase inhibitor LAQ824 induces human leukemia cell death through a process involving XIAP down-regulation, oxidative injury, and the acid sphingomyelinase-dependent generation of ceramide. *Mol Pharmacol.* 2006;69:216–225.

51. Rosato RR, Almenara JA, Grant S. The histone deacetylase inhibitor MS-275 promotes differentiation or apoptosis in human leukemia cells through a process regulated by generation of reactive oxygen species and induction of p21CIP1/WAF1 1. *Cancer Res.* 2003;63:3637–3645.

52. Zhao Y, Lu S, Wu L, Chai G, Wang H, Chen Y et al. Acetylation of p53 at lysine 373/382 by the histone deacetylase inhibitor depsipeptide induces expression of p21(Waf1/Cip1). *Mol Cell Biol.* 2006;26:2782–2790.

53. Faiola F, Liu X, Lo S, Pan S, Zhang K, Lymar E et al. Dual regulation of c-Myc by p300 via acetylation-dependent control of Myc protein turnover and coactivation of Myc-induced transcription. *Mol Cell Biol.* 2005;25:10220–10234.

54. Okabe S, Tauchi T, Nakajima A, Sashida G, Gotoh A, Broxmeyer H et al. Depsipeptide (FK228) preferentially induces apoptosis in BCR/ABL-expressing cell lines and cells from patients with chronic myelogenous leukemia in blast crisis. *Stem Cells Dev.* 2007;16:503–514.

55. Ray S, Lee C, Hou T, Boldogh I, Brasier A. Requirement of histone deacetylase1 (HDAC1) in signal transducer and activator of transcription 3 (STAT3) nucleocytoplasmic distribution. *Nucleic Acids Res.* 2008;36:4510–4520.

56. Dai Y, Rahmani M, Dent P, Grant S. Blockade of histone deacetylase inhibitor-induced RelA/p65 acetylation and NF-kappaB activation potentiates apoptosis in leukemia cells through a process mediated by oxidative damage, XIAP downregulation, and c-Jun N-terminal kinase 1 activation. *Mol Cell Biol.* 2005;25:5429–5444.

57. Krämer O, Baus D, Knauer S, Stein S, Jäger E, Stauber R et al. Acetylation of Stat1 modulates NF-kappaB activity. *Genes Dev.* 2006;20:473–485.

58. Robey RW, Chakraborty AR, Basseville A, Luchenko V, Bahr J, Zhan Z et al. Histone deacetylase inhibitors: Emerging mechanisms of resistance. *Mol Pharm.* 2011;8:2021–2031.

59. Kawaguchi Y, Kovacs J, McLaurin A, Vance J, Ito A, Yao T. The deacetylase HDAC6 regulates aggresome formation and cell viability in response to misfolded protein stress. *Cell.* 2003;115:727–738.

60. Ma X, Ezzeldin H, Diasio R. Histone deacetylase inhibitors: Current status and overview of recent clinical trials. *Drugs.* 2009;69:1911–1934.

61. Yu X, Guo ZS, Marcu MG, Neckers L, Nguyen DM, Chen GA et al. Modulation of p53, ErbB1, ErbB2, and Raf-1 expression in lung cancer cells by depsipeptide FR901228. *J Natl Cancer Inst.* 2002;94:504–513.

62. Fuino L, Bali P, Wittmann S, Donapaty S, Guo F, Yamaguchi H et al. Histone deacetylase inhibitor LAQ824 down-regulates Her-2 and sensitizes human breast cancer cells to trastuzumab, taxotere, gemcitabine, and epothilone B. *Mol Cancer Ther.* 2003;2:971–984.

63. Nimmanapalli R, Fuino L, Bali P, Gasparetto M, Glozak M, Tao J et al. Histone deacetylase inhibitor LAQ824 both lowers expression and promotes proteasomal degradation of Bcr-Abl and induces apoptosis of imatinib mesylate-sensitive or -refractory chronic myelogenous leukemia-blast crisis cells. *Cancer Res.* 2003;63:5126–5135.

64. Edwards A, Li J, Atadja P, Bhalla K, Haura E. Effect of the histone deacetylase inhibitor LBH589 against epidermal growth factor receptor-dependent human lung cancer cells. *Mol Cancer Ther.* 2007;6:2515–2524.

65. Nishioka C, Ikezoe T, Yang J, Takeuchi S, Koeffler H, Yokoyama A. MS-275, a novel histone deacetylase inhibitor with selectivity against HDAC1, induces degradation of FLT3 via inhibition of chaperone function of heat shock protein 90 in AML cells. *Leuk Res*. 2008;32:1382–1392.

66. Rosato R, Almenara J, Maggio S, Coe S, Atadja P, Dent P et al. Role of histone deacetylase inhibitor-induced reactive oxygen species and DNA damage in LAQ-824/fludarabine antileukemic interactions. *Mol Cancer Ther*. 2008;7:3285–3297.

67. Adimoolam S, Sirisawad M, Chen J, Thiemann P, Ford J, Buggy J. HDAC inhibitor PCI-24781 decreases RAD51 expression and inhibits homologous recombination. *Proc Natl Acad Sci USA*. 2007;104:19482–19487.

68. Geng L, Cuneo K, Fu A, Tu T, Atadja P, Hallahan D. Histone deacetylase (HDAC) inhibitor LBH589 increases duration of gamma-H2AX foci and confines HDAC4 to the cytoplasm in irradiated non-small cell lung cancer. *Cancer Res*. 2006;66:11298–11304.

69. Zhang F, Zhang T, Teng Z, Zhang R, Wang J, Mei Q. Sensitization to gamma-irradiation-induced cell cycle arrest and apoptosis by the histone deacetylase inhibitor trichostatin A in non-small cell lung cancer (NSCLC) cells. *Cancer Biol Ther*. 2009;8:823–831.

70. Guo F, Sigua C, Tao J, Bali P, George P, Li Y et al. Cotreatment with histone deacetylase inhibitor LAQ824 enhances Apo-2L/tumor necrosis factor-related apoptosis inducing ligand-induced death inducing signaling complex activity and apoptosis of human acute leukemia cells. *Cancer Res*. 2004;64:2580–2589.

71. Kwon S, Ahn S, Kim Y, Bae G, Yoon J, Hong S et al. Apicidin, a histone deacetylase inhibitor, induces apoptosis and Fas/Fas ligand expression in human acute promyelo-cytic leukemia cells. *J Biol Chem*. 2002;277:2073–2080.

72. Kim Y, Park J, Lee J, Kwon T. Sodium butyrate sensitizes TRAIL-mediated apoptosis by induction of transcription from the DR5 gene promoter through Sp1 sites in colon cancer cells. *Carcinogenesis*. 2004;25:1813–1820.

73. Park S, Kim M, Kim H, Sohn H, Bae J, Kang C et al. Trichostatin A sensitizes human ovarian cancer cells to TRAIL-induced apoptosis by down-regulation of c-FLIPL via inhibition of EGFR pathway. *Biochem Pharmacol*. 2009;77:1328–1336.

74. Rippo M, Moretti S, Vescovi S, Tomasetti M, Orecchia S, Amici G et al. FLIP over-expression inhibits death receptor-induced apoptosis in malignant mesothelial cells. *Oncogene*. 2004;23:7753–7760.

75. Jin Z, El-Deiry W. Overview of cell death signaling pathways. *Cancer Biol Ther*. 2005;4:139–163.

76. Zhang X, Gillespie S, Borrow J, Hersey P. The histone deacetylase inhibitor suberic bishydroxamate regulates the expression of multiple apoptotic mediators and induces mitochondria-dependent apoptosis of melanoma cells. *Mol Cancer Ther*. 2004;3:425–435.

77. Fandy T, Shankar S, Ross D, Sausville E, Srivastava R. Interactive effects of HDAC inhibitors and TRAIL on apoptosis are associated with changes in mitochondrial functions and expressions of cell cycle regulatory genes in multiple myeloma. *Neoplasia*. 2005;7:646–657.

78. Chen S, Dai Y, Pei X, Grant S. Bim upregulation by histone deacetylase inhibitors mediates interactions with the Bcl-2 antagonist ABT-737: Evidence for distinct roles for Bcl-2, Bcl-xL, and Mcl-1. *Mol Cell Biol*. 2009;29:6149–6169.

79. Hideshima T, Bradner J, Wong J, Chauhan D, Richardson P, Schreiber S et al. Small-molecule inhibition of proteasome and aggresome function induces synergistic antitumor activity in multiple myeloma. *Proc Natl Acad Sci U S A*. 2005;102:8567–8572.

80. Piekarz RL, Robey R, Sandor V, Bakke S, Wilson WH, Dahmoush L et al. Inhibitor of histone deacetylation, depsipeptide (FR901228), in the treatment of peripheral and cutaneous T-cell lymphoma: A case report. *Blood*. 2001;98:2865–2868.

81. Piekarz R, Frye R, Turner M, Wright J, Allen S, Kirschbaum M et al. Phase II multi-institutional trial of the histone deacetylase inhibitor romidepsin as monotherapy for patients with cutaneous T-cell lymphoma. *J Clin Oncol*. 2009;27:5410–5417.

82. Duvic M, Talpur R, Ni X, Zhang C, Hazarika P, Kelly C et al. Phase 2 trial of oral vorinostat (suberoylanilide hydroxamic acid, SAHA) for refractory cutaneous T-cell lymphoma (CTCL). *Blood*. 2007;109:31–39.

83. Ellis L, Pan Y, Smyth G, George D, McCormack C, Williams-Truax R et al. Histone deacetylase inhibitor panobinostat induces clinical responses with associated alterations in gene expression profiles in cutaneous T-cell lymphoma. *Clin Cancer Res*. 2008;14:4500–4510.

84. Pohlman B, Advani R, Duvic M, Hymes KB, Intragumtornchai T, Lekhakula A et al. Final Results of a phase II trial of belinostat (PXD101) in patients with recurrent or refractory peripheral or cutaneous T-cell lymphoma. *ASH Annual Meeting Abstracts*. 2009;114:920.

85. Piekarz RL, Frye R, Prince HM, Kirschbaum MH, Zain J, Allen SL et al. Phase 2 trial of romidepsin in patients with peripheral T-cell lymphoma. *Blood*. 2011;117:5827–5834.

86. Mann B, Johnson J, Cohen M, Justice R, Pazdur R. FDA approval summary: Vorinostat for treatment of advanced primary cutaneous T-cell lymphoma. *Oncologist*. 2007;12:1247–1252.

87. Olsen E, Kim Y, Kuzel T, Pacheco T, Foss F, Parker S et al. Phase IIb multicenter trial of vorinostat in patients with persistent, progressive, or treatment refractory cutaneous T-cell lymphoma. *J Clin Oncol*. 2007;25:3109–3115.

88. Kelly WK, Richon VM, O'Connor O, Curley T, MacGregor-Curtelli B, Tong W et al. Phase I clinical trial of histone deacetylase inhibitor: Suberoylanilide hydroxamic acid administered intravenously. *Clin Cancer Res*. 2003;9:3578–3588.

89. Kelly WK, O'Connor OA, Krug LM, Chiao JH, Heaney M, Curley T et al. Phase I study of an oral histone deacetylase inhibitor, suberoylanilide hydroxamic acid, in patients with advanced cancer. *J Clin Oncol*. 2005;23:3923–3931.

90. O'Connor O, Heaney M, Schwartz L, Richardson S, Willim R, MacGregor-Cortelli B et al. Clinical experience with intravenous and oral formulations of the novel histone deacetylase inhibitor suberoylanilide hydroxamic acid in patients with advanced hematologic malignancies. *J Clin Oncol*. 2006;24:166–173.

91. Crump M, Coiffier B, Jacobsen E, Sun L, Ricker J, Xie H et al. Phase II trial of oral vorinostat (suberoylanilide hydroxamic acid) in relapsed diffuse large-B-cell lymphoma. *Ann Oncol*. 2008;19:964–969.

92. Garcia-Manero G, Yang H, Bueso-Ramos C, Ferrajoli A, Cortes J, Wierda WG et al. Phase 1 study of the histone deacetylase inhibitor vorinostat (suberoylanilide hydroxamic acid [SAHA]) in patients with advanced leukemias and myelodysplastic syndromes. *Blood*. 2008;111:1060–1066.

93. Richardson P, Mitsiades C, Colson K, Reilly E, McBride L, Chiao J et al. Phase I trial of oral vorinostat (suberoylanilide hydroxamic acid, SAHA) in patients with advanced multiple myeloma. *Leuk Lymphoma*. 2008;49:502–507.

94. Marshall J, Rizvi N, Kauh J, Dahut W, Figuera M, Kang M et al. A phase I trial of depsipeptide (FR901228) in patients with advanced cancer. *J Exp Ther Oncol*. 2002;2:325–332.

95. Sandor V, Bakke S, Robey RW, Kang MH, Blagosklonny MV, Bender J et al. Phase I trial of the histone deacetylase inhibitor, depsipeptide (FR901228, NSC 630176), in patients with refractory neoplasms. *Clin Cancer Res*. 2002;8:718–728.

96. Kim Y, Whittaker S, Demierre MF, Rook AH, Lerner A, Duvic M et al. Clinically significant responses achieved with romidepsin in treatment-refractory cutaneous T-cell lymphoma: Final results from a phase 2B, international, multicenter, registration study. *ASH Annual Meeting Abstracts*. 2008;112:263.

97. Coiffier B, Pro B, Prince HM, Foss F, Sokol L, Greenwood M et al. Results from a pivotal, open-label, phase II study of romidepsin in relapsed or refractory peripheral T-cell lymphoma after prior systemic therapy. *J Clin Oncol*. 2012;30:631–636.

98. Dickinson M, Ritchie D, DeAngelo D, Spencer A, Ottmann O, Fischer T et al. Preliminary evidence of disease response to the pan deacetylase inhibitor panobinostat (LBH589) in refractory Hodgkin Lymphoma. *Br J Haematol*. 2009;147:97–101.

99. Deangelo DJ, Spencer A, Bhalla KN, Prince HM, Fischer T, Kindler T et al. Phase Ia/II, 2-arm, open-label, dose-escalation study of oral panobinostat administered via 2 dosing schedules in patients with advanced hematologic malignancies. *Leukemia*. 2013.

100. Crump M, Andreadis C, Assouline S, Rizzieri D, Wedgwood A, McLaughlin P et al. Treatment of relapsed or refractory non-hodgkin lymphoma with the oral isotype-selective histone deacetylase inhibitor MGCD0103: Interim results from a phase II study. *J Clin Oncol (Meeting Abstracts)*. 2008;26:8528.

101. Evens AM, Vose JM, Harb W, Gordon LI, Langdon R, Grant B et al. A phase II multicenter study of the histone deacetylase inhibitor (HDACi) abexinostat (PCI-24781) in relapsed/refractory follicular lymphoma (FL) and mantle cell lymphoma (MCL). *ASH Annual Meeting Abstracts*. 2012;120:55.

102. Morschhauser F, Terriou L, Coiffier B, Salles G, Kloos I, Tavernier N et al. Abexinostat (S78454/PCI-24781), an oral pan-histone deacetylas (HDAC) inhibitor in patients with refractory or relapsed Hodgkin's lymphoma, non-Hodgkin lymphoma and chronic lymphocytic leukemia. Results of a phase I dose-escalation study in 35 patients. *ASH Annual Meeting Abstracts*. 2012;120:3643.

103. Vansteenkiste J, Van Cutsem E, Dumez H, Chen C, Ricker J, Randolph S et al. Early phase II trial of oral vorinostat in relapsed or refractory breast, colorectal, or non-small cell lung cancer. *Invest New Drugs*. 2008;26:483–488.

104. Luu T, Morgan R, Leong L, Lim D, McNamara M, Portnow J et al. A phase II trial of vorinostat (suberoylanilide hydroxamic acid) in metastatic breast cancer: A California Cancer Consortium study. *Clin Cancer Res*. 2008;14:7138–7142.

105. Woyach J, Kloos R, Ringel M, Arbogast D, Collamore M, Zwiebel J et al. Lack of therapeutic effect of the histone deacetylase inhibitor vorinostat in patients with metastatic radioiodine-refractory thyroid carcinoma. *J Clin Endocrinol Metab*. 2009;94:164–170.

106. Krug L, Curley T, Schwartz L, Richardson S, Marks P, Chiao J et al. Potential role of histone deacetylase inhibitors in mesothelioma: Clinical experience with suberoylanilide hydroxamic acid. *Clin Lung Cancer*. 2006;7:257–261.

107. Galanis E, Jaeckle K, Maurer M, Reid J, Ames M, Hardwick J et al. Phase II trial of vorinostat in recurrent glioblastoma multiforme: A north central cancer treatment group study. *J Clin Oncol*. 2009;27:2052–2058.

108. Blumenschein GJ, Kies M, Papadimitrakopoulou V, Lu C, Kumar A, Ricker J et al. Phase II trial of the histone deacetylase inhibitor vorinostat (Zolinza, suberoylanilide hydroxamic acid, SAHA) in patients with recurrent and/or metastatic head and neck cancer. *Invest New Drugs*. 2008;26:81–87.

109. Klimek VM, Fircanis S, Maslak P, Guernah I, Baum M, Wu N et al. Tolerability, pharmacodynamics, and pharmacokinetics studies of depsipeptide (romidepsin) in patients with acute myelogenous leukemia or advanced myelodysplastic syndromes. *Clin Cancer Res*. 2008;14:826–832.

110. Odenike O, Alkan S, Sher D, Godwin J, Huo D, Brandt S et al. Histone deacetylase inhibitor romidepsin has differential activity in core binding factor acute myeloid leukemia. *Clin Cancer Res*. 2008;14:7095–7101.

111. Byrd JC, Marcucci G, Parthun MR, Xiao JJ, Klisovic RB, Moran M et al. A phase 1 and pharmacodynamic study of depsipeptide (FK228) in chronic lymphocytic leukemia and acute myeloid leukemia. *Blood*. 2005;105:959–967.

112. Stadler WM, Margolin K, Ferber S, McCulloch W, Thompson JA. A phase II study of depsipeptide in refractory metastatic renal cell cancer. *Clinical Genitourinary Cancer.* 2006;5:57–60.

113. Molife LR, Attard G, Fong PC, Karavasilis V, Reid AH, Patterson S et al. Phase II, two-stage, single-arm trial of the histone deacetylase inhibitor (HDACi) romidepsin in metastatic castration-resistant prostate cancer (CRPC). Ann. Oncol. 2010;21(1):109–113.

114. Whitehead R, Rankin C, Hoff P, Gold P, Billingsley K, Chapman R et al. Phase II trial of romidepsin (NSC-630176) in previously treated colorectal cancer patients with advanced disease: A Southwest Oncology Group study (S0336). *Invest New Drugs.* 2009;27:469–475.

115. Schrump DS, Fischette MR, Nguyen DM, Zhao M, Li X, Kunst TF et al. Clinical and molecular responses in lung cancer patients receiving Romidepsin. *Clin Cancer Res.* 2008;14:188–198.

116. Gore L, Rothenberg M, O'Bryant C, Schultz M, Sandler A, Coffin D et al. A phase I and pharmacokinetic study of the oral histone deacetylase inhibitor, MS-275, in patients with refractory solid tumors and lymphomas. *Clin Cancer Res.* 2008;14:4517–4525.

117. Gojo I, Jiemjit A, Trepel JB, Sparreboom A, Figg WD, Rollins S et al. Phase 1 and pharmacologic study of MS-275, a histone deacetylase inhibitor, in adults with refractory and relapsed acute leukemias. *Blood.* 2007;109:2781–2790.

118. Kummar S, Gutierrez M, Gardner ER, Donovan E, Hwang K, Chung EJ et al. Phase I trial of MS-275, a histone deacetylase inhibitor, administered weekly in refractory solid tumors and lymphoid malignancies. *Clin Cancer Res.* 2007;13:5411–5417.

119. Hauschild A, Trefzer U, Garbe C, Kaehler K, Ugurel S, Kiecker F et al. Multicenter phase II trial of the histone deacetylase inhibitor pyridylmethyl-N-{4-[(2-aminophenyl)-carbamoyl]-benzyl}-carbamate in pretreated metastatic melanoma. *Melanoma Res.* 2008;18:274–278.

120. Ramalingam S, Belani C, Ruel C, Frankel P, Gitlitz B, Koczywas M et al. Phase II study of belinostat (PXD101), a histone deacetylase inhibitor, for second line therapy of advanced malignant pleural mesothelioma. *J Thorac Oncol.* 2009;4:97–101.

121. Steele N, Plumb J, Vidal L, Tjørnelund J, Knoblauch P, Rasmussen A et al. A phase 1 pharmacokinetic and pharmacodynamic study of the histone deacetylase inhibitor belinostat in patients with advanced solid tumors. *Clin Cancer Res.* 2008;14:804–810.

122. Bates S, Zhan Z, Steadman K, Obrzut T, Luchenko V, Frye R et al. Laboratory correlates for a phase II trial of romidepsin in cutaneous and peripheral T-cell lymphoma. *Br J Haematol.* 2010;148:256–267.

123. Ryan Q, Headlee D, Acharya M, Sparreboom A, Trepel J, Ye J et al. Phase I and pharmacokinetic study of MS-275, a histone deacetylase inhibitor, in patients with advanced and refractory solid tumors or lymphoma. *J Clin Oncol.* 2005;23:3912–3922.

124. de Bono JS, Kristeleit R, Tolcher A, Fong P, Pacey S, Karavasilis V et al. Phase I pharmacokinetic and pharmacodynamic study of LAQ824, a hydroxamate histone deacetylase inhibitor with a heat shock protein-90 inhibitory profile, in patients with advanced solid tumors. *Clin Cancer Res.* 2008;14:6663–6673.

125. Iancu-Rubin C, Gajzer D, Mosoyan G, Feller F, Mascarenhas J, Hoffman R. Panobinostat (LBH589)-induced acetylation of tubulin impairs megakaryocyte maturation and platelet formation. *Exp Hematol.* 2012;40:564–574.

126. Giles F, Fischer T, Cortes J, Garcia-Manero G, Beck J, Ravandi F et al. A phase I study of intravenous LBH589, a novel cinnamic hydroxamic acid analogue histone deacetylase inhibitor, in patients with refractory hematologic malignancies. *Clin Cancer Res.* 2006;12:4628–4635.

127. Piekarz RL, Frye AR, Wright JJ, Steinberg S, Liewehr DJ, Rosing DR et al. Cardiac studies in patients treated with depsipeptide, FK228, in a phase II trial for T-cell lymphoma. *Clin Cancer Res.* 2006;12(12):3762–3773.

128. Zhang L, Lebwohl D, Masson E, Laird G, Cooper M, Prince H. Clinically relevant QTc prolongation is not associated with current dose schedules of LBH589 (panobinostat). *J Clin Oncol*. 2008;26:332–333; discussion 3–4.

129. Rowinsky EK, de Bono J, Deangelo DJ, van Oosterom A, Morganroth J, Laird GH et al. Cardiac monitoring in phase I trials of a novel histone deacetylase (HDAC) inhibitor LAQ824 in patients with advanced solid tumors and hematologic malignancies. *J Clin Oncol (Meeting Abstracts)*. 2005;23:3131.

130. Munster P, Rubin E, Van Belle S, Friedman E, Patterson J, Van Dyck K et al. A single supratherapeutic dose of vorinostat does not prolong the QTc interval in patients with advanced cancer. *Clin Cancer Res*. 2009;15:7077–7084.

131. Cabell C, Bates S, Piekarz R, Whittaker S, Kim YH, Currie M et al. Systematic assessment of potential cardiac effects of the novel histone deacetylase (HDAC) inhibitor romidepsin. *ASH Annual Meeting Abstracts*. 2009;114:3709.

132. Beck J, Fischer T, George D, Huber C, Calvo E, Atadja P et al. Phase I pharmacokinetic (PK) and pharmacodynamic (PD) study of ORAL LBH589B: A novel histone deacetylase (HDAC) inhibitor. *J Clin Oncol (Meeting Abstracts)*. 2005;23:3148.

133. Fischer T, Patnaik A, Bhalla K, Beck J, Morganroth J, Laird GH et al. Results of cardiac monitoring during phase I trials of a novel histone deacetylase (HDAC) inhibitor LBH589 in patients with advanced solid tumors and hematologic malignancies. *J Clin Oncol (Meeting Abstracts)*. 2005;23:3106.

134. Kelly WK, DeBono J, Blumenschein G, Lassen U, Zain J, O'Connor O et al. Final results of a phase I study of oral belinostat (PXD101) in patients with solid tumors. *J Clin Oncol (Meeting Abstracts)*. 2009;27:3531.

135. Kristeleit R, Fong P, Aherne G, de Bono J. Histone deacetylase inhibitors: Emerging anticancer therapeutic agents? *Clin Lung Cancer*. 2005;7 Suppl 1:S19–S30.

136. Molife R, Fong P, Scurr M, Judson I, Kaye S, de Bono J. HDAC inhibitors and cardiac safety. *Clin Cancer Res*. 2007;13:1068; author reply: 1068–1069.

137. O'Mahony D, Peikarz R, Bandettini W, Arai A, Wilson W, Bates S. Cardiac involvement with lymphoma: A review of the literature. *Clin Lymphoma Myeloma*. 2008;8:249–252.

138. Grant C, Rahman F, Piekarz R, Peer C, Frye R, Robey RW et al. Romidepsin: A new therapy for cutaneous T-cell lymphoma and a potential therapy for solid tumors. *Expert Rev Anticancer Ther*. 2010;10:997–1008.

139. Garcia-Manero G, Kantarjian H, Sanchez-Gonzalez B, Yang H, Rosner G, Verstovsek S et al. Phase 1/2 study of the combination of 5-aza-2′¢-deoxycytidine with valproic acid in patients with leukemia. *Blood*. 2006;108:3271–3279.

140. Garcia-Manero G, Yang AS, Klimek V, Luger S, Newsome WM, Berman N et al. Phase I/II study of a novel oral isotype-selective histone deacetylase (HDAC) inhibitor MGCD0103 in combination with azacitidine in patients (pts) with high-risk myelodysplastic syndrome (MDS) or acute myelogenous leukemia (AML). *J Clin Oncol (Meeting Abstracts)*. 2007;25:7062.

141. Soriano AO, Yang H, Faderl S, Estrov Z, Giles F, Ravandi F et al. Safety and clinical activity of the combination of 5-azacytidine, valproic acid, and all-trans retinoic acid in acute myeloid leukemia and myelodysplastic syndrome. *Blood*. 2007;110:2302–2308.

142. David KA, Mongan NP, Smith C, Gudas LJ, Nanus DM. Phase I trial of ATRA-IV and depakote in patients with advanced solid tumor malignancies. *Cancer Biol Ther*. 2010;9:678–684.

143. Pili R, Salumbides B, Zhao M, Altiok S, Qian D, Zwiebel J et al. Phase I study of the histone deacetylase inhibitor entinostat in combination with 13-cis retinoic acid in patients with solid tumours. *Br J Cancer*. 2012;106:77–84.

144. Juergens RA, Wrangle J, Vendetti FP, Murphy SC, Zhao M, Coleman B et al. Combination epigenetic therapy has efficacy in patients with refractory advanced non-small cell lung cancer. *Cancer Discov.* 2011;1:598–607.

145. Stathis A, Hotte SJ, Chen EX, Hirte HW, Oza AM, Moretto P et al. Phase I study of decitabine in combination with vorinostat in patients with advanced solid tumors and non-Hodgkin's lymphomas. *Clin Cancer Res.* 2011;17:1582–1590.

146. Garcia-Manero G, Tambaro FP, Bekele NB, Yang H, Ravandi F, Jabbour E et al. Phase II trial of vorinostat with idarubicin and cytarabine for patients with newly diagnosed acute myelogenous leukemia or myelodysplastic syndrome. *J Clin Oncol.* 2012;30:2204–2210.

147. Munster P, Marchion D, Thomas S, Egorin M, Minton S, Springett G et al. Phase I trial of vorinostat and doxorubicin in solid tumours: Histone deacetylase 2 expression as a predictive marker. *Br J Cancer.* 2009;101:1044–1050.

148. Fakih MG, Groman A, McMahon J, Wilding G, Muindi JR. A randomized phase II study of two doses of vorinostat in combination with 5-FU/LV in patients with refractory colorectal cancer. *Cancer Chemother Pharmacol.* 2012;69:743–751.

149. Dizon DS, Blessing JA, Penson RT, Drake RD, Walker JL, Johnston CM et al. A phase II evaluation of belinostat and carboplatin in the treatment of recurrent or persistent platinum-resistant ovarian, fallopian tube, or primary peritoneal carcinoma: A Gynecologic Oncology Group study. *Gynecol Oncol.* 2012;125:367–371.

150. Finkler NJ, Dizon DS, Braly P, Micha J, Lassen U, Celano P et al. Phase II multicenter trial of the histone deacetylase inhibitor (HDACi) belinostat, carboplatin and paclitaxel (BelCaP) in patients (pts) with relapsed epithelial ovarian cancer (EOC). *J Clin Oncol (Meeting Abstracts).* 2008;26:5519.

151. Jones SF, Bendell JC, Infante JR, Spigel DR, Thompson DS, Yardley DA et al. A phase I study of panobinostat in combination with gemcitabine in the treatment of solid tumors. *Clin Adv Hematol Oncol.* 2011;9:225–230.

152. Jones SF, Infante JR, Spigel DR, Peacock NW, Thompson DS, Greco FA et al. Phase 1 results from a study of romidepsin in combination with gemcitabine in patients with advanced solid tumors. *Cancer Invest.* 2012;30:481–486.

153. Ramalingam S, Maitland M, Frankel P, Argiris A, Koczywas M, Gitlitz B et al. Carboplatin and paclitaxel in combination with either vorinostat or placebo for first-line therapy of advanced non-small-cell lung cancer. *J Clin Oncol.* 2010;28(1):56–62.

154. Reguart N, Cardona AF, Isla D, Cardenal F, Palmero R, Carrasco-Chaumel E et al. Phase I trial of vorinostat in combination with erlotinib in advanced non-small cell lung cancer (NSCLC) patients with EGFR mutations after erlotinib progression. *J Clin Oncol (Meeting Abstracts).* 2009;27:e19057.

155. Witta SE, Jotte RM, Konduri K, Neubauer MA, Spira AI, Ruxer RL et al. Randomized phase II trial of erlotinib with and without entinostat in patients with advanced non-small-cell lung cancer who progressed on prior chemotherapy. *J Clin Oncol.* 2012;30:2248–2255.

156. Harrison SJ, Quach H, Link E, Seymour JF, Ritchie DS, Ruell S et al. A high rate of durable responses with romidepsin, bortezomib, and dexamethasone in relapsed or refractory multiple myeloma. *Blood.* 2011;118:6274–6283.

157. Dimopoulos MA, Jagannath S, Yoon S-S, Siegel DS, Lonial S, Hajek R et al. Vantage 088: Vorinostat in combination with bortezomib in patients with relapsed/refractory multiple myeloma: Results of a global, randomized phase 3 trial. *ASH Annual Meeting Abstracts.* 2011;118:811.

158. Lee JH, Choy ML, Marks PA. Mechanisms of resistance to histone deacetylase inhibitors. *Adv Cancer Res.* 2012;116:39–86.

159. Lee JS, Paull K, Alvarez M, Hose C, Monks A, Grever M et al. Rhodamine efflux patterns predict P-glycoprotein substrates in the National Cancer Institute Drug Screen. *Mol Pharmacol.* 1994;46:627–638.

160. Cerveny L, Svecova L, Anzenbacherova E, Vrzal R, Staud F, Dvorak Z et al. Valproic acid induces CYP3A4 and MDR1 gene expression by activation of constitutive androstane receptor and pregnane X receptor pathways. *Drug Metab Dispos.* 2007;35:1032–1041.

161. Kim YK, Kim NH, Hwang JW, Song YJ, Park YS, Seo DW et al. Histone deacetylase inhibitor apicidin-mediated drug resistance: Involvement of P-glycoprotein. *Biochem Biophys Res Commun.* 2008;368:959–964.

162. Piekarz RL, Robey RW, Zhan Z, Kayastha G, Sayah A, Abdeldaim AH et al. T-cell lymphoma as a model for the use of histone deacetylase inhibitors in cancer therapy: Impact of depsipeptide on molecular markers, therapeutic targets, and mechanisms of resistance. *Blood.* 2004;103:4636–4643.

163. Robey RW, Zhan Z, Piekarz RL, Kayastha GL, Fojo T, Bates SE. Increased MDR1 expression in normal and malignant peripheral blood mononuclear cells obtained from patients receiving depsipeptide (FR901228, FK228, NSC630176). *Clin Cancer Res.* 2006;12:1547–1555.

164. Yamada H, Arakawa Y, Saito S, Agawa M, Kano Y, Horiguchi-Yamada J. Depsipeptide-resistant KU812 cells show reversible P-glycoprotein expression, hyper-acetylated histones, and modulated gene expression profile. *Leuk Res.* 2006;30:723–734.

165. Ungerstedt J, Sowa Y, Xu W, Shao Y, Dokmanovic M, Perez G et al. Role of thioredoxin in the response of normal and transformed cells to histone deacetylase inhibitors. *Proc Natl Acad Sci U S A.* 2005;102:673–678.

166. Shao W, Growney JD, Feng Y, O'Connor G, Pu M, Zhu W et al. Activity of deacetylase inhibitor panobinostat (LBH589) in cutaneous T-cell lymphoma models: Defining molecular mechanisms of resistance. *Int J Cancer.* 2010;127:2199–2208.

167. Wiegmans AP, Alsop AE, Bots M, Cluse LA, Williams SP, Banks KM et al. Deciphering the molecular events necessary for synergistic tumor cell apoptosis mediated by the histone deacetylase inhibitor vorinostat and the BH3 mimetic ABT-737. *Cancer Res.* 2011;71:3603–3615.

168. Ellis L, Bots M, Lindemann RK, Bolden JE, Newbold A, Cluse LA et al. The histone deacetylase inhibitors LAQ824 and LBH589 do not require death receptor signaling or a functional apoptosome to mediate tumor cell death or therapeutic efficacy. *Blood.* 2009;114:380–393.

169. Chakraborty AR, Robey RW, Luchenko VL, Zhan Z, Piekarz RL, Gillet JP et al. MAPK pathway activation leads to Bim loss and histone deacetylase inhibitor resistance: Rationale to combine romidepsin with an MEK inhibitor. Blood. 2013;121(20):4115–4125.

170. Ozaki K, Minoda A, Kishikawa F, Kohno M. Blockade of the ERK pathway markedly sensitizes tumor cells to HDAC inhibitor-induced cell death. *Biochem Biophys Res Commun.* 2006;339:1171–1177.

171. Yu X, Wang S, Chen G, Hou C, Zhao M, Hong J et al. Apoptosis induced by depsipeptide FK228 coincides with inhibition of survival signaling in lung cancer cells. *Cancer J.* 2007;13:105–113.

172. Yu C, Friday BB, Lai JP, McCollum A, Atadja P, Roberts LR et al. Abrogation of MAPK and Akt signaling by AEE788 synergistically potentiates histone deacetylase inhibitor-induced apoptosis through reactive oxygen species generation. *Clin Cancer Res.* 2007;13:1140–1148.

173. Fantin V, Loboda A, Paweletz C, Hendrickson R, Pierce J, Roth J et al. Constitutive activation of signal transducers and activators of transcription predicts vorinostat resistance in cutaneous T-cell lymphoma. *Cancer Res.* 2008;68:3785–3794.

174. Petrij F, Dauwerse H, Blough R, Giles R, van der Smagt J, Wallerstein R et al. Diagnostic analysis of the Rubinstein-Taybi syndrome: Five cosmids should be used for microdeletion detection and low number of protein truncating mutations. *J Med Genet.* 2000;37:168–176.

175. Taki T, Sako M, Tsuchida M, Hayashi Y. The t(11;16)(q23;p13) translocation in myelodysplastic syndrome fuses the MLL gene to the CBP gene. *Blood*. 1997;89:3945–3950.

176. Borrow J, Stanton VJ, Andresen J, Becher R, Behm F, Chaganti R et al. The translocation t(8;16)(p11;p13) of acute myeloid leukaemia fuses a putative acetyltransferase to the CREB-binding protein. *Nat Genet*. 1996;14:33–41.

177. Mullighan CG, Zhang J, Kasper LH, Lerach S, Payne-Turner D, Phillips LA et al. CREBBP mutations in relapsed acute lymphoblastic leukaemia. *Nature*. 2011;471:235–239.

178. Pasqualucci L, Dominguez-Sola D, Chiarenza A, Fabbri G, Grunn A, Trifonov V et al. Inactivating mutations of acetyltransferase genes in B-cell lymphoma. *Nature*. 2011;471:189–195.

179. Koshiishi N, Chong J, Fukasawa T, Ikeno R, Hayashi Y, Funata N et al. p300 gene alterations in intestinal and diffuse types of gastric carcinoma. *Gastric Cancer*. 2004;7:85–90.

180. Mattera L, Escaffit F, Pillaire M, Selves J, Tyteca S, Hoffmann J et al. The p400/Tip60 ratio is critical for colorectal cancer cell proliferation through DNA damage response pathways. *Oncogene*. 2009;28:1506–1517.

181. Grignani F, De Matteis S, Nervi C, Tomassoni L, Gelmetti V, Cioce M et al. Fusion proteins of the retinoic acid receptor-alpha recruit histone deacetylase in promyelocytic leukaemia. *Nature*. 1998;391:815–818.

182. Wang J, Hoshino T, Redner R, Kajigaya S, Liu J. ETO, fusion partner in t(8;21) acute myeloid leukemia, represses transcription by interaction with the human N-CoR/mSin3/HDAC1 complex. *Proc Natl Acad Sci U S A*. 1998;95:10860–10865.

183. Ropero S, Fraga MF, Ballestar E, Hamelin R, Yamamoto H, Boix-Chornet M et al. A truncating mutation of HDAC2 in human cancers confers resistance to histone deacetylase inhibition. *Nat Genet*. 2006;38:566–569.

184. Sjöblom T, Jones S, Wood L, Parsons D, Lin J, Barber T et al. The consensus coding sequences of human breast and colorectal cancers. *Science*. 2006;314:268–274.

185. Ginter T, Bier C, Knauer SK, Sughra K, Hildebrand D, Münz T et al. Histone deacetylase inhibitors block IFNγ-induced STAT1 phosphorylation. *Cell Signal*. 2012;24:1453–1460.

186. Gupta M, Han JJ, Stenson M, Wellik L, Witzig TE. Regulation of STAT3 by histone deacetylase-3 in diffuse large B-cell lymphoma: Implications for therapy. *Leukemia*. 2012;26:1356–1364.

187. Gu W, Roeder RG. Activation of p53 sequence-specific DNA binding by acetylation of the p53 C-terminal domain. *Cell*. 1997;90:595–606.

188. Boutillier AL, Trinh E, Loeffler JP. Selective E2F-dependent gene transcription is controlled by histone deacetylase activity during neuronal apoptosis. *J Neurochem*. 2003;84:814–828.

189. Chen C, Wang Y, Yang H, Huang P, Kulp S, Yang C et al. Histone deacetylase inhibitors sensitize prostate cancer cells to agents that produce DNA double-strand breaks by targeting Ku70 acetylation. *Cancer Res*. 2007;67:5318–5327.

190. Bali P, Pranpat M, Bradner J, Balasis M, Fiskus W, Guo F et al. Inhibition of histone deacetylase 6 acetylates and disrupts the chaperone function of heat shock protein 90: A novel basis for antileukemia activity of histone deacetylase inhibitors. *J Biol Chem*. 2005;280:26729–26734.

191. Jin YH, Jeon EJ, Li QL, Lee YH, Choi JK, Kim WJ et al. Transforming growth factor-beta stimulates p300-dependent RUNX3 acetylation, which inhibits ubiquitination-mediated degradation. *J Biol Chem*. 2004;279:29409–29417.

192. Fu M, Rao M, Wang C, Sakamaki T, Wang J, Di Vizio D et al. Acetylation of androgen receptor enhances coactivator binding and promotes prostate cancer cell growth. *Mol Cell Biol*. 2003;23:8563–8575.

193. Wang C, Fu M, Angeletti RH, Siconolfi-Baez L, Reutens AT, Albanese C et al. Direct acetylation of the estrogen receptor alpha hinge region by p300 regulates transactivation and hormone sensitivity. *J Biol Chem.* 2001;276:18375–18383.
194. Whittaker SJ, Demierre MF, Kim EJ, Rook AH, Lerner A, Duvic M et al. Final results from a multicenter, international, pivotal study of romidepsin in refractory cutaneous T-cell lymphoma. *J Clin Oncol.* 2010;28:4485–4491.
195. Duvic M, Dummer R, Becker JC, Poulalhon N, Ortiz Romero P, Grazia Bernengo M et al. Panobinostat activity in both bexarotene-exposed and -naïve patients with refractory cutaneous T-cell lymphoma: Results of a phase II trial. *Eur J Cancer.* 2013;49:386–394.
196. Munster P, Marchion D, Bicaku E, Schmitt M, Lee JH, DeConti R et al. Phase I trial of histone deacetylase inhibition by valproic acid followed by the topoisomerase II inhibitor epirubicin in advanced solid tumors: A clinical and translational study. *J Clin Oncol.* 2007;25:1979–1985.
197. Gore S, Baylin S, Sugar E, Carraway H, Miller C, Carducci M et al. Combined DNA methyltransferase and histone deacetylase inhibition in the treatment of myeloid neoplasms. *Cancer Res.* 2006;66:6361–6369.
198. Tredaniel J, Descourt R, Moro-Sibilot D, Misset J, Gachard E, Garcia-Vargas J et al. Vorinostat in combination with gemcitabine and cisplatinum in patients with advanced non-small cell lung cancer (NSCLC): A Phase I dose-escalation study. *J Clin Oncol (Meeting Abstracts).* 2009;27:8049.
199. Fakih M, Pendyala L, Fetterly G, Toth K, Zwiebel J, Espinoza-Delgado I et al. A phase I, pharmacokinetic and pharmacodynamic study on vorinostat in combination with 5-fluorouracil, leucovorin, and oxaliplatin in patients with refractory colorectal cancer. *Clin Cancer Res.* 2009;15:3189–3195.
200. Fouladi M, Park JR, Sun J, Ingle AM, Ames MM, Stewart CF et al. A phase I trial and pharmacokinetic (PK) study of vorinostat (SAHA) in combination with 13 cis-retinoic acid (13cRA) in children with refractory neuroblastomas, medulloblastomas, primitive neuroectodermal tumors (PNETs), and atypical teratoid rhabdoid tumor. *J Clin Oncol (Meeting Abstracts).* 2008;26:10012.
201. Dummer R, Hymes K, Sterry W, Steinhoff M, Assaf C, Kerl H et al. Vorinostat in combination with bexarotene in advanced cutaneous T-cell lymphoma: A phase I study. *J Clin Oncol (Meeting Abstracts).* 2009;27:8572.
202. Badros A, Burger A, Philip S, Niesvizky R, Kolla S, Goloubeva O et al. Phase I study of vorinostat in combination with bortezomib for relapsed and refractory multiple myeloma. *Clin Cancer Res.* 2009;15:5250–5257.
203. Wilson PM, El-Khoueiry A, Iqbal S, Fazzone W, LaBonte MJ, Groshen S et al. A phase I/II trial of vorinostat in combination with 5-fluorouracil in patients with metastatic colorectal cancer who previously failed 5-FU-based chemotherapy. *Cancer Chemother Pharmacol.* 2010;65:979–988.
204. Ree AH, Dueland S, Folkvord S, Hole KH, Seierstad T, Johansen M et al. Vorinostat, a histone deacetylase inhibitor, combined with pelvic palliative radiotherapy for gastrointestinal carcinoma: The Pelvic Radiation and Vorinostat (PRAVO) phase 1 study. *Lancet Oncol.* 2010;11:459–464.
205. Chinnaiyan P, Chowdhary S, Potthast L, Prabhu A, Tsai YY, Sarcar B et al. Phase I trial of vorinostat combined with bevacizumab and CPT-11 in recurrent glioblastoma. *Neuro Oncol.* 2012;14:93–100.
206. Kadia TM, Yang H, Ferrajoli A, Maddipotti S, Schroeder C, Madden TL et al. A phase I study of vorinostat in combination with idarubicin in relapsed or refractory leukaemia. *Br J Haematol.* 2010;150:72–82.
207. Fakih MG, Pendyala L, Egorin MJ, Fetterly G, Espinoza-Delgado I, Ross M et al. A phase I clinical trial of vorinostat in combination with sFULV2 in patients with refractory solid tumors. *J Clin Oncol (Meeting Abstracts).* 2009;27:4083.

208. Schneider BJ, Kalemkerian GP, Bradley D, Smith DC, Egorin MJ, Daignault S et al. Phase I study of vorinostat (suberoylanilide hydroxamic acid, NSC 701852) in combination with docetaxel in patients with advanced and relapsed solid malignancies. *Invest New Drugs*. 2012;30:249–257.
209. Dickson MA, Rathkopf DE, Carvajal RD, Grant S, Roberts JD, Reid JM et al. A phase I pharmacokinetic study of pulse-dose vorinostat with flavopiridol in solid tumors. *Invest New Drugs*. 2011;29:1004–1012.
210. Lassen U, Molife LR, Sorensen M, Engelholm SA, Vidal L, Sinha R et al. A phase I study of the safety and pharmacokinetics of the histone deacetylase inhibitor belinostat administered in combination with carboplatin and/or paclitaxel in patients with solid tumours. *Br J Cancer*. 2010;103:12–17.
211. Hurwitz H, Nelson B, O'Dwyer PJ, Chiorean EG, Gabrail N, Li Z et al. Phase I/II: The oral isotype-selective HDAC inhibitor MGCD0103 in combination with gemcitabine (Gem) in patients (pts) with refractory solid tumors. *J Clin Oncol (Meeting Abstracts)*. 2008;26:4625.
212. Drappatz J, Lee EQ, Hammond S, Grimm SA, Norden AD, Beroukhim R et al. Phase I study of panobinostat in combination with bevacizumab for recurrent high-grade glioma. *J Neurooncol*. 2012;107:133–138.
213. Rathkopf D, Wong BY, Ross RW, Anand A, Tanaka E, Woo MM et al. A phase I study of oral panobinostat alone and in combination with docetaxel in patients with castration-resistant prostate cancer. *Cancer Chemother Pharmacol*. 2010;66:181–189.
214. Scherpereel A, Berghmans T, Lafitte JJ, Colinet B, Richez M, Bonduelle Y et al. Valproate-doxorubicin: Promising therapy for progressing mesothelioma. A phase II study. *Eur Respir J*. 2011;37:129–135.
215. Ramaswamy B, Fiskus W, Cohen B, Pellegrino C, Hershman DL, Chuang E et al. Phase I-II study of vorinostat plus paclitaxel and bevacizumab in metastatic breast cancer: Evidence for vorinostat-induced tubulin acetylation and Hsp90 inhibition in vivo. *Breast Cancer Res Treat*. 2012;132:1063–1072.
216. Munster PN, Thurn KT, Thomas S, Raha P, Lacevic M, Miller A et al. A phase II study of the histone deacetylase inhibitor vorinostat combined with tamoxifen for the treatment of patients with hormone therapy-resistant breast cancer. *Br J Cancer*. 2011;104:1828–1835.
217. Friday BB, Anderson SK, Buckner J, Yu C, Giannini C, Geoffroy F et al. Phase II trial of vorinostat in combination with bortezomib in recurrent glioblastoma: A north central cancer treatment group study. *Neuro Oncol*. 2012;14:215–221.
218. Akilov OE, Grant C, Frye R, Bates S, Piekarz R, Geskin LJ. Low-dose electron beam radiation and romidepsin therapy for symptomatic cutaneous T-cell lymphoma lesions. *Br J Dermatol*. 2012;167:194–197.

18 Compounds Targeting Androgen Pathways

Aurelius Omlin
Royal Marsden NHS Foundation Trust
The Institute of Cancer Research

Carmel Pezaro
Royal Marsden NHS Foundation Trust
The Institute of Cancer Research

Johann de Bono
Royal Marsden NHS Foundation Trust
The Institute of Cancer Research

CONTENTS

ANDROGEN SUPPRESSION: THE MAINSTAY OF PROSTATE CANCER TREATMENT

The effect of orchiectomy in patients with prostate cancer was reported in 1942 by Charles Huggins in a study of 45 patients where orchiectomy led to symptomatic improvement, decline in alkaline phosphatase and a "great decrease in the size and in the stony consistency of the primary neoplasm" [1]. Dr. Huggins was awarded the Nobel Prize in medicine for his groundbreaking research on prostate cancer treatment. The current standard treatment for patients with metastatic prostate cancer remains androgen deprivation by either orchiectomy or luteinizing hormone releasing hormone agonist (LHRH) analogue treatments [2]. An initial surge in testosterone induced by LHRH analogues, which can lead to deterioration of clinical symptoms, can be blocked by a number of agents including antiandrogens, diethylstilbestrol (DES), ketoconazole, and cyproterone acetate [3]. The precise role and clinical benefit of LHRH antagonists that decrease androgen levels without the initial surge remains to be determined [2].

The adrenal glands are the source of about 10% of androgens and cannot be suppressed by LHRH analogue treatment alone. Combined androgen blockade (CAB) with LHRH analogues and antiandrogens has been shown to result in a very small survival benefit of <5% at 5 years compared to LHRH analogue treatment alone in a meta-analysis [4]. Due to the increased rate of mainly gastrointestinal side effects and reduced quality of life, upfront CAB is not routinely offered to patients. In men with locally advanced or metastatic prostate cancer, bicalutamide 150 mg once daily was inferior when compared to castration; however, a large randomized trial with 1453 patients found a small benefit for bicalutamide with regard to quality of life, namely sexual function and physical capacity [5].

Patients on androgen deprivation therapy for metastatic disease develop progressive disease after a median of 18–24 months [6]. Once prostate cancer progresses despite castrate levels of testosterone, it is referred to as castration-resistant prostate cancer (CRPC), previously called androgen-independent prostate cancer [7]. It is now clear that both terms fail to fully characterize the complex situation of advanced prostate cancer.

In patients with rising prostate specific antigen (PSA) on LHRH analogues, addition of an antiandrogen is a standard therapeutic option [8]. PSA declines on CAB can be achieved in 20%–50% of patients with a median response of 3–6 months [9,10].

In case of rising PSA despite CAB, patients discontinue antiandrogen treatment and continue LHRH analogue therapy. An antiandrogen withdrawal syndrome, characterized by falling PSA, can be observed in 20%–30% patients 4–6 weeks after stopping antiandrogen treatment [8,11]. Further hormonal manipulations with ketoconazole, megestrol acetate, DES, and glucocorticoids can result in PSA declines for generally a limited period in the range of several months [12,13].

Ketoconazole is an antifungal and nonspecific weak inhibitor of steroid biosynthesis including inhibition of CYP17 impacting mineralocorticoids, glucocorticoids, testosterone, and estrogens. High-dose ketoconazole (1200 mg/day) alone or in combination with hydrocortisone has produced $\geq$50% PSA declines in 27%–62% of trial participants [14,15]. The unfavorable side effect profile of high-dose ketoconazole, which includes liver toxicity, fatigue/lethargy, gastrointestinal toxicity (nausea, vomiting, and diarrhea), and skin rash, has limited the use of this agent. Aminoglutethimide is another nonspecific CYP17 inhibitor with modest activity in advanced prostate cancer and a limiting side effect profile [16].

Estrogen-containing treatments, such as DES, was amongst the earliest pharmacological therapies for patients with advanced prostate cancer. The main mechanism of action of DES is thought to be the result of negative feedback on the hypothalamic–pituitary axis. However, preclinical data have shown that DES also has estrogen receptor-independent activity through modulation of tubulin isotype expression and induction of aberrant microtubule arrays [17]. Treatment with DES can result in PSA declines of ≥50% in 20%–40% of patients lasting generally for an average of 3–6 months [12]. DES treatment is associated with a significant risk of thromboembolic complications (venous thrombosis, pulmonary embolism, myocardial infarction, and stroke) in 5%–15% recipients. It is recommended that DES is administrated either with aspirin or low-dose warfarin [12,18].

In the absence of prospective randomized trials, such third-line hormonal manipulations are used at the discretion of individual treating clinicians.

In summary, prostate cancer generally responds initially to androgen withdrawal. For many years, CRPC was thought to reflect a state of resistance to further hormonal manipulations. The following sections now highlight significant advances in prostate cancer management that have been achieved by further targeting of the androgen receptor (AR).

CYP17 INHIBITION

The key enzyme of androgen biosynthesis, CYP17, has a dual function as a 17-α-hydroxylase and 17,20-lyase (see Figure 18.1). The importance of intratumoral synthesis of testosterone from adrenal androgens through CYP17 enzymes that are upregulated in CRPC supported the clinical development of novel androgen biosynthesis inhibitors [19,20].

Abiraterone

Abiraterone acetate (abiraterone; Zytiga®, Janssen) is a pregnenolone-derived 3-pyridyl steroidal drug, developed in collaboration between The Institute of Cancer Research and Cancer Research, UK. Abiraterone irreversibly inhibits both 17-α-hydroxylase and 17,20-lyase [21]. For the first clinical trials, concerns regarding adrenocortical insufficiency induced by potent CYP17 inhibition were addressed by careful clinical and biochemical monitoring of patients. Reports on teenagers with familial CYP17 deficiency, however, showed the main symptoms to be delayed puberty and hypertension [22].

Phase I and II trials in chemotherapy-naïve and docetaxel pre-treated patients reported very encouraging activity with ≥50% PSA declines in 50%–60% of patients [23–26]. Soft tissue responses were documented in 37% chemotherapy-naïve and in 27% post-chemotherapy patients. Symptoms of secondary mineralocorticoid excess due to accumulation of upstream steroids, namely hypertension, hypokalemia, and fluid retention, were the main side effects of abiraterone treatment and were successfully abrogated with the addition of low-dose glucocorticoids such as dexamethasone

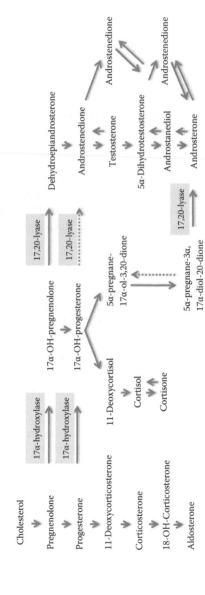

FIGURE 18.1 Androgen biosynthesis pathways with the CYP17 enzymes 17α-hydroxylase and 17,20-lyase highlighted.

(0.5 mg once daily), prednisolone (5 mg twice daily), or the mineralocorticoid receptor antagonist eplerenone. Two large phase III trials were subsequently initiated.

In the post-chemotherapy COU-301 abiraterone trial, 1195 patients with CRPC were randomized in a 2:1 ratio to treatment with prednisone/prednisolone combined with abiraterone or placebo. All patients had progressive disease after docetaxel-based chemotherapy, and about 30% of patients had received two lines of prior chemotherapy. At a planned interim analysis, the median overall survival (OS) on abiraterone was significantly longer than placebo with an absolute improvement of 3.9 months (14.8 months versus 10.9 months, hazard ratio [HR] 0.65, 95% confidence interval [CI] 0.54–0.77) [27]. The trial was then unblinded to allow crossover of patients from placebo. The updated analysis at the time of crossover confirmed an OS benefit of 4.6 months (15.8 months versus 11.2 months; HR 0.74, 95% CI 0.64–0.86) [28]. With regard to secondary endpoints, abiraterone was superior compared to placebo for confirmed ≥50% PSA decline rates (29% versus 6%), soft tissue responses (14% versus 3%), time to PSA progression (10.2 months versus 6.6 months), and median radiographic progression-free survival (PFS) (5.6 months versus 3.6 months).

Abiraterone was found to be a safe and tolerable treatment, with mainly mild to moderate drug-related side effects of fluid retention (31% versus 22%, $p = .04$), hypokalcmia (17% versus 8% $p < .001$), and hypertension (10% versus 8%). Common terminology criteria for adverse events grade 3 and 4 elevations of liver function tests were slightly more common on abiraterone (3.5% versus 3%). Preplanned subgroup analyses confirmed abiraterone benefit in elderly patients aged ≥75 years (14.9 months versus 9.3 months; HR: 0.52; 95% CI: 0.38–0.71), in patients with visceral disease (12.6 months versus 8.4 months; HR: 0.7; 95% CI: 0.52–0.94), and in patients with significant baseline pain (worst pain ≥4 on brief pain inventory: 12.9 months versus 8.9 months; HR: 0.68; 95% CI: 0.53–0.85) [27].

The analyses of circulating tumor cells (CTCs) in the COU-301 trial have been presented. Changes in CTC counts in patients with CRPC, namely the conversion from unfavorable (CTC ≥ 5/7.5 ml blood) to favorable (CTC < 5), have been associated with survival [29,30]. In the COU–301 trial, CTC counts were enumerated at baseline and at weeks 4, 8, and 12, using the CellSearch® platform. CTC conversion was associated with improved OS as early as 4 weeks after commencing treatment [31]. Further confirmation from this and other trials is awaited to determine whether CTC count changes could serve as a marker of surrogacy for survival.

The results of the COU-302 phase III trial of abiraterone in chemotherapy-naïve patients have also been presented. A total of 1088 asymptomatic or minimally symptomatic patients were randomized 1:1 to prednisone/prednisolone combined with abiraterone ($n = 546$) or placebo ($n = 542$). The primary endpoint was a composite of radiographic PFS and OS. The protocol pre-specified interim analysis was conducted after 311 deaths and showed a statistically significant improvement in radiographic PFS in patients treated with abiraterone compared to placebo (16.5 m) versus 8.3 months; HR: 0.53; 95% CI: 0.45–0.62). Also significantly improved survival with abiraterone was reported (median not reached [NR] versus 27.2 months; HR: 0.75; 95% CI: 0.61–0.93) [32]. Secondary endpoints were also in favor of abiraterone, namely ≥50% PSA declines (62% versus 24%) and soft tissue responses (36% versus 16%).

Based on these results, the independent data monitoring committee recommended that the trial be unblinded to allow crossover for placebo patients. The decision to stop the trial early was criticized because at the interim analysis, the OS p value of .0097 failed to meet the pre-specified p value of .0008 to achieve statistical significance (O'Brien Fleming boundary). Final results of this trial are awaited; however, it is likely that abiraterone will become a new standard therapy for chemotherapy-naïve patients.

Practical Considerations

Although abiraterone is a well-tolerated oral therapy, it does require regular review and active management of toxicities related to mineralocorticoid excess. Routine monitoring should include measurements of blood pressure, weight, potassium levels, and liver function tests. The co-administration of prednisone or prednisolone may also have implications, especially in patients who remain on treatment for a long time, such as weight gain, bone loss, or unmasking of a diabetic condition, and importantly long-term corticosteroid treatment may eventually lead to AR activation.

Early discontinuation of abiraterone treatment should be avoided especially in view of the described incidence of radiographic bone flares [33]. Both phase III trials recommended that, in the absence of clinical progression, patients with rising PSA should continue on treatment until radiographic evidence of progression was documented.

Abiraterone in Breast Cancer

ARs can be expressed in breast cancer tissue, usually associated with negative estrogen receptor expression and overexpression of human epidermal growth factor receptor 2 (HER2). AR can activate HER2 and Wnt signaling through direct induction [34]. Results of a phase I trial in estrogen receptor (ER)+ or ER–/AR+ patients with advanced breast cancer resistant to >2 lines of hormone therapies were presented at American Society of Clinical Oncology (ASCO) 2011. Of 25 enrolled patients, one patient achieved a radiological partial response and 80% reduction in serum CA15.3 from baseline [35]. The phase II part of this clinical trial is ongoing (NCT00755885), and a randomized phase II clinical trial is evaluating abiraterone plus prednisone compared to abiraterone with prednisone and exemestane (NCT01381874).

OTHER CYP17 INHIBITORS

A number of novel CYP17 inhibitor compounds are in clinical development that are, when compared to abiraterone, more specific for the CYP17,20-lyase, which might in theory result in less mineralocorticoid excess toxicity and may not require concomitant corticosteroid treatment.

Orteronel (TAK-700, Takeda Pharmaceuticals) is a novel inhibitor of androgen biosynthesis and compared to abiraterone is a more potent inhibitor of the CYP17,20-lyase. The selectivity of orteronel has been postulated to allow treatment without concomitant steroid use, although ongoing phase III clinical trials administered this agent with steroids. Results of a phase II expansion of the original phase I/II trial were presented at the ASCO 2012 Genitourinary Cancers

Symposium. A total of 97 chemotherapy-naïve patients were treated in four cohorts with orteronel 300 mg BID (twice daily), 400 mg and 600 mg BID with prednisone, and 600 mg QD (once daily). PSA declines of ≥50% were observed in 63%, 50%, 41%, and 60% of participants in the respective cohorts. Soft tissue responses by RECIST were reported in 20% (10/51) evaluable patients. The most common grade ≥ 3 side effects were fatigue (12%) and hypokalemia (8%). Three phase III trials with orteronel are currently ongoing (see Table 18.1) [36].

Galeterone (TOK-001, Tokai Pharmaceuticals) is a selective CYP17,20-lyase inhibitor with additional antiandrogen properties. The preliminary results of a phase I trial were presented at ASCO 2012. A total of 49 chemotherapy-naïve patients received escalating doses of galeterone, although the maximum tolerated dose was not reached. Overall 22% (11/49) patients had PSA declines of ≥50% and soft tissue responses were seen in two patients. Transient liver function test elevations were seen in 15 patients (30%), five of whom had suspected or confirmed Gilbert's disease [37]. Further results including the phase II component of this trial are awaited.

Another novel compound in clinical phase I testing is *VT-464* (Viamet Pharmaceuticals), which is a highly potent and lyase-selective CYP17 inhibitor. *CFG920* (Novartis Pharmaceuticals) is a novel CYP17 inhibitor that will be tested in a phase I/II clinical trial shortly (NCT01647789).

NEXT-GENERATION ANTIANDROGENS

Antiandrogens are agents that compete with endogenous androgens for the ligand-binding pocket of the AR. Overexpression or mutations in the AR can cause "first-generation" antiandrogens such as flutamide or bicalutamide to become partial agonists, contributing to cancer progression. Such agonist activity is also responsible for the androgen withdrawal syndrome. In contrast, second-generation AR antagonists have been rationally designed and selected to avoid agonist activity even in models overexpressing AR.

Enzalutamide

Enzalutamide (MDV3100, XTANDI®, Medivation) is a second-generation nonsteroidal AR antagonist. It was selected for development after demonstrating high affinity for AR [38]. In preclinical models, enzalutamide inhibited AR nuclear translocation, DNA binding, and recruitment of coactivator peptides, leading to apoptosis. Encouraging activity was seen in a phase I–II clinical trial involving 140 men with metastatic CRPC [39]. Antitumor activity was observed in all dose cohorts from 30 to 600 mg/day, with ≥50% PSA declines in 56% in the population overall, supported by radiological evidence of benefit and declines in the number of CTCs. The maximum tolerated dose was defined as 240 mg, taking into account increasing rates of severe fatigue as well as concern about a possible link between higher dose enzalutamide and seizures.

The pivotal phase III AFFIRM trial recruited 1199 men with metastatic CRPC progressing after docetaxel treatment and randomized them in a 2:1 ratio to receive enzalutamide 160 mg/day or matched placebo. The study was unblinded following a preplanned analysis after 520 deaths. Enzalutamide treatment resulted in a 4.8 month improvement in survival, with median OS of 18.4

TABLE 18.1
Completed and Open Phase III Trials of Novel Compounds Targeting the Androgen Receptor Signaling Pathway

Mechanism of Action	Drug	Trial	Patient Population	Primary Endpoint	Reference (From Main Reference List)
17α-hydroxylase and 17,20-lyase (CYP17) inhibitor	Abiraterone	III (COU-301 trial)	1195 CRPC patients, post-chemotherapy	Overall survival 14.8 months versus 10.9 months (HR: 0.65; 95% CI: 0.54–0.77) Updated survival analysis (ECCO 2011): 15.8 months versus 11.2 (HR: 0.74; 95% CI: 0.64–0.86)	[27]
17α-hydroxylase and 17,20-lyase (CYP17) inhibitor	Abiraterone	III (COU-302)	1088 CRPC patients, asymptomatic or minimally symptomatic, pre-chemotherapy	Composite primary endpoint: OS and radiographic progression-free survival. Radiographic progression free survival (16.5 versus 8.3 months; HR: 0.53; 95% CI: 0.45–0.62); overall survival (NR versus 27.2 months, HR 0.75, 95% CI 0.61–0.93).	[32]
17α-hydroxylase and 17,20-lyase (CYP17) inhibitor	Abiraterone	II/III STAMPEDE	Ongoing, planned 4000 patients. Multiple arms: metastatic prostate cancer. Arm A: androgen suppression (AS) ±radiotherapy Arm B: AS+zoledronic acid; Arm C: AS+docetaxel; Arm D: AS+abiraterone.	Overall survival	NCT00268476

Class	Compound	Phase/Trial	Patients	Endpoint/Results	Reference
Antiandrogen	Enzalutamide	III AFFIRM	1199 CRPC patients, post-chemotherapy	Overall survival 18.4 months versus 13.6 months (HR: 0.631; 95% CI: 0.529–0.752)	[40]
Antiandrogen	Enzalutamide	III PREVAIL	Planned 1680 CRPC patients, pre-chemotherapy	Composite primary endpoint: Overall survival and progression-free survival	NCT01212991
Selective 17, 20-lyase inhibitor	Orteronel (TAK700)	III	1083 CRPC patients planned, post-chemotherapy	Overall survival	NCT01193257
Selective 17, 20-lyase inhibitor	Orteronel (TAK700)	III	1454 CRPC patients planned, chemotherapy naïve	Composite primary endpoint: Overall survival and radiographic progression-free survival	NCT01193244
Selective 17, 20-lyase inhibitor	Orteronel (TAK700)	III	900 patients planned: Dose escalated RT and ADT with a GNRH agonist versus dose escalated RT and enhanced ADT with a GNRH agonist and TAK-700 for men with high-risk prostate cancer	Overall survival	NCT01546987

months in the enzalutamide arm compared to 13.6 months in the placebo arm, giving an estimated HR of 0.631 (95% CI: 0.53–0.75) [40]. The survival advantage was maintained in all examined subgroups including notably patients with visceral metastases at baseline (13.4 months versus 9.5 months; HR: 0.78; 95% CI: 0.56–1.09). Enzalutamide was also superior for the reported secondary efficacy endpoints. PSA declines of more than 50% were reported in 54% of patients on enzalutamide compared to 2% on placebo. Radiological soft tissue responses (29% versus 4%), time to first skeletal-related event (16.7 months versus 13.3 months), and quality of life using the functional assessment of cancer therapy—prostate all favored enzalutamide treatment. Of note, although corticosteroids may be used concurrently with enzalutamide, they were not mandated in the AFFIRM trial. Patients who received corticosteroids on this trial had a worse outcome with a median survival of 12.3 months on enzalutamide compared to 9.3 months on placebo (HR: 0.7, $p = .0116$), whereas patients without concomitant corticosteroid use had a median survival on enzalutamide that was NR compared to 15.8 months on placebo (HR: 0.59, $p < .0001$). This finding may be due to the fact that physicians treat poorer prognosis patients with corticosteroids as supportive care. However, preclinical studies indicate that CRPC cells can have aberrant AR that may be driven by corticosteroids [41,42].

Side effects were generally mild to moderate with a low frequency of grade ≥ 3 events in both arms including fatigue (6% versus 7%), diarrhea (1% versus <1%), and hot flushes (no grade 3 events). Seizure rate did appear higher on enzalutamide, despite the exclusion of men with a seizure history or known CNS metastases. Overall, five men (0.6%) in the enzalutamide arm had a seizure compared to none in the placebo arm. Several of the cases were associated with diagnosis of CNS metastases or with concomitant medications known to act centrally to lower the seizure threshold.

There are a number of ongoing enzalutamide trials, including the phase III PREVAIL study in men with chemotherapy-naïve CRPC (NCT01212991). In earlier stage disease, enzalutamide is being evaluated as a single agent in men with hormone-naïve prostate cancer (NCT01302041) against bicalutamide (NCT01288911) and in combination with docetaxel chemotherapy (NCT01565928). A study of neoadjuvant enzalutamide is also planned (NCT01547299). Combination testing with abiraterone has commenced (NCT01650194) and other combinations are planned.

Practical Considerations

Generally enzalutamide is well tolerated and dose reduction is rarely required, allowing for outpatient administration with regular clinic reviews. Due to the possibility that enzalutamide might lower the threshold for seizures, it is recommended to avoid enzalutamide in men with a history of seizures, strokes, or unexplained loss of consciousness and to consider carefully the concomitant medications.

As with abiraterone, the AFFIRM trial recommended continued treatment for rising PSA in the absence of clinical or radiological progression. If possible, patients who remain well despite PSA progression should therefore be continued on enzalutamide.

Novel Antiandrogens in Development

ARN-509 (Aragon Pharmaceuticals, Inc.) is another second-generation AR antagonist that has structural similarity to enzalutamide. In preclinical models, ARN-509 exhibited superior characteristics compared to related agents [43]. Phase I testing showed evidence of durable PSA declines at doses between 30 and 300 mg/day [44]. An optimal biological dose of 240 mg daily was selected for further clinical development. The risk of seizures with novel antiandrogens was associated with blockade of the GABA$_\underline{A}$ receptor. ARN-509, however, has a very low affinity in radioligand binding assays and, when compared to enzalutamide, a significantly decreased penetrance of the blood–brain barrier [43]. ARN-509 is currently in early-phase testing in men who are either treatment-naïve or following abiraterone (NCT01171898).

Other novel agents: *BMS-641988* (Bristol-Myers Squibb) is a novel antiandrogen with increased binding affinity for AR compared to bicalutamide. A phase I study was initiated, but limited antitumor activity and an episode of seizure in a trial participant led to trial discontinuation [45]. *EPI-001* is a small molecule AR antagonist, purported to target the AR aminoterminal domain, with encouraging preclinical evidence of activity in CRPC [46]. *MEL-3* was identified during an in vitro screening program and utilizes a novel nonsteroidal scaffold. Preclinical testing of MEL-3 demonstrated inhibition of prostate cancer growth, activity against mutant AR, and reduced expression of androgen-related genes, PSA, and the co-chaperone FK506 binding protein 5 (FKBP5) [47]. Concerns, however, remain about the selectivity of this compound.

Novel Strategies Targeting Androgen Signaling

A number of novel strategies are being employed to target androgen synthesis or the AR, including compounds with encouraging clinical activity in early-phase clinical trials.

Selective AR degraders (SARD) are designed to bind to the AR and induce a conformational change, leading to proteasomal degradation. One such agent is AZD3514 (AstraZeneca), and although there are as yet no published data, preliminary evidence from preclinical studies suggests encouraging activity, and a multicenter phase I clinical trial is in progress (NCT01162395 and NCT01351688) [48]. Aragon Pharmaceuticals also have a discovery program for SARD.

EZN-4176 (Enzon Pharmaceuticals, Inc.) is an antisense oligonucleotide targeting AR. Antisense oligonucleotides are synthetic strands of nucleic acids that bind messenger RNA (mRNA) for a target gene, either directly inactivating the mRNA by preventing translation, or binding to a splicing site, modifying the exon content. EZN-4176 utilizes a third-generation locked nucleic acid structure, providing higher binding affinity and increased potency for target mRNA downregulation compared to early-generation antisense compounds. Preclinical data demonstrated down regulation of AR mRNA and protein and inhibited growth of CRPC cells in vitro and in xenograft models [49]. No effect was observed with a control antisense not targeting AR, or in AR-negative cell lines. A phase I clinical trial is currently in progress (NCT01337518).

Heat shock proteins (HSPs) are a class of functionally related proteins, named according to molecular weight, which function as intracellular chaperones for other proteins. Expression of HSPs is increased by exposure to stressful stimuli. HSP-90 is one of the most common of the HSPs. HSP-90 folds and stabilizes client proteins such as AR and is commonly overexpressed in prostate cancer cells [50]. HSP-27 regulates cell signaling and survival pathways. In prostate cancer models, androgen-bound AR induced HSP-27 phosphorylation, which then complexed with AR and enhanced AR stability, shuttling, and transcriptional activity [51]. Expression of HSP-27 protein in diagnostic prostate cancer biopsies was shown to be an independent predictor of poorer clinical outcome, and HSP-27 has also been implicated in gamma radiation resistance [52,53].

HSP-90 inhibitors include naturally occurring products such as geldanamycin, semisynthetic derivatives, and synthetic compounds. Preclinical and phase I testing has suggested potential antitumor activity in CRPC with semisynthetic derivatives, although notably preclinical data suggested that the derivative 17-AAG (tanespimycin) caused activation of osteoclast c-Src kinase signaling and promoted growth within bone metastases [54–56]. A number of synthetic HSP-90 inhibitors are in clinical testing, including AUY922 (Novartis Pharmaceuticals), which is currently being investigated in a number of phase I trials, and AT13387 (ASTEX Pharmaceuticals), which is currently being tested in a phase II trial in men with CRPC following docetaxel and abiraterone.

HSP-27 inhibitors: OGX-427 (OncoGenex Technologies) is a second-generation antisense oligonucleotide against HSP-27. OGX-427 is administered intravenously, with three loading doses followed by maintenance weekly treatment. A phase I study was conducted in patients with advanced solid malignancies and tested OGX-427 both as a single agent and combined with docetaxel. At the maximum tolerated dose of 1000 mg, treatment was well tolerated, with toxicities mainly due to infusion reactions and transient coagulation changes related to elevation in partial thromboplastin time [57]. Evidence of single agent and combination activity was reported including $\geq$30% PSA declines in 3 of 16 and 5 of 9 eligible patients in single agent and combination cohorts, respectively, as well as radiographic responses and CTC conversions. Preliminary data from a randomized phase II study were reported at ASCO 2012. The study was conducted in the chemotherapy-naïve CRPC setting and randomized men between OGX-427 with prednisone or prednisone alone [58]. Encouraging activity was observed in 32 evaluable men, including $\geq$50% PSA declines in 41% of men who received OGX-427, compared to 20% with prednisone alone, and CTC conversion in 50% and 30%, respectively. OGX-427 treatment was associated with radiographic partial responses in 3 of 8 evaluable men.

Novel combination strategies: Further examination of the biological basis for cancer progression on novel androgen targeting therapies is likely to lead to better therapeutic strategies. One such example is the translational observation that mutant AR can be activated by prednisolone at plasma levels achieved during concomitant dosing with abiraterone, with in vitro evidence that the activation could be reversed using enzalutamide [42]. Preclinical evidence of synergy has been reported using the combination of enzalutamide and the clusterin antisense oligonucleotide, OGX-011 [59]. Preclinical synergy has also been reported using bicalutamide in combination with carbidopa (Lodosyn®, Valeant Pharmaceuticals), which inhibits the AR coactivator L-dopa decarboxylase [60].

MECHANISMS OF RESISTANCE TO TARGETING THE AR

The phase III trials of abiraterone and enzalutamide have generated strong evidence that CRPC is still driven by signaling through the AR [27,32,61]. However, primary refractory disease and secondary resistance after initial response occur with both agents. An increasing number of mechanisms of resistance to targeting the AR and androgen biosynthesis are being recognized, including the following:

- AR mutations
- AR amplification
- AR splice variants
- Tissue steroidogenesis
- Activation of alternative pathways
- Ligand independent AR activation

AR MUTATIONS

Resistance to AR antagonists can occur through mutations in the ligand-binding domain of the AR [62]. However, mutations can also increase sensitivity and promiscuity of the AR so that AR antagonists are turned into stimulating agents and promote prostate cancer cell growth. With AR targeting treatments, the frequency of "gain of function" AR mutations increases. Mutations can be found infrequently in treatment naïve patients, mainly in the NH2-terminal domain, but are more commonly observed in castration-resistant disease where they occur in the ligand-binding domain [63]. The clinical relevance of these data is that several steroidal compounds including prednisolone, eplerenone, and spironolactone have been shown to bind and activate mutant AR [42,64]. Spironolactone should be avoided in patients with advanced prostate cancer and eplerenone used with caution.

AR AMPLIFICATION

AR overexpression was shown in preclinical models to result in increased sensitivity to low levels of androgens [65]. Furthermore, overexpression of AR resulted in increased transcription of AR-regulated genes through an enhanced binding to chromatin [66].

AR SPLICE VARIANTS

Several key domains of the AR protein have been identified to play a role in mechanisms of resistance. The ligand-binding domain (COOH-terminal) is followed by a central DNA-binding domain, a hinge region, and the NH2-terminal transactivation domain [67]. Alternative AR products as a result of splicing are called splice variants (AR-V) and are AR proteins that generally lack the ligand-binding domain. Increased activation of AR-V has been associated with prostate cancer progression through ligand independent constitutive activation mechanisms [68]. Resistance to abiraterone has been postulated to be meditated by increased expression of truncated AR-V [69]. Since AR-V can be found in normal and malignant prostate tissue with highest concentrations in castration-resistant tissue, the clinical importance of AR-V needs to be further investigated.

There is preclinical evidence that enzalutamide may overcome AR-V mediated growth, raising the hypothesis that AR-V requires the full-length AR for signaling [70].

TISSUE STEROIDOGENESIS

The intratumoral conversion of weak androgens (e.g., dehydroepiandrosterone and androstenedione), primarily sourced from the adrenal glands, has been recognized as a mechanism of continued AR activation [71]. Furthermore, in patients treated with CYP17 inhibitors, intratumoral expression of CYP17A1 increased significantly whilst on therapy. In T877A AR mutant cell lines which are not CYP17A1 dependent, continued activity was mediated by upstream CYP11A1 steroid synthesis from pregnenolone/progesterone [72].

Dihydrotestosterone (DHT) is the main AR ligand and is synthesized by 5α-reduction of testosterone. There is increasing evidence of an alternative or so-called backdoor pathway of androgen synthesis where the inactive DHT metabolite androstanediol is oxidized to DHT through the 17-beta-hydroxysteroid dehydrogenase type 6 enzyme [73,74]. Inhibitors of the 5α-reductase enzymes such as finasteride or dutasteride could potentially block androgen synthesis through the backdoor pathway, and further research will have to evaluate whether combination strategies of 5α-reductase inhibitors and novel androgen biosynthesis inhibitors are of clinical importance [73,75].

OTHER MECHANISMS OF AR ACTIVATION

The AR can also be activated as a result of up- or downregulation in co-factors including the HSP chaperones. Other chaperone proteins that regulate the binding of ligands to the AR are the co-chaperones FKBP51 and FKBP52 [76]. A number of nuclear receptor coactivators have been shown to be upregulated in CRPC and to contribute to continued AR activation [77,78].

Another important preclinical advance was the discovery of reciprocal feedback mechanisms between the AR and the critical Phosphatase and tensin homolog (PTEN), Phosphatidylinositide 3-kinases (PI3K), mammalian target of rapamycin (mTOR) (PI3K–AKT–mTOR) signaling pathway. These findings suggest that AR blockade may result in AKT activation and conversely that blockade of the PI3K–AKT–mTOR pathway may result in AR activation through activation of HER2/3 [79].

UNDERSTANDING RESISTANCE MECHANISMS

More than ever, characterizing metastatic tissue is of considerable importance because of the heterogeneity that occurs within tumors, between primary and metastatic sites, and during treatment. Examination of serial bone marrow biopsies is feasible and has demonstrated ongoing testosterone suppression at the time of progression on abiraterone without an increase in steroid synthesis [80]. In addition to tumor biopsies, CTCs, free nucleic acids in plasma, and urine represent potential sources for molecular characterization of patients. CTCs have been assayed for AR gene amplification, PTEN deletion, epidermal growth factor receptor expression, and chromosomal rearrangements (e.g., TMPRSS2-ERG rearrangements) [81,82].

CONCLUSIONS

Until very recently, docetaxel was the only CRPC treatment option with a proven survival benefit. Abiraterone has been approved for treatment of patients progressing after docetaxel-based chemotherapy in both the United States and Europe and is now considered a new standard therapy option. The recently presented positive results of abiraterone in chemotherapy-naïve patients resulted in the approval of abiraterone earlier in the disease. Enzalutamide was also granted approval for chemotherapy pre-treated patients by the US Food and Drug Administration with approval in Europe pending. Both drugs target AR signaling by different mechanisms of action and have led to significant improvements in OS of patients with advanced prostate cancer.

With cabazitaxel (Jevtana®, Sanofi Aventis) approved as second-line chemotherapy and possible further treatment options, including sipuleucel-T (Provenge®, Dendreon) and radium-223 (Xofigo®, Algeta ASA), new challenges will need to be addressed. Clinical trials will have to target the questions of combination strategies of these novel agents and sequencing to achieve maximal clinical benefit. Even more importantly, molecular characterization of prostate cancer is needed to further dissect this disease, and robust predictive biomarkers for patient selection are urgently needed. CTCs may serve as surrogate markers for future phase III combination or sequencing trials.

In summary, significant advances have been achieved for the benefit of patients with advanced prostate cancer, by ongoing targeting of AR signaling. Future research efforts will address the increasing complexity of selecting the right patients for different treatments. Inclusion of patients into clinical trial protocols is therefore recommended.

Disclosure

All authors are ICR employees. The ICR has a commercial interest in abiraterone and PI3K and AKT inhibitors. JS de Bono has served as a paid consultant for J&J, Sanofi Aventis, Medivation, Astellas, AstraZeneca, Dendreon, Genentech, Pfizer, and GSK.

ACKNOWLEDGMENT

Aurelius Omlin's work is supported by a grant by the Swiss Cancer League (BIL KLS-02592–02–2010).

REFERENCES

1. Huggins C. Effect of orchiectomy and irradiation on cancer of the prostate. *Annals of Surgery*. 1942;115(6):1192–1200. Epub 1942/06/01.
2. Weckermann D, Harzmann R. Hormone therapy in prostate cancer: LHRH antagonists versus LHRH analogues. *European Urology*. 2004;46(3):279–283; discussion 83–84. Epub 2004/08/13.
3. Thompson IM. Flare associated with LHRH-agonist therapy. *Reviews in Urology*. 2001;3 (Suppl 3):S10–S14. Epub 2006/09/21.

4. Mottet N, Bellmunt J, Bolla M, Joniau S, Mason M, Matveev V et al. EAU guidelines on prostate cancer. Part II: Treatment of advanced, relapsing, and castration-resistant prostate cancer. *European Urology.* 2011;59(4):572–583. Epub 2011/02/15.

5. Tyrrell CJ, Kaisary AV, Iversen P, Anderson JB, Baert L, Tammela T et al. A randomised comparison of 'Casodex' (bicalutamide) 150 mg monotherapy versus castration in the treatment of metastatic and locally advanced prostate cancer. *European Urology.* 1998;33(5):447–456. Epub 1998/06/27.

6. Lam JS, Leppert JT, Vemulapalli SN, Shvarts O, Belldegrun AS. Secondary hormonal therapy for advanced prostate cancer. *The Journal of Urology.* 2006;175(1):27–34. Epub 2006/01/13.

7. Scher HI, Halabi S, Tannock I, Morris M, Sternberg CN, Carducci MA et al. Design and end points of clinical trials for patients with progressive prostate cancer and castrate levels of testosterone: Recommendations of the Prostate Cancer Clinical Trials Working Group. *Journal of Clinical Oncology: Official Journal of the American Society of Clinical Oncology.* 2008;26(7):1148–1159. Epub 2008/03/04.

8. Small EJ, Vogelzang NJ. Second-line hormonal therapy for advanced prostate cancer: A shifting paradigm. *Journal of Clinical Oncology: Official Journal of the American Society of Clinical Oncology.* 1997;15(1):382–388. Epub 1997/01/01.

9. Fossa SD, Slee PH, Brausi M, Horenblas S, Hall RR, Hetherington JW et al. Flutamide versus prednisone in patients with prostate cancer symptomatically progressing after androgen-ablative therapy: A phase III study of the European organization for research and treatment of cancer genitourinary group. *Journal of Clinical Oncology: Official Journal of the American Society of Clinical Oncology.* 2001;19(1):62–71. Epub 2001/01/03.

10. Fowler JE, Jr., Pandey P, Seaver LE, Feliz TP. Prostate specific antigen after gonadal androgen withdrawal and deferred flutamide treatment. *The Journal of Urology.* 1995;154(2 Pt 1):448–453. Epub 1995/08/01.

11. Sartor AO, Tangen CM, Hussain MH, Eisenberger MA, Parab M, Fontana JA et al. Antiandrogen withdrawal in castrate-refractory prostate cancer: A Southwest Oncology Group Trial (SWOG 9426). *Cancer.* 2008;112(11):2393–2400. Epub 2008/04/03.

12. Bosset PO, Albiges L, Seisen T, de la Motte Rouge T, Phe V, Bitker MO et al. Current role of diethylstilbestrol in the management of advanced prostate cancer. *BJU International.* 2012;110(11 Pt C):E826–E829. Epub 2012/05/15.

13. Ryan CJ. Secondary hormonal manipulations in prostate cancer. *Hematology/Oncology Clinics of North America.* 2006;20(4):925–934. Epub 2006/07/25.

14. Small EJ, Halabi S, Dawson NA, Stadler WM, Rini BI, Picus J et al. Antiandrogen withdrawal alone or in combination with ketoconazole in androgen-independent prostate cancer patients: A phase III trial (CALGB 9583). *Journal of Clinical Oncology: Official Journal of the American Society of Clinical Oncology.* 2004;22(6):1025–1033. Epub 2004/03/17.

15. Small EJ, Baron AD, Fippin L, Apodaca D. Ketoconazole retains activity in advanced prostate cancer patients with progression despite flutamide withdrawal. *The Journal of Urology.* 1997;157(4):1204–1207. Epub 1997/04/01.

16. Figg WD, Dawson N, Middleman MN, Brawley O, Lush RM, Senderowicz A et al. Flutamide withdrawal and concomitant initiation of aminoglutethimide in patients with hormone refractory prostate cancer. *Acta Oncologica.* 1996;35(6):763–765. Epub 1996/01/01.

17. Montgomery RB, Bonham M, Nelson PS, Grim J, Makary E, Vessella R et al. Estrogen effects on tubulin expression and taxane mediated cytotoxicity in prostate cancer cells. *The Prostate.* 2005;65(2):141–150. Epub 2005/06/01.

18. Clemons J, Glode LM, Gao D, Flaig TW. Low-dose diethylstilbestrol for the treatment of advanced prostate cancer. *Urologic Oncology.* 2011. Epub 2011/07/29.

19. Stanbrough M, Bubley GJ, Ross K, Golub TR, Rubin MA, Penning TM et al. Increased expression of genes converting adrenal androgens to testosterone in androgen-independent prostate cancer. *Cancer Research*. 2006;66(5):2815–2825. Epub 2006/03/03.

20. Dillard PR, Lin MF, Khan SA. Androgen-independent prostate cancer cells acquire the complete steroidogenic potential of synthesizing testosterone from cholesterol. *Molecular and Cellular Endocrinology*. 2008;295(1–2):115–120. Epub 2008/09/11.

21. Barrie SE, Potter GA, Goddard PM, Haynes BP, Dowsett M, Jarman M. Pharmacology of novel steroidal inhibitors of cytochrome P450(17) alpha (17 alpha-hydroxylase/C17–20 lyase). *The Journal of Steroid Biochemistry and Molecular Biology*. 1994; 50(5–6):267–273. Epub 1994/09/01.

22. Auchus RJ. The genetics, pathophysiology, and management of human deficiencies of P450c17. *Endocrinology and Metabolism Clinics of North America*. 2001;30(1): 101–119, vii. Epub 2001/05/10.

23. Attard G, Reid AH, Yap TA, Raynaud F, Dowsett M, Settatree S et al. Phase I clinical trial of a selective inhibitor of CYP17, abiraterone acetate, confirms that castration-resistant prostate cancer commonly remains hormone driven. *Journal of Clinical Oncology: Official Journal of the American Society of Clinical Oncology*. 2008;26(28):4563–4571. Epub 2008/07/23.

24. Ryan CJ, Smith MR, Fong L, Rosenberg JE, Kantoff P, Raynaud F et al. Phase I clinical trial of the CYP17 inhibitor abiraterone acetate demonstrating clinical activity in patients with castration-resistant prostate cancer who received prior ketoconazole therapy. *Journal of Clinical Oncology: Official Journal of the American Society of Clinical Oncology*. 2010;28(9):1481–1488. Epub 2010/02/18.

25. Reid AH, Attard G, Danila DC, Oommen NB, Olmos D, Fong PC et al. Significant and sustained antitumor activity in post-docetaxel, castration-resistant prostate cancer with the CYP17 inhibitor abiraterone acetate. *Journal of Clinical Oncology: Official Journal of the American Society of Clinical Oncology*. 2010;28(9):1489–1495. Epub 2010/02/18.

26. Danila DC, Morris MJ, de Bono JS, Ryan CJ, Denmeade SR, Smith MR et al. Phase II multicenter study of abiraterone acetate plus prednisone therapy in patients with docetaxel-treated castration-resistant prostate cancer. *Journal of Clinical Oncology: Official Journal of the American Society of Clinical Oncology*. 2010;28(9):1496–1501. Epub 2010/02/18.

27. de Bono JS, Logothetis CJ, Molina A, Fizazi K, North S, Chu L et al. Abiraterone and increased survival in metastatic prostate cancer. *The New England Journal of Medicine*. 2011;364(21):1995–2005. Epub 2011/05/27.

28. Fizazi K, Scher HI, Molina A, Logothetis CJ, Chi KN, Jones RJ et al. Abiraterone acetate for treatment of metastatic castration-resistant prostate cancer: final overall survival analysis of the COU-AA-301 randomised, double-blind, placebo-controlled phase 3 study. *Lancet Oncol*. 2012;13(10):983–992. doi: 10.1016/S1470-2045(12)70379-0. Epub 2012 Sep 18. Erratum in: *Lancet Oncol*. 2012;13(11):e464.

29. Scher HI, Jia X, de Bono JS, Fleisher M, Pienta KJ, Raghavan D et al. Circulating tumour cells as prognostic markers in progressive, castration-resistant prostate cancer: A reanalysis of IMMC38 trial data. *The Lancet Oncology*. 2009;10(3):233–239. Epub 2009/02/14.

30. de Bono JS, Scher HI, Montgomery RB, Parker C, Miller MC, Tissing H et al. Circulating tumor cells predict survival benefit from treatment in metastatic castration-resistant prostate cancer. *Clinical Cancer Research: An official journal of the American Association for Cancer Research*. 2008;14(19):6302–6309. Epub 2008/10/03.

31. Scher HI, Heller G, Molina A, Kheoh TS, Attard G, Moreira J et al. Evaluation of circulating tumor cell (CTC) enumeration as an efficacy response biomarker of overall survival (OS) in metastatic castration-resistant prostate cancer (mCRPC): Planned final analysis (FA) of COU-AA-301, a randomized double-blind, placebo-controlled phase III

study of abiraterone acetate (AA) plus low-dose prednisone (P) post docetaxel. *Journal of Clinical Oncology: Official Journal of the American Society of Clinical Oncology.* 2011;29 (Suppl; abstr LBA4517^).

32. Ryan CJ, Smith MR, de Bono JS, Molina A, Logothetis CJ, de Souza P et al. Abiraterone in metastatic prostate cancer without previous chemotherapy. *N Engl J Med.* 2013;368(2):138–148. doi: 10.1056/NEJMoa1209096. Epub 2012 Dec 10. Erratum in: *N Engl J Med.* 2013;368(6):584.

33. Ryan CJ, Shah S, Efstathiou E, Smith MR, Taplin ME, Bubley GJ et al. Phase II study of abiraterone acetate in chemotherapy-naive metastatic castration-resistant prostate cancer displaying bone flare discordant with serologic response. *Clinical Cancer Research: An Official Journal of the American Association for Cancer Research.* 2011;17(14): 4854–4861. Epub 2011/06/03.

34. Ni M, Chen Y, Lim E, Wimberly H, Bailey ST, Imai Y et al. Targeting androgen receptor in estrogen receptor-negative breast cancer. *Cancer Cell.* 2011;20(1):119–131. Epub 2011/07/12.

35. Basu B, Ang JE, Crawley D, Folkerd E, Sarker D, Blanco-Codesido M et al. Phase I study of abiraterone acetate (AA) in patients (pts) with estrogen receptor (ER) or androgen receptor (AR) positive advanced breast carcinoma resistant to standard endocrine therapies. *Journal of Clinical Oncology: Official Journal of the American Society of Clinical Oncology.* 2011;29 (Suppl; abstr 2525).

36. Agus DB, Stadler WM, Shevrin DH, Hart L, MacVicar GR, Hamid O et al. Safety, efficacy, and pharmacodynamics of the investigational agent orteronel (TAK-700) in metastatic castration-resistant prostate cancer (mCRPC): Updated data from a phase I/II study. *Journal of Clinical Oncology: Official Journal of the American Society of Clinical Oncology.* 2012;30 (Suppl 5; abstr 98).

37. Montgomery RB, Eisenberger MA, Rettig M, Chu F, Pili R, Stephenson J et al. Phase I clinical trial of galeterone (TOK-001), a multifunctional antiandrogen and CYP17 inhibitor in castration resistant prostate cancer (CRPC). *Journal of Clinical Oncology: Official Journal of the American Society of Clinical Oncology.* 2012;30 (Suppl; abstr 4665).

38. Tran C, Ouk S, Clegg NJ, Chen Y, Watson PA, Arora V et al. Development of a second-generation antiandrogen for treatment of advanced prostate cancer. *Science.* 2009; 324(5928):787–790. Epub 2009/04/11.

39. Scher HI, Beer TM, Higano CS, Anand A, Taplin ME, Efstathiou E et al. Antitumour activity of MDV3100 in castration-resistant prostate cancer: A phase 1–2 study. *Lancet.* 2010;375(9724):1437–1446. Epub 2010/04/20.

40. Scher HI, Fizazi K, Saad F, Taplin ME, Sternberg CN, Miller MD et al. Increased survival with enzalutamide in prostate cancer after chemotherapy. *The New England Journal of Medicine.* 2012;367(13):1187–1197. Epub 2012/08/17.

41. Scher HI, Fizazi K, Saad F, Chi K, Taplin M-E, Sternberg CN et al. Association of baseline corticosteroid with outcomes in a multivariate analysis of the Phase 3 affirm study of enzalutamide (ENZA), an androgen receptor signaling inhibitor (ARSI). *ESMO Conference 2012.* Abstract 899PD. 2012.

42. Richards J, Lim AC, Hay CW, Taylor AE, Wingate A, Nowakowska K et al. Interactions of abiraterone, eplerenone, and prednisolone with wild-type and mutant androgen receptor: A rationale for increasing abiraterone exposure or combining with MDV3100. *Cancer Research.* 2012;72(9):2176–2182. Epub 2012/03/14.

43. Clegg NJ, Wongvipat J, Joseph JD, Tran C, Ouk S, Dilhas A et al. ARN-509: A novel antiandrogen for prostate cancer treatment. *Cancer Research.* 2012;72(6):1494–1503. Epub 2012/01/24.

44. Rathkopf DE, Morris MJ, Danila DC, Slovin SF, Steinbrecher JE, Arauz G et al. A phase I study of the androgen signaling inhibitor ARN-509 in patients with metastatic castration-resistant prostate cancer (mCRPC). *Journal of Clinical Oncology: Official Journal of the American Society of Clinical Oncology.* 2012;30 (Suppl; abstr 4548).

45. Rathkopf D, Liu G, Carducci MA, Eisenberger MA, Anand A, Morris MJ et al. Phase I dose-escalation study of the novel antiandrogen BMS-641988 in patients with castration-resistant prostate cancer. *Clinical Cancer Research: An Official Journal of the American Association for Cancer Research.* 2011;17(4):880–887. Epub 2010/12/07.

46. Andersen RJ, Mawji NR, Wang J, Wang G, Haile S, Myung JK et al. Regression of castrate-recurrent prostate cancer by a small-molecule inhibitor of the amino-terminus domain of the androgen receptor. *Cancer Cell.* 2010;17(6):535–546. Epub 2010/06/15.

47. Helsen C, Marchand A, Chaltin P, Munck S, Voet A, Verstuyf A et al. Identification and characterization of MEL-3, a novel AR antagonist that suppresses prostate cancer cell growth. *Molecular Cancer Therapeutics.* 2012;11(6):1257–1268. Epub 2012/04/13.

48. Loddick SA, Bradbury R, Broadbent N, Campbell H, Gaughan L, Growcott J et al. AZD3514: Targeting androgen receptor function with a novel mechanism of action and the potential to treat castration-resistant prostate cancer. *AACR Advances in Prostate Cancer,* Meeting Abstracts C32 2012. 2012.

49. Zhang Y, Castaneda S, Dumble M, Wang M, Mileski M, Qu Z et al. Reduced expression of the androgen receptor by third generation of antisense shows antitumor activity in models of prostate cancer. *Molecular Cancer Therapeutics.* 2011;10(12):2309–2319. Epub 2011/10/27.

50. Cardillo MR, Ippoliti F. IL-6, IL-10 and HSP-90 expression in tissue microarrays from human prostate cancer assessed by computer-assisted image analysis. *Anticancer Research.* 2006;26(5A):3409–3416. Epub 2006/11/11.

51. Zoubeidi A, Zardan A, Beraldi E, Fazli L, Sowery R, Rennie P et al. Cooperative interactions between androgen receptor (AR) and heat-shock protein 27 facilitate AR transcriptional activity. *Cancer Research.* 2007;67(21):10455–10465. Epub 2007/11/03.

52. Aloy MT, Hadchity E, Bionda C, Diaz-Latoud C, Claude L, Rousson R et al. Protective role of Hsp27 protein against gamma radiation-induced apoptosis and radiosensitization effects of Hsp27 gene silencing in different human tumor cells. *International Journal of Radiation Oncology, Biology, Physics.* 2008;70(2):543–553. Epub 2007/11/06.

53. Foster CS, Dodson AR, Ambroisine L, Fisher G, Moller H, Clark J et al. Hsp-27 expression at diagnosis predicts poor clinical outcome in prostate cancer independent of ETS-gene rearrangement. *British Journal of Cancer.* 2009;101(7):1137–1144. Epub 2009/08/27.

54. Pacey S, Wilson RH, Walton M, Eatock MM, Hardcastle A, Zetterlund A et al. A phase I study of the heat shock protein 90 inhibitor alvespimycin (17-DMAG) given intravenously to patients with advanced solid tumors. *Clinical Cancer Research: An Official Journal of the American Association for Cancer Research.* 2011;17(6):1561–1570. Epub 2011/02/01.

55. Yano A, Tsutsumi S, Soga S, Lee MJ, Trepel J, Osada H et al. Inhibition of Hsp90 activates osteoclast c-Src signaling and promotes growth of prostate carcinoma cells in bone. *Proceedings of the National Academy of Sciences of the United States of America.* 2008;105(40):15541–15546. Epub 2008/10/09.

56. Saporita AJ, Ai J, Wang Z. The Hsp90 inhibitor, 17-AAG, prevents the ligand-independent nuclear localization of androgen receptor in refractory prostate cancer cells. *The Prostate.* 2007;67(5):509–520. Epub 2007/01/16.

57. Hotte SJ, Yu EY, Hirte HW, Higano CS, Gleave ME, Chi KN. Phase I trial of OGX-427, a 2'methoxyethyl antisense oligonucleotide (ASO), against heat shock protein 27 (Hsp27): Final results. *Journal of Clinical Oncology: Official Journal of the American Society of Clinical Oncology.* 2010;28:15s (Suppl; abstr 3077).

58. Chi KN, Hotte SJ, Ellard S, Gingerich JR, Joshua AM, Yu EY et al. A randomized phase II study of OGX-427 plus prednisone (P) versus P alone in patients (pts) with metastatic castration resistant prostate cancer (CRPC). *Journal of Clinical Oncology: Official Journal of the American Society of Clinical Oncology.* 2012;30 (Suppl; abstr 4514).

59. Matsumoto H, Kuruma H, Zoubeidi A, Fazli L, Gleave ME. An evaluation of clusterin antisense inhibitor OGX-011 in combination with the second-generation antiandrogen MDV3100 in a castrate-resistant prostate cancer model. *Journal of Clinical Oncology: Official Journal of the American Society of Clinical Oncology.* 2011;29 (Suppl; abstr 4502).

60. Thomas C, Wafa LA, Lamoureux F, Cheng H, Fazli L, Gleave ME et al. Carbidopa enhances antitumoral activity of bicalutamide on the androgen receptor-axis in castration-resistant prostate tumors. *The Prostate.* 2012;72(8):875–885. Epub 2011/11/11.

61. De Bono JS, Fizazi K, Saad F, Taplin ME, Sternberg CN, Miller K et al. Primary, secondary, and quality-of-life endpoint results from the phase III AFFIRM study of MDV3100, an androgen receptor signaling inhibitor. *Journal of Clinical Oncology: Official Journal of the American Society of Clinical Oncology.* 2012;30:4519.

62. Taplin ME, Bubley GJ, Ko YJ, Small EJ, Upton M, Rajeshkumar B et al. Selection for androgen receptor mutations in prostate cancers treated with androgen antagonist. *Cancer Research.* 1999;59(11):2511–2515. Epub 1999/06/11.

63. Steinkamp MP, O'Mahony OA, Brogley M, Rehman H, Lapensee EW, Dhanasekaran S et al. Treatment-dependent androgen receptor mutations in prostate cancer exploit multiple mechanisms to evade therapy. *Cancer Research.* 2009;69(10):4434–4442. Epub 2009/04/16.

64. Sundar S, Dickinson PD. Spironolactone, a possible selective androgen receptor modulator, should be used with caution in patients with metastatic carcinoma of the prostate. *BMJ Case Reports.* 2012;2012. Epub 2012/06/06.

65. Kawata H, Ishikura N, Watanabe M, Nishimoto A, Tsunenari T, Aoki Y. Prolonged treatment with bicalutamide induces androgen receptor overexpression and androgen hypersensitivity. *The Prostate.* 2010;70(7):745–754. Epub 2010/01/09.

66. Urbanucci A, Sahu B, Seppala J, Larjo A, Latonen LM, Waltering KK et al. Overexpression of androgen receptor enhances the binding of the receptor to the chromatin in prostate cancer. *Oncogene.* 2012;31(17):2153–2163. Epub 2011/09/13.

67. Guo Z, Yang X, Sun F, Jiang R, Linn DE, Chen H et al. A novel androgen receptor splice variant is up-regulated during prostate cancer progression and promotes androgen depletion-resistant growth. *Cancer Research.* 2009;69(6):2305–2313. Epub 2009/02/27.

68. Hornberg E, Ylitalo EB, Crnalic S, Antti H, Stattin P, Widmark A et al. Expression of androgen receptor splice variants in prostate cancer bone metastases is associated with castration-resistance and short survival. *PloS One.* 2011;6(4):e19059. Epub 2011/05/10.

69. Mostaghel EA, Marck BT, Plymate SR, Vessella RL, Balk S, Matsumoto AM et al. Resistance to CYP17A1 inhibition with abiraterone in castration-resistant prostate cancer: Induction of steroidogenesis and androgen receptor splice variants. *Clinical Cancer Research: An Official Journal of the American Association for Cancer Research.* 2011;17(18):5913–5925. Epub 2011/08/03.

70. Watson PA, Chen YF, Balbas MD, Wongvipat J, Socci ND, Viale A et al. Constitutively active androgen receptor splice variants expressed in castration-resistant prostate cancer require full-length androgen receptor. *Proceedings of the National Academy of Sciences of the United States of America.* 2010;107(39):16759–16765. Epub 2010/09/09.

71. Locke JA, Guns ES, Lubik AA, Adomat HH, Hendy SC, Wood CA et al. Androgen levels increase by intratumoral de novo steroidogenesis during progression of castration-resistant prostate cancer. *Cancer Research.* 2008;68(15):6407–6415. Epub 2008/08/05.

72. Cai C, Chen S, Ng P, Bubley GJ, Nelson PS, Mostaghel EA et al. Intratumoral de novo steroid synthesis activates androgen receptor in castration-resistant prostate cancer and is upregulated by treatment with CYP17A1 inhibitors. *Cancer Research.* 2011;71(20):6503–6513. Epub 2011/08/27.

73. Mohler JL, Titus MA, Bai S, Kennerley BJ, Lih FB, Tomer KB et al. Activation of the androgen receptor by intratumoral bioconversion of androstanediol to dihydrotestosterone in prostate cancer. *Cancer Research.* 2011;71(4):1486–1496. Epub 2011/02/10.

74. Attard G, Reid AH, Auchus RJ, Hughes BA, Cassidy AM, Thompson E et al. Clinical and biochemical consequences of CYP17A1 inhibition with abiraterone given with and without exogenous glucocorticoids in castrate men with advanced prostate cancer. *The Journal of Clinical Endocrinology and Metabolism.* 2012;97(2):507–516. Epub 2011/12/16.

75. Mohler JL, Titus MA, Wilson EM. Potential prostate cancer drug target: Bioactivation of androstanediol by conversion to dihydrotestosterone. *Clinical Cancer Research: An Official Journal of the American Association for Cancer Research.* 2011;17(18): 5844–5849. Epub 2011/06/28.

76. Ni L, Yang CS, Gioeli D, Frierson H, Toft DO, Paschal BM. FKBP51 promotes assembly of the Hsp90 chaperone complex and regulates androgen receptor signaling in prostate cancer cells. *Molecular and Cellular Biology.* 2010;30(5):1243–1253. Epub 2010/01/06.

77. Gregory CW, He B, Johnson RT, Ford OH, Mohler JL, French FS et al. A mechanism for androgen receptor-mediated prostate cancer recurrence after androgen deprivation therapy. *Cancer Research.* 2001;61(11):4315–4319. Epub 2001/06/05.

78. Karpf AR, Bai S, James SR, Mohler JL, Wilson EM. Increased expression of androgen receptor coregulator MAGE-11 in prostate cancer by DNA hypomethylation and cyclic AMP. *Molecular Cancer Research.* 2009;7(4):523–535. Epub 2009/04/18.

79. Carver BS, Chapinski C, Wongvipat J, Hieronymus H, Chen Y, Chandarlapaty S et al. Reciprocal feedback regulation of PI3K and androgen receptor signaling in PTEN-deficient prostate cancer. *Cancer Cell.* 2011;19(5):575–586. Epub 2011/05/18.

80. Efstathiou E, Titus M, Tsavachidou D, Tzelepi V, Wen S, Hoang A et al. Effects of abiraterone acetate on androgen signaling in castrate-resistant prostate cancer in bone. *Journal of Clinical Oncology: Official Journal of the American Society of Clinical Oncology.* 2012;30(6):637–643. Epub 2011/12/21.

81. Shaffer DR, Leversha MA, Danila DC, Lin O, Gonzalez-Espinoza R, Gu B et al. Circulating tumor cell analysis in patients with progressive castration-resistant prostate cancer. *Clinical Cancer Research: An Official Journal of the American Association for Cancer Research.* 2007;13(7):2023–2029. Epub 2007/04/04.

82. Attard G, Swennenhuis JF, Olmos D, Reid AH, Vickers E, A'Hern R et al. Characterization of ERG, AR and PTEN gene status in circulating tumor cells from patients with castration-resistant prostate cancer. *Cancer Research.* 2009;69(7):2912–2918. Epub 2009/04/03.

19 Targeting DNA Repair
PARP and Chk1 Inhibitors

Peter Stephens
Newcastle University

Ruth Plummer
Newcastle University
Freeman Hospital

CONTENTS

INTRODUCTION TO DNA DAMAGE RESPONSE PATHWAYS AND POTENTIAL TARGETS FOR DRUG MODULATION

Repair of DNA and thus preservation of the genetic code is critical for normal cellular function, and over the past three decades, significant advances have been made in understanding the components of the pathways, which signal or "respond" to DNA damage and thus protect the genome. Various elements within the DNA damage response (DDR) pathways have subsequently been evaluated as targets for drug discovery and clinical drug development. This chapter will focus on the development of agents targeting two such elements—poly(ADP-ribose)polymerase (PARP) and checkpoint 1 kinase (Chk1).

There are five recognized pathways that protect the genome by signaling specific types of DNA damage and carrying out repair (reviewed in[1-3]). In cancer cells, it is recognized that mutations in DDR pathways can predispose to cancer and are hallmarks of many of the hereditary cancer syndromes.[4-6] Additionally, it is felt that in many situations, once a tumor cell has developed, the DDR pathways can be used by the tumor cell to overcome many standard anticancer treatments and hence are a cause of treatment resistance. There is increasing evidence in the literature that tumor tissue has high levels of some elements of the DNA repair pathways,[7-11] potentially enhancing the ability to use these pathways to repair damage caused by anticancer therapies. These two features of cancer cells present opportunities for the development of treatments using inhibitors of the DDR pathways. Blocking a second pathway in a tumor cell deficient in a key oncogenic pathway can cause tumor cell death by synthetic lethality, and the combination of inhibitors with DNA-damaging drugs or radiation is a potential mechanism to increase cytotoxicity.

The major DNA repair pathways are direct repair, mismatch repair (MMR), base excision repair (BER), nucleotide excision repair (NER), and double-strand break (DSB) recombinational repair, which includes both non-homologous end joining (NHEJ) and homologous recombinational repair (HRR).[1,2,12] The direct repair, MMR and NER pathways appear to function independently to repair specific DNA lesions and will not be discussed further in this chapter. There is significant interaction between the single-strand break (SSB) and DSB repair pathways, and it is known that blockade of SSB repair will activate DSB signaling and repair.[13,14]

PARP and Chk1 are enzymes that play key roles in the signaling of DNA SSB and DSB, and cell cycle checkpoint control to allow accurate repair of these cytotoxic and mutagenic forms of DNA damage (Figure 19.1). BER is involved in the repair of SSBs, contributing to resistance to ionizing radiation and alkylating agents. Recombinational repair has two pathways, the error-free HRR in dividing cells and error-prone NHEJ active in G1. These two pathways repair much of the damage caused by radiotherapy and chemotherapeutic agents such as cisplatin and mitomycin C.[2] Chk1 plays a key role in the signaling of cell cycle checkpoint control to allow DSB repair via the HRR pathway (Figure 19.2).

Role of PARP in DNA Damage Response

Poly(ADP-ribose) polymerase (PARP) enzymes, when activated, catalyze the formation of ADP-ribose polymers using nicotinamide adenine dinucleotide (NAD) as a substrate. The product, poly(ADP-ribose), and the first PARP enzymes were discovered independently by scientists in France and Japan in the 1960s.[15-20] PARP-1 is the most abundant form of the enzyme and, along with PARP-2, is found in the nucleus, acting as a "molecular nick sensor" to signal DNA SSBs and assist in their repair.[21] PARP-1 knockout animals are viable,[22] but the double knockout of PARP-1 and PARP-2 is embryologically lethal.[23]

PARP-1 (EC. 2.4.2.30) is encoded by the *ADPRT-1* gene on chromosome 1q41-q42, consisting of 23 exons spanning 43 kb.[24,25] It has a molecular weight of 113 kDa and consists of three major domains. The DNA-binding domain occupies the 42 kDa NH_2-terminal region, which includes two zinc-finger motifs that bind DNA breaks[26]

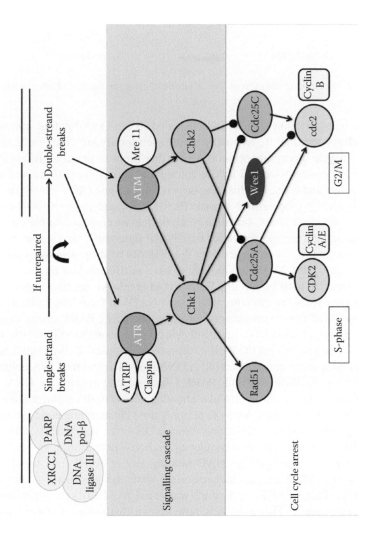

FIGURE 19.1 Simplified diagram showing the interaction of DNA DSB and SSB repair, indicating the roles of PARP and Chk1 and other key members of the pathway.

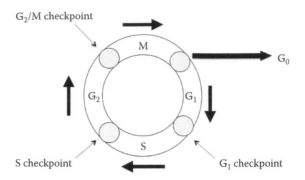

FIGURE 19.2   Schematic diagram of the cell cycle illustrating the key check points.

and a nuclear localization signal.[27] Also located in the DNA-binding domain is a BRCA1 carboxy-terminal (C-terminal) motif; such motifs are commonly found in DDR and cell cycle checkpoint proteins, where they promote protein–protein interactions. There is a centrally located 16 kDa automodification domain that contains conserved glutamate and lysine residues, the targets for auto-poly(ADP-ribosyl)ation.[28,29] The 55 kDa catalytic domain of human PARP is located in the COOH-terminal region of the enzyme.[30] This C-terminal catalytic domain contains the region of highest conservation between species called the "PARP signature"[21] and is also the region of the enzyme that has been targeted by the majority of drug discovery programs, with only iniparib (BSI-201) being thought to have a different drug target.

PARP is inactive until bound to a DNA strand break via the zinc-finger domain. This binding activates the enzyme, which uses NAD^+ to form long branched polymers of poly (ADP-ribose) on acceptor proteins, including PARP itself. This auto-poly(ADP-ribosyl)ation creates a negatively charged target at the SSB, which recruits the enzymes required to form the BER multi-protein complex. This complex is made up of X-ray repair cross-complementing 1, DNA ligase III, and the DNA polymerase pol β. Following ADP-ribosylation, PARP-1 has reduced affinity for DNA and is released, opening up the chromatin and allowing access to the damaged site to the other repair complex proteins. Many commonly used chemotherapeutic agents, such as alkylating agents and camptothecins, damage DNA by causing SSBs, and for this reason, PARP inhibitors were first developed as chemo-potentiating agents.[31,32]

The "PARP signature" in the NAD-binding site of PARP-1 is highly (92%) conserved across plant and animal species,[21] with the greatest homology seen with PARP-2. This "PARP signature" was used to identify a superfamily of 16 "PARP enzymes."[33] However, it is now known that some of these have only mono ADP-ribosyltransferase activity and some have no known catalytic activity. Nevertheless, vault PARP, tankyrase-1 and 2, and probably PARP-3, are bona-fide PARPs, but PARP-1 and PARP-2 are the only DNA damage activated PARPs. As the majority of PARP inhibitors in the clinic target this conserved region, it would be expected that there will also be some inhibitors of non-nuclear PARPs with clinical use of these agents. A recent publication has demonstrated that this is indeed the case in vitro.

Role of Chk1 in DNA Damage Response

Chk1 is essential for normal development and cell cycle control; Chk1 deficiency is embryonic lethal.[34] Chk1 is activated by both ataxia telangiectasia and Rad 3 related (ATR) and ataxia telangiectasia mutated (ATM). ATR is recruited to chromatin during S-phase within the normal cell cycle in the absence of DNA damage.[35] DNA damage leads to stalling of replication forks as DNA polymerase and other associated enzymes are prevented from completing normal replication. ATR forms nuclear foci at stalled replication forks. ATR activates Chk1 by phosphorylation at Ser317 and Ser345.[36]

ATM is a key in the response to DNA DSBs.[37] ATM acts at the G_1 checkpoint via an activating phosphorylation of Chk2, which subsequently performs an activating phosphorylation of p53, arresting the cell cycle in G_1.[38] ATM also phosphorylates Chk1[Ser317] and Chk1[Ser345], leading to G_2 cell cycle checkpoint arrest.

Activated phosphorylated Chk1 acts at both the S and G_2/M checkpoints.[39] Cyclin-dependent kinases (CDKs) act as downstream effectors of checkpoint control. Activated Chk1 promotes the degradation of Cdc25A, leading to S-phase arrest, whilst phosphorylation of Cdc25C[Ser216] leads to G2 arrest via the cyclin B/Cdc2 mitotic kinase complex. Activated Chk1 also recruits Rad51 to chromatin and phosphorylates the C-terminal domain of hBRCA2, promoting its association with Rad51.

SUMMARY OF PRECLINICAL DATA SUPPORTING CLINICAL DEVELOPMENT OF PARPi

Chemo- and Radio-Potentiation

There is abundant in vitro and in vivo evidence demonstrating a role for PARP-1/2 in the repair of DNA damage and cell survival following exposure to DNA-methylating agents, topoisomerase I poisons and ionizing radiation, and anticancer agents. There are numerous reviews on these inhibitors,[40–48] and this section will outline briefly the salient observations that have guided the clinical development of PARP inhibitors.

Monofunctional DNA-methylating agents are the most potent activators of PARP-1 (and 2), and all conventional PARP inhibitors can be considered modulators of resistance to anticancer DNA-methylating agents such as 5-(3,3-dimethyl-1-triazeno)imidazole-4-carboxamide and temozolomide. These drugs methylate DNA at the O^6- and N^7-position of guanine and the N^3-position of adenine.[49] Although a minor lesion, the most cytotoxic lesion is O^6-methylguanine, because, unless it is repaired by methylguanine methyltransferase prior to replication, it will mispair triggering the MMR proteins to initiate futile repair cycles, resulting in apoptosis.[50,51] The N-methylpurines, which are much more numerous (~80% of the methylation species), are targets for BER, and hence PARP-1 and 2 play a role in their repair. A number of preclinical studies have investigated temozolomide chemosensitization by PARP inhibitors, PD128763 and NU1025 increased temozolomide-induced DNA strand breakage and caused a four to seven-fold potentiation of temozolomide cytotoxicity.[52] CEP-6800 and GPI 15427 increased temozolomide-induced DNA damage and cytotoxicity or growth inhibition in human glioblastoma cells and enhanced the antitumor activity of temozolomide in mice bearing gliomas, including intracranially implanted tumors.[53–55]

In preclinical models, PARP inhibitors have also been shown to potentiate the topoisomerase I poisons[55–57] both in vitro and in vivo, with also evidence that PARP inhibition might reduce normal organ toxicity.[55] This potential protective effect in normal tissues has also been observed with cisplatin[58,59] and doxorubicin[60] and may open up future avenues for clinical research.

Radiotherapy, an anticancer treatment used in almost 50% of all patients, causes tumor cell death by the induction of SSB and DSB. PARP inhibitors have been shown to potentiate radiotherapy in preclinical models,[61–63] and it is expected that this will also be a clinical area where these agents may be beneficial, although no clinical trials of PARP inhibitors with radiotherapy have been reported to date.

SYNTHETIC LETHALITY: SINGLE-AGENT USE OF PARP INHIBITORS

The publication in 2005 of paired preclinical papers in *Nature*, demonstrating hypersensitivity of *BRCA*-deficient cancer cells to single-agent PARP inhibitors, opened the door to clinical research into these agents as monotherapy[25,26] and has provided the clearest demonstration to date of a class effect in the clinic. Before this groundbreaking research was published, it had been argued that PARP inhibitors would have no activity when used alone, and drug developers continued to chase the elusive goal of chemo-potentiation in tumors without an increase in toxicity in normal tissue.

Initial preclinical experiments in cell lines and xenografts demonstrated that cells with loss of the homologous recombination repair pathway for DNA DSB are hypersensitive to blockade of SSB repair with a PARP inhibitor. The key to this mechanism of action is the role that *BRCA1* and *BRCA2* play in signaling DSB (*BRCA1*) and the repair of such breaks via the homologous recombination pathway (*BRCA2*).[27]

The proposed mechanism for the cytotoxicity of PARP inhibition is that blockade of SSB repair leads to the formation of unrepaired DSB at the replication fork. In normal or *BRCA*-heterozygous cells, the lesion can be repaired by DSB mechanisms, and DNA replication and cell division continue. However, in cells that lack functional DSB repair, such as those with a homozygous mutation in *BRCA1* or *BRCA2*, loss of two DNA repair pathways causes synthetic lethality and cell death[25,26] (Figure 19.3).

CLINICAL DEVELOPMENT OF PARP INHIBITORS

Based on the preclinical data summarized earlier, the clinical development of PARP inhibitors has been on two fronts, in combination with chemotherapy in an attempt to improve tumor cytotoxicity and thus patient outcomes, and also as single agents in HR-defective cancers based on the preclinical evidence of hypersensitivity of these tumors. This is a rapidly evolving clinical field with nine agents in the clinic (Table 19.1), the current status of clinical trials is summarized in the subsequent sections. As yet, no phase III registration study has reported positive data, so there is no licensed PARP inhibitor. The key translational data, which have informed the clinical development paths and the current trials, are summarized in the subsequent sections.

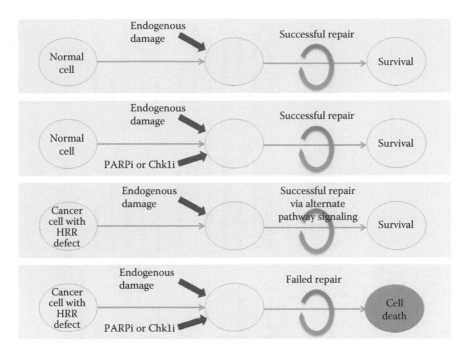

FIGURE 19.3 Synthetic lethality—endogenous DNA damage is repaired in normal cells using the DDR pathways. In the presence of a DDR inhibitor, damage can still be repaired using alternate pathways. In cancer cells where defects on DDR pathways are common, repair can occur via the alternative pathways but blocking a second pathway causes cell death, even in the absence of a DNA-damaging agent due to these intrinsic strand breaks.

Chemotherapy Combination Trials

On the basis of the preclinical activity of AG014361 and AG-014699 (rucaparib) in combination with temozolomide, resulting in durable complete tumor regressions,[61,64] the first clinical trial of a PARP inhibitor for the treatment of cancer was initiated in 2003. This phase 0/I trial involved dose escalation of the PARP inhibitor (PARPi) in combination with temozolomide (phase I component) combined with a predose of the PARPi alone so as to establish pharmacokinetics (PK) and pharmacodynamics (PD) (phase 0 component). PARP inhibition in surrogate normal tissues (peripheral blood lymphocytes [PBL]) was a primary endpoint of the study with a >50% inhibition for 24 h being the target based on the preclinical efficacy studies. As this was a first-in-class clinical trial, safety and toxicity endpoints were also included.[65] Rucaparib was escalated from 1 to 12 mg/m^2 in combination with 50% of the recommended maximum dose of temozolomide (100 mg/m^2/day for 5 days every 28 days) to establish a PARP inhibitory dose endpoint. A reduced dose of temozolomide was used due to concerns that the combination might enhance normal tissue toxicity of temozolomide, similar to the clinical experience with other DNA damage repair modulating agents, O^6-benzyl guanine, and lomaguatrib.[66–70] The PARP inhibitory dose (PID) was defined as 12 mg/m^2 based on 74%–97%

TABLE 19.1
PARP Inhibitors in Clinical Development

Agent (Company) & Date First into Clinic	Route	Disease	Single Agent/Combination	Clinical Status
AG014699/PF0367338/CO338/Rucaparib (Pfizer/Clovis) 2003	IV and oral	Solid tumors Melanoma BRCA-related tumors	Various combinations Single agent	Phase I/II ongoing
KU59436/AZD2281/Olaparib (AstraZeneca) 2005	Oral	BRCA-related cancers Solid tumors	Single agent Various combinations	Phase I complete Several Phase II
ABT888/Veliparib (Abbott) 2006	Oral	Solid and lymphoblastoid	Single agent Various combinations	Ph 0/I complete Several Phase II
BSI-201/Iniparib (BiPar/Sanofi) 2006	IV	TNBC	Gem-carbo/TMZ combinations	Phase II complete Phase III complete
INO-1001 (Inotek/Genentek) 2003/6	IV	Melanoma, GBM	TMZ combinations	Phase II
MK4827 (Merck/Tesaro) 2008	Oral	Solid BRCA ovarian	Single agent	Phase I complete
CEP-9722 (Cephalon) 2009	Oral	Solid tumors	TMZ combinations and single agent	Phase I complete
GPI 21016/E7016 (E7449 2011)(MGI Pharma/Eisai) 2010	Oral	Solid tumors	TMZ combinations	Phase I
LT763/BM763 (Biomarin) 2011	Oral	Solid tumors and hematological malignancies	Single agent	Phase I

inhibition of PBL PARP activity in samples taken 24 h after a single dose of rucaparib, and tumor PARP inhibition was also demonstrated in paired biopsies in patients with metastatic melanoma. Mean tumor PARP inhibition at 5 h was 92% (range 46%–97%), and rucaparib was detected in tumor samples, proving that the novel agent was delivered to the tumor. In this study, it proved possible to give full dose temozolomide with the PID. However, increasing the PARP inhibitor dose further by 50% to 18 mg/m²/day did cause dose-limiting myelosuppression. It was already known that the dose–toxicity relationship for temozolomide is steep, 200 mg/m²/day being well tolerated but 225 mg/m²/day causing clinically significant myelosuppression.[71] As all patients also received a test dose of this first-in-class compound, it was possible to start evaluating single-agent toxicity. No toxicity attributable to rucaparib alone was observed, and the agent demonstrated linear pharmacokinetics with no interaction with temozolomide. The complete absence of any symptomatic or laboratory toxicities as a result of PARP inhibition on its own is also encouraging for the future use of PARP inhibitors in indications when they are given as single agents, so overall, this first study significantly informed the clinical development field for PARP inhibitors.

FURTHER CLINICAL STUDIES IN COMBINATION WITH CHEMOTHERAPY

The combination of rucaparib and temozolomide was taken into a phase II study in metastatic melanoma. However, this second trial demonstrated enhanced temozolomide-induced myelosuppression when full dose temozolomide was combined with a PARP inhibitory dose of AG014699 to a wider range of patients. Following a 25% dose reduction of the temozolomide dose, the regimen was well tolerated, and this small phase II study reported a modest increase in the response rate and median time to progression compared to temozolomide alone.[72] These encouraging data need to be confirmed in a phase III setting, and similar studies have been performed with the Abbott PARP inhibitor ABT-888 (veliparib) in a randomized phase II setting, and the results of this were reported in 2011. This larger randomized phase II study also did not show a significant improvement in response rate and overall survival, but there was a trend toward these endpoints.[73] Another combination study of a PARP inhibitor (INO-101, Inotech/Genetech) and temozolomide was also recently reported.[74] INO-101 is an intravenous PARP inhibitor given 12 hourly via a central venous catheter. This study established the maximum tolerated dose (MTD) in combination with full dose temozolomide (200 mg/m² daily times 5q 4 weekly) as 200 mg/m². Dose-limiting toxicities were myelosuppression and liver enzyme elevations (transaminitis). No pharmacodynamic data are reported, so it is not clear what degree of PARP inhibition is achieved. A total of 12 patients with metastatic melanoma were treated across the dose ranges, and it is not possible to comment of any improved efficacy.

Phase I chemotherapy combination studies of a range of other PARP inhibitors have also been performed (www.clinicaltrials.gov). A common theme that is emerging, particularly with the oral PARP inhibitors that are dosed continuously, of enhanced normal tissue toxicity, especially myelosuppression, is a predictable but common dose-limiting problem. An National Cancer Institute (NCI) sponsored combination study of olaparib (KU59436, AZD2281; KuDos/AstraZeneca) with cisplatin and gemcitabine reported dose-limiting toxicity (DLT) of myelosuppression at the first dose level explored. The investigators de-escalated to establish an MTD of a PARP inhibitory dose of olaparib with gemcitabine 400 mg/m^2 and cisplatin 40 mg/m^2 as tolerable in non-heavily pretreated patients.[75,76] Likewise, veliparib in combination with topotecan, also investigated by the NCI, dose-limiting myelosuppression was again observed at the first dose level, and the MTD established with the PARP inhibitory dose was topotecan 0.6 mg/m^2 days 1–5.[77] Enhanced normal tissue toxicity has also been reported with olaparib in combination with dacarbazine,[78] cyclophosphamide,[79,80] and paclitaxel.[81] For the latter agent, it may be that inhibition of telomerase (PARP-4) is responsible as inhibition of SSB repair would not be expected to increase the myelosuppression caused by an antimitotic agent.

A fascinating contradiction to this trend of enhanced normal tissue toxicity is the intravenous agent iniparib (BSI-201, BiPar, Sanofi Aventis), initially reported as a PARP inhibitor. Clinical trials with this agent have explored an intermittent twice-weekly schedule, and no increase in normal tissue toxicity has been reported.[82,83] A dramatic improvement in antitumor activity was reported in a randomized phase II study of a total 120 triple-negative breast cancer patients where treatment with BSI-201 on the biweekly schedule (days 1, 4, 8, and 11) combined with carboplatin (AUC2) and gemcitabine 1000 mg/m^2, days 1 and 8, was compared to treatment with carboplatin and gemcitabine alone. This study showed an increased objective response rate (48% vs 16%, $p = .002$), median progression-free survival (6.9 months vs 3.3 months, $p < .0001$), and overall survival (9.6 months vs 7.5 months, $p = .0005$); however, these results were not confirmed in a subsequent phase III study,[84] and recent publications suggest that iniparib should not be considered as a PARP inhibitor.[85,86]

SUMMARY OF SINGLE-AGENT CLINICAL TRIALS

The exciting promise of synthetic lethality to HR-defective tumors was first tested clinically with olaparib. The phase I study of this agent had an expanded cohort of patients with known germ line mutations in *BRCA1* or *BRCA2* genes, and presumed loss of the second allele as a tumor-forming event.[87] This study used an oral formulation of the compound and explored dosing from 10 mg daily for 2 of 3 weeks, increasing to 600 mg twice daily on a continuous dosing schedule to achieve optimal PK and PD parameters. Dose-limiting toxicities were myelosuppression and central nervous system side effects. The recommended phase II dose was 400 mg twice daily as continuous dosing. Nine patients developed confirmed partial responses in this phase I study, all of them had confirmed BRCA mutations, and this represented a 39% response rate (9/23) in this population. Toxicities were similar in the *BRCA* mutated and normal population, so there was no suggestion that normal tissue toxicity might be worse in germ line mutation carriers. The investigators also demonstrated an increase in γH2AX foci in plucked eyebrow hair follicles 6 h after olaparib treatment. These foci indicate the accumulation of DNA DSBs, indicating a proof of mechanism of the process of *synthetic lethality* where preservation of SSB by PARP inhibition leads to the formation of DNA DSB. It must be noted that this mechanistic proof was demonstrated in normal tissue, not in the tumor. The data do raise a concern over the potential dangers of continuous dosing over a long period if there is accumulation of DNA damage within normal tissue.

Two phase II studies of olaparib in *BRCA1* or *BRCA2* mutant carriers in breast and ovarian cancer, respectively, have confirmed these data. Both these studies explored response and toxicity in two sequential cohorts of patients treated with 400 and 100 mg twice daily. The activity as a single agent was confirmed in the 400 mg cohorts, but there was less activity and toxicity in the lower dose cohort, suggesting that the degree of PARP inhibition is important for response. In the study reported by Dr. Tutt and colleagues, 27 patients with metastatic breast cancer were treated at each of the doses. The response rate in the 400 mg cohort was 41%, falling to 22% with the lower dose.[88] Toxicities were mild overall, with fatigue, nausea, and vomiting being the commonest toxicities. This dose response was confirmed in the ovarian study where 33 patients were treated at 400 mg bd and 24 at 100 mg bd with a 33% confirmed partial response rate at the higher dose and 13% at the lower dose.[89] Responses were seen in both *BRCA1* and *BRCA2* mutation carriers, and in patients with both platinum-sensitive and platinum-resistant disease. There is evidence in the literature that loss of platinum sensitivity in ovarian cancer is associated with regain of BRCA function[90,91]; however, these findings were not borne out in the study described earlier. Clearly, the findings in these small non-randomized studies require confirmation in the phase III trial, but they do represent an exciting indication that PARP inhibitors will be of benefit in these patients with low observed toxicity. It is to be hoped that this is the area where the clinical development of olaparib will move forward when the ongoing trials exploring dose and formulation are completed. Phase II studies in this indication are also ongoing with rucaparib and veliparib.

It is clear that mutations in *BRCA1/2* are just the "tip of the iceberg" when it comes to HR defects in cancer. Epigenetic silencing of BRCA1 through promoter methylation and upregulation of inhibitors of BRCA2 have been shown to contribute to a "BRCAness" phenotype in breast and ovarian cancer.[92] However, this term is too narrow, implying that HR depends principally on BRCA1 and 2 and is largely restricted to breast and ovarian cancer, when, in fact, it is a complex pathway, involving a panoply of proteins that include damage signaling and checkpoint kinases (e.g., ATR and Chk1), the Fanconi and Rad51 homologues, and many other components, some of which remain to be identified, and is defective in a wide variety of cancers. The first clinical evidence that there are indeed patients where their tumor does display this biological phenotype is in high-grade serous ovarian cancer, where there has been reported activity with single-agent olaparib[93] and initial promising data as a maintenance treatment following response to platinum-based chemotherapy in this tumor type[94] suggest that this may also be a clinical area where a homologous repair deficiency (HRD) phenotype exists as predicted by the emerging predictive biomarker data.[95,96] For many investigators, the current focus of clinical development of PARP inhibitors involves the development of appropriate biomarker assays such that patient's tumors may undergo molecular profiling to identify this HRD phenotype. It is to be hoped that this area of clinical investigation will also lead to a pivotal phase III study and the registration of one of the agents in this powerful class of drugs.

SUMMARY OF PRECLINICAL DATA SUPPORTING
CLINICAL DEVELOPMENT OF CHK1 INHIBITORS

The focus of the preclinical development of the Chk1 inhibitors has been in their role as chemo-potentiating agents. The data for the leading compounds in this class are summarized in the subsequent sections.

UCN-01, a staurosporine analogue, was the first drug identified to inhibit Chk1 as well as other kinases including the protein kinase C inhibitor.[97,98] UCN-01 reduces radiation-induced degradation of Cdc25A in U2OS (osteosarcoma) and abrogates doxorubicin-induced G_2/M phase arrest.[99] The synergism of UCN-01 with chemotherapy was demonstrated in non-small-cell lung carcinoma cell lines (A549 and H596) with cisplatin and in colorectal cancer cell line (HCT116) with camptothecin.[100,101]

Small "second-generation" ATP-competitive inhibitors of Chk1 have been developed. These have a greater specificity and potency than UCN-01. PD321852 (Pfizer) is a UCN-01 analogue; its IC_{50} for Chk1 inhibition is 5 nM.[102] All the remaining potential Chk1 candidates in development are novel compounds. PF00477736 (Pfizer) is a diazepinoindolone with a K_i of 0.49 nM for Chk1 and 100-fold selectivity for Chk1 vs Chk2. The cellular EC_{50} of PF00477736 is 45 nM; this was measured by examining the mitotic entry rate (histone H3 phosphorylation by a spectral dot-blot assay).[103] As a monoagent, PF00477736 did not change the cell cycle, but when used in combination with gemcitabine abrogates S-phase arrest with an increase in the number of cells G_2–M and G_0–G_1. PF00477736 has also been shown to abrogate camptothecin-mediated G_2 cell cycle arrest in CA46 cells (p53-mutated human lymphoma) and HeLa (cervical cancer—p53-null) cells.

AZD7762 (AstraZeneca) is a thiophene carboxamide urea that inhibits both Chk1 (K_i=3.6 nM, IC_{50}=5 nM) and Chk2 (IC_{50}< 10 nM) with similar potency.[104] As with PF00477736, AZD7762 abrogates the camptothecin-induced arrest of cells in G_2 as determined by staining for phospho-histone H3. The effect of AZD7762 on cell lines (HCT116—colorectal cancer) has shown that AZD7762 as a monoagent does not effect cell proliferation in HCT116 cells, but the addition of AZD7762 potentiates the cytotoxicity of gemcitabine.[105] Zabludoff et al demonstrated that AZD7762 has a greater potency in HCT116 p53 mutant cells that have lost their G_1 cell cycle checkpoint when compared to wild-type HCT116 cells.[104] Chk1 inhibitors have been postulated to be potential radiosensitizers. Mitchell et al exposed DU145 (human prostate cancer cells) and HT29 (colon carcinoma) cells to radiation.[106] Chk1 was upregulated for up to 3 h after radiation exposure. When cell lines were exposed to a Chk1 inhibitor, AZD7762, for 1 h before and 24 h after radiation exposure, there was marked increased radiation cytotoxicity compared to untreated controls. This effect was greatest in p53 mutated cell lines but remained significant in p53 wild-type cell lines. This has been replicated in pancreatic cancer cell lines (MiaPaCa-2 and Mpanc96) where AZD7762 has been shown to sensitize cells to radiation sensitized pancreatic cell lines.[107] In MiaPaCa-2 and Mpanc96 cells, following radiation exposure with AZD7762, Rad51 failed to form new foci. There was no corresponding promotion of the dissociation of Rad51 foci.

SCH900776 (Schering) is a pyrazolo[1,5-a]pyrimidine inhibitor of Chk1 (K_d=2 nM, IC_{50}=60 nM); it does not inhibit Chk2 and is a weak CDK2 inhibitor.[108]

SCH900776 causes a concentration-dependent inhibition of hydroxyurea-induced Chk1 serine[296] autophosphorylation in U2OS cells. The potentiation of gamma-H2AX by SCH900776 correlates with the potentiation seen in U2OS cells following treatment with Chk1 small interfering RNA (siRNA), but not Chk2 siRNA. Flow cytometric analysis showed an increasing proportion of cells accumulating in G_2 with increasing doses of SCH900776 and an increasing sub-G_1 population. Mouse studies with A2780 (ovarian) and MiaPaCa (pancreatic) xenografts showed negligible SCH900776 single-agent activity, but potentiation of gemcitabine cytotoxicity with dose-dependent tumor regression with doses of more than 8 mg/Kg of SCH900776. There was no potentiation of gemcitabine-related myelotoxicity (doses of SCH900776 up to 32 mg/Kg).

SAR-020106 (Sareum) is a pyrazolo[1,5-a]pyrimidine too (IC_{50} of 13.3 nM).[109] SAR-020106 abrogates etoposide-induced G_2 cell cycle arrest of HT29 (colorectal cancer) cells with an IC_{50} of 55 nM. SAR-020106 potentiates gemcitabine and SN38 cytotoxicity in HT29, SW620, and Colo205 cells. When repeated in an isogenic pair of A2780 cells, cells with p53$^{-/-}$ showed 2.3-fold (gemcitabine) and 4.5-fold (SN38) selectivity compared to the wild type. Combination treatment with SAR-020106 and gemcitabine for 24 h is associated with increased expression of gamma-H2AX and PARP cleavage.

XL9844 (EXEL-9844) is an oral aminopyrazine inhibitor of both Chk1 and Chk2 (K_i 2.2 nM and 0.07 nM, respectively).[110] XL9844 has nonsignificant single-agent activity but potentiates gemcitabine-mediated cytotoxicity in PANC-1, AsPC-1 (pancreatic), SKOV3 (ovarian), and HeLa cells. In PANC-1 cells, XL9844 abrogated the reduction in Cdc25A expression seen with gemcitabine treatment and increased γH2AX expression in a dose-dependent fashion.

Given this wealth of preclinical data, this class of compounds has also entered early-phase clinical testing (Table 19.2), although limited fully published data are available at present.

SINGLE-AGENT CLINICAL TRIALS WITH CHK1 INHIBITORS

UCN-01, as the first Chk1 inhibitor, was tested in two single-agent phase I trials. UCN-01 has avid plasma binding and long variable half-life. This probably led to the early cessation of the first trial of a 72 h infusion of UCN-01 due to significant DLT with symptomatic hypotension and hyperglycemia at 53 mg/m^2/day.[111] Patient tolerance was improved in the subsequent trial of a short 3 h infusion, but again DLT of symptomatic hypotension at 95 mg/m^2 stopped the trial.[112] The only second-generation Chk1 inhibitor in a single-agent phase I trial is LY2606368; this has not been published but includes an expansion cohort of patients with squamous cell head and neck cancer.

CLINICAL TRIALS OF CHK1 INHIBITORS WITH CHEMOTHERAPY

UCN-01 was used as a short infusion in combination with cisplatin, topotecan, and irinotecan in phase I trials[113–115] and in phase II trials with topotecan for ovarian cancer. Further development has been halted due to toxicity and lack of efficacy.

TABLE 19.2

Chk1 Inhibitors in Clinical and Late Preclinical Development

Agent (Company) & Date First into Clinic	Route	Disease	Single Agent/ Combination	Clinical Status
UCN-01 1995	IV	Solid tumors Ovarian tumors	Single agent and combination with topotecan/cisplatin	Phase I complete
			Combination with topotecan	Phase II complete
AZD7762 (AstraZeneca) 2006	IV	Solid tumors	Combination with gemcitabine and irinotecan	Phase I complete
PF00477736 (Pfizer) 2006	IV	Solid tumors	Combination with gemcitabine	Phase I complete
XL844 (Exelixis) 2007	Oral	Solid tumors and lymphoma	Combination with gemcitabine	Phase I terminated
SCH900776 (Schering-Plough) 2008	IV	Solid tumors Leukemia	Combination with gemcitabine	Phase I complete
			Combination with cytarabine	Phase I complete
LY2606368 (Lily) 2010	IV	Solid tumors	Single agent	Phase I recruiting
SAR020106 (Sareum)	IV	Preclinical		
GDC-0245 (Roche/ Genentech)	IV	Solid tumors	Combination with gemcitabine	Phase I recruiting
CEP3891 (Cephalon)	IV	Preclinical		
ARRY575 (Array Pharma)	Oral	Preclinical		
V158411 (Vernalis)	IV	Preclinical		

Six phase I trials of second-generation Chk1 inhibitors in combination with chemotherapy have been completed or are ongoing, some of which are published in abstract form. The combinations that have been examined include AZD7762 with gemcitabine and AZD7762 with irinotecan in advanced solid tumors[116,117]; SCH900776 with gemcitabine or hydroxyurea in advanced solid tumors and with cytarabine in leukemias[118]; and PF00477736 with gemcitabine.[119] Hematological toxicity, neutropenia and thrombocytopenia, has been reported in all the published abstracts. Reversible myocardial ischemia was a DLT with AZD7762 in combination with both irinotecan and gemcitabine.[116,117]

No clinical trials of Chk1 inhibitors with radiotherapy have been started.

SUMMARY AND FUTURE DIRECTIONS

For both the PARP and Chk1 inhibitors, the initial focus of clinical development has been in combination with cytotoxic chemotherapeutic agents. These trials investigating the possibility of effective chemo-potentiation within the tumor have been challenged by the enhancement of normal tissue toxicity. This inability to find the therapeutic window in which the enhanced tumor cell kill observed in preclinical models can be translated into clinical benefit for patients has dogged the field of chemo-potentiation for many years.[66,70,120]

There are three emerging areas where it is to be hoped that the true benefit of these classes of agents may be realized, single-agent activity or chemo-potentiation in appropriately selected patients, where tumor vulnerability due to HRD allows advantage to be taken of this therapeutic window, and radio-potentiation, where the newer image-guided or image-modulated radiotherapy techniques are already minimizing normal tissue exposure and hence may allow enhanced tumor cell kill without a further increase in normal tissue toxicity. The clinical development of both these classes of compounds will remain an interesting and evolving field over the next few years.

REFERENCES

1. Hoeijmakers JH. Genome maintenance mechanisms for preventing cancer. *Nature*. 2001;411(6835):366–374.
2. Bernstein C, Bernstein H, Payne CM et al. DNA repair/pro-apoptotic dual-role proteins in five major DNA repair pathways: Fail-safe protection against carcinogenesis. *Mutat Res*. 2002;511(2):145–178.
3. Christmann M, Tomicic MT, Roos WP et al. Mechanisms of human DNA repair: An update. *Toxicology*. 2003;19:3–34.
4. Heinen CD, Schmutte C, Fishel R. DNA repair and tumorigenesis: Lessons from hereditary cancer syndromes. *Cancer Biol Ther*. 2002;1(5):477–485.
5. Risinger MA, Groden J. Crosslinks and crosstalk: Human cancer syndromes and DNA repair defects. *Cancer Cell*. 2004;6(6):539–545.
6. de la Chapelle A. Genetic predisposition to colorectal cancer. *Nat Rev Cancer*. 2004;4(10):769–780.
7. Staibano S, Pepe S, Lo Muzio L et al. Poly(adenosine diphosphate-ribose) polymerase 1 expression in malignant melanomas from photoexposed areas of the head and neck region. *Hum Pathol*. 2005;36(7):724–731.
8. Wharton SB, McNelis U, Bell HS et al. Expression of poly(ADP-ribose) polymerase and distribution of poly(ADP-ribosyl)ation in glioblastoma and in a glioma multicellular tumour spheroid model. *Neuropath Appl Neuro*. 2000;26:528–535.
9. Hoglund A, Nilsson LM, Muralidharan SV et al. Therapeutic implications for the induced levels of Chk1 in Myc-expressing cancer cells. *Clin Cancer Res*. 2011;17(22):7067–7079.
10. Madoz-Gurpide J, Canamero M, Sanchez L et al. A proteomics analysis of cell signaling alterations in colorectal cancer. *Mol Cell Proteomics*. 2007;6(12):2150–2164.
11. Speers C, Tsimelzon A, Sexton K et al. Identification of novel kinase targets for the treatment of estrogen receptor-negative breast cancer. *Clin Cancer Res* 2009;15(20):6327–6340.
12. Hansen K, Kelly M. Review of mammalian DNA repair and translational implications. *J Pharm Exp Ther*. 2000;295(1):1–9.
13. Farmer H, McCabe N, Lord CJ et al. Targeting the DNA repair defect in BRCA mutant cells as a therapeutic strategy. *Nature*. 2005;434(7035):917–921.
14. Bryant HE, Helleday T. Inhibition of poly (ADP-ribose) polymerase activates ATM which is required for subsequent homologous recombination repair. *Nucleic Acids Res*. 2006;34(6):1685–1691.

15. Chambon P, Weil J, Mandel P. Nicotinamide mononucleotide activation of a new DNA-dependent polyadenylic acid sythesizing nuclear enzyme. *Biochem Biophy Res Communcations.* 1963;11:39–43.
16. Sugimura T, Fujimura S, Hasegawa S et al. Polymerization of the adenosine 5′¢-diphosphate ribose moiety of NAD by rat liver nuclear enzyme. *Biochim Biophys Acta.* 1967;138(2):438–441.
17. Nishizuka Y, Ueda K, Nakazawa K et al. Studies on the polymer of adenosine diphosphate ribose. I. Enzymic formation from nicotinamide adenine dinuclotide in mammalian nuclei. *J Biol Chem.* 1967;242(13):3164–3171.
18. Doly J, Petek F. Etude de la structure d-un compose "poly(ADP-ribose) synthetise par des extraits nucleares de foie de poulet. *C R Hebd Sciences Acad Sci Ser D Sci Nat.* 1966;263:1341–1344.
19. Fujimura S. NMN-activated poly(A)polymerase in nuclei from rat liver and hepatoma cells. *J Jap Biochem Soc.* 1965;37:584.
20. Chambon P, Weill JD, Doly J et al. On the formation of a novel adencyclic compound by enzymatic extracts of liver nuclei. *Biochem Biophy Res Communications.* 1966;25:638–643.
21. de Murcia G, Menissier de Murcia J. Poly(ADP-ribose) polymerase: A molecular nick-sensor. *Trends Biochem Sci.* 1994;19(4):172–176.
22. Masutani M, Nozaki T, Nishiyama E et al. Function of poly(ADP-ribose) polymerase in response to DNA damage: Gene-disruption study in mice. *Mol Cell Biochem.* 1999;193(1–2):149–152.
23. Shall S, de Murcia G. Poly(ADP-ribose) polymerase-1: What have we learned from the deficient mouse model? *Mutat Res.* 2000;460(1):1–15.
24. Roitt IM. The inhibition of carbohydrate metabolism in ascites-tumour cells by ethyleneimines. *Biochem J.* 1956;63(2):300–307.
25. Auer B, Nagl U, Herzog H et al. Human nuclear NAD + ADP-ribosyltransferase(polym erizing): Organization of the gene. *DNA* 1989;8(8):575–580.
26. Menissier-de Murcia J, Molinete M, Gradwohl G et al. Zinc-binding domain of poly(ADP-ribose)polymerase participates in the recognition of single strand breaks on DNA. *J Mol Biol.* 1989;210(1):229–233.
27. Gradwohl G, Menissier de Murcia JM, Molinete M et al. The second zinc-finger domain of poly(ADP-ribose) polymerase determines specificity for single-stranded breaks in DNA. *Proc Natl Acad Sci.* 1990;87(8):2990–2994.
28. Tao Z, Gao P, Liu HW. Identification of the ADP-ribosylation sites in the PARP-1 automodification domain: Analysis and implications. *J Am Chem Soc.* 2009;131(40): 14258–14260.
29. Altmeyer M, Messner S, Hassa PO et al. Molecular mechanism of poly(ADP-ribosyl) ation by PARP1 and identification of lysine residues as ADP-ribose acceptor sites. *Nucleic Acids Res.* 2009;37(11):3723–3738.
30. Cherney BW, McBride OW, Chen DF et al. cDNA sequence, protein structure, and chromosomal location of the human gene for poly(ADP-ribose) polymerase. *Proc Natl Acad Sci.* 1987;84(23):8370–8374.
31. Canan Koch SS, Thoresen LH, Tikhe JG et al. Novel tricyclic poly(ADP-ribose) polymerase-1 inhibitors with potent anticancer chemopotentiating activity: Design, synthesis, and X-ray cocrystal structure. *J Med Chem.* 2002;45(23):4961–4974.
32. Curtin N. PARP inhibitors for Cancer Therapy. *Expert Rev Mol Med.* 2005;7(4):1–20.
33. Schreiber V, Dantzer F, Ame JC et al. Poly(ADP-ribose): Novel functions for an old molecule. *Nat Rev.* 2006;7(7):517–528.
34. Liu Q, Guntuku S, Cui XS et al. Chk1 is an essential kinase that is regulated by Atr and required for the G(2)/M DNA damage checkpoint. *Genes Dev.* 2000;14(12): 1448–1459.

35. Dart DA, Adams KE, Akerman I et al. Recruitment of the cell cycle checkpoint kinase ATR to chromatin during S-phase. *J Biol Chem*. 2004;279(16):16433–16440.

36. Jamil S, Mojtabavi S, Hojabrpour P et al. An essential role for MCL-1 in ATR-mediated CHK1 phosphorylation. *Mol Biol Cell*. 2008;19(8):3212–3220.

37. Shiloh Y. ATM and related protein kinases: Safeguarding genome integrity. *Nat Rev Cancer*. 2003;3(3):155–168.

38. Kastan MB, Zhan Q, el-Deiry WS et al. A mammalian cell cycle checkpoint pathway utilizing p53 and GADD45 is defective in ataxia-telangiectasia. *Cell*. 1992;71(4):587–597.

39. Zhao H, Piwnica-Worms H. ATR-mediated checkpoint pathways regulate phosphorylation and activation of human Chk1. *Mol Cell Biol*. 2001;21(13):4129–4139.

40. Curtin N. Therapeutic potential of drugs to modulate DNA repair in cancer. *Expert Opin Ther Targets*. 2007;11(6):783–799.

41. Drew Y, Calvert H. The potential of PARP inhibitors in genetic breast and ovarian cancers. *Ann N Y Acad Sci*. 2008;1138:136–145.

42. Ferraris DV. Evolution of poly(ADP-ribose) polymerase-1 (PARP-1) inhibitors. From concept to clinic. *J Med Chem*. 2010;53:4561–4584.

43. Rouleau M, Patel A, Hendzel MJ et al. PARP inhibition: PARP1 and beyond. *Nat Rev Cancer*. 2010;10:293–301.

44. Drew Y, Plummer R. PARP inhibitors in cancer therapy: Two modes of attack on the cancer cell widening the clinical applications. *Drug Resist Updat*. 2009; 12(6):153–156.

45. Mangerich A, Burkle A. How to kill tumor cells with inhibitors of poly(ADP-ribosyl) ation. *Int J Cancer*. 2011;128(2):251–265.

46. Zaremba T, Curtin NJ. PARP inhibitor development for systemic cancer targeting. *Anticancer Agents Med Chem*. 2007;7(5):515–523.

47. Jagtap P, Szabo C. Poly(ADP-Ribose)polymerase and the therapeautic effects of its inhibitors. *Nat Rev Drug Disc*. 2005;4:421–440.

48. Tentori L, Portarena I, Graziani G. Potential clinical applications of poly(ADP-ribose) polymerase (PARP) inhibitors. *Pharmacol Res*. 2002;45(2):73–85.

49. Denny BJ, Wheelhouse RT, Stevens MF et al. NMR and molecular modeling investigation of the mechanism of activation of the antitumor drug temozolomide and its interaction with DNA. *Biochemistry*. 1994;33(31):9045–9051.

50. Bignami M, O'Driscoll M, Aquilina G et al. Unmasking a killer: DNA O(6)-methylguanine and the cytotoxicity of methylating agents. *Mutat Res*. 2000;462(2–3):71–82.

51. Karran P. Mechanisms of tolerance to DNA damaging therapeutic drugs. *Carcinogenesis*. 2001;22(12):1931–1937.

52. Boulton S, Pemberton LC, Porteous JK et al. Potentiation of temozolomide-induced cytotoxicity: A comparative study of the biological effects of poly(ADP-ribose) polymerase inhibitors. *Br J Cancer*. 1995;72(4):849–856.

53. Miknyoczki SJ, Jones-Bolin S, Pritchard S et al. Chemopotentiation of temozolomide, irinotecan, and cisplatin activity by CEP-6800, a poly(ADP-ribose) polymerase inhibitor. *Mol Cancer Ther*. 2003;2(4):371–382.

54. Tentori L, Leonetti C, Scarsella M et al. Systemic administration of GPI 15427, a novel poly(ADP-ribose) polymerase-1 inhibitor, increases the antitumor activity of temozolomide against intracranial melanoma, glioma, lymphoma. *Clin Cancer Res*. 2003;9(14):5370–5379.

55. Tentori L, Leonetti C, Scarsella M et al. Inhibition of poly(ADP-ribose) polymerase prevents irinotecan-induced intestinal damage and enhances irinotecan/temozolomide efficacy against colon carcinoma. *Faseb J*. 2006;20(10):1709–1711.

56. Bowman KJ, Newell DR, Calvert AH et al. Differential effects of the poly(ADP-ribose) polymerase (PARP) inhibitor NU1025 on topoisomerase I and II inhibitor cytotoxicity in L1210 cells in vitro. *Br J Cancer*. 2001;84(1):106–112.

57. Malanga M, Althaus FR. Poly(ADP-ribose) reactivates stalled DNA topoisomerase I and induces DNA strand break resealing. *J Biol Chem*. 2004;279(7):5244–5248.

58. Mayer F, Mueller M, Malenke E et al. Polyadenosine diphosphate-ribose polymerase (PARP) inhibition as a means of protecting the inner ear from cisplatin (CDDP)-mediated ototoxicity without affecting antitumor efficacy in vitro. *J Clin Oncol*. 2010;28 (Suppl):Abstract e13501.

59. Racz I, Tory K, Gallyas F, Jr. et al. BGP-15—A novel poly(ADP-ribose) polymerase inhibitor—protects against nephrotoxicity of cisplatin without compromising its antitumor activity. *Biochem Pharmacol*. 2002;63(6):1099–1111.

60. Szenczi O, Kemecsei P, Holthuijsen MF et al. Poly(ADP-ribose) polymerase regulates myocardial calcium handling in doxorubicin-induced heart failure. *Biochem Pharmacol*. 2005;69(5):725–732.

61. Calabrese CR, Almassy R, Barton S et al. Anticancer chemosensitization and radio-sensitization by the novel poly(ADP-ribose) polymerase-1 inhibitor AG14361. *J Natl Cancer Inst*. 2004;96(1):56–67.

62. Donawho CK, Luo Y, Luo Y et al. ABT-888, an orally active poly(ADP-ribose) poly-merase inhibitor that potentiates DNA-damaging agents in preclinical tumor models. *Clin Cancer Res*. 2007;13(9):2728–2737.

63. Khan K, Araki K, Wang D et al. Head and neck cancer radiosensitization by the novel poly(ADP-ribose) polymerase inhibitor GPI-15427. *Head & Neck*. 2010;32(3):381–391.

64. Thomas HD, Calabrese CR, Batey MA et al. Preclinical selection of a novel poly (ADP-ribose) polymerase inhibitor for clinical trial. *Mol Cancer Ther*. 2007;6(3):945–956.

65. Plummer R, Jones C, Middleton M et al. Phase I study of the poly(ADP-ribose) poly-merase inhibitor, AG014699, in combination with temozolomide in patients with advanced solid tumors. *Clin Cancer Res*. 2008;14(23):7917–7923.

66. Ranson M, Middleton MR, Bridgewater J et al. Lomeguatrib, a potent inhibitor of O6-alkylguanine-DNA-alkyltransferase: Phase I safety, pharmacodynamic, and phar-macokinetic trial and evaluation in combination with temozolomide in patients with advanced solid tumors. *Clin Cancer Res*. 2006;12(5):1577–1584.

67. Ranson M, Hersey P, Thompson D et al. A randomised trial of the combination of lomeguatrib and temozolomide alone in patients with advanced melanoma. *J Clin Oncol*. 2007;25(18):2540–2545.

68. Gajewski TF, Sosman J, Gerson SL et al. Phase II trial of the O6-alkylguanine DNA alkyltransferase inhibitor O6-benzylguanine and 1,3-bis(2-chloroethyl)-1-nitrosourea in advanced melanoma. *Clin Cancer Res*. 2005;11(21):7861–7865.

69. Quinn JA, Desjardins A, Weingart J et al. Phase I trial of temozolomide plus O6-benzylguanine for patients with recurrent or progressive malignant glioma. *J Clin Oncol*. 2005;23(28):7178–7187.

70. Quinn JA, Pluda J, Dolan ME et al. Phase II trial of carmustine plus O(6)-benzylguanine for patients with nitrosourea-resistant recurrent or progressive malignant glioma. *J Clin Oncol*. 2002;20(9):2277–2283.

71. Brada M, Judson I, Beale P et al. Phase I dose-escalation and pharmacokinetic study of temozolomide (SCH 52365) for refractory or relapsing malignancies. *Br J Cancer*. 1999;81(6):1022–1030.

72. Plummer ER, Lorigan P, Evans J et al. First and final report of a phase II study of the poly(ADP-ribose) polymerase (PARP) inhibitor, AG014699, in combination with temo-zolomide (TMZ) in patients with metastatic malignant melanoma (MM). *J Clin Oncol*. 2006;24(18s):456s.

73. Middleton M, Friedberg EC, Hamid O et al. Veliparib (ABT-888) plus temozolomide versus temozolomide alone: Efficacy and safety in patients with metastatic melanoma in a randomized double-blind placebo-controlled trial. *Pigment Cell Melanoma Res*. 2011;24(5):1022–1023.

74. Bedikian AY, Papadopoulos NE, Kim KB et al. A phase IB trial of intravenous INO-1001 plus oral temozolomide in subjects with unresectable stage-III or IV melanoma. *Cancer Invest*. 2009;27:756–763.

75. Rajan A, Carter CA, Gutierrez M et al. A phase I combination study of olaparib (AZD2281; KU-0059436) and cisplatin plus gemcitabine in adults with solid tumors. *J Thoracic Oncol*. 2009;4(9):S598–S599.

76. Rajan A, Gutierrez M, Kummar S et al. A phase I combination study of AZD2281 and cisplatin plus gemcitabine in adults with solid tumors. *Ann Oncol*. 2009;20:42–43.

77. Kummar S, Ji J, Zhang Y, Simmons D et al. A phase I combination study of Abt-888 and topotecan hydrochloride in adults with refractory solid tumors and lymphomas. *Ann Oncol*. 2009;20:42.

78. Khan OA, Gore M, Lorigan P et al. A phase I study of the safety and tolerability of olaparib (AZD2281, KU0059436) and dacarbazine in patients with advanced solid tumours. *Br J Cancer*. 104(5):750–755.

79. Kummar S, Chen AP, Ji JJ et al. A phase I study of ABT-888 (A) in combination with metronomic cyclophosphamide (C) in adults with refractory solid tumors and lymphomas. *J Clin Oncol*. 2010;28 (Suppl):Abstract 2605.

80. Tan AR, Gibbon D, Stein MN et al. Preliminary results of a phase I trial of ABT-888, a poly(ADP-ribose) polymerase (PARP) inhibitor, in combination with cyclophosphamide. *J Clin Oncol*. 2010;28 (Suppl):Abstract 3000.

81. Dent RA, Lindeman GJ, Clemons M et al. Safety and efficacy of the oral PARP inhibitor olaparib (AZD2281) in combination with paclitaxel for the first- or second-line treatment of patients with metastatic triple-negative breast cancer: Results from the safety cohort of a phase I/II multicenter trial. *J Clin Oncol*. 2010;28 (Suppl):Abstract 1018.

82. Kopetz S, Mita M, Mok I et al. First in human phase I study of BSI-201, a small molecule inhibitor of poly ADP-ribose polymerase (PARP) in subjects with advanced solid tumors. *J Clin Oncol*. 2008;26(Suppl):3577.

83. Mahany J, Lewis N, Heath E et al. A phase IB study evaluating BSI-201 in combination with chemotherapy in subjects with advanced solid tumors. *J Clin Oncol*. 2008;26(Suppl):3579.

84. Metzger-Filho O, Tutt A, de Azambuja E et al. Dissecting the heterogeneity of triple-negative breast cancer. *J Clin Oncol*. 2012;30(15):1879–1887.

85. Liu X, Shi Y, Maag DX et al. Iniparib nonselectively modifies cysteine-containing proteins in tumor cells and is not a bona fide PARP inhibitor. *Clin Cancer Res*. 2012;18(2):510–523.

86. Patel AG, De Lorenzo SB, Flatten KS et al. Failure of iniparib to inhibit poly(ADP-Ribose) polymerase in vitro. *Clin Cancer Res*. 2012;18(6):1655–1662.

87. Fong P, Boss D, Yap T et al. Inhibition of poly(ADP-ribose) polymerase in tumors from BRCA mutation carriers. *N Engl J Med*. 2009;361(2):123–134.

88. Tutt A, Robson M, Garber J et al. Phase II trial of the oral PARP inhibitor olaparib in BRCA-deficient advanced breast cancer. *J Clin Oncol*. 2009;27(18s):CRA501.

89. Audeh M, Penson R, Friedlander M et al. Phase II trial of the oral PARP inhibitor olaparib (AZD2281) in BRCA-deficient advanced ovarian cancer. *J Clin Oncol*. 2009;27(15s):5500.

90. Edwards S, Brough R, Lord C et al. Resistance to therapy caused by intragenic deletion in BRCA2. *Nature*. 2008;451:1111–1115.

91. Sakai W, Swisher E, Karlan B, Agarwal M, Higgins J, Friedman C et al. Secondary mutations as a mechanism of cisplatin resistance in BRCA2-mutated cancers. *Nature*. 2008;451:1116–1120.

92. Ashworth A. What has and does DNA repair biology tell us? *Ann Oncol*. 2010;21 (Suppl 4):Abstract 41N.

93. Gelmon KA, Tischkowitz M, Mackay H et al. Olaparib in patients with recurrent high-grade serous or poorly differentiated ovarian carcinoma or triple-negative breast cancer: A phase 2, multicentre, open-label, non-randomised study. *Lancet Oncol.* 2011;12(9):852–861.

94. Ledermann J, Harter P, Gourley C et al. Olaparib maintenance therapy in platinum-sensitive relapsed ovarian cancer. *N Engl J Med.* 2012;366(15):1382–1392.

95. Mukhopadhyay A, Elattar A, Cerbinskaite A et al. Development of a functional assay for homologous recombination status in primary cultures of epithelial ovarian tumor and correlation with sensitivity to poly(ADP-ribose) polymerase inhibitors. *Clin Cancer Res.* 2010;16:2344–2351.

96. Graeser M, McCarthy A, Lord CJ et al. A marker of homologous recombination predicts pathologic complete response to neoadjuvant chemotherapy in primary breast cancer. *Clin Cancer Res.* 2010;16(24):6159–6168.

97. Courage C, Budworth J, Gescher A. Comparison of ability of protein kinase C inhibitors to arrest cell growth and to alter cellular protein kinase C localisation. *Br J Cancer.* 1995;71(4):697–704.

98. Sorensen CS, Syljuasen RG, Falck J et al. Chk1 regulates the S phase checkpoint by coupling the physiological turnover and ionizing radiation-induced accelerated proteolysis of Cdc25A. *Cancer Cell.* 2003;3(3):247–258.

99. Luo Y, Rockow-Magnone SK, Kroeger PE et al. Blocking Chk1 expression induces apoptosis and abrogates the G2 checkpoint mechanism. *Neoplasia.* 2001;3(5):411–419.

100. Mack PC, Gandara DR, Lau AH et al. Cell cycle-dependent potentiation of cisplatin by UCN-01 in non-small-cell lung carcinoma. *Cancer Chemother Pharmacol.* 2003;51(4):337–348.

101. Furuta T, Hayward RL, Meng LH et al. p21CDKN1A allows the repair of replication-mediated DNA double-strand breaks induced by topoisomerase I and is inactivated by the checkpoint kinase inhibitor 7-hydroxystaurosporine. *Oncogene.* 2006;25(20):2839–2849.

102. Parsels LA, Morgan MA, Tanska DM et al. Gemcitabine sensitization by checkpoint kinase 1 inhibition correlates with inhibition of a Rad51 DNA damage response in pancreatic cancer cells. *Mol Cancer Ther.* 2009;8(1):45–54.

103. Blasina A, Hallin J, Chen E et al. Breaching the DNA damage checkpoint via PF-00477736, a novel small-molecule inhibitor of checkpoint kinase 1. *Mol Cancer Ther.* 2008;7(8):2394–2404.

104. Zabludoff SD, Deng C, Grondine MR et al. AZD7762, a novel checkpoint kinase inhibitor, drives checkpoint abrogation and potentiates DNA-targeted therapies. *Mol Cancer Ther.* 2008;7(9):2955–2966.

105. McNeely S, Conti C, Sheikh T et al. Chk1 inhibition after replicative stress activates a double strand break response mediated by ATM and DNA-dependent protein kinase. *Cell Cycle.* 2010;9(5):995–1004.

106. Mitchell JB, Choudhuri R, Fabre K et al. in vitro and in vivo radiation sensitization of human tumor cells by a novel checkpoint kinase inhibitor, AZD7762. *Clin Cancer Res.* 2010;16(7):2076–2084.

107. Morgan MA, Parsels LA, Zhao L et al. Mechanism of radiosensitization by the Chk1/2 inhibitor AZD7762 involves abrogation of the G2 checkpoint and inhibition of homologous recombinational DNA repair. *Cancer Res.* 2010;70(12):4972–4981.

108. Guzi TJ, Paruch K, Dwyer MP et al. Targeting the replication checkpoint using SCH 900776, a potent and functionally selective CHK1 inhibitor identified via high content screening. *Mol Cancer Ther.* 2011;10(4):591–602.

109. Walton MI, Eve PD, Hayes A et al. The preclinical pharmacology and therapeutic activity of the novel CHK1 inhibitor SAR-020106. *Mol Cancer Ther.* 2010;9(1):89–100.

110. Matthews DJ, Yakes FM, Chen J et al. Pharmacological abrogation of S-phase checkpoint enhances the anti-tumor activity of gemcitabine in vivo. *Cell Cycle.* 2007;6(1):104–110.

111. Sausville EA, Arbuck SG, Messmann R et al. Phase I trial of 72-hour continuous infusion UCN-01 in patients with refractory neoplasms. *J Clin Oncol.* 2001;19(8):2319–2333.
112. Dees EC, Baker SD, O'Reilly S et al. A phase I and pharmacokinetic study of short infusions of UCN-01 in patients with refractory solid tumors. *Clin Cancer Res.* 2005;11:664–671.
113. Perez RP, Lewis LD, Beelen AP et al. Modulation of cell cycle progression in human tumors: A pharmacokinetic and tumor molecular pharmacodynamic study of cisplatin plus the Chk1 inhibitor UCN-01 (NSC 638850). *Clin Cancer Res.* 2006;12(23): 7079–7085.
114. Hotte SJ, Oza A, Winquist EW et al. Phase I trial of UCN-01 in combination with topotecan in patients with advanced solid cancers: A Princess Margaret Hospital Phase II Consortium study. *Ann Oncol.* 2006;17(2):334–340.
115. Fracasso PM, Williams KJ, Chen RC et al. A Phase 1 study of UCN-01 in combination with irinotecan in patients with resistant solid tumor malignancies. *Cancer Chemo Pharm.* 2011;67(6):1225–1237.
116. Sausville E, LoRosso P, Carducci MA et al. Phase 1 dose-escalation study of AZD7762 in combination with gemcitabine (gem) in patients (pts) with advanced solid tumours. *J Clin Oncol.* 2011;29(S):3058.
117. Ho AL, Bendell JC, Cleary JM et al. Phase 1, open-label, dose-escalation study of AZD7762 in combination with irinotecan (irino) in patients (pts) with advanced solid tumours. *J Clin Oncol.* 2011;29(S):3033.
118. Daud A, Springett G, Mendleson D et al. A Phase I dose-escalation study of SCH-900776, a selective inhibitor of checkpoint 1 (CHK1), in combination with gemcitabine (Gem) in subjects with advanced solid tumours. *J Clin Oncol.* 2010;28(15S):3064.
119. Brega N, McArthur C, Britten S et al. Phase 1 clinical trial of gemcitabine (GEM) in combination with PF-00477736 (PF-736), a selective inhibitor of CHK1 kinase. *J Clin Oncol.* 2010;28(15S):3062.
120. Schilsky RL, Dolan ME, Bertucci D et al. Phase I clinical and pharmacological study of O6-benzylguanine followed by carmustine in patients with advanced cancer. *Clin Cancer Res.* 2000 Aug;6(8):3025–3031.

20 Inhibitors Targeting Mitosis

Dan L. Sackett
National Institutes of Health

Edina Komlodi-Pasztor
National Institutes of Health

Tito Fojo
National Institutes of Health

CONTENTS

INTRODUCTION

Mitosis, the process whereby a eukaryotic cell separates its replicated chromosomes into identical sets and segregates them to two offspring, has long been an attractive chemotherapy target. The past decade has seen the development of drugs targeting proteins crucial in cell division. Among these, drugs targeting mitotic kinases have received special attention (Harrison et al., 2009). The clinical efficacy of agents targeting microtubules (MTs) and the belief tumors harbor a large fraction of actively dividing cells provided support for this focus. However, as our knowledge and appreciation of the complexities of a cell have increased, we recognize a more nuanced view than targeting of cell division is more appropriate. In this chapter, we describe the basic science that supported the development of drugs targeting mitosis and review their clinical fate.

UNDERSTANDING MITOSIS

Mitosis is the stage of the cell cycle ("M phase") during which the contents of the cytoplasm and nucleus of a cell are divided into two (usually) equal daughter cells (Williams et al., 2012). It consists of karyokinesis, partition of the nuclear contents, and the subsequent cytokinesis, division of the whole cell body. Preparing the cell for mitosis actually starts in the G2 phase that precedes mitosis proper and involves such events as maturation and initial separation of centrosomes and changes in post-translational modifications on histones, as well as other events. The beginning of mitosis itself (in mammalian cells) is usually taken as the point at which the nuclear envelope breaks down, allowing free mixing between the formerly separated contents of the nucleus and the cytoplasm. The end of M phase is signaled by cytokinesis and the release of two daughter cells (Rieder, 2011).

Drugs that target mitosis, collectively referred to as "mitotic inhibitors," include the classical MT-targeting agents (MTAs) and a new class of agents that have targets that are only found in mitosis, which we will refer to as mitosis-specific agents (MSAs) (for recent reviews, see Manchado et al., 2012; Campos and Dizon, 2012). The MTAs include agents such as vincristine, combretastatin, and paclitaxel (Taxol®) and others, including many not yet in the clinic. These agents all bind to tubulin, the structural subunit of MTs, and alter the dynamics and/or quantity of a cell's MTs. MTs are found in all phases of the cell cycle, although they have a special role in mitosis as the main structural elements of the mitotic spindle. MTAs therefore have effects throughout the cell cycle and are more properly thought of as anti-MT, as opposed to antimitosis, in action. The MSAs have as targets a variety of proteins that are present or active only in mitosis, including spindle-specific motor proteins such as kinesin-5 (also known as KSP or kinesin spindle protein), and a variety of kinases that regulate progression of mitosis, notably from the aurora and polo families.

What all of the mitotic inhibitors have in common is that they affect the *process* of mitosis. When viewed this way, as a process, it is clear that mitosis involves structures, as well as regulation. Mitotic inhibitors can almost be neatly divided between these two aspects of the process, so the two are briefly discussed.

MTAs AND THEIR EFFECTS ON MITOTIC STRUCTURES

Effects on *mitotic structures* include both the breakdown of interphase structures and the construction of mitotic ones. Breakdown or rearrangement of interphase structures includes disruption and dispersal of the Golgi apparatus, breakdown of the nuclear envelope, and rearrangement of the single centrosome-focused interphase MT array. Construction of structures that are only used in mitosis includes assembly of the mitotic spindle and, later, assembly of the contractile ring apparatus that mediates cytokinesis. The mitotic apparatus is arguably the largest and most complex mechanochemical machine in cell biology and is a bipolar structure based on two centrosome-centered arrays of MT. It is these MT arrays that allow MTAs to exert antimitotic action, by targeting the dynamic MTs that are the core of the mitotic spindle. However, the MTs that make up this bipolar array are essentially identical to those that make up the unipolar MT array found in ≥95% of the cell cycle, that is, interphase. Hence, the MTAs, which bind to tubulin, can therefore target MTs throughout the cell cycle and not only in mitosis. In addition to these interphase effects, these agents cause robust mitotic disruption in rapidly dividing cells. A small subset of all known MTAs has found application and success in the clinic. The notable success of these agents against human cancers is often attributed to their ability to induce mitotic arrest, although this attribution may be incorrect and may be inhibiting identification of responsible pathways (Komlodi-Pasztor et al., 2011; Mitchison, 2012).

MTAs AND THEIR EFFECTS ON MITOTIC REGULATION

Mitotic regulation consists of the control and coordination of entry into, progression through, and termination of, mitosis. Changes in post-translational modifications of many proteins comprise this regulatory program. Many but not all of the post-translational modifications involved are phosphorylation and dephosphorylation (Johnson and Kornbluth, 2012), and many critical phosphorylation events are due to kinases that are active only, or predominantly, in mitosis (Johnson, 2011). These include Cdk1/cyclin B; aurora family kinases, especially A and B; and polo-like kinase (Plk) family members, especially Plk1 (Lens et al., 2010). Cdk1/cyclin B is the master regulator of mitosis, promoting the G2 to M transition, phosphorylating downstream proteins including aurora and polo kinases, and maintaining the mitotic state until anaphase (Manchado et al., 2012). Aurora A action drives centrosome maturation and separation and hence is involved in assembling a properly functioning bipolar mitotic spindle. Aurora B regulates the checkpoint mechanism that prevents or corrects misattachment of chromosomes to spindle MT. Plk 1 action regulates multiple points in mitosis including centrosome maturation and spindle formation, maintenance of MT-chromosome (kinetochore) junction, and cytokinesis.

The actions of these and other kinases that function in mitosis are not cleanly separate. Rather, their activities may be redundant, additive, or even antagonistic. In addition, these may act sequentially. For example, aurora A can activate Plk1, which can phosphorylate cyclin B and thereby regulate Cdk1/cyclin B activity; Cdk1/cyclin B in turn can activate aurora A and close a cycle (Johnson, 2011; Lens et al., 2010). If kinase activities are antagonistic, effects on cell division caused by inhibition of one kinase may be reversed by simultaneous inhibition of a second kinase, whether by a second drug or by a single drug with overlapping targeting (Lens et al., 2010).

MITOSIS-SPECIFIC AGENTS

Many *MSAs* have been described in the past decade, and of these, a number have progressed to clinical trials (see recent reviews in Campos and Dizon, 2012; Komlodi-Pasztor et al., 2011). Targeting the beginning of mitosis, the Cdk1-cyclin B-dependent transition from G2 to M, was attempted with pan-Cdk inhibitors such as flavopiridol and UCN-01, but this was not successful due to side effects and possibly due to induction of quiescence rather than the desired cell death (Manchado et al., 2012). Inhibitors of aurora A and/or B, as well as inhibitors of Plk1, comprise the largest group of MSAs that have progressed to clinical trials (Figure 20.1). These agents

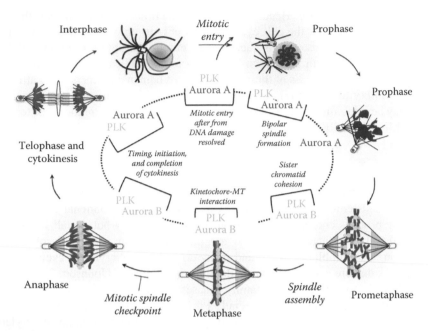

FIGURE 20.1   The mammalian mitotic cycle. The cell cycle of a mammalian cell is shown, with the majority of the cycle (G1, S, G2) compressed into the one figure labeled "Interphase." Cells enter mitosis from interphase as the centrosomes begin to separate from each other. The centrosomes begin maturation during G2 and complete this process as they move apart, the nuclear envelope breaks down, and chromatin condenses. During prophase and prometaphase, the centrosomes move to opposite poles of the cell as MTs nucleate from and organize between them, forming a bipolar spindle. Chromosomes are captured by MT binding to the chromosomes' kinetochores, after which the chromosomes become aligned on the spindle equator at metaphase. Following satisfaction of the spindle checkpoint, the sister chromatids separate and are drawn to the opposite poles. Completion of separation triggers completion of mitosis by cytokinesis. Mitotic kinases regulate many aspects of this process. Steps where the action of particular mitotic kinases has been demonstrated are indicated by the names of the kinases next to the affected step.

vary in specificity, and as discussed earlier, overlapping targeting likely alters efficacy. Furthermore, as discussed earlier, all of these agents target mitosis in progress, disrupting regulation of steps in the mitotic process that must occur after mitosis has begun, although Plk1 and aurora A contribute to regulation of mitotic entry as well through feedback control loops. These agents all disrupt mitosis and inhibit cell growth in vitro and in xenograft models. Clinical trials as single agents have not yet revealed significant activity, however, and this is discussed in greater detail in the subsequent sections.

   A number of tumor types have been suggested as suitable targets for MSAs, often based on overexpression of mitotic kinases in patient samples or in patient-derived cell lines. Three recent examples are prostate and thyroid cancer and gliomas. Androgen-refractory prostate cancer targeting was examined using transgenic murine androgen-sensitive or androgen depletion-independent (ADI) prostate cancer cell lines to demonstrate significant upregulation of aurora kinases (AKs) A and B in vitro as well as in mouse tumors derived from ADI cells. Additionally, ADI with the largest increase in upregulation showed increased sensitivity to a pan-AK inhibitor (Jeet et al., 2012). Similarly, a study of patient samples of small cell (neuroendocrine) prostate cancer (NEPC) found upregulation of aurora A as well as N-myc and suggested that the two proteins cooperate in development of the neuroendocrine character. Increased sensitivity of NEPC cell models to the AK inhibitor, danusertib (PHA-739358), led to the suggestion that this or other MSAs may show activity in patients with NEPC (Beltran et al., 2011). A study of medullary thyroid carcinoma (MTC) tissues from different tumor stages found measureable levels but no correlation of tumor stage with levels of AKs A, B, or C. A pan-aurora inhibitor, MK-0457, showed significant activity against an MTC cell line, and based on these results, further evaluation of MSA treatment of patients with MTC has been suggested (Baldini et al., 2011). Finally, a study of aurora A expression in major glioma types found lineage-specific patterns of expression by quantitative western blots and by reverse transcription polymerase chain reaction. The results indicated that lower aurora A expression level was significantly correlated with poorer patient survival in glioblastoma, while in other types, increased expression correlated with increased tumor aggressiveness. The aurora A inhibitor MLN8237 showed strong cytotoxicity against glioblastoma cell lines, and the combined results suggested to the authors that aurora A may be a potential target for therapy in glioblastoma (Lehman et al., 2012).

CLINICAL RESULTS WITH MSAs

The large number of MSAs developed against targets in mitosis including the AKs, Plks, and KSPs is evidence of their appeal as chemotherapy agents. Their development was seen as attractive given the success of MT-targeting agents. It was envisioned that MSAs would target mitosis while avoiding the neurotoxicity that so often accompanies the taxanes and the vinca alkaloids. But while many thought the clinical efficacy of MTAs could be ascribed to the induction of mitotic arrest, in humans, a more complex paradigm is likely applicable and interference with intracellular trafficking on MTs is likely the principal mechanism of action. The preclinical data for the MSAs, both in vitro and in vivo, were robust, but as we will review, this robustness was not seen when these agents were explored clinically, at least in solid tumors. While development is still ongoing, and the final word has not been written, examination of the preclinical and clinical data for these inhibitors targeting mitosis sheds light as to why they have thus far not delivered on their promise and what we have learned that may help us going forward.

Let us begin with positing why MSAs have not performed as well in the clinic. Their development, like that of most other anticancer agents, relied on commonly used in vitro and in vivo platforms. Countless preclinical studies demonstrated the activity of these agents but, importantly, almost exclusively in models with doubling times measured in less than one to at most a few days (Arbitrario et al., 2010; Benten et al., 2009; Fletcher et al., 2011; Harrington et al., 2004; Huck et al., 2010; Wilkinson et al., 2007). Unfortunately, tumors in humans, especially solid tumors, do not divide as rapidly, and herein one can find one explanation for the results we have witnessed as these agents advanced to the clinic (Komlodi-Pasztor et al., 2012). A simple, but important, lesson we knew long before the "era of targeted therapies" and have seen reinforced time and again is that targeted therapies require the presence of the target. In the case of the mitotic targets, numerous studies have shown that expression of the AKs, the Plks, and the KSPs does not occur or occurs only at levels that are very low during G1 (and G0) as well as during the S phase. These proteins (targets) are expressed primarily in the M phase of the cell cycle and to a lesser extent in G (Crosio et al., 2002; Dutertre et al., 2002; Jackson et al., 2007; Kishi et al., 2009; Lens et al., 2010; Sasai et al., 2004). Because mitosis represents only a fraction and in many cells only a small fraction of the cell cycle, the required target will be found and in turn drug effect will occur only in cells that are rapidly dividing (cycling) and hence likely to be in or passing through G2 or M while drug is present. This highly restricted, cycle-specific expression likely explains why these agents have had difficulty affecting tumor growth in patients whose solid tumors divide much less rapidly.

But can we really be sure? Might there be other explanations? Let us consider the data. Agents targeting the AKs, Plk, and KSP have been developed, and in Tables 20.1 through 20.3, we summarize the clinical results in 66 studies conducted with 25 different mitotic inhibitors. One can see that to date the response rate recorded against solid tumors has been low. While a majority of these studies have been reported as phase 1 studies, in fact with an average enrollment of 40 patients in each study, the majority of these trials sought to look at expanded cohorts in search of some evidence of activity. Further studies might uncover heretofore undetected activity, but if we accept that the low level of activity reported to date in solid tumors will not increase in a meaningful way, might there be explanations other than the slow(er) growth of solid tumors and the absence of target? None stand out. The reason for failure in solid tumors is unlikely to have been low bioavailability, since many of these agents were given intravenously; and for many, pharmacokinetics demonstrated that desired concentrations had been achieved. In numerous studies, biomarkers for "mitotic arrest" (mitotic index or histone H3 phosphorylation most often in skin biopsies) demonstrated target engagement (Dees et al., 2010; Kristeleit et al., 2009). One interesting study carefully looked for inhibition of aurora A by MLN8054 both in skin and in tumors (Chakravarty et al., 2011). In addition to estimating the "mitotic index," the investigators quantitated two "hallmark phenotypes" of aurora A inhibition—the percent of mitotic cells in which misaligned chromosomes were detected and the percent of mitotic cells without properly formed bipolar mitotic spindles (Hoar et al., 2007; Marumoto et al., 2003). In several patients in the highest dose cohorts, the mitotic index in the skin showed marked increases after dosing. However, a more variable outcome was observed in tumors with both increases and decreases in mitotic cells (mitotic index) seen after dosing; a variable outcome the authors felt was consistent with the induction of either mitotic arrest or mitotic slippage, both of which have been reported in tumors with agents targeting mitosis. In contrast they observed, primarily in the highest dose cohorts, marked decreases in the percentage of mitotic cells with aligned chromosomes and bipolar spindles; biomarkers the authors noted act independently of mitotic arrest or slippage. This study, as did others, demonstrated evidence of target engagement, albeit in a small fraction of cells.

TABLE 20.1

Clinical Trials with Aurora Kinase Inhibitors

Drug [Company]	Disease	Treatment	Trial Design	Number Enrolled	Response	DLT/AE	Reference
MK-0457/ VX-680 [Vertex/Merck]	CML/ALL	5 day CIV q2–3 weeks	—	3	1 PHR 1 CHR	↓BM	Giles et al. (2007)
	ST	5 day CIV q28d	Phase 1	16	3 SD	↓ANC, F/N, and allergic reaction	Rubin (2006)
	ST	24 h CIV q21d	Phase 1	27	1 SD	↓ANC, N/V/diarrhea, and fatigue	Traynor et al. (2011)
	Hem/CML	5 day CIV q28d	Phase 1/2	77	8/18 BcrAbl T315I PR; 1/3 Ph+ALL CR	Mucositis and alopecia	Giles et al. (2013)
AZD1152/ Barasertib [Astra Zeneca]	AML	7 day CIV q21d	Phase 1	16	2 CR, 1 PR, 6 SD	↓ANC, F/N, ↓WBC, ↓Plt, fatigue, pneumonia, ARDS, and sepsis	Tsuboi et al. (2011)
	ST	2 h IV q7d; 2 h IV q14d	Phase 1	59	15 SD	↓ANC and F/N	Boss et al. (2011)
	AML	7 day CIV q21d	Phase 1	32	8 hematologic R	F/N, stomatitis, and mucosal inflammation	Löwenberg et al. (2011)
	AML	7 day CIV q21d	Phase 2	32	8 hematologic R		
	AML	7 day CIV q28d	Phase 1	5	1 CR	Nausea and stomatitis	Dennis et al. (2012)
PHA 739358/ Danusertib [Nerviano]	ST	6 h CIV	Phase 1	42	7 SD	↓ANC, HTN, fatigue, anorexia, and N/diarrhea	De Jonge et al. (2008)
	ST	24 h CIV q14d ± GCSF	Phase 1	56	1 PR; 18 SD, 4 PSD	F/N, fatigue, anorexia, N/V/diarrhea mucositis, ↑LFTs, ↓K+, HTN, and fever	Cohen et al. (2009)
	ST	3 week CIV q28d	Phase 1	50	9 SD	↓ANC, ↓WBC, ↓Hgb N/diarrhea anorexia, and fatigue	Steeghs et al. (2009)
MLN8054 [Millenium]	ST	PO d1–5+d8–12 q28d or PO QID d1–14 q28d	Phase 1	43	3 SD	↓MS, ↑LFTs, and mucositis	Macarulla et al. (2010)
	ST	PO×7d q21d; PO×14d q28d; PO×21d q35d	Phase 1	61	9 SD	↓MS, N/V, confusion, cognitive disorder, hallucination, and fatigue	Dees et al. (2011)

(continued)

TABLE 20.1 (continued)
Clinical Trials with Aurora Kinase Inhibitors

Drug [Company]	Disease	Treatment	Trial Design	Number Enrolled	Response	DLT/AE	Reference
MLN8237 [Millenium]	ST	PO×7d q21d; PO×14d q28d; PO×21d q35d	Phase 1	65	1 PR, 8 SD	↓ANC, ↓Plt, sepsis, mucositis, N/D, fatigue, and alopecia	Dees et al. (2010)
	NHM	PO bid×7 days q21d	Phase 1	17	ND	F/N, ↓ANC, and fatigue	Sharma et al. (2011)
	Ped Onc	PO qd/bid×7 days q21	Phase 1	33	1 PR	↓ANC and hand–foot syndrome	Mossé et al. (2012)
	OvCa	PO bid×7 days q21d	Phase 2	31	3 PR	↓ANC, ↓WBC, ↓Plt, and stomatitis	Matulonis et al. (2012)
R763 [Merck/Serono]	ST	PO d1, 8 q21d; PO d1–3 q21d	Phase 1	15	2 SD	ND	Renshaw et al. (2007)
AT9283 [Astex]	Leuk	72 h CIV q3wk	Phase 1	29	2 PHR; 1 PCR	↓ANC, ↓BM, ↑LFTs, and alopecia	Foran et al. (2008)
	ST	72 h CIV q3wk	Phase 1	22	3 SD	F/N	Plummer et al. (2008)
	ST	72 h CIV q3wk	Phase 1	33	1 PR, 4 SD	F/N, GI disturbance, and fatigue	Kristeleit et al. (2009)
	ST	72 h CIV q3wk	Phase 1	40	4 SD>6 months	↓ANC, GI, fatigue, and alopecia,	Arkenau et al. (2012)
SNS-314 [Sunesis]	ST	3 h CIV d1, 8 and 15 q28d	Phase 1	32	6 SD	N/V, fatigue, constipation, and pain	Robert et al. (2009)
SU6668 [Sugen/Pfizer]	ST	PO bid, 28d	Phase 1	35	4 SD	↓Plt, pericarditis, pleuritis, and fatigue	Britten et al. (2002)
	ST	PO bid, 28d	Phase 1	19	3 SD	GI, fatigue, pleuritis, SOB, pericardial effusion	Brahmer et al. (2002)
ENMD-2076 [EntreMed]	ST	PO qd, 28d	Phase 1	14	4 SD	HTN, fatigue, proteinuria, and diarrhea	Bastos et al. (2009)
	ST	PO qd×21d, q28d	Phase 1	67	2 PR, 49 SD	↓ANC, HTN, N/V/D, fatigue, and ↑LFTs	Diamond et al. (2011)
	OvCa	PO	Phase 2	64	3 PR, 27 SD	↓BM, fatigue, HTN, mucositis, ↑LFTs, HFS, thromboembolic event, subarachnoid hemorrhage, ↓LV function, and PRES	Matulonis et al. (2011)

				No			
BI 811283 [Boehringer Ingelheim]	ST	24 h CIV q21d	Phase 1	57	33% SD	↓ANC, F/N, and ↓WBC	Mross et al. (2010)
	ST	24 h CIV q2wk	Phase 1	52	29% SD	↓ANC and ↓WBC	Scheulen et al. (2010)
PF-03814735 [Pfizer]	ST	1–5 or 1–10 q21d	Phase 1	57	19 SD; 4 prolonged SD	F/N; ↑LFTs [AST], left ventricular dysfunction, diarrhea, fatigue, and N/V	Schöffski et al. (2011)
AS703569 [EMD Serono]	Heme	1–3 and 8–10 or 1–6 q21d	Phase 1	45	AML: 3/7 response, 2/7 no progression	↓ANC, F/N, ↓Plts, mucositis, diarrhea, and GI bleeding	Sonet et al. (2008)
GSK1070916 [Glaxo Smith Kline]	Aurora B/C kinase inhibitor GSK1070916A in treating patients with advanced solid tumors [recruiting]						
MK-5108/ VX-689 [Vertex/Merck]	Treatment of participants with advanced and/or refractory solid tumors (MK-5108–001 AM4)—MK-5108 and docetaxel [completed accrual]						

No, Number of patients enrolled; Cycles, median number of cycles administered; CML/ALL, T315I abl-mutated CML or (Ph)+ALL or other CML/ALL; ST, advance solid tumors or advanced and refractory solid tumors or refractory solid tumors; NHM, non-hematologic malignancies; Leuk, refractory leukemia; OvCa, platinum-resistant ovarian cancer; CIV, continuous intravenous infusion; GCSF, granulocyte colony-stimulating factor; CML, chronic myeloid/myelogenous leukemia; AML, acute myeloid/myelogenous leukemia; ALL, acute lymphoblastic leukemia; Heme, hematologic malignancies; PR, partial response; SD, stable disease; PHR, partial hematologic response; CHR, complete hematologic response; PCR, partial cytogenetic response; DLT/AE, dose-limiting toxicity/adverse event; ↓ANC, neutropenia; ↓WBC, leucopenia; ↓BM, pancytopenia; ↓Plt, thrombocytopenia; ↓Hgb, anemia; ↓K+, hypokalemia; ↑LFTs, elevated liver function tests; ↓MS, reduced mental status/ somnolence; ARDS, acute respiratory distress syndrome; F/N, febrile neutropenia; GI, GI disturbance; HFS, hand–foot syndrome; HTN, hypertension; N/V, nausea/ vomiting; PRES, reversible posterior leukoencephalopathy syndrome; and SOB, shortness of breath.

TABLE 20.2
Clinical Trials with Polo-like Kinase Inhibitors

Drug [Company]	Disease	Treatment	Trial Design	Number Enrolled	Response	DLT/AE	Reference
ON 01910.Na [Onconova]	ST	72-h CIV q14d	Phase 1	5	2 SD	↓ANC and fatigue	Ohnuma et al. (2006)
	ST	24-h CIV q7d	Phase 1	23	1 SD	Fatigue and anorexia	Vainshtein et al. (2008)
	ST	2-h infusion d1, 4, 8, 11, 15, 18 q28d	Phase 1	20	1 PR	N/V/D, flatulence, fatigue, and skeletal/abdominal/tumor pain	Jimeno et al. (2008)
BI2536 [Boehringer]	NSCLC	1 h IV, + 500 mg/m^2 pemetrexed q21d	Phase 1 dose escalation	33	2 PR 7 SD	↓ANC, rash, pruritus, nausea, stomatitis, anorexia, ARF, and confusion	Ellis et al. (2008)
	ST	1 h IV d1 q21d	Phase 1 dose escalation	40	14 SD	↓ANC, ↓WBC, fatigue, N/V, anorexia, alopecia, and mucositis	Mross et al. (2008)
	SCLC	1 h IV q21d	Phase 2	23	7 SD	↓ANC, ↓Plt, ↓Hgb, Fatigue N/V, constipation, and ARDS	Gandhi et al. (2009)
	NSCLC	d1 q21d or d1–3 q21d	Phase 2	95	4 PR	↓ANC, F/N, fatigue, nausea, and two deaths	Sebastian et al. (2010)
	ST	1 h IV d 1, 8 q21d or 24 h IV d1 q21d	Phase 1	44 26	14 SD	↓ANC, ↓WBC, ↓Plt, fatigue, and N/V	Hofheinz et al. (2010)
	Pancreatic CA	200 mg q21 60 mg d1–3 q21	Phase 2	86	2 PR, 21 SD	↓ANC, ↓WBC, ↓Plt, fatigue, and nausea	Mross et al. (2012)

GSK 461364 [GlaxoSmithKline]	ST	4 h IV, d1, 8, 15 q28 or 4 h IV d1, 2, 8, 9, 15, 16 q28	Phase 1	40	2 SD	↓ANC, ↓Plt, ↓Hgb, VTE, ARF, and infusion site reaction	Olmos et al. (2011)
HMN-214 [D. Western Therapeutics Institute]	ST	PO d1–5 q28d	Phase 1	32	1 MR, 3 SD	↓ANC, F/N, electrolyte disturbance, neuropathy, and myalgia	Patnaik et al. (2003)
	ST	PO qd×21d q 28d	Phase 1	33	7 SD	↑Gluc, chest pain, and bone pain/myalgia	Garland et al. (2006)
BI 6727 [Boehringer]	ST	1 h IV q21d	Phase 1	65	3 PR, 26 SD	↓ANC, ↓Plt, ↓Hgb, F/N, and fatigue	Schöffski et al. (2012)

No, Number of patients enrolled; Cycles, median number of cycles administered; ST, advance solid tumors or advanced and refractory solid tumors; NSCLC, Relapsed, advanced or metastatic NSCLC; SCLC, sensitive relapse SCLC; IV, intravenous infusion; PR, partial response; SD, stable disease; DLT/AE, dose-limiting toxicity/adverse event; ↓ANC, neutropenia; ↓WBC, leucopenia; ↓Plt, thrombocytopenia; ↓Hgb, anemia; ↓K+, hypokalemia; ↑LFTs, elevated liver function tests; ↑Gluc, hyperglycemia; ↓MS, reduced mental status/somnolence; ARDS, acute respiratory distress syndrome; ARF, acute renal failure; VTE, venous thromboembolic events; F/N, febrile neutropenia; HTN, hypertension; and N/V, nausea/vomiting.

TABLE 20.3

Clinical Trials with Kinesin Spindle Protein Inhibitors

Drug [Company]	Disease	Treatment	Trial Design	Number Enrolled	Response	DLT/AE	Reference
Ispinesib (SB-715992) [Cytokinetics]	ST	IV q21d	Phase 1	42	4 SD	↓ANC, ↓WBC, ↓Hgb, F/N, and fatigue	Chu et al. (2004)
	ST	IV 1 h, q21d+carboplatin	Phase 1	24	3 uMR	↓ANC, ↓Hgb, ↓Plt, F/N, N/V, and fatigue	Jones et al. (2006)
	ST	IV 1 h, d1, 2, 3 q21d	Phase 1	27	2 SD, 1 MR	↓ANC, ↓WBC, fatigue, and infusion reaction	Heath et al. (2006)
	RCC	IV 1 h, d1, 8, and 15 q28d	Phase 2	20	6 SD	↓ANC, ↓Hgb, ↓Lymphs, ↑LFTs, fatigue, anorexia, ↓Na$^+$, dyspnea, headache, ↑creatinine, fatigue, ↑glucose, and skin infection	Lee RT et al. (2008)
	Melanoma	IV 1 h q28d	Phase 2	17	6 SD	↓ANC, ↓WBC, injection site reaction, fatigue, and N/V	Lee CW et al. (2008)
	RMHNSC	IV 1 h q28d	Phase 2	20	5 SD	↓ANC and ↓WBC	Tang et al. (2008)
	HCC	IV 1 h q28d	Phase 2	15	7 SD	↓ANC, ↓WBC, ↑LFTs, and diarrhea	Knox et al. (2008)
	ST	IV 1 h, q21d+Docetaxel 50–75 mg/m^2	Phase 1	24	7 SD	↓ANC, F/N, ↓WBC, F/N, lethargy, and diarrhea	Blagden et al. (2008)
	AIPC	IV 1 h, q21d	Phase 2	21	NR	↓ANC, ↓WBC, weakness, and fatigue	Beer et al. (2008)
	Pediatric	IV 1 h, d1, 8, 15 q28d	Phase 1	24	4 SD	↓ANC and ↑bilirubin	Souid et al. (2010)
	ST	IV 1 h d1, 8, 15 q28d	Phase 1	30	9 SD	↓ANC, N/V, diarrhea, and fatigue	Burris et al. (2011)
	ABC	IV 1 h, d1, 15 q28d	Phase 1	16	1 PR, 2uPR, 9 SD	↓ANC, ↓WBC, ↓Plt, GI, and ↑LFTs	Gomez et al. (2012)

Drug	Indication	Schedule	N	Response	Adverse events	Reference
SB-743921 [Cytokinetics]	NHL/HL	IV d1, 15 q28d	32	1 PR, 1 SD	↓ANC, infection, dehydration, and dyspnea	O'Connor et al. (2008)
	NHL/HL	IV d1, 15 q28d	51	2 PR	↓ANC, ↑LFTs, and neutropenia with sepsis	Gerecitano et al. (2009)
	ST NHL/HL	IV 1 h, d1 q21d	64	1 PR, 6 SD	↓ANC, ↓PO$_4$, PE, ↑LFTs,↓Na$^+$, and ↑bilirubin	Holen et al. (2011)
MK-0731 [MRK]	ST	24 h CIV q21d ± GCSF	43	4 SD	↓ANC, ↓*Hgb*, ↓ *Lymph*, N/V, fatigue, and anorexia Syncope	Holen et al. (2012)
ARRY-520 [Array Biopharma]	ST	IV d1 q21 IV d1, 2 q14d ± G-CSF	34	3 SD	↓*WBC*, ↓ *Lymphs*, *F/N*, sepsis, ↑*LFTs*, ↓Na$^+$, anorexia, N/V, and fatigue	Goncalves et al. (2010)
	MM/PCL	IV d1, 2 q14d ± G-CSF	13	1 PR	↓ANC, ↓*Hgb*, ↓*Plt*, and fatigue	Shah et al. (2010)
	AML/MDS	IV d1 or d1, 3, 5 q21d	36	1 PR, 10SD	↓ANC, ↓*Hgb*, ↓*Plt*, mucositis, exfoliative rash, hand–foot syndrome, and ↑bilirubin	Khoury et al. (2012)
AZD4877 [AstraZeneca]	ST	IV 1 h, d1, 8, 15 q28d	43	11 SD	↓ANC, *F/N*, and mucositis	Infante et al. (2012)
	AML	IV 1 h, d1, 2, 3 q14d	39	None	↓ANC, mucositis, palmar-plantar erythrodysesthesia, ↑bilirubin, diarrhea, fatigue, ↓K$^+$, and ↓Ca$^+$	Kantarjian et al. (2012)

ST, advance solid tumors or advanced and refractory solid tumors or refractory solid tumors; RCC, advance/metastatic renal cell carcinoma; RMHNSC, recurrent or metastatic head and neck squamous cell carcinoma; HCC, hepatocellular carcinoma; ABC, advanced breast cancer; NHL/HL, non–Hodgkin lymphoma/Hodgkin lymphoma; MM/PCL, relapsed/refractory multiple myeloma or plasma cell leukemia; AML, acute myeloid leukemia; MDS, myeloproliferative disorder; IV, intravenous infusion; CIV, continuous intravenous infusion; GCSF, granulocyte colony-stimulating factor; ND, not determined; PR, partial response; SD, stable disease; MR, minor response; uMR, unconfirmed MR; uPR, unconfirmed PR; DLT/AE, dose-limiting toxicity/adverse events; ↓ANC, neutropenia; ↓WBC, leucopenia; ↓Hgb, anemia; ↓ Lymphs, lymphopenia; ↓Plt, thrombocytopenia; ↓Na+, hyponatremia; ↑LFTs, elevated liver function tests; AIPC, androgen-independent prostate cancer; PE, pulmonary embolus; N/V, nausea/vomiting; F/N, febrile neutropenia; and GI, GI disturbance.

Importantly, it also confirmed the presence of only a small percentage of cells—mitotic cells—vulnerable to their drug. As the authors noted, they assessed aurora A inhibition in tumor biopsies by quantifying accumulation of "mitotic cells within proliferative tumor regions." By staining tumor sections for pHistH3, KI67, and DNA, the "mitotic index" was evaluated in tumor biopsies by "calculating the percentage of total cells (nuclei count) that were mitotic (pHistH3 immunopositive) within the proliferative tumor regions (KI67 immunopositive)." Mitotic indices of less than 5% were found in the majority of tumors, even though the analysis that had focused only on "proliferative regions of tumors" underscores the slow doubling times of tumors in humans and the presence of target in only a small fraction of cells.

Moreover, one can argue that the febrile neutropenia, often scored as the principal toxicity observed in many of the treated patients, is further evidence these drugs hit their target and inhibited mitosis in humans. While the majority of human tumors do not divide rapidly enough to be susceptible to these mitotic poisons, the same cannot be said of vulnerable marrow elements. With the doubling times of 17 h for myeloblasts, 63 h for promyelocytes, and 55 h for myelocytes (Boll and Fuchs, 1970), the occurrence of reversible neutropenia with an agent targeting a mitotic kinase or KSP is not surprising, since at any one time, one-fourth or more of marrow neutrophils are in mitosis. Indeed, one can argue that the emergence of neutropenia as a dose-limiting toxicity, in most trials, provides evidence of successfully designed drugs engaging their targets in humans.

Finally, as shown in Tables 20.1 through 20.3, with stable disease rates of 17.3% (Plk inhibitors), 17.8% (KSP inhibitors) and 19.2% (AK inhibitors), we would argue that this measure more likely reflects the inherent biology of the tumors being treated. For example, stable disease rates of 55%–67% have been reported with placebos in renal cell and hepatocellular carcinomas (Escudier et al., 2007; Llovet et al., 2008). Because mitotic arrest can only be sustained for about 1–2 days, one cannot envision how antimitotic agents could arrest cells in mitosis for any period of time that might be scored clinically as "stable disease."

We have restricted our comments thus far primarily to solid tumors, but we would note that in the subset of patients with hematologic malignancies, AK inhibitors have had a tabulated response rate of 10.9%. Two principal categories of responders have been observed. Thirty-eight percent (14/37) have been observed in patients with chronic myeloid/myelogenous leukemia (CML) with AT9283 and MK-0457/VX680, drugs that we know are potent inhibitors of *BCR-Abl* harboring a T315I mutation (Giles et al., 2013; Foran et al., 2008). These represent an "off-target" effect inhibiting a kinase other than a mitotic kinase—in this case, BCR-ABL harboring a T315I mutation—and while clinically valuable, are cell-cycle-independent effects that do not require inhibition of AK. We would note here that the approval of ponatinib for the treatment of just such CML patients establishes this "unmet need" and supports further development of such drugs, albeit as inhibitors of BCR-ABL, not as inhibitors of mitotic kinases (Cortes et al., 2012). It is most interesting that in these cases, the "mitotic kinase inhibitors" achieved activity in one of the least "mitotic," that is, most indolent, diseases oncologists treat.

The other 62% (23/37) of responses in hematologic malignancies have been reported in patients with acute myeloid leukemia (AML) (Foran et al., 2008;

Löwenberg et al., 2011; Sonet et al., 2008). Because these malignancies have doubling times that are faster than those of solid tumors, ranging from a few days to a few weeks, one could envision a potential role for agents targeting mitosis in these malignancies (Blanco et al., 2001; Riccardi et al., 1989). Preliminary activity in AML has been described with three agents developed as inhibitors of the AKs: AT9283 (Astex) (Foran et al., 2008), AS703569 (EMD Serono) (Sonet et al., 2008), and AZD1152/ barasertib (Astra Zeneca) (Löwenberg et al., 2011). However, the extent to which the activity in these more rapidly proliferating malignancies is due to the inhibition of the AKs remains to be established. Neither AT9283 nor AS703569 is selective for AKs, leaving unresolved the extent to which the observed activity is an "off-target effect" or a consequence of an effect on the AKs. Furthermore, while the efficacy observed with AZD1152/barasertib in AML is more likely because of inhibition of aurora B kinase, this too remains to be determined. We do know that AZD1152/ barasertib is a prodrug and that the more active barasertib-hQPA is highly potent and predominantly inhibits aurora B kinase compared with aurora A kinase and a panel of 50 other kinases (Keen et al., 2009). Although the duration of the responses achieved with AZD1152/barasertib was limited—the investigators noted durations of CR of 23, 58, and 115 days and CRi of 7, 23, 25, 27, 29, and 206 days, with the duration of response censored at 23, 27, and 115 days for three patients who voluntarily discontinued from the study while still in remission, and at 206 days for one patient who was still in remission at data cutoff—activity in a malignancy as lethal as AML where progress has been difficult to achieve should not be ignored. There is no doubt mitotic inhibitors will not be used as single agents in AML, and their development in combinations, already in progress, will determine their value, if any (Kantarjian et al., 2010). Indeed, inhibitors targeting mitosis could prove effective in rapidly growing (rapidly dividing) leukemias or lymphomas (i.e., Burkitt's lymphoma) and maybe even anaplastic thyroid carcinomas, and their value in these malignancies should be further explored.

LESSONS LEARNED, INSIGHT GLEANED

MSAs, developed as "non-neurotoxic" alternatives to MTAs, continue to be developed clinically, as we continue to hope they will deliver on their promise. While preclinical models with doubling times of one to at most a few days proved vulnerable to therapies that target crucial mitosis associated proteins, it is not surprising that they have struggled in the clinic, most notably with solid tumors. In the latter, S-phase fraction of at most a few percent and tumor doubling times of 30–60 days or greater meant that only a small, insignificant fraction of cells were vulnerable to a drug aimed at a target that is expressed only transiently during a very specific phase of the cell cycle.

Reversible neutropenia, the dose-limiting toxicity observed with these agents, demonstrates the sophistication of pharmaceutical drug development. Unfortunately, one could argue this pharmaceutical prowess led to the overdevelopment of drugs aimed at targets that had not yet been validated (AKs, Plks, and KSP). Increasingly, it appears that the preclinical models used in drug development—models we know to be imperfect—may have been especially misleading with these drugs where doubling time is a critical factor in the drug's activity. Finally, the results achieved to date in the clinic ratify the paradigm that MTAs do not kill cancer cells in humans primarily by inhibiting mitosis. We have proposed the inhibition of trafficking on MTs as the principal mechanism of action of MTAs (Komlodi-Pasztor et al., 2011).

REFERENCES

Arbitrario JP, Belmont BJ, Evanchik MJ et al. SNS-314, a pan-Aurora kinase inhibitor, shows potent anti-tumor activity and dosing flexibility in vivo. *Cancer Chemother Pharmacol.* 2010; 65:707–717.

Arkenau HT, Plummer R, Molife LR, Olmos D, Yap TA, Squires M, Lewis S, Lock V, Yule M, Lyons J, Calvert H, Judson I. A phase I dose escalation study of AT9283, a small molecule inhibitor of aurora kinases, in patients with advanced solid malignancies. *Ann Oncol.* 2012; 23:1307–1313.

Baldini E, Arlot-Bonnemains Y, Sorrenti S, Mian C, Pelizzo MR, De Antoni E, Palermo S, Morrone S, Barollo S, Nesca A, Moretti CG, D'Armiento M, Ulisse S. Aurora kinases are expressed in medullary thyroid carcinoma (MTC) and their inhibition suppresses in vitro growth and tumorigenicity of the MTC derived cell line TT. *BMC Cancer.* 2011; 11:411.

Bastos BR, Diamond J, Hansen R, Gustafson D, Arnott J, Bray M, Sidor C, Messersmith W, Shapiro G. An open-label, dose escalation, safety, and pharmacokinetic study of ENMD-2076 administered orally to patients with advanced cancer. *J Clin Oncol.* 2009; 27:15s, (suppl; abstr 3520).

Beer TM, Goldman B, Synold TW, Ryan CW, Vasist LS, Van Veldhuizen PJ Jr, Dakhil SR, Lara PN Jr, Drelichman A, Hussain MH, Crawford ED. Southwest Oncology Group phase II study of ispinesib in androgen-independent prostate cancer previously treated with taxanes. *Clin Genitourin Cancer.* 2008; 6:103–109.

Beltran H, Rickman DS, Park K Chae SS, Sboner A, MacDonald TY, Wang Y et al. Molecular characterization of neuroendocrine prostate cancer and identification of new drug targets. *Cancer Discov.* 2011; 1:487–495.

Benten D, Keller G, Quaas A et al. Aurora kinase inhibitor PHA-739358 suppresses growth of hepatocellular carcinoma in vitro and in a xenograft mouse model. *Neoplasia.* 2009; 11:934–944.

Blagden SP, Molife LR, Seebaran A, Payne M, Reid AH, Protheroe AS, Vasist LS et al. A phase I trial of ispinesib, a kinesin spindle protein inhibitor, with docetaxel in patients with advanced solid tumours. *Br J Cancer.* 2008; 98:894–899.

Boll IT, Fuchs G. A kinetic model of granulocytopoiesis. *Exp Cell Res.* 1970; 61:147–152.

Boss DS, Witteveen PO, van der Sar J, Lolkema MP, Voest EE, Stockman PK, Ataman O, Wilson D, Das S, Schellens JH. Clinical evaluation of AZD1152, an i.v. inhibitor of Aurora B kinase, in patients with solid malignant tumors. *Ann Oncol.* 2011; 22:431–437.

Brahmer JR, Kelsey S, Scigalla P, Hill G, Bello C, Elza-Brown K, Donehower R. A phase I study of SU6668 in patients with refractory solid tumors. *Proc Am Soc Clin Oncol.* 2002; 21:2002 (abstr 335).

Britten CD, Rosen L, Kabbinavar F, Rosen P, Mulay M, Hernandez L, Brown J, Bello C, Kelsey SM, Scigalla P. Phase I trial of SU6668, a small molecule receptor tyrosine kinase inhibitor, given twice daily in patients with advanced cancers. *Proc Am Soc Clin Oncol.* 2002; 21:28b (abstr 1922).

Burris HA 3rd, Jones SF, Williams DD, Kathman SJ, Hodge JP, Pandite L, Ho PT, Boerner SA, Lorusso P. A phase I study of ispinesib, a kinesin spindle protein inhibitor, administered weekly for three consecutive weeks of a 28-day cycle in patients with solid tumors. *Invest New Drugs.* 2011; 29:467–472.

Campos SM, Dizon DS. Antimitotic inhibitors. *Hematol Oncol Clin North Am*. 2012; 26:607–628.

Chakravarty A, Shinde V, Tabernero J, Cervantes A, Cohen RB, Dees EC, Burris H et al. The Phase I assessment of new mechanism-based pharmacodynamic biomarkers for MLN8054, a small-molecule inhibitor of Aurora A kinase. *Cancer Res*. 2011; 71:675–685.

Chu QS, Holen KD, Rowinsky EK, Wilding G, Volkman JL, Orr JB, Williams DD, Hodge JP, Sabry J. Phase I trial of novel kinesin spindle protein (KSP) inhibitor SB-715992 IV Q 21 days [abstract]. *J Clin Oncol*. 2004; 22 (14 suppl; abstr 2078).

Cohen RB, Jones SF, Aggarwal C, von Mehren M, Cheng J, Spigel DR, Greco FA. A phase I dose-escalation study of danusertib (PHA-739358) administered as a 24-hour infusion with and without granulocyte colony-stimulating factor in a 14-day cycle in patients with advanced solid tumors. *Clin Cancer Res*. 2009; 15:6694–6701.

Cortes JE, Kantarjian H, Shah NP, Bixby D, Mauro MJ, Flinn I, O'Hare T et al. Ponatinib in refractory Philadelphia chromosome-positive leukemias. *N Engl J Med*. 2012; 367: 2075–2088.

Crosio C, Fimia GM, Loury R et al. Mitotic phosphorylation of histone H3: Spatio-temporal regulation by mammalian Aurora kinases. *Mol Cell Biol*. 2002; 22:874–885.

De Jonge M, Steeghs N, Verweij J, Nortier JW, Eskens F, Ouwerkerk J, Laffranchi B, Mariani M, Rocchetti M, Gelderblom H. Phase I study of the aurora kinases (AKs) inhibitor PHA-739358 administered as a 6 and 3-h IV infusion on Days 1, 8, 15 every 4 wks in patients with advanced solid tumors. *J Clin Oncol*. 2008; 26:2008 (May 20 suppl; abstr 3507).

Dees C IJ, Burris HA, Astsaturov IA, Stinchcombe T, Liu H, Galvin K, Venkatakrishnan K, Fingert HJ, Cohen RB. Phase I study of the investigational drug MLN8237, an Aurora A kinase (AAK) inhibitor, in patients (pts) with solid tumors. *J Clin Oncol*. 2010; 28:15s.

Dees EC, Infante JR, Cohen RB, O'Neil BH, Jones S, von Mehren M, Danaee H et al. Phase 1 study of MLN8054, a selective inhibitor of Aurora A kinase in patients with advanced solid tumors. *Cancer Chemother Pharmacol*. 2011; 67:945–954.

Dennis M, Davies M, Oliver S, D'Souza R, Pike L, Stockman P. Phase I study of the Aurora B kinase inhibitor barasertib (AZD1152) to assess the pharmacokinetics, metabolism and excretion in patients with acute myeloid leukemia. *Cancer Chemother Pharmacol*. 2012; 70:461–469.

Diamond JR, Bastos BR, Hansen RJ, Gustafson DL, Eckhardt SG, Kwak EL, Pandya SSet al. Phase I safety, pharmacokinetic, and pharmacodynamic study of ENMD-2076, a novel angiogenic and Aurora kinase inhibitor, in patients with advanced solid tumors. *Clin Cancer Res*. 2011; 17:849–860.

Dutertre S, Descamps S, Prigent C. On the role of aurora-A in centrosome function. *Oncogene*. 2002; 21:6175–6183.

Ellis PM, Chu QS, Leighl NB, Laurie SA, Trommeshauser D, Hanft G, Munzert G, Gyorffy S. A phase I dose escalation trial of BI 2536, a novel Plk1 inhibitor, with standard dose pemetrexed in previously treated advanced or metastatic non-small cell lung cancer (NSCLC) [abstract]. *J Clin Oncol*. 2008; 26 (suppl; abstr 8115).

Escudier B, Eisen T, Stadler WM et al. Sorafenib in advanced clear-cell renal-cell carcinoma. *N Engl J Med*. 2007; 356:125–134.

Fletcher GC, Brokx RD, Denny TA et al. ENMD-2076 is an orally active kinase inhibitor with antiangiogenic and antiproliferative mechanisms of action. *Mol Cancer Ther*. 2011; 10:126–137.

Foran JM, Ravandi F, O'Brien SM, Borthakur G, Rios M, Boone P, Worrell J, Mallett KH, Squires M, Fazal LH, Kantarjian HM. Phase I and pharmacodynamic trial of AT9283, an aurora kinase inhibitor, in patients with refractory leukemia. *J Clin Oncol*. 2008; 26: May 20 suppl; abstr 2518.

Gandhi L, Chu QS, Stephenson J, Johnson BE, Govindan R, Bonomi P, Eaton K, Fritsch H, Munzert G, Socinski; M. An open label phase II trial of the Plk1 inhibitor BI 2536, in patients with sensitive relapse small cell lung cancer (SCLC) [abstract]. *J Clin Oncol.* 2009; 27 (15 suppl; abstr 8108).

Garland LL, Taylor C, Pilkington DL, Cohen JL, Von Hoff DD. A phase I pharmacokinetic study of HMN-214, a novel oral stilbene derivative with polo-like kinase-1-interacting properties, in patients with advanced solid tumors. *Clin Can Res.* 2006; 12:5182–5189.

Gerecitano JF et al. A phase I/II trial of the kinesin spindle protein (KSP) inhibitor SB-743921 dosed q14d without and with prophylactic G-CSF in non-Hodgkin lymphoma (NHL) or Hodgkin lymphoma (HL) [abstract]. *J Clin Oncol.* 2009; 27 (15 suppl; abstr 8578).

Giles FJ, Cortes J, Jones D, Bergstrom D, Kantarjian H, Freedman SJ. MK-0457, a novel kinase inhibitor, is active in patients with chronic myeloid leukemia or acute lympho-cytic leukemia with the T315I BCR-ABL mutation. *Blood.* 2007; 109:500–502.

Giles FJ, Swords RT, Nagler A, Hochhaus A, Ottmann OG, Rizzieri DA, Talpaz M et al. MK-0457, an Aurora kinase and BCR-ABL inhibitor, is active in patients with BCR-ABL T315I leukemia. *Leukemia.* 2013; 27:113–117.

Gomez HL, Philco M, Pimentel P, Kiyan M, Monsalvo ML, Conlan MG, Saikali KG, Chen MM, Seroogy JJ, Wolff AA, Escandon RD. Phase I dose-escalation and pharmacoki-netic study of ispinesib, a kinesin spindle protein inhibitor, administered on days 1 and 15 of a 28-day schedule in patients with no prior treatment for advanced breast cancer. *Anticancer Drugs.* 2012; 23:335–341.

Goncalves PH, Sausville EA, Edelman MJ, Pandya NB, Houlehan MM, Freeman BB, Simmons HM, Stallings JS, Ptaszynski AM LoRusso P. A phase I study of ARRY-520 in solid tumors [abstract]. *J Clin Oncol.* 2010; 28 (15 suppl; abstr 2570).

Harrington EA, Bebbington D, Moore J et al. VX-680, a potent and selective small-molecule inhibitor of the Aurora kinases, suppresses tumor growth in vivo. *Nat Med.* 2004; 10:262–267.

Harrison MR, Holen KD, Liu G. Beyond taxanes: A review of novel agents that target mitotic tubulin and microtubules, kinases, and kinesins. *Clin Adv Hematol Oncol.* 2009; 7:54–64.

Heath EI, Aloiusi A, Eder JP, Valdivieso M, Vasist LS, Appleman L, Bhargava P, Colevas AD, Lorusso PM, Shapiro G. A phase I dose escalation trial of ispinesib (SB-715992) admin-istered days 1–3 of a 21-day cycle in patients with advanced solid tumors [abstract]. *J Clin Oncol.* 2006; 24 (18 suppl; abstr 2026).

Hoar K, Chakravarty A, Rabino C, Wysong D, Bowman D, Roy N, Ecsedy JA. MLN8054, a small-molecule inhibitor of Aurora A, causes spindle pole and chromosome congression defects leading to aneuploidy. *Mol Cell Biol.* 2007; 27:4513–4525.

Hofheinz RD, Al-Batran SE, Hochhaus A, Jäger E, Reichardt VL, Fritsch H, Trommeshauser D, Munzert G. An open-label, phase I study of the polo-like kinase-1 inhibitor, BI 2536, in patients with advanced solid tumors. *Clin Cancer Res.* 2010; 16:4666–4674.

Holen K, Dipaola R, Liu G, Tan AR, Wilding G, Hsu K, Agrawal N, Chen C, Xue L, Rosenberg E, Stein M. A phase I trial of MK-0731, a Kinesin Spindle Protein (KSP) inhibitor, in patients with solid tumors. *Invest New Drugs.* 2012; 30:1088–1095.

Holen KD, Belani CP, Wilding G, Ramalingam S, Volkman JL, Ramanathan RK, Vasist LS, Bowen CJ, Hodge JP, Dar MM, Ho PT. A first in human study of SB-743921, a kinesin spindle protein inhibitor, to determine pharmacokinetics, biologic effects and establish a recommended phase II dose. *Cancer Chemother Pharmacol.* 2011; 67:447–454.

Huck JJ, Zhang M, McDonald A et al. MLN8054, an inhibitor of Aurora A kinase, induces senes-cence in human tumor cells both in vitro and in vivo. *Mol Cancer Res.* 2010; 8:373–384.

Infante JR, Kurzrock R, Spratlin J, Burris HA, Eckhardt SG, Li J, Wu K, Skolnik JM, Hylander-Gans L, Osmukhina A, Huszar D, Herbst RS. A Phase I study to assess the safety, tolerability, and pharmacokinetics of AZD4877, an intravenous Eg5 inhibitor in patients with advanced solid tumors. *Cancer Chemother Pharmacol.* 2012; 69:165–172.

Jackson JR, Patrick DR, Dar MM, Huang PS. Targeted anti-mitotic therapies: Can we improve on tubulin agents? *Nat Rev Cancer*. 2007; 7:107–117.

Jeet V, Russell PJ, Verma ND, Khatri A. Targeting aurora kinases: A novel approach to curb the growth & chemoresistance of androgen refractory prostate cancer. *Curr Cancer Drug Targets*. 2012; 12:144–163.

Jimeno A, Li J, Messersmith WA, Laheru D, Rudek MA, Maniar M, Hidalgo M, Baker SD, Donehower RC. Phase I study of ON 01910.Na, a novel modulator of the Polo-like kinase 1 pathway, in adult patients with solid tumors. *J Clin Oncol*. 2008; 26: 5504–5510.

Johnson ES, Kornbluth S. Phosphatases driving mitosis: Pushing the gas and lifting the brakes. *Prog Mol Biol Transl Sci*. 2012; 106:327–341.

Johnson LN. Substrates of mitotic kinases. *Sci Signal*. 2011; 4(179):pe31.

Jones SF, Plummer ER, Burris HA, Razak AR, Meluch AA, Bowen CJ, Williams DH, Hodge JP, Dar MM, Calvert AH. Phase I study of ispinesib in combination with carboplatin in patients with advanced solid tumors [abstract]. *J Clin Oncol*. 2006; 24 (18 suppl; abstr 2027).

Kantarjian HM, Padmanabhan S, Stock W, Tallman MS, Curt GA, Li J, Osmukhina et al. Phase I/II multicenter study to assess the safety, tolerability, pharmacokinetics and pharmacodynamics of AZD4877 in patients with refractory acute myeloid leukemia. *Invest New Drugs*. 2012; 30:1107–1115.

Kantarjian HM, Sekeres MA, Ribrag V et al. Phase I study to assess the safety and tolerability of AZD1152 in combination with low dose cytosine arabinoside in patients with acute myeloid leukemia (AML) [abstract]. *Blood*. 2010;116(21):656.

Khoury HJ, Garcia-Manero G, Borthakur G, Kadia T, Foudray MC, Arellano M, Langston A et al. A phase 1 dose-escalation study of ARRY-520, a kinesin spindle protein inhibitor, in patients with advanced myeloid leukemias. *Cancer*. 2012; 118:3556–3564.

Kishi K, van Vugt MA, Okamoto K, Hayashi Y, Yaffe MB. Functional dynamics of Polo-like kinase 1 at the centrosome. *Mol Cell Biol*. 2009; 29:3134–3150.

Knox JJ, Gill S, Synold TW, Biagi JJ, Major P, Feld R, Cripps C, Wainman N, Eisenhauer E, Seymour L. A phase II and pharmacokinetic study of SB-715992, in patients with metastatic hepatocellular carcinoma: A study of the National Cancer Institute of Canada Clinical Trials Group (NCIC CTG IND.168). *Invest New Drugs*. 2008; 26:265–272.

Komlodi-Pasztor E, Sackett D, Wilkerson J, Fojo T. Mitosis is not a key target of microtubule agents in patient tumors. *Nat Rev Clin Oncol*. 2011; 8:244–250.

Komlodi-Pasztor E, Sackett DL, Fojo AT. Inhibitors targeting mitosis: Tales of how great drugs against a promising target were brought down by a flawed rationale. *Clin Cancer Res*. 2012; 18:51–63.

Kristeleit R, Calvert H, Arkenau H, Olmos D, Adam J, Plummer ER, Lock V, Squires M, Fazal L, Judson I. A phase I study of AT9283, an aurora kinase inhibitor, in patients with refractory solid tumors. *J Clin Oncol*. 2009; 27:15s (suppl; abstr 2566).

Lee CW, Bélanger K, Rao SC, Petrella TM, Tozer RG, Wood L, Savage KJ, Eisenhauer EA, Synold TW, Wainman N, Seymour L. A phase II study of ispinesib (SB-715992) in patients with metastatic or recurrent malignant melanoma: A National Cancer Institute of Canada Clinical Trials Group trial. *Invest New Drugs*. 2008; 26:249–255.

Lee RT, Beekman KE, Hussain M, Davis NB, Clark JI, Thomas SP, Nichols KF, Stadler WM. A University of Chicago consortium phase II trial of SB-715992 in advanced renal cell cancer. *Clin Genitourin Cancer*. 2008; 6:21–24.

Lehman NL, O'Donnell JP, Whiteley LJ, Stapp RT, Lehman TD, Roszka KM, Schultz LR et al. Aurora A is differentially expressed in gliomas, is associated with patient survival in glioblastoma and is a potential chemotherapeutic target in gliomas. *Cell Cycle*. 2012; 11:489–502.

Lens SM, Voest EE, Medema RH. Shared and separate functions of polo-like kinases and aurora kinases in cancer. *Nat Rev Cancer*. 2010; 10:825–841.

Llovet JM, Ricci S, Mazzaferro V et al. Sorafenib in advanced hepatocellular carcinoma. *N Engl J Med.* 2008; 359:378–390.

Löwenberg B, Muus P, Ossenkoppele G, Rousselot P, Cahn JY, Ifrah N, Martinelli et al. Phase 1/2 study to assess the safety, efficacy, and pharmacokinetics of barasertib (AZD1152) in patients with advanced acute myeloid leukemia. *Blood.* 2011; 118:6030–6036.

Macarulla T, Cervantes A, Elez E, Rodríguez-Braun E, Baselga J, Roselló S, Sala G et al. Phase I study of the selective Aurora A kinase inhibitor MLN8054 in patients with advanced solid tumors: Safety, pharmacokinetics, and pharmacodynamics. *Mol Cancer Ther.* 2010; 9:2844–2852.

Manchado E, Guillamot M, Malumbres M. Killing cells by targeting mitosis. *Cell Death Differ.* 2012; 19:369–377.

Marumoto T, Honda S, Hara T, Nitta M, Hirota T, Kohmura E, Saya H. Aurora-A kinase maintains the fidelity of early and late mitotic events in HeLa cells. *J Biol Chem.* 2003; 278:51786–51795.

Matulonis U, Tew W, Matei D, Behbakht K, Fleming GF, Oza AM. A phase II study of ENMD-2076 in platinum-resistant ovarian cancer. *J Clin Oncol.* 2011; 29:2011 (suppl; abstr 5021).

Matulonis UA, Sharma S, Ghamande S et al. Phase II study of MLN8237 (alisertib), an investigational Aurora A kinase inhibitor, in patients with platinum-resistant or -refractory epithelial ovarian, fallopian tube, or primary peritoneal carcinoma. *Gynecol Oncol.* 2012; 127:63–69.

Mitchison TJ. The proliferation rate paradox in antimitotic chemotherapy. *Mol Biol Cell.* 2012; 23:1–6.

Mossé YP, Lipsitz E, Fox E, Teachey DT, Maris JM, Weigel B, Adamson PC, Ingle MA, Ahern CH, Blaney SM. Pediatric phase I trial and pharmacokinetic study of MLN8237, an investigational oral selective small-molecule inhibitor of Aurora kinase A: A Children's Oncology Group Phase I Consortium study. *Clin Cancer Res.* 2012; 18:6058–6064.

Mross K, Dittrich C, Aulitzky WE, Strumberg D, Schutte J, Schmid RM, Hollerbach S, Merger M, Munzert G, Fleischer F, Scheulen ME. A randomised phase II trial of the Polo-like kinase inhibitor BI 2536 in chemo-naïve patients with unresectable exocrine adenocarcinoma of the pancreas—A study within the Central European Society Anticancer Drug Research (CESAR) collaborative network. *Br J Cancer.* 2012; 107:280–286.

Mross K, Frost A, Steinbild S, Hedbom S, Rentschler J, Kaiser R, Rouyrre N, Trommeshauser D, Hoesl CE, Munzert G. Phase I dose escalation and pharmacokinetic study of BI 2536, a novel Polo-like kinase 1 inhibitor, in patients with advanced solid tumors. *J Clin Oncol.* 2008; 26:5511–5517.

Mross KB, Scheulen M, Frost A, Scharr D, Richly H, Nokay B, Lee K, Hilbert J, Fleischer F, Fietz O. A phase I dose-escalation study of BI 811283, an Aurora B inhibitor, administered every three weeks in patients with advanced solid tumors. *J Clin Oncol.* 2010; 28:15s, (suppl; abstr 3011).

O'Connor OA et al. A phase I-II trial of the kinesin spindle protein (KSP) inhibitor SB-743921 on days 1 and 15 every 28 days in non-Hodgkin or Hodgkin lymphoma [abstract]. *J Clin Oncol.* 2008; 26 (suppl; abstr 8539).

Ohnuma T, Cho SY, Roboz J, Jiang JD, Lehrer D, Silverman L, Schwartz JD, Reddy EP. Phase I study of ON 01910.Na by 3-day continuous infusion (CI) in patients (pts) with advanced cancer [abstract]. *J Clin Oncol.* 2006; 24 (18 suppl; abstr 13137).

Olmos D, Barker D, Sharma R, Brunetto AT, Yap TA, Taegtmeyer AB, Barriuso J et al. Phase I study of GSK461364, a specific and competitive Polo-like kinase 1 inhibitor, in patients with advanced solid malignancies. *Clin Cancer Res.* 2011; 17:3420–3430.

Patnaik A, Forero L, Goetz A, Tolcher AW, Beeram M, De Bono JS, Weiss G, Wood L, Takimoto C, Rowinsky EK. HMN-214, a novel oral antimicrotubular agent and inhibitor of polo-like- and cyclin-dependent kinases: Clinical, pharmacokinetic (PK) and pharmacodynamic (PD) relationships observed in a phase I trial of a daily X 5 schedule every 28 days. *J Clin Oncol.* 2003; 22 (suppl; abstr 514).

Plummer ER, Calvert H, Arkenau H, Mallett KH, Squires M, Smith D, Lewis S, Judson I. A dose-escalation and pharmacodynamic study of AT9283 in patients with refractory solid tumours. *J Clin Oncol.* 2008; 26: (May 20 suppl; abstr 2519).

Renshaw JS Patnaik A, Gordon M, Beeram M, Fischer D, Gianella-Borradori A. A phase I two arm trial of AS703569 (R763), an orally available aurora kinase inhibitor, in subjects with solid tumors: Preliminary results. *J Clin Oncol.* 2007; 25:18S.

Rieder CL. Mitosis in vertebrates: The G2/M and M/A transitions and their associated checkpoints. *Chromosome Res.* 2011; 19:291–306.

Robert F, Verschraegen C, Hurwitz H, Uronis H, Advani R, Chen A, Taverna P, Wollman M, Fox J, Michelson G. A phase I trial of sns-314, a novel and selective pan-aurora kinase inhibitor, in advanced solid tumor patients. *J Clin Oncol.* 2009; 27:15s, (suppl; abstr 2536).

Rubin EH, Watson P, Bergstrom D, Xiao A, Clark JB, Freedman SJ, Eder JP. A phase I clinical and pharmacokinetic (PK) trial of the aurora kinase (AK) inhibitor MK-0457 in cancer patients. *J Clin Oncol.* 2006; Part I. 24(18S).

Sasai K, Katayama H, Stenoien DL et al. Aurora-C kinase is a novel chromosomal passenger protein that can complement Aurora-B kinase function in mitotic cells. *Cell Motil Cytoskeleton.* 2004; 59:249–263.

Scheulen ME, Mross K, Richly H, Nokay B, Frost A, Scharr D, Lee K, Saunders O, Hilbert J, Fietz O. A phase I dose-escalation study of BI 811283, an Aurora B inhibitor, administered days 1 and 15, every four weeks in patients with advanced solid tumors. *J Clin Oncol.* 2010; 28, (suppl; abstr e13065).

Schöffski P, Awada A, Dumez H, Gil T, Bartholomeus S, Wolter P, Taton M, Fritsch H, Glomb P, Munzert G. A phase I, dose-escalation study of the novel Polo-like kinase inhibitor volasertib (BI 6727) in patients with advanced solid tumours. *Eur J Cancer.* 2012; 48:179–186.

Schöffski P, Jones SF, Dumez H Infante JR, Van Mieghem E, Fowst C, Gerletti P et al. Phase I, open-label, multicentre, dose-escalation, pharmacokinetic and pharmacodynamic trial of the oral aurora kinase inhibitor PF-03814735 in advanced solid tumours. Oncotarget 2011; 2:599–609. *Eur J Cancer.* 2011; 47:2256–2264.

Sebastian M, Reck M, Waller CF, Kortsik C, Frickhofen N, Schuler M, Fritsch H, Gaschler-Markefski B, Hanft G, Munzert G, von Pawel J. The efficacy and safety of BI 2536, a novel Plk-1 inhibitor, in patients with stage IIIB/IV non-small cell lung cancer who had relapsed after, or failed, chemotherapy: Results from an open-label, randomized phase II clinical trial. *J Thorac Oncol.* 2010; 5:1060–1067.

Shah JJ, Cohen AD, Zonder JA, Kaufman JL, Burt SM, Freeman BB, Rush S, Ptaszynski AM, Orlowski RZ, Lonial S. Phase I trial of ARRY-520 in relapsed/refractory multiple myeloma (RR MM) [abstract]. *J Clin Oncol.* 2010; 28 (15 suppl; abstr 8132).

Sharma SKR, Gouw L, Hong DS, Jones K, Zhou X, Shi H, Fingert H, Falchook GS. Phase I dose-escalation study of the investigational Aurora A kinase (AAK) inhibitor MLN8237 as an enteric-coated tablet (ECT) formulation in patients with nonhematologic malignancies. *J Clin Oncol.* 2011; 29:2011 (suppl; abstr 3094).

Sonet A, Graux C, Maertens J, Hartog C-M, Duyster J, Götze K, Greiner J et al. Phase I, dose-escalation study of 2 dosing regimens of AS703569, an inhibitor of Aurora and other kinases, administered orally in patients with advanced hematological malignancies [abstract]. *Blood.* 2008; 112:2963.

Souid AK, Dubowy RL, Ingle AM, Conlan MG, Sun J, Blaney SM, Adamson PC. A pediatric phase I trial and pharmacokinetic study of ispinesib: A Children's Oncology Group phase I consortium study. *Pediatr Blood Cancer.* 2010; 55:1323–1328.

Steeghs N, Eskens FA, Gelderblom H et al. Phase I pharmacokinetic and pharmacodynamic study of the aurora kinase inhibitor danusertib in patients with advanced or metastatic solid tumors. *J Clin Oncol.* 2009; 27:5094–5101.

Tang PA, Siu LL, Chen EX, Hotte SJ, Chia S, Schwarz JK, Pond GR et al. Phase II study of ispinesib in recurrent or metastatic squamous cell carcinoma of the head and neck. *Invest New Drugs*. 2008; 26:257–264.

Traynor AM, Hewitt M, Liu G, Flaherty KT, Clark J, Freedman SJ, Scott BB et al. Phase I dose escalation study of MK-0457, a novel Aurora kinase inhibitor, in adult patients with advanced solid tumors. *Cancer Chemother Pharmacol*. 2011; 67:305–314.

Tsuboi K, Yokozawa T, Sakura T, Watanabe T, Fujisawa S, Yamauchi T, Uike N et al. A Phase I study to assess the safety, pharmacokinetics and efficacy of barasertib (AZD1152), an Aurora B kinase inhibitor, in Japanese patients with advanced acute myeloid leukemia. *Leuk Res*. 2011; 35:1384–1389.

Vainshtein, JM, Ghalib MH, Kumar M, Chaudhary I, Maniar M, Taft DR, Cosenza S, Reddy EP, Goel S, Mani S. Phase I study of ON 01910.Na, a novel polo-like kinase 1 pathway modulator, administered as a weekly 24-hour continuous infusion in patients with advanced cancer [abstract]. *J Clin Oncol*. 2008; 26 (suppl; abstr 2515).

Wilkinson RW, Odedra R, Heaton SP et al. AZD1152, a selective inhibitor of Aurora B kinase, inhibits human tumor xenograft growth by inducing apoptosis. *Clin Cancer Res*. 2007; 13:3682–3688.

Williams GH, Stoeber K. The cell cycle and cancer. *J Pathol*. 2012; 226:352–364.

Index

A

Abiraterone acetate
 breast cancer, 406
 COU-302 phase III trial, 405
 CTCs, 405
 oral therapy, 406
 phase I and II trials, 403
 placebo patients, 406
 post-chemotherapy COU-301, 405
 prednisone/prednisolone, 406
 3-pyridyl steroidal drug, 403
 radiographic bone flares, 406
 safe and tolerable treatment, 405
Acute myeloid leukemia (AML)
 aurora kinase inhibitors, 451–453
 hematologic malignancies, 458–459
 inhibitors, AKs, 459
 mitotic inhibitors, 459
 Oxi4503, 319
 tumor suppressor p53, 265
ADCC, *see* Antibody-dependent cellular
      cytotoxicity (ADCC)
Adenoid cystic carcinomas, 147
ADI, *see* Androgen depletion-independent (ADI)
Aggressive fibromatosis (AF)
 and desmoid tumors (DT), 147
 KIT protein, 130
ALCL, *see* Anaplastic large-cell
      lymphoma (ALCL)
ALPS, *see* Autoimmune lymphoproliferative
      syndrome (ALPS)
AML, *see* Acute myeloid leukemia (AML)
Anaplastic large-cell lymphoma (ALCL)
 ALK rearrangement-positive, 175–176, 179
 children, 180
 definition, 173
 gene rearrangements, 178
 *TFG-, ATIC-*and *CLTC-ALK,* 174, 175
Anaplastic lymphoma kinase (ALK)
 ALCL and NSCLC, 173
 amino acid tyrosine kinase, 174
 crizotinib, 179–181
 downstream effectors, 174
 Drosophila melanogaster, 174
 EML4-ALK, 174
 Hsp90 inhibitors, 183
 and LDK378, 182
 malignancy, *see* Malignancy, ALK

optimal methods, 183
 Phase 1 trial, 182
 physiological function, 174
 resistance to crizotinib, 181–182
 toxicity, myalgia, 183
 tyrosine kinase inhibitor, 179
 tyrosine-phosphorylated protein
      component, 174
Androgen depletion-independent (ADI)
 mouse tumors, 448–449
 pan-AK inhibitor, 449
 prostate cancer, 448–449
Androgen receptor (AR)
 abiraterone, *see* Abiraterone
 activation, 414
 amplification, 413
 enzalutamide, *see* Enzalutamide
 and EZN-4176, 411
 mutations, 413
 and SARD, 411
 splice variants, 413–414
 tissue steroidogenesis, 414
Androgen suppression
 antiandrogens, *see* Antiandrogens
 and CRPC, 402
 CYP17 inhibition, *see* CYP17 inhibition
 estrogen, treatments, 403
 ketoconazole, 402
 LHRH analogue treatment, 402
Angiogenesis
 agents, VEGF–VEGFR pathway,
      see VEGF–VEGFR pathway
 "angiogenic switch," 283
 anticancer therapies, 283
 bone marrow-derived cells, 284
 drug-related toxicities, 307
 functional vasculature, 284
 neuropilins (NRP-1 and 2), 285
 predictive biomarkers, 303–306
 resistance, antiangiogenic agents, 301–303
 tumor neoangiogenesis, 307
 types, tumor, 286
 VEGF pathway and therapeutic
      agents, 286
Antiandrogens
 ARN-509, 411
 BMS-641988, 411
 enzalutamide, *see* Enzalutamide
 target, signals, 411–412